Medical Immunology

Sixth Edition

Edited by
Gabriel Virella

Medical University of South Carolina
Charleston, South Carolina, U.S.A.

informa
healthcare

New York   London

Informa Healthcare USA, Inc.
270 Madison Avenue
New York, NY 10016

© 2007 by Informa Healthcare USA, Inc.
Informa Healthcare is an Informa business

No claim to original U.S. Government works
Printed in the United States of America on acid-free paper
10 9 8 7 6 5 4 3 2 1

International Standard Book Number-10: 0-8493-9696-4 (Hardcover)
International Standard Book Number-13: 978-0-8493-9696-0 (Hardcover)

Library of Congress Cataloging-in-Publication Data

Medical immunology / edited by Gabriel Virella. -- 6th ed.
        p. ; cm.
    Includes bibliographical references and index.
    ISBN-13: 978-0-8493-9696-0 (hardcover : alk. paper)
    ISBN-10: 0-8493-9696-4 (hardcover : alk. paper)
    1. Clinical immunology. 2. Immunology. I. Virella, Gabriel, 1943-
    [DNLM: 1. Immunity. 2. Immune System Diseases. QW 504 M4893 2007]

RC582.I59 2007
616.07'9--dc22   2007004930

Visit the Informa Web site at
www.informa.com

and the Informa Healthcare Web site at
www.informahealthcare.com

Preface

Twenty years ago, in 1986, the first edition of *Introduction to Medical Immunology* was published. I could not have imagined then that 20 years later I would be publishing the sixth edition (for which we adopted a shorter title—*Medical Immunology*). This is a classic text in a traditional format, ideal for presenting clinically relevant and updated content from the overwhelming flow of information from the primary literature.

As a matter of principle, I have always avoided trendiness in favor of time-tested knowledge for which there is a clear clinical application (or at the very least a clear experimental proof of concept). I believe that this approach is best suited for the education of physicians of the 21st century. The book provides a good balance between basic and clinical science, and should be a valuable addition to the personal book selections of students, young professionals, specialists, and nonspecialists.

This new edition of *Medical Immunology* has been thoroughly revised and reorganized. I have maintained the emphasis on the clinical application of immunology. The scientific basis of immunology is clearly conveyed without allowing details to obscure concepts. The application to medicine is clearly presented, and the text contains a general and succinct overview, including coverage of important emerging topics. The book should stimulate readers to seek more information and further develop their own education.

The book starts with basic immunology followed by diagnostic immunology. I give special attention to diagnostic immunology because this area has fertile applications and has been the basis for important new knowledge. Part III is dedicated to clinical immunology, and the chapters have been thoroughly revised and updated. The final section on immunodeficiency diseases reflects their extraordinary significance in clinical immunology. The study of primary immune deficiencies gives the best perspective about the intimate works of the human immune system, and secondary immunodeficiencies (including those caused iatrogenically as well as the acquired immune deficiency syndrome) are encountered in virtually all fields of medicine.

I have been lucky in securing authors for this edition who have written excellent chapters for previous editions. I was also able to recruit new authors who bring fresh perspectives to key chapters, such as "Immune Response: Antigens, Lymphocytes and Accessory Cells," "Cell-Mediated Immunity," "Infections and Immunity," "Immunohematology," and "Tumor Immunology." The result is a concise book that conveys our collective intrinsic fascination with a discipline that seeks understanding of fundamental biological knowledge, with the goal of applying that knowledge to the diagnosis and treatment of human diseases. We hope you find this new edition a worthy successor to the previous five editions.

Gabriel Virella

Acknowledgments

I wish to acknowledge my wife and children, whose support during the laborious phase of preparation of each one of the six editions of this book was essential for completing the task; all my former students, the best reviewers and proofreaders that one can ever ask for; the publishers, for their willingness to continue publishing this book for two decades; and last, but not least, I wish to acknowledge the excellent work of Mr. John Lucas, one of our students, who generously spent many hours redrawing several figures in the book. My most deeply felt appreciation goes to all.

Contents

Contributors

Robert J. Boackle   Department of Stomatology and Department of Microbiology and Immunology, Medical University of South Carolina, Charleston, South Carolina, U.S.A.

Kenneth D. Chavin   Department of Surgery, Division of Transplant, Medical University of South Carolina, Charleston, South Carolina, U.S.A.

Justin D. Ellett   Department of Surgery, Division of Transplant, Medical University of South Carolina, Charleston, South Carolina, U.S.A.

Donna L. Farber   Department of Surgery, Division of Transplantation, University of Maryland School of Medicine, Baltimore, Maryland, U.S.A.

Albert F. Finn, Jr.   National Allergy, Asthma, and Urticaria Centers of Charleston, Medical University of South Carolina, Charleston, South Carolina, U.S.A.

Sebastiano Gattoni-Celli   Department of Radiation Oncology, Medical University of South Carolina, Charleston, South Carolina, U.S.A.

Armand Glassman   Department of Microbiology and Immunology, Medical University of South Carolina, Charleston, South Carolina, U.S.A.

Philip D. Hall   Department of Pharmacy and Clinical Sciences, South Carolina College of Pharmacy, Medical University of South Carolina, Charleston, South Carolina, U.S.A.

Deanne M. R. Lathers   Ralph H. Johnson VAMC and Department of Otolaryngology, Medical University of South Carolina, Charleston, South Carolina, U.S.A.

Virginia M. Litwin   MDS Pharma Services, Central Lab, North Brunswick, New Jersey, U.S.A.

Janardan P. Pandey   Department of Microbiology and Immunology, Medical University of South Carolina, Charleston, South Carolina, U.S.A.

John W. Sleasman   Department of Pediatrics, Division of Allergy, Immunology, and Rheumatology, University of South Florida, St. Petersburg, Florida, U.S.A.

Stephen Tomlinson   Department of Microbiology and Immunology, Medical University of South Carolina, Charleston, South Carolina, U.S.A.

George C. Tsokos   Beth Israel Deaconess Medical Center, Harvard Medical School, Boston, Massachusetts, U.S.A.

Gabriel Virella   Department of Microbiology and Immunology, Medical University of South Carolina, Charleston, South Carolina, U.S.A.

Part I: BASIC IMMUNOLOGY

1 | Introduction

Gabriel Virella
*Department of Microbiology and Immunology, Medical University of South Carolina,
Charleston, South Carolina, U.S.A.*

HISTORICAL OVERVIEW

The fundamental observation that led to the development of immunology as a scientific discipline was that an individual might become resistant for life to a certain disease after having contracted it only once. The term immunity, derived from the Latin "immunis" (exempt), was adopted to designate this naturally acquired protection against diseases such as measles or smallpox.

The emergence of immunology as a discipline was closely tied to the development of microbiology. The work of Pasteur, Koch, Metchnikoff, and many other pioneers of the golden age of microbiology resulted in the rapid identification of new infectious agents. This was closely followed by the discovery that infectious diseases could be prevented by exposure to killed or attenuated organisms, or to compounds extracted from the infectious agents. The impact of immunization against infectious diseases such as tetanus, measles, mumps, poliomyelitis, and smallpox, to name just a few examples, can be grasped when we reflect on the fact that these diseases, which were significant causes of mortality and morbidity, are now either extinct or very rarely seen. Indeed, it is fair to state that the impact of vaccination and sanitation on the welfare and life expectancy of humans has had no parallel in any other developments of medical science.

In the second part of this century, immunology started to transcend its early boundaries and become a more general biomedical discipline. Today, the study of immunological defense mechanisms is still an important area of research, but immunologists are involved in a much wider array of problems, such as self–nonself discrimination, control of cell and tissue differentiation, transplantation, cancer immunotherapy, and so on. The focus of interest has shifted toward the basic understanding of how the immune system works in the hope that this insight will allow novel approaches to its manipulation.

GENERAL CONCEPTS
Specific and Nonspecific Defenses

The protection of our organism against infectious agents involves many different mechanisms: some nonspecific (i.e., generically applicable to many different pathogenic organisms) and others specific (i.e., their protective effect is directed to one single organism).

Nonspecific defenses, which as a rule are innate (i.e., all normal individuals are born with them), include:

1. Mechanical barriers such as the integrity of the epidermis and mucosal membranes;
2. Physicochemical barriers, such as the acidity of the stomach fluid;
3. The antibacterial substances (e.g., lysozyme, defensins) present in external secretions;
4. Normal intestinal transit and normal flow of bronchial secretions and urine, which eliminate infectious agents from the respective systems; and
5. Nonimmune mechanisms for ingestion of bacteria and particulate matter by a variety of cells, but particularly well developed in granulocytes.

TABLE 1   A Simplified Overview of the Three Main Stages of the Immune Response

Stage of the immune response	Induction	Amplification	Effector
Cells/molecules involved	Antigen-presenting cells; lymphocytes	Antigen-presenting cells; helper T lymphocytes	Antibodies (+ complement or cytotoxic cells); cytotoxic T lymphocytes; macrophages
Mechanisms	Processing and/or presentation of antigen; recognition by specific receptors on lymphocytes	Release of cytokines; signals mediated by interaction between membrane molecules	Complement-mediated lysis; opsonization and phagocytosis; cytotoxicity
Consequences	Activation of T and B lymphocytes	Proliferation and differentiation of T and B lymphocytes	Elimination of nonself; neutralization of toxins and viruses

Specific defenses, as a rule, are induced during the life of the individual as part of the complex sequence of events designated as the immune response. The immune response has two unique characteristics:

1. Specificity for the eliciting antigen. For example, immunization with inactivated poliovirus only protects against poliomyelitis, not against viral influenza. The specificity of the immune response is due to the existence of exquisitely discriminative antigen receptors on lymphocytes. Only a single or a very limited number of similar structures can be accommodated by the receptors of any given lymphocyte. When those receptors are occupied, an activating signal is delivered to the lymphocytes. Therefore, only those lymphocytes with specific receptors for the antigen in question will be activated.
2. Memory, meaning that repeated exposure to a given antigen elicits progressively more intense specific responses. Most immunizations involve repeated administration of the immunizing compound, with the goal of establishing a long-lasting, protective response. The increase in the magnitude and duration of the immune response with repeated exposure to the same antigen is due to the proliferation of antigen-specific lymphocytes after each exposure. The numbers of responding cells will remain increased even after the immune response subsides. Therefore, whenever the organism is exposed again to that particular antigen, there is an expanded population of specific lymphocytes available for activation. As a consequence, the time needed to mount a response is shorter and the magnitude of the response is higher.

Stages of the Immune Response

To better understand how the immune response is generated, it is useful to consider it as divided into separate sequential stages (Table 1). The first stage (induction) involves a small lymphocyte population with specific receptors able to recognize an antigen or antigen fragments generated by specialized cells known as antigen-presenting cells (APC). The second stage (amplification) is mediated by activated APCs and by specialized T cell subpopulations (T helper cells, defined below) which enhance each other's proliferation and differentiation. This is followed by the production of effector molecules (antibodies) or by the differentiation of effector cells (cells which directly or indirectly mediate the elimination of undesirable elements). The final outcome, therefore, is the elimination of the organism or compound that triggered the reaction by means of activated immune cells or by reactions triggered by mediators released by the immune system.

THE CELLS OF THE IMMUNE SYSTEM
Lymphocytes and Lymphocyte Sub-Populations

The peripheral blood contains two large populations of cells: the red cells, whose main physiological role is to carry oxygen to tissues, and the white blood cells, which have as their main physiological role the elimination of potentially harmful organisms or compounds. Among the white blood cells, lymphocytes are particularly important because of their central role in the immune response. Several subpopulations of lymphocytes have been defined:

1. B lymphocytes, which are the precursors of antibody-producing cells, known as plasma cells.
2. T lymphocytes, which can be divided into several subpopulations:
    *   Helper T lymphocytes (Th), which play a very significant amplification role in the immune responses. Two functionally distinct subpopulations of Th lymphocytes emerging from a precursor population (Th0) have been defined. The Th1 population assists the differentiation of cytotoxic cells and also activates macrophages. Activated macrophages, in turn, play a role as effectors of the immune response. The Th2 lymphocytes are mainly involved in the amplification of B lymphocyte responses. The amplifying effects of Th lymphocytes are mediated in part by soluble mediators—cytokines— and in part by signals delivered as a consequence of cell–cell interactions.
    *   Cytotoxic T lymphocytes, which are the main immunologic effector mechanism involved in the elimination of non-self or infected cells.
    *   Immunoregulatory T lymphocytes, which have the ability to downregulate the immune response through the release of cytokines such as interleukin-10 (IL-10) and through the expression of membrane molecules such as CTLA4, whose interaction with the corresponding receptors delivers a downregulatory signal.

Antigen-Presenting Cells

APC, such as the macrophages, macrophage-related cells, and dendritic cells play a very significant role in the induction stages of the immune response by trapping and presenting both native antigens and antigen fragments in a most favorable way for the recognition by lymphocytes. In addition, these cells also deliver activating signals to lymphocytes engaged in antigen recognition, both in the form of soluble mediators (interleukins, such as IL-1, IL-12, and IL-18) and in the form of signals delivered by cell–cell contact.

Phagocytic Cells

Phagocytic cells, such as monocytes, macrophages, and granulocytes, also play significant roles as effectors of the immune response. One of their main functions is to eliminate antigens that have elicited an immune response. This is achieved by means of antibodies and complement, as discussed in the section on antigens and antibodies. However, if the antigen is located on the surface of a cell, antibody induces the attachment of cytotoxic cells that cause the death of the antibody-coated cell [antibody-dependent cellular cytotoxicity (ADCC)].

Natural Killer Cells

Natural killer cells play a dual role in the elimination of infected and malignant cells. These cells are unique in that they have two different mechanisms of recognition: they can identify malignant or viral-infected cells by their decreased expression of histocompatibility antigens (HLA), and they can recognize antibody-coated cells and mediate ADCC.

ANTIGENS AND ANTIBODIES

Antigens are usually exogenous substances (cells, proteins, and polysaccharides), which are recognized by receptors on lymphocytes, thereby eliciting the immune response. The receptor molecules located on the membrane of lymphocytes interact with small portions of those foreign cells or proteins that are designated as antigenic determinants or epitopes. An adult human being has the capability to recognize millions of different antigens, producing antibodies, proteins that appear in circulation after infection or immunization and that have the ability to react specifically with epitopes of the antigen introduced in the organism. Because antibodies are soluble and are present in virtually all body fluids ("humors"), the term humoral immunity was introduced to designate the immune responses in which antibodies play the principal role as effector mechanism. Antibodies are also generically designated as immunoglobulins. This term derives from the fact that antibody molecules structurally belong to the family of proteins known as globulins (globular proteins) and from their involvement in immunity.

Antigen–Antibody Reactions, Complement, and Opsonization

The knowledge that the serum of an immunized animal contained protein molecules able to bind specifically to the antigen led to exhaustive investigations of the characteristics and consequences of the antigen–antibody reactions. At a morphological level, two types of reactions were defined:

1. If the antigen is soluble, the reaction with specific antibody under appropriate conditions results in precipitation of large antigen–antibody aggregates.
2. If the antigen is expressed on a cell membrane, the cell will be cross-linked by antibody and form visible clumps (agglutination).

Functionally, antigen–antibody reactions can be classified by their biological consequences:

1. Viruses and soluble toxins released by bacteria lose their infectivity or pathogenic properties after reaction with the corresponding antibodies (neutralization).
2. Antibodies complexed with antigens can activate the complement system. Nine major proteins or components that are sequentially activated constitute this system. Some of the complement components are able to promote ingestion of microorganisms by phagocytic cells, while others are inserted into cytoplasmic membranes and cause their disruption, leading to lysis of the offending microbial cell.
3. Antibodies can cause the destruction of microorganisms by promoting their ingestion by phagocytic cells or their destruction by cells mediating ADCC. Phagocytosis is particularly important for the elimination of bacteria and involves the binding of antibodies and complement components to the outer surface of the infectious agent (opsonization) and recognition of the bound antibody and/or complement components as a signal for ingestion by the phagocytic cell.
4. Antigen–antibody reactions are the basis of certain pathological conditions, such as allergic reactions. Antibody-mediated allergic reactions have a very rapid onset, in a matter of minutes, and are known as immediate hypersensitivity reactions.

LYMPHOCYTES AND CELL-MEDIATED IMMUNITY

Lymphocytes play a significant role as effector cells in three main types of situations, all of them considered as an expression of cell-mediated immunity; that is, immune reactions in which T lymphocytes are the predominant effector cells.

Immune Elimination of Intracellular Infectious Agents

Viruses, bacteria, parasites, and fungi have developed strategies that allow them to survive inside phagocytic cells or cells of other types. Infected cells are generally not amenable to destruction by phagocytosis or complement-mediated lysis. The study of how the immune system recognizes and eliminates infected cells resulted in the definition of the biological role of the HLA that has been described as responsible for graft rejection (see next). Those membrane molecules have a peptide-binding pouch that needs to be occupied, either with peptides derived from endogenous or from exogenous proteins. The immune system does not recognize self-peptides associated with self-HLA molecules. In the case of infected cells, peptides split from microbial proteins synthesized by the infected cell as part of the microbial replication cycle become associated with HLA molecules. The HLA-peptide complexes are presented to the immune system and activate specific cytotoxic T lymphocytes as well as specific Th1 lymphocytes. Both cytotoxic T cells and Th1 lymphocytes can mediate killing of the infected cells against which they became sensitized. Cytotoxic T cells kill the infected cells directly, stopping the replication of the intracellular organism, whereas activated Th1 cells release cytokines, such as interferon-γ, which activate macrophages and increase their ability to destroy the intracellular infectious agents.

Transplant (Graft) Rejection

As stated earlier, the immune system does not respond (i.e., is tolerant) to self-antigens, including antigens of the major histocompatibility complex (MHC), which includes the HLA molecules. However, transplantation of tissues among genetically different individuals of the same species or across species is followed by rejection of the grafted organs or tissues. The rejection reaction is triggered by the presentation of peptides generated from nonself MHC molecules. The MHC system is highly polymorphic (hundreds of alleles have defined and new ones are added on a regular basis to the known repertoire) and this leads to the generation of millions of peptides that differ in structure from individual to individual.

Delayed Hypersensitivity

Although the elimination of intracellular infectious agents can be considered as the main physiological role of cell-mediated immunity and graft rejection is an unexpected and undesirable consequence of a medical procedure, other lymphocyte-mediated immune reactions can be considered as pathological conditions arising spontaneously in predisposed individuals. The most common example are skin reactions described as cutaneous hypersensitivity, induced by direct skin contact or by intradermal injection of antigenic substances. These reactions express themselves 24 to 48 hours after exposure to an antigen to which the patient had been previously sensitized and, because of this timing factor, received the designation of delayed hypersensitivity reactions.

SELF VERSUS NONSELF DISCRIMINATION

The immune response is triggered by the interaction of an antigenic determinant with specific receptors on lymphocytes. It is calculated that there are several millions of different receptors in lymphocytes—10^{15} to 10^{18} on T cells and 10^{11} on B cells—sufficient to respond to a wide diversity of epitopes presented by microbial agents and potentially noxious exogenous compounds. At the same time, the immune system has the capacity to generate lymphocytes with receptors able to interact with epitopes expressed by self-antigens. During embryonic differentiation and adult life, the organism uses a variety of mechanisms to ensure that potentially autoreactive lymphocytes are eliminated or turned off. This lack of response to self-antigens is known as tolerance to self.

When the immune system is exposed to exogenous compounds, it tends to develop a vigorous immune response. The discrimination between self and nonself is based on the fact that the immune system has the ability to recognize a wide variety of structural differences on exogenous compounds. For example, infectious agents have marked differences in their chemical structure, easily recognizable by the immune system. Cells, proteins, and polysaccharides from animals of different species have differences in chemical constitution which, as a rule, are directly related to the degree of phylogenetic divergence between species. Those also elicit potent immune responses. Finally, many polysaccharides and proteins from individuals of any given species show antigenic heterogeneity, reflecting the genetic diversity of individuals within a species. Those differences are usually minor (relative to differences between species), but can still be recognized by the immune system. Transfusion reactions, graft rejection, and hypersensitivity reactions to exogenous human proteins are clinical expressions of the recognition of this type of differences between individuals.

A GENERAL OVERVIEW

One of the most difficult intellectual exercises in immunology is to try to understand the global organization and control of the immune system. Its extreme complexity and the wide array of

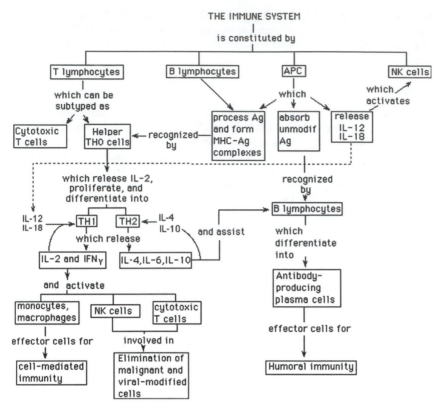

FIGURE 1   Diagrammatic representation of the major elements involved in the adaptive immune response.

regulatory circuits involved in fine-tuning the immune response pose a formidable obstacle to our understanding. A diagrammatic depiction of the main elements and steps involved in the adaptive immune response is reproduced in Figure 1.

If we use as an example the activation of the immune system by an infectious agent that has managed to overcome the innate anti-infectious defenses, the first step must be the uptake of the infectious agent by a cell capable of presenting it to the immune system in favorable conditions for the induction of an immune response. In the case of T lymphocytes, APCs expressing MHC-II molecules play this role. A variety of cells can function as APCs, including tissue macrophages, B cells, and dendritic cells. Those cells adsorb the infectious agent to their surface, ingest some of the absorbed microorganism, and process it into small antigenic subunits. These subunits become intracellularly associated with HLA, and the resulting complex is transported to the cytoplasmic membrane, allowing stimulation of Th lymphocytes. The interaction between surface proteins expressed by APCs and T lymphocytes as well as cytokines released by the APCs act as costimulants of the Th cells. How antigen is presented to B cells is not very clear, but it is well-established that the activation of an immune response takes place in a lymphoid organ (lymph node, peri-intestinal lymphoid tissues, spleen). All cellular elements necessary for the inductive and effector stages of an immune response are present on the lymphoid tissues, where there is ample opportunity for interactions and cooperation between those different cells.

Once stimulated to proliferate and differentiate, Th cells become able to assist the differentiation of effector cells. However, not all Th cells seem to assist all types of effector cells that require their help. Activated Th1 lymphocytes secrete cytokines that act on a variety of cells, including macrophages (further increasing their level of activation and enhancing their ability to eliminate infectious agents that may be surviving intracellularly) and cytotoxic T cells, which are very efficient in the elimination of virus-infected cells. In contrast, activated Th2 lymphocytes secrete a different set of cytokines that will assist the proliferation and differentiation of antigen-stimulated B lymphocytes, which then differentiate into plasma cells. The plasma cells are engaged in the synthesis of large amounts of antibody.

As stated earlier, antibodies are the main effector molecules of the humoral immune response. As specific antibodies bind to a microorganism and the complement system is activated, the microorganisms will either be ingested and destroyed by phagocytic cells or will be killed by complement-mediated lysis or by leukocytes able to mediate ADCC.

Once the microorganism is removed, negative feedback mechanisms become predominant, turning off the immune response. The downregulation of the immune response appears to result from the combination of several factors, such as the elimination of the positive stimulus that the microorganism represented, and the activation of lymphocytes with immunoregulatory activity that secrete cytokines that deliver inactivating signals to other lymphocytes.

At the end of the immune response, a residual population of long-lived lymphocytes specific for the offending antigen will remain. This is the population of memory cells that is responsible for protection, after natural exposure or immunization. It is also the same generic cell subpopulation that may cause accelerated graft rejections in recipients of multiple grafts. As discussed in greater detail next, the same immune system that protects us can be responsible for a variety of pathological conditions.

IMMUNOLOGY AND MEDICINE

Immunological concepts have found ample applications in medicine, in areas related to diagnosis, treatment, prevention, and pathogenesis.

The exquisite specificity of the antigen-antibody reaction has been extensively applied to the development of diagnostic assays for a variety of substances. Such applications received a strong boost when experiments with malignant plasma cell lines and normal antibody-producing cells resulted serendipitously in the discovery of the technique of hybridoma production, the basis for the production of monoclonal antibodies, which have had an enormous impact in the fields of diagnosis and immunotherapy.

Immunotherapy is a field with enormous potential. Efforts to stimulate the immune system of patients with acquired immunodeficiency syndrome (AIDS) with cytokines (particularly IL-2) have met with some success. Other areas of interest are the treatment of malignancies with monoclonal antibodies and immunotoxins, and induction of tolerance to grafts, but the excellent results obtained in studies with animal models have not been replicated in humans. The main clinical successes have been obtained in the prevention and treatment of graft rejection with monoclonal antibodies and on the therapeutic downregulation of hypersensitivity and inflammatory reactions using anti-cytokine antibodies or recombinant soluble receptors.

1. The study of children with deficient development of their immune system (immunodeficiency diseases) has provided the best tools for the study of the immune system in humans, while at the same time giving us ample opportunity to devise corrective therapies. AIDS underscored the delicate balance that is maintained between the immune system and infectious agents in the healthy individual and has stimulated a considerable amount of basic research into the regulation of the immune system.
2. The importance of maintaining self-tolerance in adult life is obvious when we consider the consequences of the loss of tolerance. Several diseases, some affecting single organs, others of a systemic nature, have been classified as autoimmune diseases. In those diseases, the immune system reacts against cells and tissues, and this reactivity can either be the primary insult leading to the disease, or may represent a factor contributing to the evolution and increasing severity of the disease. Considerable effort has been dedicated to the study of conditions that could reconstitute the state of tolerance in these patients, but so far without clinical translation.
3. Not all reactions against nonself are beneficial. If and when the delicate balance that keeps the immune system from overreacting is broken, hypersensitivity diseases may become

manifest. The common allergies, such as asthma and hay fever, are prominent examples of diseases caused by hypersensitivity reactions. The manipulation of the immune response to induce a protective rather than harmful immunity was first attempted with success in this type of disease.

4. Research into the mechanisms underlying the normal state of tolerance against nonself attained during normal pregnancy continues to be intensive, since this knowledge could be the basis for more effective manipulations of the immune response in patients needing organ transplants and for the treatment or prevention of infertility.

5. The concept that malignant mutant cells are constantly being eliminated by the immune system (immune surveillance) and that malignancies develop when the mutant cells escape the protective effects of the immune system has been extensively debated, but not quite proven. However, anticancer therapies directed at the enhancement of antitumoral responses continue to be evaluated, and some have met with encouraging results.

In the following chapters of this book, we illustrate the productive interaction that has always existed in immunology between basic concepts and clinical applications. In fact, no other biological discipline illustrates better the importance of the interplay between basic and clinical scientists; in this lies probably the main reason for the prominence of immunology as a biomedical discipline.

2 | Cells and Tissues Involved in the Immune Response

Gabriel Virella
Department of Microbiology and Immunology, Medical University of South Carolina, Charleston, South Carolina, U.S.A.

INTRODUCTION

The fully developed immune system of humans and most mammalians is constituted by a variety of cells and tissues whose different functions are remarkably well-integrated. Among the cells, the lymphocytes play the key roles in the control and regulation of immune responses as well as in the recognition of infected or heterologous cells, which the lymphocytes can recognize as undesirable and promptly eliminate. Among the tissues, the thymus is the site of differentiation for T lymphocytes and, as such, directly involved in critical steps in the differentiation of the immune system.

Cells of the Immune System

Lymphocytes

Lymphocytes (Fig. 1A) occupy a very special place among the leukocytes that participate in one way or another in immune reactions due to their ability to interact specifically with antigenic substances and to react to nonself antigenic determinants. Lymphocytes differentiate from stem cells in the fetal liver, bone marrow, and thymus into two main functional classes. They are found in the peripheral blood and in all lymphoid tissues.

B Lymphocytes

B lymphocytes or B cells are so designated because the Bursa of Fabricius, a lymphoid organ located close to the caudal end of the gut in birds, plays a key role in their differentiation. Removal of this organ, at or shortly before hatching, is associated with lack of differentiation, maturation of B lymphocytes, and the inability to produce antibodies. A mammalian counterpart to the avian bursa has not yet been found. Some investigators believe that the bone marrow is the most likely organ for B lymphocyte differentiation, while others propose that the peri-intestinal lymphoid tissues play this role.

B lymphocytes carry immunoglobulins on their cell membrane, which function as antigen receptors. After proper stimulation, B cells undergo blastogenic transformation and after several rounds of division differentiate into antibody producing cells (plasma cells). Activated B lymphocytes may also play the role of antigen-presenting cells (APC), which is usually attributed to cells of monocytic/macrophagic lineage (see Chapters 3 and 4).

T Lymphocytes

T lymphocytes or T cells are so designated because the thymus plays a key role in their differentiation. The functions of the T lymphocytes include the regulation of immune responses, and various effector functions (cytotoxicity and lymphokine production being the main ones) that are the basis of cell-mediated immunity. T lymphocytes also carry an antigen-recognition unit on their membranes, known as T cell receptors (TcR). TcR and immunoglobulin molecules are structurally unrelated.

Several subpopulations of T lymphocytes with separate functions have been recognized. The main two populations are the helper T lymphocytes, involved in the induction and regulation of immune responses, and the cytotoxic T lymphocytes, involved in the destruction of infected cells. It is also known that at specific stages of the immune response, T lymphocytes

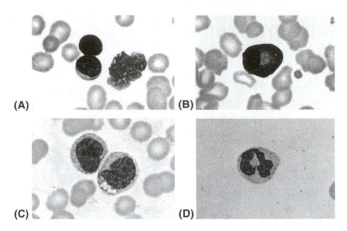

FIGURE 1   Morphology of the main types of human leukocytes. (**A**) Lymphocyte; (**B**) plasma cell; (**C**) monocyte; (**D**) granulocyte. *Source*: Reproduced from Reich PR. Manual of Hematology. Kalamazoo, MI: Upjohn, 1976.

can have regulatory functions, and it appears that there are several subpopulations of T lymphocytes with the capacity to suppress immune responses (regulatory T cells or Tregs).

Membrane markers have been used to define T lymphocyte subpopulations, although it seems obvious that the phenotype can only be correlated with a predominant function, not to the exclusion of others. For example, it is possible to differentiate cells with predominant helper function from those with predominant cytotoxic function, but it is well-known that phenotypically helper T lymphocytes can also behave as cytotoxic effector cells.

T lymphocytes have a longer life span than B lymphocytes. Long-lasting lymphocytes are particularly important because of their involvement on immunological memory.

T Lymphocyte activation requires the interaction of the T cell receptor with an antigen-derived polypeptide and additional costimulatory signals from auxiliary cells. When properly stimulated, a small, resting T lymphocyte rapidly undergoes blastogenic transformation into a large lymphocyte (13–15 μm). This large lymphocyte (lymphoblast) then divides several times to produce an expanded population of medium (9–12 μm) and small lymphocytes (5–8 μm) with the same antigenic specificity. Activated and differentiated T lymphocytes are morphologically indistinguishable from a small, resting lymphocyte.

Plasma Cells

Plasma cells are morphologically characterized by their eccentric nuclei with clumped chromatin, and a large cytoplasm with abundant rough endoplasmic reticulum (Fig. 1B). Plasma cells produce and secrete large amounts of immunoglobulins, but do not express membrane immunoglobulins. Plasma cells seldom divide, if at all. Plasma cells are usually found in the bone marrow and in the perimucosal lymphoid tissues.

Natural Killer Cells

Natural killer (NK) cells morphologically are described as large granular lymphocytes. These cells do not carry antigen receptors of any kind, but can recognize antibody molecules bound to target cells and destroy those cells, using the same general mechanisms involved on T lymphocyte cytotoxicity (antibody-dependent cellular cytotoxicity). They also have a recognition mechanism that allows them to destroy tumor cells and viral-infected cells.

A related lymphocyte subpopulation are the NK T cells that express the TcR/CD3 complex. This is a heterogeneous group of cells, which share the ability to recognize and kill tumor cells with NK cells, but also appear involved in immunoregulation.

Antigen-Presenting Cells: Monocytes, Macrophages, and Dendritic Cells

Monocytes and macrophages are believed to be closely related. The monocyte (Fig. 1C) is considered a leukocyte in transit through the blood, which, when fixed in a tissue, will become a macrophage. Monocytes and macrophages, as well as granulocytes (see the next section), are able to ingest particulate matter (microorganisms, cells, and inert particles) and for this reason are said to have phagocytic functions. The phagocytic activity is greater in macrophages (particularly after activation by soluble mediators released during immune responses) than in monocytes.

Macrophages and monocytes play an important role in the inductive stages of the immune response by processing complex antigens and concentrating antigen fragments on the cell membrane. In this form, the antigen is recognized by helper T lymphocytes, as discussed in detail in Chapters 3 and 4. For this reason, these cells are known as antigen-presenting cells (APCs). The most specialized and efficient APCs are the dendritic cells, which are also heterogenous, including at least two populations, one of myeloid origin and the other of lymphoid origin. Some dendritic cells tend to be present in tissues such as the kidney, brain (microglia), capillary walls, and mucosae. In the resting state, they seem very inefficient as APCs, but after activation by microbial substance or other stimuli they migrate to the lymphoid tissues, where they differentiate into efficient APCs, able to stimulate naive T cells. The Langerhans cells of the epidermis are of myeloid origin and are the prototype for migrating dendritic cells. When they reach the lymph nodes, Langerhans cells assume the morphological characteristics of dendritic cells and interact with T lymphocytes (Fig. 2).

A defining property of all APCs is the expression of a special class of histocompatibility antigens, designated as class-II major histocompatibility complex (MHC) antigens (see Chapter 3). The expression of MHC-II molecules is essential for the interaction with helper T lymphocytes. APCs also release cytokines, which assist the proliferation of antigen-stimulated lymphocytes, including interleukins-1, -6, and -12.

Another type of cell involved in the inductive stages of the immune response is the follicular dendritic cell, present in the spleen and lymph nodes, particularly in follicles and germinal centers. This cell, apparently of monocytic lineage, is not phagocytic and does not express MHC-II molecules on the membrane, but appears particularly suited to carry out the antigen-presenting function in relation to B lymphocytes. Follicular dendritic cells concentrate unprocessed antigen on the membrane and keep it there for relatively long periods of time—a factor that may be crucial for a sustained B cell response. The follicular dendritic cells form a network in the germinal centers, known as the antigen-retaining reticulum.

Granulocytes

Granulocytes are a collection of white blood cells with segmented or lobulated nuclei and granules in their cytoplasm, which are visible with special stains. Because of their segmented nuclei, which assume variable sizes and shapes, these cells are generically designated as polymorphonuclear

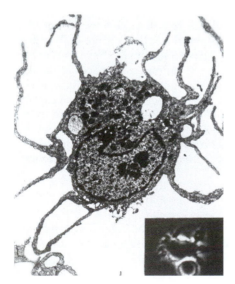

FIGURE 2   Electron microphotograph of a follicular dendritic cell isolated from a rat lymph node (×5000). The inset illustrates the in vitro interaction between a dendritic cell and a lymphocyte as seen in phase contrast microscopy (×300). *Source*: Reproduced from Klinkert WEF, Labadie JH, O'Brien JP, Beyer LF, Bowers WE. Proc Natl Acad Sci USA 1980; 77:5414.

(PMN) leukocytes (Fig. 1D). Different subpopulations of granulocytes (neutrophils, eosinophils, and basophils) can be distinguished by differential staining of the cytoplasmic granules, reflecting their different chemical constitution.

Neutrophils

Neutrophils are the largest subpopulation of white blood cells and have two types of cytoplasmic granules containing compounds with bactericidal activity. Their biological importance derives from their phagocytic activity. Similar to most other phagocytic cells, they ingest with greatest efficiency microorganisms and particulate matter coated by antibody and complement (see Chapter 9). However, nonimmunological mechanisms have also been shown to lead to phagocytosis by neutrophils, perhaps reflecting phylogenetically more primitive mechanisms of recognition.

Neutrophils are attracted by chemotactic factors to areas of inflammation. Those factors may be released by microbes (particularly bacteria) or may be generated during complement activation as a consequence of an antigen–antibody reaction. The attraction of neutrophils is especially intense in bacterial infections. Great numbers of neutrophils may die trying to eliminate the invading bacteria. Dead PMN and their debris become the primary component of pus, characteristic of many bacterial infections. Bacterial infections associated with the formation of pus are designated as purulent.

Eosinophils

Eosinophils are PMN leukocytes with granules that stain orange–red with cytological stains containing eosin. These cells are found in high concentrations in allergic reactions and during parasitic infections, and their roles in both areas will be discussed in later chapters.

Basophils

Basophils have granules that stain metachromatically due to their contents of histamine and heparin. The tissue-fixed mast cells are very similar to basophils, even though they appear to evolve from different precursor cells. Both basophils and mast cells are involved in antiparasitic immune mechanisms and play a key pathogenic role in allergic reactions.

LYMPHOID TISSUES AND ORGANS

The immune system is organized on several special tissues, collectively designated as lymphoid or immune tissues. These tissues, as shown in Figure 3, are distributed throughout the entire body. Some lymphoid tissues achieve a remarkable degree of organization and can be designated as lymphoid organs. The most ubiquitous of the lymphoid organs are the lymph nodes that are located in groups along major blood vessels and loose connective tissues. Other mammalian lymphoid organs are the thymus and the spleen (white pulp). Lymphoid tissues include the gut-associated lymphoid tissues (GALT)—tonsils, Peyer's patches, and appendix—as well as aggregates of lymphoid tissue in the submucosal spaces of the respiratory and genitourinary tracts. The distribution of T and B lymphocytes within human lymphoid tissues is not homogeneous. As shown in Table 1, T lymphocytes predominate in the lymph, peripheral blood, and, above all, in the thymus. B lymphocytes predominate in the bone marrow and perimucosal lymphoid tissues. Furthermore, lymphoid tissues can be subdivided into primary and secondary lymphoid tissues based on the ability to produce progenitor cells of the lymphocytic lineage, which is characteristic of primary lymphoid tissues (thymus and bone marrow).

Lymph Nodes

The lymph nodes are extremely numerous and disseminated all over the body. They measure 1 to 25 mm in diameter and play a very important and dynamic role in the initial or inductive states of the immune response.

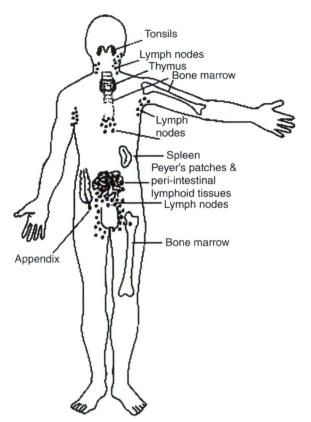

FIGURE 3 Diagrammatic representation of the distribution of lymphoid tissues in humans. *Source*: Modified from Mayerson HS. Sci Am 1963; 208:80.

Anatomical Organization

The lymph nodes are circumscribed by a connective tissue capsule. Afferent lymphatics draining peripheral interstitial spaces enter the capsule of the node and open into the subcapsular sinus. The lymph node also receives blood from the systemic circulation through the hilar arteriole. Two main regions can be distinguished in a lymph node: the cortex and the medulla. The cortex and the deep cortex (also known as paracortical area) are densely populated by lymphocytes, in constant traffic between the lymphatic and systemic circulation. In the cortex, at low magnification, one can distinguish roughly spherical areas containing densely packed lymphocytes, termed follicles or nodules (Fig. 4).

T and B lymphocytes occupy different areas in the cortex. B lymphocytes predominate in the follicles (hence, the follicles are designated as T-independent area), which also contain

TABLE 1 Distribution of T and B Lymphocytes in Humans

Immune tissue	Lymphocyte distribution (%)[a]	
	T lymphocyte	B lymphocyte
Peripheral blood	80	10[b]
Thoracic duct	90	10
Lymph node	75	25
Spleen	50	50
Thymus	100	<5
Bone marrow	<25	>75
Peyer's patch	10–20	70

[a]Approximate values.
[b]The remaining 10% would correspond to non-T, non-B lymphocytes.

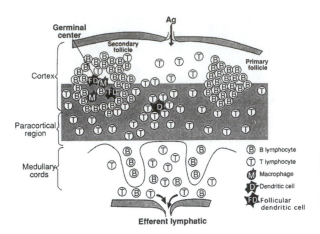

FIGURE 4 Diagrammatic representation of the lymph node structure. B lymphocytes are predominantly located on the lymphoid follicles and medullary cords (B-dependent areas), while T lymphocytes are mostly found in the paracortical area (T-dependent area).

macrophages, dendritic cells, and some T lymphocytes. The follicles can assume two different morphologies:

1. The primary follicles are very densely packed with small naive B lymphocytes.
2. In a lymph node draining, an area in which an infection has taken place, one will find larger, less dense follicles, termed secondary follicles, containing a dark, packed mantle, where naive B cells predominate, and clear germinal centers, where B lymphocytes are actively dividing as a result of antigenic stimulation.

Nonstimulated B cells enter the germinal center by the mantle area of the basal dark zone. In the light zone, B cells interact with antigens retained by the follicular dendritic cells, and start to proliferate. The proliferation of B cells in germinal centers is associated with phenotypic changes (membrane IgD ceases to be expressed) and with somatic mutations affecting the genes coding for the variable regions of the immunoglobulin molecule (see Chapters 5 and 7). The proliferation and differentiation of B cells continues on the apical light zone, where B lymphocytes eventually differentiate into plasma cells and memory B cells. In humans, both plasmablasts and memory B cells leave the lymph node through the medullary cords. Memory B cells enter recirculation patterns, which are described later in this chapter. Plasmablasts are home to the bone marrow, where they fully differentiate into plasma cells.

In the deep cortex or paracortical area, which is not as densely populated as the follicles, T lymphocytes are the predominant cell population, and for this reason, the paracortical area is designated as T-dependent. Dendritic cells are also present in this area, where they present antigen to T lymphocytes.

The medulla, less densely populated, is organized into medullary cords draining into the hilar efferent lymphatic vessels. Plasmablasts can be easily identified in the medullary cords.

Physiological Role

The lymph nodes can be compared to a network of filtration and communication stations, where antigens are trapped and messages are interchanged between the different cells involved in the immune response. This complex system of interactions is made possible by the dual circulation in the lymph nodes. Lymph nodes receive both lymph and arterial blood flow. The afferent lymph, with its cellular elements, percolates from the subcapsular sinus to the efferent lymphatics via cortical and medullary sinuses, and the cellular elements of the lymph have ample opportunity to migrate into the lymphocyte-rich cortical structures during their transit through the nodes. The artery that penetrates through the hilus brings peripheral blood lymphocytes into the lymph node; these lymphocytes can leave the vascular bed at the level of the high endothelial venules located in the paracortical area.

Thus, lymph nodes can be considered as the anatomical fulcrum of the immune response. Soluble or particulate antigens reach the lymph nodes primarily through the lymphatic circulation. Once in the lymph nodes, antigen is concentrated on the antigen-retaining reticulum formed by the follicular dendritic cells. The antigen is retained by these cells in its unprocessed form, often associated with antibody (particularly during secondary immune responses), and is efficiently presented to B lymphocytes. The B lymphocytes recognize specific epitopes, but are also able to internalize and process the antigen, presenting antigen-derived peptides associated to MHC-II molecules to helper T lymphocytes, whose "help" is essential for the proper activation and differentiation of the B cells presenting the antigen (see Chapter 3).

Spleen

The spleen is an organ with multiple functions. Its protective role against infectious diseases is related both to its filtering functions and to the presence of lymphoid structures—able to support the initial stages of the immune response.

Anatomical Organization

Surrounded by a connective tissue capsule, the parenchyma of this organ is heterogeneous, constituted by white and red pulp. The white pulp is rich in lymphocytes, arranged in periarteriolar lymphatic sheaths that surround the narrow central arterioles derived from the splenic artery after multiple branchings, and follicles, which lie more peripherally relative to the arterioles (Fig. 5). T cells are concentrated in the periarteriolar lymphatic sheaths, whereas B lymphocytes are concentrated in the follicles. The follicles may or may not show germinal centers depending on the state of activation of the resident cells.

The red pulp surrounds the white pulp. Blood leaving the white pulp through the central arterioles flows into the penicillar arteries and from there flows directly into the venous sinuses. The red pulp is formed by these venous sinuses that are bordered by the splenic cords (cords of Billroth), where macrophages abound. From the sinuses, blood re-enters the systemic circulation through the splenic vein.

Between the white and the red pulp lies an area known as the marginal zone, more sparsely cellular than the white pulp but very rich in macrophages and B lymphocytes.

Physiological Role

The spleen is the lymphoid organ associated with the clearing of particulate matter, infectious organisms, and aged or defective formed elements (e.g., spherocytes, ovalocytes) from the peripheral blood. The main filtering function is performed by the macrophages lining up the splenic cords. In the marginal zone, circulating antigens are trapped by the macrophages, which will then be able to trap and process the antigen, migrate deeper into the white pulp, and initiate the immune response by interacting with T and B lymphocytes.

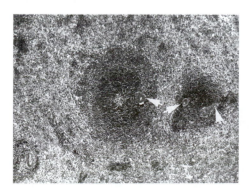

FIGURE 5 Morphology of the white pulp of the spleen. Lymphoid cells are concentrated around small arterioles (*arrows*), forming a diffuse periarteriolar lymphoid sheet, where T cells predominate, and large follicles (as seen in the picture) where B cells predominate. *Source*: Courtesy of Professor Robert W. Ogilvie, Department of Cell Biology and Anatomy, Medical University of South Carolina, Charleston, South Carolina, U.S.A.

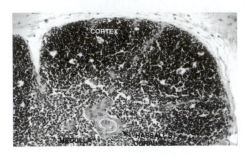

FIGURE 6 Morphology of a thymic lobe. The densely packed cortex is mostly populated by T lymphocytes and by some cortical dendritic epithelial cells and cortical epithelial cells. The more sparsely populated medulla contains epithelial and dendritic cells, macrophages, T lymphocytes and Hassall's corpuscles. *Source*: Courtesy of Professor Robert W. Ogilvie, Department of Cell Biology and Anatomy, Medical University of South Carolina, Charleston, South Carolina, U.S.A.

Thymus

The thymus is the only clearly individualized primary lymphoid organ in mammals. It is believed to play a key role in determining the differentiation of T lymphocytes.

Anatomical Organization

The thymus, whose microscopic structure is illustrated in Figure 6, is located in the superior mediastinum, anterior to the great vessels. It has a connective tissue capsule from which emerge the trabeculae, which divide the organ into lobules. Each lobule has a cortex and medulla, and the trabeculae are coated with epithelial cells.

The cortex, an area of intense cell proliferation, is mainly populated by immunologically immature T lymphocytes. A small number of macrophages and plasma cells are also present. In addition, the cortex contains two subpopulations of epithelial cells, the epithelial nurse cells and the cortical epithelial cells that form a network within the cortex.

Not as densely populated as the cortex, the medulla contains predominantly mature T lymphocytes, and has a larger epithelial cell to lymphocyte ratio than the cortex. Unique to the medulla are concentric rings of squamous epithelial cells known as Hassall's corpuscles.

Physiological Role

The thymus is believed to be the organ where T lymphocytes differentiate during embryonic life and thereafter, although for how long the thymus remains functional after birth is unclear (recent data shows that 30% of individuals of 40 years of age or older retain substantial thymic tissue and function). The thymic cortex is an area of intense cell proliferation and death (only 1% of the cells generated in the thymus eventually mature and migrate to the peripheral tissues).

The mechanism whereby the thymus determines T lymphocyte differentiation is believed to involve the interaction of T lymphocyte precursors with thymic epithelial cells. These interactions result in the elimination or inactivation of self-reactive T-cell clones and in the differentiation of two separate lymphocyte subpopulations with different membrane antigens and different functions. The thymic epithelial cells are also believed to produce hormonal factors (e.g., thymosin and thymopoietin) that may play an important role in the differentiation of T lymphocytes. Most T-lymphocyte precursors appear to reach full maturity in the medulla.

Mucosal-Associated Lymphoid Tissues

Mucosal-associated lymphoid tissues (MALT) encompass the lymphoid tissues of the intestinal tract, genitourinary tract, tracheobronchial tree, and mammary glands. All of the MALT are unencapsulated and contain both T and B lymphocytes, the latter predominating. GALT, on the other hand, is the designation proposed for all lymphatic tissues found along the digestive tract. Three major areas of GALT that can be identified are the tonsils, the Peyer's patches, located on the submucosa of the small intestine, and the appendix. In addition, scanty lymphoid tissue is present in the lamina propria of the gastrointestinal tract.

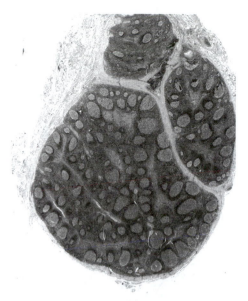

FIGURE 7 Morphology of the tonsils. The lymphoid tissue of these lymphoid organs is mostly constituted by primary and secondary follicles (characterized by the pale germinal centers), the latter predominating as seen in this picture. The predominant cell population in the tonsillar follicles is B cells. *Source*: Courtesy of Professor Robert W. Ogilvie, Department of Cell Biology and Anatomy, Medical University of South Carolina, Charleston, South Carolina, U.S.A.

Tonsils

Tonsils, localized in the oropharynx, are predominantly populated by T lymphocytes and are the site of intense antigenic stimulation, as reflected by the presence of numerous secondary follicles with germinal centers in the tonsilar crypts (Fig. 7).

Peyer's Patches

Peyer's patches are lymphoid structures disseminated through the submucosal space of the small intestine (Fig. 8). The follicles of the intestinal Peyer's patches are extremely rich in B cells, which differentiate into IgA-producing plasma cells. Specialized epithelial cells, known as M cells, abound in the dome epithelia of Peyer's patches, particularly at the ileum. These cells take up small particles, virus, bacteria, and so on and deliver them to submucosal macrophages, where the engulfed material will be processed and presented to T and B lymphocytes.

T lymphocytes are also diffusely present in the intestinal mucosa, the most abundant of them expressing membrane markers which are considered typical of memory helper T cells. This population appears to be critically involved in the induction of humoral immune responses. A special subset of T cells, with a different type of T cell receptor (γ/δ T lymphocytes), is well-represented on the mucosa of the small intestine. These lymphocytes appear to recognize and destroy infected epithelial cells by a nonimmunological mechanism (i.e., not involving the TcR).

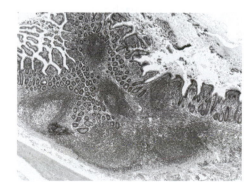

FIGURE 8 Morphology of a Peyer's patch. Well-developed follicles with obvious germinal centers are characteristic of the normal Peyer's patch. B lymphocytes are the predominant cell population. *Source*: Courtesy of Professor Robert W. Ogilvie, Department of Cell Biology and Anatomy, Medical University of South Carolina, Charleston, South Carolina, U.S.A.

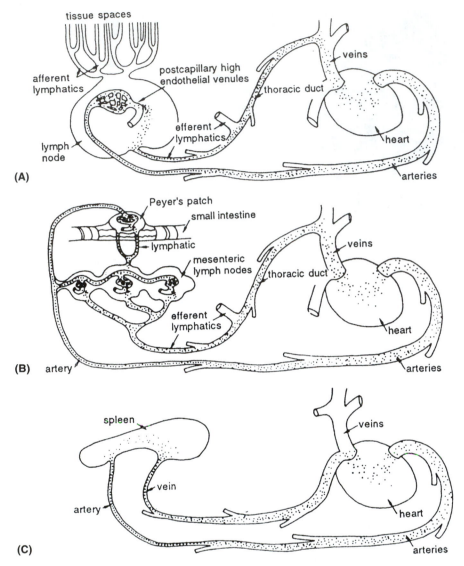

FIGURE 9 Pathways of lymphocyte circulation: (**A**) blood lymphocytes enter lymph nodes, adhere to the walls of specialized postcapillary venules, and migrate to the lymph node cortex. Lymphocytes then percolate through lymphoid fields to medullary lymphatic sinuses and on to efferent lymphatics, which in turn collect in major lymphatic ducts in the thorax that empty into the superior vena cava; (**B**) the gut-associated lymphoid tissues (Peyer's patches and mesenteric lymph nodes) drain into the thoracic duct, which also empties into the superior vena cava; (**C**) the spleen receives lymphocytes and disburses them mainly via the blood vascular system (inferior vena cava). *Source*: Reproduced from Hood LE, Weissman IL, Wood WB, Wilson JH. Immunology. 2nd Ed. Menlo Park, CA: Benjamin/Cummings, 1984.

LYMPHOCYTE TRAFFIC

The lymphatic and circulatory systems are intimately related (Fig. 9), and there is a constant traffic of lymphocytes throughout the body, moving from one system to another. Afferent lymphatics from interstitial spaces drain into lymph nodes, which "filter" these fluids, removing foreign substances. "Cleared" lymph from below the diaphragm and the upper left half of the body drains via efferent lymphatics, emptying into the thoracic duct for subsequent drainage into the left innominate vein. "Cleared" lymph from the right side above the diaphragm drains into the right lymphatic duct with subsequent drainage into the origin of the right innominate vein. The same routes are traveled by lymphocytes stimulated in the lymph nodes or peripheral lymphoid tissues, which eventually reach the systemic circulation.

Peripheral blood, in turn, is "filtered" by the spleen and liver, the spleen having organized lymphoid areas while the liver is rich in Kupffer's cells, which are macrophage-derived phagocytes. Organisms and antigens that enter directly into the systemic circulation will be trapped in these two organs, of which the spleen plays the most important role as a lymphoid organ.

Lymphocyte Recirculation and Extravascular Migration

One of the most important biological characteristics of B and T lymphocytes is their constant recirculation—entering the lymphoid tissues to circulate through the vascular system, just to enter the lymphoid tissues again or to exit into the interstitial tissues if an inflammatory reaction is taking place.

Lymphocytes circulating in the systemic circulation eventually enter a lymph node, exit the systemic circulation at the level of the high endothelial venules, leave the lymph node with the efferent lymph, and eventually re-enter the systemic circulation.

B lymphocytes of mucosal origin circulate between different segments of the MALT, including the GALT, the mammary gland-associated lymphoid tissue, and the lymphoid tissues associated with the respiratory tree and urinary tract.

Cell Adhesion Molecules

The crucial step in the traffic of lymphocytes from the systemic circulation to a lymphoid tissue or to interstitial tissues is the crossing of the endothelial barrier by diapedesis at specific locations. Under physiological conditions, this seems to take place predominantly at the level of the high endothelial venules of lymphoid tissues. These specialized endothelial cells express surface molecules—cell adhesion molecules (CAMs)—that interact with ligands, including other CAMs, expressed on the membrane of T and B lymphocytes. The interplay between endothelial and lymphocyte CAMs determines the traffic and homing of lymphocytes. CAMs are also upregulated during inflammatory reactions and determine the extravascular migration of lymphocytes and other white blood cells.

Three main families of CAMs have been defined (Table 2). The addressins or selectins are expressed on endothelial cells and leukocytes, and mediate leukocyte adherence to the endothelium. The immunoglobulin superfamily of CAMs includes a variety of molecules expressed by leukocytes, endothelial cells, and other cells. The integrins are defined as molecules that interact with the cytoskeleton and tissue matrix compounds. The following CAMs have been reported to be involved in lymphocyte traffic and homing:

1. LAM-1 (L-selectin), intercellular adhesion molecules (ICAM)-1, CD34, and CD44 are primarily involved in controlling lymphocyte traffic and homing in peripheral lymphoid tissues.
2. MadCAM-1 is believed to control lymphocyte homing to the mucosal lymphoid tissues.

The interaction between adhesion molecules and their ligands takes place in several stages. First, the cells adhere to the endothelial cells at the level of the high endothelium venules (HEV), and the adhering lymphocyte is then able to migrate through endothelial slits into the lymphoid organ parenchyma. Different CAMs and ligands are involved in this sequence of events.

Regulation of Lymphocyte Traffic and Homing

The way in which CAMs regulate lymphocyte traffic and homing seems to be a result both of differences in the level of their expression and in the nature of the CAMs expressed in different segments of the microcirculation. The involvement of HEV as the primary site for lymphocyte egress from the systemic circulation is a consequence of the interaction between CD34, a specific CAM expressed in HEV, and L-selectin, expressed by naive T lymphocytes. Because CD34 is predominantly expressed by HEV, the opportunity for cell adhesion and extravascular

TABLE 2 Main Adhesion Molecules, Their Families, Ligands, and Functions

Family	Members	Ligand	Function
Selectins			
	Endothelial-Leukocyte adhesion molecule (E-selectin)	Sialylated/fucosylated molecules	Mediates leukocyte adherence to endothelial cells in inflammatory reactions
	LAM-1, L-Selectin	Immunoglobulin superfamily CAMs; mucins and sialomucins	Interaction with HEV (lymphocyte homing); leukocyte adherence to endothelial cells in inflammatory reactions
Immunoglobulin Superfamily CAMs			
	ICAM-1	LFA-1 (CD11a/CD18), Mac-1 (CD11b)	Expressed by leukocytes, endothelial cells, dendritic cells, etc.; mediates leukocyte adherence to endothelial cells in inflammatory reactions
	ICAM-2	LFA-1	Expressed by leukocytes, endothelial cells, and dendritic cells; involved in control of lymphocyte recirculation and traffic
	VCAM-1	VLA-4	Expressed primarily by endothelial cells; mediates leukocyte adherence to activated endothelial cells in inflammatory reactions
	MadCAM-1	$\beta7$, $\alpha4$, L-Selectin	Expressed by mucosal lymphoid HEV; mediates lymphocyte homing to mucosal lymphoid tissues
	PECAM-1	PECAM-1	Expressed by platelets, leukocytes, and endothelial cells; involved in leukocyte transmigration across the endothelium in inflammation
Integrins			
VLA family	VLA-1 to 6	Fibronectin, laminin, collagen	Ligands mediating cell-cell and cell-substrate interaction
LEUCAM family	LFA-1	ICAM-1, ICAM-2, ICAM-3	Ligands mediating cell-cell and cell-substrate interaction
	Mac-1	ICAM-1, Fibrinogen, C3bi	
Other			
	CD34	L-selectin	HEV/lymphocyte interactions in the lymph nodes
	CD44	Hyaluronate, collagen, fibronectin	Expressed on leukocytes; mediates cell-cell and cell-matrix interactions; involved in lymphocyte homing

Abbreviations: CAM, cell adhesion molecules; HEV, high endothelium venules; ICAM, intercellular adhesion molecules; LAM, leukocyte adhesion molecule; LFA, leukocyte function antigen; Mac-1, a synonym of complement receptor 3 (CR3); MadCAM-1, Mucosal addressin CAM-1; PECAM, platelet/endothelial cell adhesion molecules; VCAM, vascular cell adhesion molecules; VLA, very late antigen.

migration is considerably higher in HEV than on segments of the venous circulation covered by flat endothelium.

It is known that the lymphocyte constitution of lymphoid organs is variable (Table 1). T lymphocytes predominate in the lymph nodes, but B lymphocytes and IgA-producing plasma cells predominate in the Peyer's patches and the GALT, in general. This differential homing is believed to be the result of the expression of specific addressins such as MadCAM-1 on the HEV of the perimucosal lymphoid tissues that are specifically recognized by the B cells and plasma cells resident in those tissues. Most B lymphocytes recognize specifically the GALT-associated HEV and do not interact with the lymph node-associated HEV, while most naive T lymphocytes recognize both the lymph node-associated HEV and the GALT-associated HEV.

The differentiation of T-dependent and B-dependent areas in lymphoid tissues is a poorly understood aspect of lymphocyte "homing." It appears likely that the distribution of T and B lymphocytes is determined by their interaction with nonlymphoid cells. For example, the interaction between interdigitating cells and T lymphocytes may determine the predominant location of T lymphocytes in the lymph node paracortical areas and periarteriolar sheets of the spleen, while the interaction of B lymphocytes with follicular dendritic cells may determine the organization of lymphoid follicles in the lymph node, spleen, and GALT.

The modulation of CAMs at different states of cell activation explains changing patterns in lymphocyte recirculation seen during immune responses. Immediately after antigen stimulation, the recirculating lymphocyte appears to transiently lose its capacity to recirculate. This loss of recirculating ability is associated with a tendency to self-aggregate (perhaps explaining why antigen-stimulated lymphocytes are trapped at the site of maximal antigen density), due to the upregulation of CAMs involved in lymphocyte–lymphocyte and lymphocyte-accessory cell interactions.

After the antigenic stimulus ceases, a population of memory T lymphocytes carrying distinctive membrane proteins can be identified. This population seems to have a different recirculation pattern than that of the naive T lymphocyte, leaving the intravascular compartment at sites other than the HEV, and reaching the lymph nodes via the lymphatic circulation. This difference in migration seems to result from the downregulation of the CAMs, which mediate the interaction with HEV selectins and upregulation of other CAMs, which interact with selectins located in other areas of the vascular tree.

B lymphocytes also change their recirculation patterns after antigenic stimulation. Most B cells differentiate into plasma cells after stimulation, and this differentiation is associated with marked changes in the antigenic composition of the cell membrane. Consequently, the plasma-cell precursors (plasmablasts) exit the germinal centers, move into the medullary cords, and, eventually, to the bone marrow, where most of the antibody production in humans takes place. Another B cell subpopulation—the memory B cells—retain B cell markers and re-enter the circulation to migrate back to specific territories of the lymphoid tissues.

All memory lymphocytes, T or B, appear to home preferentially in the type of lymphoid tissue where the original antigen encounter took place, that is, a lymphocyte that recognized an antigen in a peripheral lymph node will recirculate to another peripheral lymph node, while a lymphocyte that was stimulated at the GALT level will recirculate to the GALT. Memory B lymphocytes remain in the germinal centers while memory T lymphocytes "home" in T cell areas.

Inflammatory and immune reactions often lead to the release of mediators that upregulate the expression of CAMs in venules or in other segments of the microvasculature near the area where the reaction takes place. This results in a sequence of events that is mediated by different sets of CAMs at the respective ligands.

First, the leukocytes slow down and start rolling along the endothelial surface. This stage is mediated primarily by selections. Next, leukocytes adhere to endothelial cells expressing integrins, such as VLA and CAMs of the immunoglobulin superfamily, such as ICAM and vascular cell adhesion molecules (VCAM). Finally, the adherent leukocytes squeeze between two adjoining endothelial cells and move to the extravascular space.

The end result of this process is an increase in leukocyte migration to specific areas where those cells are needed to eliminate some type of noxious stimulus or to initiate an immune response. As a corollary, there is great interest in developing compounds that are able to block upregulated CAMs to be used as anti-inflammatory agents.

BIBLIOGRAPHY

Agnello D, Lankford CS, Bream J, et al. Cytokines and transcription factors that regulate T helper cell differentiation: new players and new insights. J Clin Immunol 2003; 23:147–146.

Bevilaqua MP. Endothelial-leucocyte adhesion molecules. Annu Rev Immunol 1993; 11:767.

Camerini V, Panwala C, Kronenberg M. Regional specialization of the mucosal immune system. Intraepithelial lymphocytes of the large intestine have a different phenotype and function than those of the small intestine. J Immunol 1993; 151:1765.

Collins T. Adhesion molecules and leukocyte emigration. Sci Med 1995; 2(6):28–37.

Dustin ML, Springer TA. Role of lymphocyte adhesion receptors in transient interactions and cell locomotion. Annu Rev Immunol 1991; 9:27.

Garside P, Ingulli E, Merica RR, et al. Visualization of specific B and T interactions in the lymph node. Science 1998; 281:96.

Jankovic D, Liu Z, Gause WC. Th1- and Th2-cell commitment during infectious disease: asymmetry in divergent pathways. Trends Immunol 2001; 22:450–457.

Jiang H, Chess L. An integrated view of suppressor T cell subsets in immunoregulation. J Clin Invest 2004; 114:1198–1208.

JunMichl J, Qiu QY, Kuerer HM. Homing receptors and addressins. Curr Opin Immunol 1991; 3:373.

Klaus GGB, Humphrey JH, Kunkl A, Dongworth DW. The follicular dendritic cell: its role in antigen presentation in the generation of immunological memory. Immunol Rev 1980; 53:3.

MacLennan ICM. Germinal centers. Annu Rev Immunol 1994; 12:117.

Moll H. Antigen delivery by dendritic cells. Int J Med Microbiol 2004; 294:337–344.

O'Garra A, Vieira P. Regulatory T cells and mechanisms of immune system control. Nat Med 2004; 10:891–804.

Picker LJ, Butcher EC. Physiological and molecular mechanisms of lymphocyte homing. Annu Rev Immunol 1992; 10:561.

3 | Major Histocompatibility Complex

Janardan P. Pandey
Department of Microbiology and Immunology, Medical University of South Carolina, Charleston, South Carolina, U.S.A.

INTRODUCTION

Grafting of tissues or organs between genetically unrelated individuals is usually followed by rejection of the grafted tissue or organ. On the other hand, if tissues or organs are transplanted between genetically identical individuals, rejection does not take place. Development of inbred strains of mice was a prerequisite to designing experiments to advance our understanding of the factors controlling graft rejection or acceptance. Inbred strains are obtained after 20 or more generations of brother/sister mating, and all individuals of a strain are virtually identical genetically. Skin-grafting experiments using inbred mice have shown that ability to accept or reject a graft is under genetic control, and that it is subject to the general immunological rules of specificity and memory. When skin was grafted among animals of the same inbred strain, no rejection was observed. When grafting involved mice of different strains, the recipients rejected the graft; the speed and intensity of the rejection reaction were clearly dependent on the degree of genetic relatedness between the strains used in the experiment.

Further understanding of the genetic regulation of graft rejection/acceptance was obtained in studies involving first-generation hybrids (F1) produced by mating animals of two genetically different strains. Such hybrids did not reject tissues from either parent, while the parents rejected the skin graft from the hybrids. The acceptance of tissues from both parental strains by F1 hybrids was explained by the development of tolerance in these animals to all paternal and maternal antigens during embryonic differentiation. The animals of the parental strains rejected the tissues from the hybrids because the grafts express histocompatibility antigens of the other nonidentical strain to which they were not tolerant. Another important conclusion from these experiments was that the histocompatibility determinants are codominantly expressed.

Further studies, diagrammatically summarized in Figure 1, showed that graft rejection shares two important characteristics with the classical immune responses: specificity and memory. Animals repeatedly grafted with skin from a donor of one given strain show accelerated rejection, but if they receive a skin graft from an unrelated strain the rejection time is as long as that observed in a first graft.

MAJOR HISTOCOMPATIBILITY COMPLEX
General Concepts

The genetic system that determines the outcome of a transplant is complex and highly polymorphic. It encodes for antigens of variable immunogenic strength. The major antigens are responsible for most graft rejection responses, and trigger a stronger immune response than the others, which are designated as minor. The aggregate of major histocompatibility antigens is known as major histocompatibility complex (MHC). It includes numerous components of widely diverse and related structure and function.

Human Major Histocompatibility Complex: Human Leukocyte Antigens

Historically, the human histocompatibility antigens were defined after investigators observed that the serum of multiparous women contained antibodies that agglutinated their husbands lymphocytes. These leukoagglutinins were also present in the serum of multitransfused

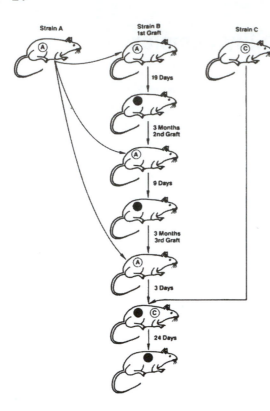

FIGURE 1 Diagrammatic representation of an experiment designed to demonstrate the memory and specificity of graft rejection. Memory is demonstrated by the progressive shortening of the time that takes a mouse of strain B to reject consecutive skin grafts from a strain A. Specificity is demonstrated by the fact that the mouse of strain B is already able to reject a graft from strain A in an accelerated fashion, and if given a graft from a third, unrelated strain (C), rejection will take as long as the rejection of the first graft from strain A. In other words, sensitization of mouse B to strain A was strain-specific and did not extend to unrelated strains.

individuals, even when the donors were compatible with the transfused individual for all known blood groups. The antigens responsible for the appearance of these antibodies were thus present on leukocytes and received the designation of human leukocyte antigen (HLA).

It is immune responsiveness to these antigens that underlies the rejection of tissues grafted between genetically unrelated individuals (see Chapter 27). The study of HLA antigens received its initial impetus from the desire to transplant tissues with minimal risk of rejection and from their interest to geneticists as the most polymorphic genetic system in humans. (Polymorphism is the presence of more than one allele at the same locus. A locus is considered polymorphic if the least frequent allele is present in more than 1% of the individuals in a population.)

It took several decades for a wider picture of the biological significance of HLA antigens to become obvious. Today, we know that these molecules are at the very core of the immune response and are the basis of the establishment of immune tolerance (lack of response) to self-antigens, as discussed later in this chapter, as well as in Chapters 4, 10, 11, and 16.

CLASSIFICATION, STRUCTURE, AND DETECTION OF HLA GENES AND GENE PRODUCTS
Major Histocompatibility Complex and Human Leukocyte Antigen Classes

Six major loci of the human MHC (HLA) have been identified and are divided in two classes: class I (HLA-A, HLA-B, and HLA-C) and class II (HLA-DP, HLA-DQ, and HLA-DR). All loci are polymorphic at varying degrees, and the number of alleles identified at each locus is growing rapidly. For instance, at the end of 2005, 414 A, 728 B, and 210 C alleles have been identified. The class II loci are similarly polymorphic. In addition to these major loci, there are some minor loci in the HLA region that are not as well-defined: E, F, G, and H for class I and DM, DN, and DO for class II. Homologous MHC classes have been defined in other mammalian species (Table 1).

TABLE 1 Main Characteristics of Major Histocompatibility Complex Antigen Classes

Characteristics	Class I	Class II
Major loci (mouse)	K, D, L	I (-A,-E)
Major loci (man)	A, B, C	D class (DP, DQ, DR)
Nonclassic loci (man)	E, G, F	
No. of alleles[a]	>100	>100
No. of specificities[a]	100	>100
Bound peptides	7–15 AA	10–30 AA
Distribution of products	Classical: all nucleated cells; nonclassical: extravillous trophoblasts	APCs: Monocytes, dendritic cells, macrophages, B cells; activated T cells

[a]For major loci.
Abbreviation: APCs, antigen-presenting cells.

Structure of the Major Histocompatibility Complex Antigens
Class I Major Histocompatibility Complex Molecules

The HLA or H2 (MHC of mice) molecules are heterodimers formed by two nonidentical polypeptide chains: an α chain and a β chain. The heavier α chain of 43,000 to 48,000 daltons, encoded by genes in the MHC region on chromosome 6, has a long extracellular region folded in three domains, named α_1, α_2 and α_3. β_2-microglobulin, a 12,000-dalton protein coded by a gene located on chromosome 15, is postsynthetically and noncovalently associated with the major polypeptide chain.

Comparison of amino acid and nucleotide sequences of various domains of class I MHC shows that the α_1 and α_2 domains are highly variable, and that most of the amino acid and nucleotide changes responsible for the differences between alleles occur in these domains. It also shows areas in these domains that are relatively constant and closely related in different alleles. This explains why polyclonal antibodies raised against MHC molecules can recognize several epitopes, an occurrence designated as the existence of "public" specificities as opposed to the "private" specificities unique to each allele.

X-ray crystallography studies have determined the three-dimensional structure of HLA class I molecules (Fig. 2), and clarified the relation between the structure and the function of this molecule. The most polymorphic areas of the molecule are located within and on the edges of a groove formed at the junction of the helical α_1 and α_2 domains. This groove is usually occupied by a short peptide (10–11 residues), usually of endogenous origin. The α_3 domain shows much less genetic polymorphism and, together with β_2-microglobulin, is like a frame supporting the deployment in space of the more polymorphic α_1 and α_2 domains. In addition, the α_3 domain has a binding site for the CD8 molecule characteristic of cytotoxic T cells (see Chapters 4, 10, and 11).

Class II Major Histocompatibility Complex Molecules

Although a remarkable degree of tertiary structure homology exists between class I and class II gene products (Fig. 3), there are important differences in their primary structure. First, class II gene products are not associated with β_2-microglobulin. The MHC-II molecules consist of two distinct polypeptide chains, a β chain (MW 28,000) that is highly polymorphic, and a less polymorphic, heavier chain, α chain (MW 33,000). Each polypeptide chain has two extracellular domains (α_1 and α_2; β_1 and β_2). The NH2 terminal ends of the α_1 and β_1 domains contain hypervariable regions. Both chains are encoded by genes in the MHC region on chromosome 6.

The three-dimensional structure of class II antigens has also been established. The β_1 domains of class II MHC antigens resemble the α_2 domain of their class I counterparts. The junction of α_1 and β_1 domains forms a groove similar to the one formed by the α_1 and α_2 domains of class I MHC antigens, and it also binds antigen-derived peptides (usually of exogenous origin), but it is larger than the groove of MHC-1 indicating that the peptides bound to it are longer.

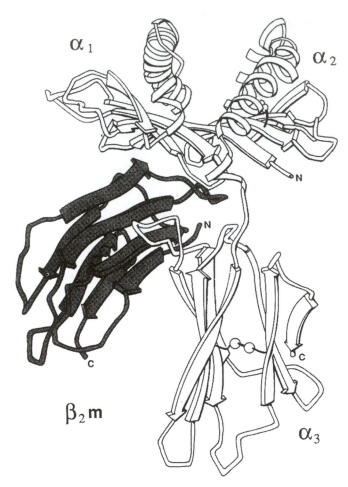

FIGURE 2 Schematic representation of the spatial configuration of the HLA-A2 molecule, based on X-ray crystallography data. The diagram shows the immunoglobulin-like domains (α_3, β_2m) at the bottom and the polymorphic domains (α_1, α_2) at the top. The indicated C terminus corresponds to the site of papain cleavage; the native molecule has additional intramembrane and intracellular segments. The α_1 and α_2 domains form a deep groove, which is identified as the antigen recognition site. *Source*: Modified from Bjorkman PJ, et al. Nature 1987; 329:506.

The β_1 domain also contains two important sites located below the antigen-binding site. The first acts as a receptor for the CD4 molecule of helper T lymphocytes (see Chapters 4, 10, and 11). The second site, which overlaps the first, is a receptor for the envelope glycoprotein (gp 120) of the human immunodeficiency virus (HIV).

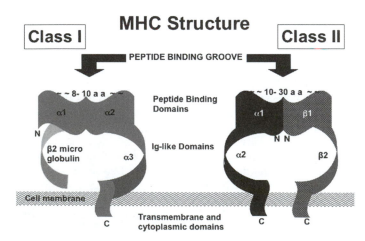

FIGURE 3 Diagrammatic representation of the structure of human class I and class II histocompatibility antigens. *Source*: From Dr JA Sleasman.

Identification of Human Leukocyte Antigen Antigens

HLA alleles are recognized by two main types of assays—serological technique and hybridization with sequence-specific oligonucleotides.

Serological Technique

The serological technique, which is the oldest and most widely used, is based on the lymphocytotoxicity of anti-HLA antibodies of known specificity in the presence of complement. The antibodies used for HLA typing were initially obtained from multiparous women or from recipients of multiple transfusions. Such antibodies are still in use, but monoclonal antibodies (see Chapter 10) are now available for most HLA specificities. These antibodies identify a broad constellation of HLA epitopes, designated as serologically defined antigens.

Some individuals express unknown specificities at some loci, which the typing laboratory reports as "blank." Investigation of these "blank" specificities often leads to the discovery of new HLA antigens. To avoid confusion, they are assigned a numerical designation by regularly held workshops of the World Health Organization. At first, the designation is preceded by a w, indicating a provisional assignment. For example, DQw3 designates an antigenic specificity of the DQ locus that has been tentatively designated as w3 by a workshop. When worldwide agreement is reached that it is a new specificity, the w is dropped.

Hybridization with Sequence-Specific Oligonucleotides

Hybridization with sequence-specific oligonucleotides is particularly useful for typing MHC-II specificities. The MHC region has been completely sequenced. In case of MHC-I molecules, all alleles correspond to variations in the α chains; the β chain (β-2 microglobulin) is monomorphic. In case of HLA-DR molecules, the α chain is invariant, but the β chain genes are extremely polymorphic. In contrast, HLA-DP and DQ molecules have polymorphic α and β chains, and thus are much more diverse than the DR molecules. As the sequences of HLA genes became known, it became possible to produce specific probes for different alleles. Typing usually involves DNA extraction, denaturation into single-stranded DNA, fragmentation with restriction enzymes, amplification by PCR, and finally hybridization with labeled cDNA probes specific for different alleles of the corresponding genes.

Such molecular typing has further subdivided the serologically defined alleles into more refined specificities based on their nucleotide sequences. For instance, serologically defined HLA-A2 antigen now has more than 56 members based on DNA sequence analyses. All these are collectively known as HLA-*A02 alleles that code for the serologically defined HLA-A2 antigen. Similarly, nucleotide-defined alleles of HLA-B7 are designated as HLA-B*0702-*0706. In the case of DQ and DP the nomenclature identifies both the polypeptide chain where the nucleotide sequence has been identified and the serological corresponding marker, if defined. For example, two DQ haplotypes, one of DQ03 (HLADQA1*0301-DQB1*0302) and the other of DQ05 (DQA1*0501-DQB1*0201), are often mentioned in the literature because they are generally associated with susceptibility to develop type-1 diabetes (see Chapter 17).

Cellular Distribution of the Major Histocompatibility Complex Antigens

Class I MHC molecules (HLA-A, B, and C alleles in humans and H2-K, D, and L alleles in mice) are expressed on all nucleated cells. They are particularly abundant on the surface of lymphocytes (1000 to 10,000 molecules/cell).

Class II MHC molecules (The I-A and I-E alleles of the mouse H2 complex and the DP, DQ, and DR alleles of the human HLA system) are primarily expressed in two groups of leukocytes: B lymphocytes and cells of the monocyte-macrophage family. The latter includes all antigen-presenting cells (Langerhans cells in the skin, Kupffer cells in the liver, microglial cells in the central nervous system, and dendritic cells in the spleen and lymph nodes). While resting T lymphocytes do not express MHC-II molecules, these antigens can be detected after cell activation.

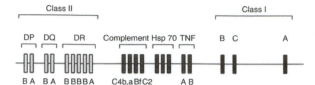

FIGURE 4 Simplified map of the region of human chromosome 6, where the human leukocyte antigen (HLA) locus is located. The genes for 21 α and 21 β hydroxylase and for tumor necrosis factor α and β (lymphotoxin-α) have also been located to chromosome 6, but are not considered as part of the HLA complex.

Chromosomal Localization and Arrangement of the Major Histocompatibility Complex Genes

The MHC genes are located on chromosome 6 of humans and chromosome 17 of the mouse. A simplified map of human chromosome 6 is shown in Figure 4. The MHC genes can be grouped in the same classes as the antigens detected in cell membranes, that is, MHC class I and class II genes. The MHC region in humans spans about four million base pairs, whereas in mice it is only about two million base pairs long. In mice, the H2-K, D, and L loci (class Ia genes) are the most polymorphic; in contrast, class Ib genes, which include H2M3 and Qa1, are much less polymorphic. They are followed by the I region that includes two loci: I-A and I-E (class II genes). One related locus (locus S), located between the H-2K and H-2D loci, codes for the complement components C4, C2, and Bf.

The organization of the HLA gene complex in man is similar (Fig. 5). The class-I genes are also divided into two groups: Ia, which includes the polymorphic HLA-A, B, and C genes and Ib, which includes HLA-E, F, and G that are almost monomorphic. Class II genes (DP, DQ, and DR) in humans, located proximal to the centromere, are followed by genes coding for proteins related to the complement cascade such as Bf, C2, and C4. There are two C4 loci (C4A and C4B) separated from each other by the gene coding for the enzyme 21-α hydroxylase, which is involved in the synthesis of steroid hormones. This region also includes genes for tumor necrosis factor-α (TNF-α) and TNF-β, also known as lymphotoxin α.

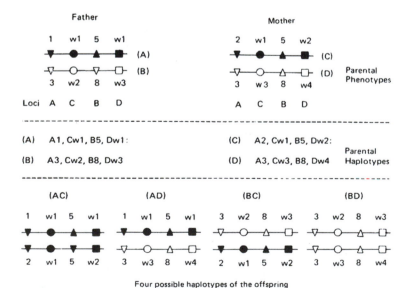

Four possible haplotypes of the offspring

FIGURE 5 Diagrammatic representation of the genetic transmission of HLA halotypes. Each parent has two haplotypes (one in each chromosome). Paternal haplotypes are designated A and B and maternal haplotypes C and D. Each offspring has to receive one paternal haplotype and one maternal haplotype. In a large family, 25% of the children share both haplotypes, 50% share one haplotype, and 25% have no haplotype in common. *Source*: Reproduced from Hokama Y, Nakamura RM. Immunology and Immunopathology. Boston: Little Brown, 1982.

GENETICS OF THE MAJOR HISTOCOMPATIBILITY COMPLEX

HLA antigens are inherited as autosomal codominant (both alleles are expressed in a hetero-zygote) genes according to Mendelian laws. As mentioned before, the HLA system is extremely polymorphic, making it unlikely for two unrelated individuals to share all their HLA alleles. This is the basis for their use as genetic markers, which found a major practical application in paternity studies before DNA analysis became routine. Extensive HLA polymorphism, however, also presents a major obstacle to organ and tissue transplantation. As expected, related individuals share their HLA genes, and the proportion of shared genes depends on the degree of relatedness. For instance, there is a 25% chance of two siblings being HLA identical, making them ideal donor-recipient candidates for organ and tissue transplantation.

Because of the close proximity of HLA loci, the set of alleles present on a maternal or paternal chromosome 6 is usually transmitted *en bloc*, and such a group of closely linked alleles is called a haplotype. There are infrequent exceptions to this intact transmission of a hap-lotype from a parent to the child because of occasional (approximately 1%) meiotic crossing over between the loci in paternal or maternal chromosome 6 homologues.

Because all alleles of an individual are codominant, it follows that both haplotypes that form an individual genotype will be expressed in the cells of that individual. The sum of all the specificities coded by the genome of the individual is known as that individual's HLA type. An example of the notation of a given individual's phenotype is as follows: HLA- Al,2; B8,27; Dw3,-; DR23,-. The hyphen indicates that only one antigen of a particular locus can be typed; this can signify that the individuals are homozygous or they possesses an antigen that cannot be typed because appropriate reagents are not yet available.

Population genetics theory predicts that in a panmictic population (random mating), given enough time in evolution, alleles of a locus will be randomly associated with alleles of other loci (linkage equilibrium), and the probability of co-occurrence of any two alleles will be the product of their individual frequencies. For the HLA loci, however, this is not the case: certain alleles are found together more often than would be expected from the product of their individual frequencies in the population. This phenomenon is termed linkage disequi-librium. As an example, the HLA-A1 allele is found in the Caucasian population with a frequency of 0.158, and the HLA-B8 allele is found with a frequency of 0.092. The A1, B8 haplotype should, therefore, be found with a frequency of $0.158 \times 0.092 = 0.015$. In reality, it is found with a frequency of 0.072. The linkage disequilibrium is expressed as the difference (Δ) between the observed and expected frequencies of the alleles, that is, $0.072 - 0.015 = 0.057$. The reasons for the extensive polymorphism and linkage disequilibrium in the HLA system are not known. It is possible that during our evolutionary history new alleles and par-ticular combination of alleles have been differentially selected because of their role in confer-ring immunity to infectious pathogens.

MAJOR HISTOCOMPATIBILITY COMPLEX AND THE IMMUNE RESPONSE

A major advance in immunology occurred with the observation that $CD8^+$ cytotoxic T lympho-cytes would only kill virus-infected cells if both (the cytotoxic T cell and the infected cell) shared identical class I MHC antigens. The T cells recognize a specific determinant formed by the association of a viral peptide with an autologous MHC-I molecule. Cells infected by the same virus, but expressing different MHC-I molecules will present a different MHC-I-peptide complex, not recognizable by a cytotoxic T cell from an animal expressing different set of MHC-I molecules. Thus, cytotoxicity mediated by T lymphocytes is MHC-restricted and the MHC-I molecules are the "restricting elements." This discovery provided a physiologi-cal function (recognition of self from nonself) for MHC molecules, which until then had been known only as major barriers to transplantation. The restriction of cytotoxic reactions rep-resents an adaptation of the immune system to the need to differentiate "normal" cells from cells altered as a consequence of intracellular infections. The elimination of "nonself" material requires the recognition of nonself antigenic structures and the induction of an immune response through a set of cell–cell interactions involving macrophages, T lymphocytes and B lymphocytes. The effector mechanisms responsible for elimination of "nonself" may be mediated by antibodies or by cytotoxic T cells. Viruses and other intracellular parasites present a special problem to the immune system due to their shielding from contact with immunocompetent cells recognizing antigenic structures on the infectious agents. To circumvent this, the immune system developed the ability to recognize and destroy the infected cells themselves.

The loading of peptides into MHC-I molecules is a complex process. To reach the cell membrane in a stable configuration, the MHC molecule must always be loaded with a peptide. In the absence of intracellular infection, peptides derived from autologous proteins occupy the peptide-binding groove and these fail to elicit an immune response due to the fact that they are self-peptides. During an infection, proteins synthesized by a replicating intracellular infectious agent are first cut by a proteasome, a multi-subunit proteolytic enzyme that yields fragments of 7 to 15 amino acids. The peptides are subsequently transported to the endoplasmic reticulum (ER) by molecules known as transporters associated with antigen-processing (TAP) that are located within the MHC. Once in the ER, the transported peptides replace endogenous peptides bound to newly synthesized MHC molecules and the complex is transported to the cell membrane allowing the immune system to recognize the self MHC-I/nonself peptide complex.

Major Histocompatibility Complex -II and Antigen Presentation to Helper T Lymphocytes

T lymphocytes cannot respond to unmodified antigens. Their activation requires endocytosis and processing of the antigen by a specialized antigen-presenting cell. During "processing," soluble antigens are broken down into peptides of 12 to 23 amino acids that become associated in the cytoplasm with the newly synthesized MHC-II molecules (the groove of the HLA-class-II dimer is longer than the groove of MHC-I molecules and accommodates slightly larger peptides). The peptide-MHC-II complex is then transported across the cytoplasm and inserted in the cell membrane. The MHC-II associated peptides can be recognized by $CD4^+$ helper T lymphocytes carrying a peptide-specific T cell receptor (TCR), but are not recognized by TCR on $CD8^+$ lymphocytes. This is because the CD4 coreceptor binds to the $\beta2$ domain of MHC-II molecules, while the CD8 coreceptor binds to the $\alpha3$ domain of the MHC-I heavy chain.

Regulation of Major Histocompatibility Complex Expression

Cellular restrictions concerning the expression of MHC-I and MHC-II molecules apply mainly to the resting cells. Activated leukocytes and nonleukocyte cells may express MHC molecules at higher levels than resting cells, or even express MHC molecules normally not expressed in their resting counterparts. Interferons play a crucial role in upregulating MHC expression. Class I Interferons (α/β) primarily increase the expression of MHC-I molecules, whereas the Class II interferon (γ) upregulates the expression of MHC-II as well as MHC-I molecules.

Increased expression of MHC molecules on cell membranes requires prior peptide loading of these molecules. Interferons seem to stimulate the synthesis of the components needed to ensure the overexpression of MHC molecules, including the MHC molecules, proteasomes, and transport proteins (TAP1 and 2). The consequences of MHC upregulation may be both beneficial and harmful: on the one hand, it facilitates the induction of helper and cytotoxic T cell responses against pathogens; on the other hand, it may create optimal conditions for the activation of autoreactive T-cell clones (see Chapter 16).

Major Histocompatibility Complex Binding and the Immune Response

It appears that a limited number of MHC molecules are sufficient to bind a vast repertoire of peptides (on the order of 10^8–10^{10}). The peptides presented to T lymphocytes are helical structures with two parts (Fig. 6). The part of the peptide that protrudes above the surface of the groove and is accessible to the TCR is known as the "epitope." The rest of the peptide interacts with the groove of the MHC molecule. This interaction is mediated by "anchoring residues," shared by many peptides. Thus, a given peptide can bind to much different class I or class II HLA molecules, and a limited repertoire of these molecules can accommodate a wide diversity of peptides.

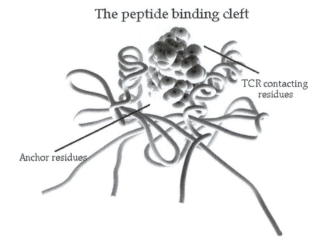

The peptide binding cleft

TCR contacting residues

Anchor residues

FIGURE 6 Diagrammatic representation of the interaction between an immunogenic peptide and an MHC-II molecule. The peptide binds to the major histocompatibility complex (MHC) molecule pouch through its "anchor residues," enabling the interaction between the T cell receptors (TCR) binding residues, which form the epitope, and the TCR. *Source*: Modified from Lernmark A. Selecting culprits in type 1 diabetes β-cell killing. J Clin Invest 1999; 104:1487.

The anchoring residues determine the binding affinity of a given peptide to specific MHC alleles, which varies over two or three orders of magnitude between different alleles. These differences in binding affinity are believed to determine the strength of the response. A peptide bound with high affinity will be presented to the T cells in optimal conformation determining a high response to this epitope. In contrast, if the binding is of low affinity the individual will be a low responder or a nonresponder. Thus, the magnitude of the immune response is determined by the close fit between peptides and MHC molecules.

Importance of Antigen Complexity and Major Histocompatibility Complex Heterozygosity

Even with a limited MHC repertoire, the probability of mounting a good response to a complex antigen is high. Such antigens are likely to generate many different peptides during processing, increasing the odds of generating some peptide(s) that are able to bind to the MHC molecules of an individual. Heterozygous individuals, with twice as many peptide-binding MHC motifs, can generate a more effective immune response than homozygotes.

Additional Antigen-Presenting Molecules

MHC molecules are not designed to bind strongly hydrophobic antigens such as lipids or carbohydrates. While the response to carbohydrates is elicited with minimal or no cooperation from helper T cells (thus circumventing the need for MHC presentation to helper T cells), the response to lipids and glycolipids involves presentation by a different set of molecules, generically designated as CD1. The CD1 molecules are structurally similar to the MHC-1 molecules, but are not coded by genes in the MHC region. The human CD1 molecules are coded by five closely linked genes on chromosome 1. A CD1 molecule consists of a large polypeptide chain with three domains (α1, α2, α3) that is noncovalently associated with β2 microglobulin. The α1 and α2 domains form a groove much deeper than the MHC-I groove. It is formed by hydrophobic residues likely to bind very hydrophobic ligands such as compounds derived from *Mycobacterium tuberculosis*, including mycolic acids, lipoarabinomannan, and glucose monomycolate. Lipopolysaccharides from gram-negative bacteria and lipotechoic acid from gram-positive bacteria are also likely to be presented by CD1.

HUMAN LEUKOCYTE ANTIGEN—DISEASE ASSOCIATIONS
General Considerations

There are two major approaches to determining the genetic etiology of a disease: linkage analysis and association analysis. The terms linkage and association are often mistakenly used synonymously. Linkage implies that the gene under consideration and the putative gene responsible for the disease are on the same chromosome. It is determined by cosegregation of the disease with a particular genetic variant in families consisting of affected and unaffected individuals. This approach has been useful in the identification of genes for diseases that follow simple Mendelian inheritance, like cystic fibrosis (autosomal recessive) and Huntington's chorea (autosomal dominant), but not for complex diseases like diabetes and heart disease. Association implies that a specific allele is found more often (associated with susceptibility) or less often (associated with resistance) in a group of unrelated individuals with a disease than in subjects without that disease. This approach is more powerful than linkage in detecting the genes for complex diseases.

The Associations

Numerous diseases have been associated with particular HLA alleles, some more strongly than others. Most of the diseases associated with HLA are autoimmune in nature; some are infectious (e.g., malaria). A list of strong HLA-disease associations, which have been confirmed by many studies, is given in Table 2. Some HLA-disease associations are strong enough to be of diagnostic assistance. For instance, virtually all narcolepsy patients are positive for the HLA-DQB1*0602

TABLE 2 Some Human Leukocyte Antigen and Disease Associations

Disease	HLA allele(s)	Relative risk of developing the disease[a]	Description of the disease
Inflammatory diseases			
Ankylosing spondylitis	B27	100–200	Inflammation of the spine, leading to stiffening of vertebral joints
Reiter's syndrome	B27	40	Inflammation of the spine, prostate, and parts of eye (conjunctiva, uvea)
Juvenile rheumatoid arthritis	B27	10–12	A multisystem inflammatory disease of children characterized by rapid onset of joint lesions and fever
Adult rheumatoid arthritis	DR4	9	Autoimmune inflammatory disease of the joints often associated with vasculitis
Psoriasis	Cw6	7	An acute, recurrent, localized inflammatory disease of the skin (usually scalp, elbows, associated with arthritis
Celiac disease	DQ2, DQ8	30	A chronic inflammatory disease of the small intestine; probably a food allergy to a protein in grains (gluten)
Multiple sclerosis	DQ6	12	A progressive chronic inflammatory disease of brain and spinal cord that destroys the myelin sheath
Endocrine diseases			
Addison's disease	DR3	5	A deficiency in production of adrenal gland cortical hormones
Diabetes mellitus	DQ8	14	A deficiency of insulin production; pancreatic islet cells usually absent or damaged
	DQ6	0.02	
Miscellaneous diseases			
Narcolepsy	DQ6	>40	A condition characterized by the tendency to fall asleep unexpectedly

[a]Numerical indicator of how many more times a disease is likely to occur in individuals possessing a given HLA allele relative to those who do not express the marker, determined by the following formula:

$$\text{Relative risk} = \frac{\text{No. of patients with the marker} \times \text{No. of controls without the marker}}{\text{No. of patients without the marker} \times \text{No. controls with the marker}}$$

Epidemiologists term this value odds ratio (OR), which is usually accompanied by a 95% confidence interval (CI). The OR is considered significant if the CI does not include 1. *Source*: Modified from Hood LE, Weissman IL, Wood WB, Wilson JH. Immunology. 2nd Ed. Menlo Park, CA: Benjamin/Cummings, 1984.

allele. Hence, a diagnosis of narcolepsy can be excluded in a patient who does not have this allele. One cannot, however, predict the development of narcolepsy by typing for this allele, as it is frequently present in the general population in the absence of the disease.

Mechanisms Underlying Human Leukocyte Antigen—Disease Associations

The mechanisms underlying most HLA-disease associations are not known. Several possible mechanisms (not mutually exclusive) have been proposed over the years, and some of these are briefly discussed below:

1. Molecular mimicry between antigenic determinants in infectious agents and HLA antigens. This mechanism has been postulated to explain the relationship between *Yersinia pseudotuberculosis* and ankylosing spondylitis. This bacterium has been shown to contain epitopes cross-reactive with HLA-B27. Therefore, it could be speculated that an immune response directed against *Y. pseudotuberculosis* could lead to an autoimmune reaction against self. However, why this reaction would affect specific joints remains to be explained.
2. MHC molecules may act as receptors for intracellular pathogens. Such pathogens would interact with specific HLA antigens in the cell membrane, and as a result infect the cells carrying those antigens. The infected cell would undergo long-lasting changes in cell functions, which would eventually result in disease. This could be the case in ankylosing spondylitis and related disorders (acute anterior uveitis, Reiter's syndrome). Over 90% of the individuals with ankylosing spondylitis are HLA-B27 and about 75% of the patients developing Reiter's syndrome are HLA-B27 positive. Reiter's syndrome frequently follows an infection with *Chlamydia trachomatis*, and some evidence of persistent infection with this intracellular organism has been obtained, but it still remains controversial.
3. Linkage disequilibrium between HLA genes and disease-causing genes. Some HLA and disease associations involve diseases that have no immunological basis. Examples in this category include hemochromatosis and congenital adrenal hyperplasia. Genes responsible for these diseases are linked to the HLA loci. Significant association between these diseases and HLA arises because of linkage disequilibrium between particular HLA alleles and those of the genes causing the diseases.

BIBLIOGRAPHY

Frodsham AJ, Hill AV. Genetics of infectious diseases. Hum Mol Genet 2004; 13:R187.

Hill AVS. Immunogenetics and genomics. Lancet 2001; 357:2037.

Hughes AL, Packer B, Welch R, Chanock SJ, Yeager M. High level of functional polymorphism indicates a unique role of natural selection at human immune system loci. Immunogenetics 2005; 57:821.

Khakoo SI, Thio CL, Martin MP, et al. HLA and NK cell inhibitory receptor genes in resolving hepatitis C virus infection. Science 2004; 305:872.

Kumanovics A, Takada T, Lindahl KF. Genomic organization of the mammalian MHC. Annu Rev Immunol 2003; 21:629.

Margulies DH, McCluskey J. The major histocompatibility complex and its encoded proteins. In: Paul WE, ed. Fundamental Immunology Fifth Edition. Philadelphia: Lippincot-Raven, 2003.

McDevitt H. The discovery of linkage between the MHC and genetic control of the immune response. Immunol Rev 2002; 185:78.

Miretti MM, Walsh EC, Ke X, et al. A high-resolution linkage-disequilibrium map of the human major histocompatibility complex and first generation of tag single-nucleotide polymorphisms. Am J Hum Genet 2005; 76:634.

Porcelli SA, Modlin RL. The CD1 system: antigen presenting molecules for T cell recognition of lipids and glycolipids. Annu Rev Immunol 1999; 17:297.

Siebold C, Hansen BE, Wyer JR, et al. Crystal structure of HLA-DQ0602 that protects against type 1 diabetes and confers strong susceptibility to narcolepsy. Proc Natl Acad Sci U S A 2004; 101:1999.

Thorsby E, Benedicte AE. HLA associated genetic predisposition to autoimmune diseases: Genes involved and possible mechanisms. Transpl Immunol 2005; 14:175.

Trowsdale J. HLA genomics in the third millennium. Curr Opin Immunol 2005; 17:498.

Zernich D, Purcell AW, Macdonald WA, et al. Natural HLA class I polymorphism controls the pathway of antigen presentation and susceptibility to viral evasion. J Exp Med 2004; 200:13.

4 | Immune Response: Antigens, Lymphocytes, and Accessory Cells

Donna L. Farber
Department of Surgery, Division of Transplantation, University of Maryland School of Medicine, Baltimore, Maryland, U.S.A.

John W. Sleasman
Department of Pediatrics, Division of Allergy, Immunology, and Rheumatology, University of South Florida, St. Petersburg, Florida, U.S.A.

Gabriel Virella
Department of Microbiology and Immunology, Medical University of South Carolina, Charleston, South Carolina, U.S.A.

INTRODUCTION

The immune system has evolved to ensure constant surveillance of "nonself" structures. Both T and B lymphocytes have cell-surface receptors that are able to recognize structures not normally presented or expressed by the organism. Once that recognition takes place, a complex series of events is triggered, leading to the proliferation and differentiation of immune competent cells and to the development of immunological memory. These events will be directly or indirectly responsible for the elimination of the organism, cells, or molecules presenting nonself structures. Considerable effort has been applied to the study of in vitro and animal models, allowing a detailed insight into the steps involved in the generation of an immune response.

ANTIGENICITY AND IMMUNOGENICITY

Antigenicity is defined as the property of a substance (antigen) that allows it to react with the products of a specific immune response (antibody or T cell receptor). On the other hand, immunogenicity is defined as the property of a substance (immunogen) that endows it with the capacity to provoke a specific immune response. From these definitions it follows that all immunogens are antigens; the reverse, however, is not true, as shall be discussed later.

B cell immunogens are usually complex, large molecules, able to interact with B cell-surface receptors (membrane immunoglobulins) and deliver the initial activating signal leading to clonal expansion and differentiation of antibody-producing cells. T cell immunogens can be best defined as compounds that can be processed by antigen-presenting cells (APCs) into short polypeptide chains that combine with major histocompatibility complex (MHC) molecules; the peptide/MHC complexes are able to interact with specific T cell receptors (TcR) and deliver activating signals to the T cells carrying such receptors.

Landsteiner, Pauling, and others discovered in the 1930s and 1940s that small aromatic groups, such as sulfonate, arsenate, and carboxylate of amino-benzene that are unable to induce antibody responses by themselves, could be chemically coupled to immunogenic proteins. The injection of these complexes into laboratory animals resulted in the production of antibodies specific to the different aromatic groups. The aromatic groups were designated as "haptens" and the immunogenic proteins as "carriers." The immune response induced by a hapten–carrier conjugate included antibodies able to recognize the hapten and the carrier as separate entities. The hapten-specific antibodies are also able to react with soluble hapten molecules, free of carrier protein. Thus, a hapten is an antigen but not an immunogen. In practical terms, it must be noted that the designations of antigen and immunogen are often used interchangeably.

Experiments comparing the specificity of hapten-specific antibodies induced with isomers of aromatic groups were critical for the definition of antibody specificity (see Chapter 8). Experiments comparing the effects of different hapten–carrier combinations or preimmunization with carrier proteins on hapten-specific responses helped to define T-B lymphocyte cooperation, as discussed later in this chapter. Later, the principles established with hapten-carrier conjugates were expanded to the induction of immune responses directed against many small molecular weight compounds and polysaccharides, all of which may induce strong responses after conjugation to an immunogenic carrier protein. This knowledge helped explain the pathogenesis of some hypersensitivity disorders and was the basis for the development of improved immunization protocols (see subsequently).

ANTIGENIC DETERMINANTS

As noted earlier, most immunogens are complex molecules (mostly proteins and polysaccharides). However, only a restricted portion of the antigen molecule—known as an antigenic determinant or epitope—is able to interact with the specific binding site of a B lymphocyte membrane immunoglobulin, a soluble antibody, or a T lymphocyte antigen receptor.

While B-lymphocytes recognize epitopes expressed by unmodified, native, molecules, T-lymphocytes recognize short peptides generated by antigen processing (i.e., intracellular cleaving of large proteins into short peptides) or derived from newly synthesized proteins cleaved in the cytoplasm. These oligopeptides are newly formed and have little or no three-dimensional homology with the epitopes expressed on native proteins.

Studies with X-ray crystallography and two-dimensional nuclear magnetic resonance have resulted in the detailed characterization of B cell epitopes presented by some small proteins, such as lysozyme, in their native configuration. From such studies the following rules have been derived for antibody-antigen recognition:

1. Most epitopes are defined by a series of 15 to 22 amino acids located on discontinuous segments of the polypeptide chain, forming a roughly flat area with peaks and valleys that establish contact with the folded hypervariable regions of the antibody heavy and light chains.
2. Specific regions of the epitope constituted by a few amino acids bind with greater affinity to specific areas of the antibody-binding site, and thus are primarily responsible for the specificity of antigen-antibody interaction. On the other hand, the antibody-binding site has some degree of flexibility that optimizes the fit with the corresponding epitope.
3. A polypeptide with 100 amino acids may have as many as 14 to 20 nonoverlapping epitopes. However, a typical 100 amino acid globular protein is folded over itself, and most of its structure is hidden from the outside. Only surface epitopes will usually be accessible for recognition by B lymphocytes and for interactions with antibodies (Fig. 1).

DETERMINANTS OF IMMUNOGENICITY

Many different substances can induce immune responses. The following characteristics influence the ability for a substance to behave as an immunogen:

1. Foreignness: As a rule, only substances recognized as "nonself" will trigger the immune response. Microbial products and exogenous molecules are obviously "nonself" and may be strongly immunogenic.
2. Molecular size: The most potent immunogens are macromolecular proteins (MW >100,000 daltons). Molecules smaller than 10,000 daltons are often only weakly immunogenic, unless coupled to an immunogenic carrier protein.

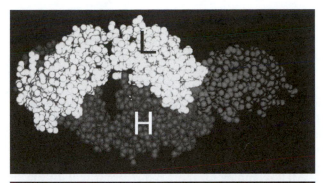

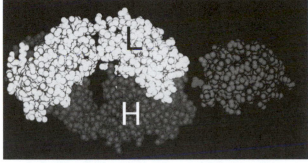

FIGURE 1 Diagrammatic representation of a space-filling model showing the fit between an epitope of lysozyme and the antigen-binding site on an Fab fragment obtained from an anti-lysozyme antibody. *Source*: Reproduced from Amit AG, Mariuzza RA, Phillips SEV, Poljack RJ. Science 1984; 233:747.

3. Chemical structure: Proteins and polysaccharides are among the most potent immunogens, although relatively small polypeptide chains, nucleic acids, and even lipids can, given the appropriate circumstances, be immunogenic.

   Heterologous proteins of high MW express a wide diversity of antigenic determinants and are potent immunogens. It must be noted that the immunogenicity of a protein is strongly influenced by its chemical composition. Positively charged (basic) amino acids, such as lysine, arginine, and histidine are repeatedly present in the antigenic sites of lysozyme and myoglobin, while aromatic amino acids (such as tyrosine) are found in two of six antigenic sites defined in albumin. Therefore, it appears that basic and aromatic amino acids may contribute more strongly to immunogenicity than other amino acids. Thus, basic proteins with clusters of positively charged amino acids are strongly immunogenic.

   Polysaccharides are among the most important antigens, because of their abundant representation in nature. Pure polysaccharides, the sugar moieties of glycoproteins, lipopolysaccharides (LPS), glycolipid-protein complexes, and so on, are all immunogenic. Many microorganisms have polysaccharide-rich capsules or cell walls, and a variety of mammalian antigens, such as the erythrocyte antigens (A, B, Le, H) and short-chain polysaccharides (oligosaccharides). As noted later in this chapter, polysaccharides and oligosaccharides stimulate B cells without promoting T cell help. This is probably a result of the lack of binding of oligosaccharides to MHC-II molecules, resulting in the inability to activate helper T cells.

   Nucleic acids (RNA and DNA) usually are not immunogenic, but can induce antibody formation if coupled to a protein to form a nucleoprotein. The autoimmune responses characteristic of some of the so-called autoimmune diseases (e.g., systemic lupus erythematosus) are often directed to DNA and RNA.

   Polypeptides, such as insulin and other hormones, relatively small in size (MW 1500 for insulin), are usually able to induce antibody formation when isolated from one species and administered over long periods of time to an individual of a different species.

4. Chemical complexity: There appears to be a direct relationship between antigenicity and chemical complexity—aggregated or chemically polymerized proteins are much stronger immunogens than their soluble monomeric counterparts.

FACTORS ASSOCIATED WITH THE INDUCTION OF AN IMMUNE RESPONSE

In addition to the chemical nature of the immunogen, other factors strongly influence the development and potency of an immune response, including:

Genetic Background

Different animal species and different strains of one given species may show different degrees of responsiveness to a given antigen. In humans, different individuals can behave as "high responders" or "low responders" to any given antigen. The genetic control of the immune response is poorly understood, but involves the repertoire of MHC molecules that bind antigen fragments and present them to the responding T cell population. The affinity of the peptide for the MHC and of the peptide/MHC complex for the T cell receptor will dictate, at least in part, the T cell response. Other factors that promote or suppress the immune response must exist, but they are less well understood.

Method of Antigen Administration

The method of antigen administration has a profound effect on the immune response. A given dose of antigen may elicit no detectable response when injected intravenously, but a strong immune response is observed if injected intradermally. The presence of dendritic cells in the dermis (where they are known as Langerhans cells) may be a critical factor determining the enhanced immune responses when antigens are injected intradermally. This route of administration results in slow removal from the site of injection, and in uptake and processing of the antigen by dendritic cells. The dendritic cells may present antigen to migrating T cells or may themselves migrate to the lymph node follicles, where the initial stages of the immune response take place. Thus, intradermal administration promotes prolonged antigenic stimulation and facilitates the involvement of one of the most specialized populations of APCs.

Use of Adjuvants

Adjuvants are agents that, when administered along with antigens enhance the specific response. In contrast to carrier proteins, adjuvants are often nonimmunogenic and are never chemically coupled to the antigens. Several factors seem to contribute to the enhancement of immune responses by adjuvants, including delayed release of antigen, nonspecific inflammatory effects, and the activation of monocytes and macrophages. Several microbial and inorganic compounds have been used effectively as adjuvants both clinically and as investigational agents.

One of the most effective adjuvants is complete Freund's adjuvant; a water-in-oil emulsion with killed mycobacteria in the oil phase. This is the adjuvant of choice for production of antisera in laboratory animals. Bacillus Calmette-Guérin (BCG), an attenuated strain of *Mycobacterium bovis* used as a vaccine against tuberculosis and muramyl-dipeptide, the active moiety of *Mycobacterium tuberculosis* and of BCG, also have adjuvant properties. BCG has also been used as an immunotherapeutic agent to boost the immune system in patients with special types of cancer (e.g., superficial bladder cancer). Their use is limited, however, by side effects such as intense inflammatory reactions and discomfort. Recently, growth factors such as granulocyte macrophage colony stimulating factor (GM-CSF) have been found to have adjuvant properties that may be clinically useful for the induction of cancer-specific immune responses (see Chapter 26).

Aluminum hydroxide, an inert compound that absorbs the immunogen, stimulates phagocytosis, and delays removal from the inoculation side, is an adjuvant frequently used with human vaccines. Aluminum hydroxide is not as effective as many of the adjuvants listed earlier, but is also considerably less toxic.

EXOGENOUS AND ENDOGENOUS ANTIGENS

Most antigens to which we react are of exogenous origin, and include microbial antigens, environmental antigens (such as pollens and pollutants), and medications. The objective of the immune response is the elimination of foreign antigens, but in some instances, the immune response itself may have a deleterious effect, resulting in hypersensitivity or in autoimmune disease, discussed in later chapters of this book.

Endogenous antigens, by definition, are part of self, and the immune system is usually tolerant to them. The response to self-antigens may have an important role in normal catabolic processes (i.e., antibodies to denatured IgG may help in eliminating antigen-antibody complexes from circulation; antibodies to oxidized low density lipoprotein (LDL) may help in eliminating a potentially toxic lipid). The loss of tolerance to self-antigens, however, can also have pathogenic implications (autoimmune diseases).

Special type of endogenous antigens are those that distinguish one individual from another within the same species and are termed "alloantigens." Alloantigens elicit immune responses when cells or tissues of one individual are introduced into another. The alloantigens that elicit the strongest immune response are alleles of highly polymorphic systems, such as the erythrocyte of blood group antigens A, B, and O: some individuals carry the polysaccharide that defines the A specificity, others have B positive red cells, AB positive red cells, or red cells that do not express neither A nor B (O). Other alloantigenic systems that elicit strong immune responses are histocompatibility antigens of nucleated cells and tissues, the platelet antigens, and the Rh erythrocyte blood group antigens. Examples of sensitization to exogenous alloantigens include:

1. Women sensitized to fetal red cell antigens during pregnancy.
2. Polytransfused patients who become sensitized against cellular alloantigens from the donor(s).
3. Recipients of organ transplants who become sensitized against histocompatibility alloantigens, expressed in the transplanted organ.

T-B CELL COOPERATION IN ANTIBODY RESPONSES

Experiments carried out with hapten-carrier complexes have contributed significantly to our understanding of T-B lymphocyte cooperation. A specific example is illustrated in Figure 2. Mice primed with a hapten–carrier conjugate prepared by chemically coupling the 2-dinitrophenyl (2-DNP) radical to egg albumin [ovalbumin (OVA)] produced antibodies both to DNP

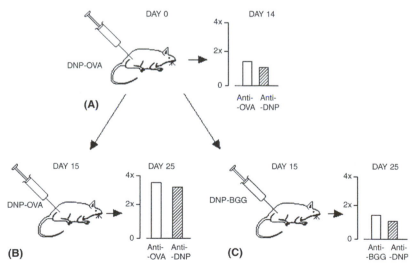

FIGURE 2 The hapten–carrier effect: In order to obtain a secondary immune response to the hapten (DNP), the animal needs to be immunized (**A**) and challenged (**B**) with the same DNP-carrier combination. Boosting with a different DNP-carrier conjugate (**C**) will result in an anti-DNP response of identical magnitude to that obtained after the initial immunization. The memory response, therefore, appears to be carrier-dependent. *Abbreviations*: BGG, bovine gamma globulin; DNP, dinitrophenyl; OVA, ovalbumin.

and OVA. Antibodies to the hapten (DNP) were not observed when mice were immunized with DNP alone or with a mixture of nonchemically linked DNP and OVA. Secondary challenge of mice primed with DNP–OVA with the same hapten–carrier conjugate triggered an anamnestic or "recall" response of higher magnitude against both hapten and carrier. In contrast, if the DNP–OVA primed animals were challenged with the same hapten coupled to a different carrier, such as bovine gamma globulin (DNP–BGG), the ensuing response to DNP was of identical magnitude to that observed after the first immunization with DNP–OVA. The conclusion from these observations is that a "recall" response to the hapten can only be observed when the animal is repeatedly immunized with the same hapten–carrier conjugate.

It was further observed that if mice were primed with the carrier OVA alone, and then challenged with DNP–OVA, the response to DNP was as high as that observed when mice had been primed with DNP–OVA (Fig. 3). When OVA-primed mice were challenged with a mixture of nonchemically linked DNP and OVA, no response to DNP was observed. Thus, it was concluded that immunologic "memory" (defined in this case as a response of the magnitude characteristic of a secondary response) to the hapten moiety of a hapten–carrier conjugate is exclusively dependent on a previous exposure to the carrier moiety. In other words, the factors responsible for the secondary immune response were effective in enhancing the response to any hapten coupled to the immunizing carrier.

The hapten–carrier experiments were later repeated using sublethally irradiated inbred mice reconstituted with different cell subpopulations from immunocompetent animals of the same strain. In a classical study reproduced in Figure 4, four groups of animals were used as a source of reconstituting cells. Mice were immunized with DNP or with two different immunogenic proteins, such as keyhole limpet hemocyanin (KLH) and OVA; a fourth group was injected with saline. T and B lymphocytes were purified from the immunized animals and transferred to the sublethally irradiated mice of the same strain. Several observations were made:

1.   If both DNP-primed B lymphocytes and OVA-primed T lymphocytes were transferred to sublethally irradiated recipients, the reconstituted mice produced relatively large amounts of anti-DNP antibody upon challenge with DNP–OVA.

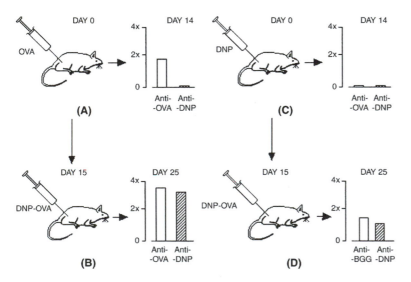

FIGURE 3   Further proof of the carrier dependency of the memory response to a hapten–carrier conjugate was obtained by studying the effects of primary immunization with carrier [e.g., ovalbumin (OVA)] or hapten [e.g., dinitrophenyl (DNP)] alone on a booster response with the hapten–carrier conjugate. A primary immunization with OVA (**A**) was followed by a "secondary" response to both hapten and carrier when the animals were challenged with OVA–DNP (**B**). A primary immunization with DNP (**C**) did not induce anti-DNP antibodies and the animal reacted to a challenge with OVA–DNP (**D**) as if it was a primary immunization to either carrier or hapten. *Abbreviations*: BGG, bovine gamma globulin; DNP, dinitrophenyl; OVA, ovalbumin.

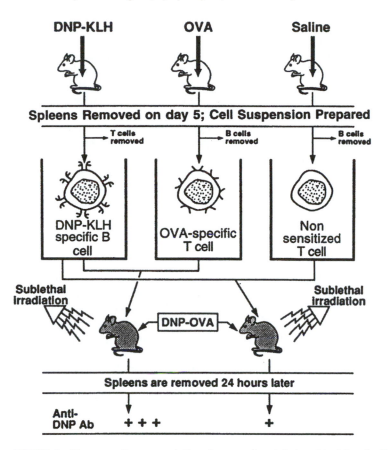

FIGURE 4 Diagrammatic representation of an experiment designed to determine the nature of T cell help in a classical hapten–carrier response. Sublethally irradiated mice were reconstituted with different combinations of T and B cells obtained from nonimmune mice or from mice immunized with dinitrophenyl (DNP)–ovalbumin (OVA). T cells from mice preimmunized with OVA "helped" B cells from animal preimmunized with DNP–keyhole limpet hemocyanin (KLH) to produce large amounts of anti-DNP antibodies, but the same B cells did not receive noticeable help from T cells separated from nonimmune mice. Thus, T cells with "carrier" memory efficiently help B cells. *Abbreviations*: DNP, dinitrophenyl; KLH, keyhole limpet hemocyanin; OVA, ovalbumin.

2. If nonimmune or KLH-primed T lymphocytes were cotransferred with DNP primed B lymphocytes, only a minimal anti-DNP antibody response was obtained after challenge with DNP–OVA.
3. If DNP-specific B lymphocytes were transferred with OVA-specific T-lymphocytes, robust anti-DNP antibody responses were observed upon challenge with DNP–OVA. However, only suboptimal anti-DNP responses were observed upon challenge with DNP–KLH and no anti-DNP antibody response was observed when the mice were challenged with an unconjugated mixture of OVA and DNP.

These experiments demonstrated that the amplification of the B cell response required T cells. Additionally, both carrier and hapten-specific antibody-producing cells were "helped" by carrier-specific T-lymphocytes. In other words, T lymphocyte "help" is not antigen-specific, since the T and B lymphocytes collaborating in the immune response may recognize antigenic determinants from totally unrelated compounds (hapten and carrier).

A consistent observation in all hapten–carrier observations is that the efficient collaboration between T and B lymphocytes requires the antigenic determinants for each cell type to be on the same molecule. This suggests that the helper effect is most efficient if the collaborating B and T lymphocytes are brought into intimate, cell-to-cell contact, with each cell reacting to distinct determinants on the same molecule.

In the last two decades, the hapten–carrier concept has found significant applications in medicine. Hapten–carrier systems have been developed to raise antibodies to a variety of non-immunogenic chemicals that are the basis for a variety of drug level assays (e.g., plasma cyclosporine levels). Lastly, the immune response to haptens coupled to autologous carriers has been demonstrated to be the pathological basis for some abnormal immune reactions, including some drug allergies. For instance, the spontaneous coupling of the penicilloyl derivative of penicillin to a host protein is believed to be the first step toward developing hypersensitivity to penicillin. Hypersensitivity reactions to a number of drugs, chemicals, and metals are believed to result from spontaneous coupling of these nonimmunogenic compounds to endogenous proteins, which are modified as a consequence of the chemical reaction with the hapten. As a consequence, the conditions necessary for the elicitation of immune responses to nonimmunogenic compounds are created.

T-DEPENDENT AND T-INDEPENDENT ANTIGENS

The studies with hapten–carrier complexes were followed by many others in which inbred rodents were sublethally irradiated to render them immunoincompetent, and their immune systems were then reconstituted with T lymphocytes, B lymphocytes, or mixtures of T and B lymphocytes, obtained from normal animals of the same strain. After reconstitution of the immune system, the animals were challenged with a variety of antigens, and their antibody responses were measured.

For most antigens, including complex proteins, heterologous cells, and viruses, a measurable antibody response was only observed in animals reconstituted with mixtures of T and B lymphocytes. In other words, for most antigens, proper differentiation of antibody-producing cells required T cell "help." The antigens that could not induce immune responses in T cell-deficient animals were designated as T-dependent antigens. Structurally, T-dependent antigens are usually complex proteins with large numbers of different, nonrepetitive, antigenic determinants.

Other antigens, particularly polysaccharides, can induce antibody synthesis in animals depleted of T lymphocytes, and are known as T-independent antigens. It should be noted that, in many species, there may be a continuous gradation of antigenic responses from T dependence to T independence, rather than two discrete groups of antigens. However, this differentiation is useful as a working classification.

Biological Basis of T-Independence

The basic fact that explains the inability of polysaccharides to behave as T-dependent antigens is that these compounds do not bind to MHC-II molecules, and, therefore, cannot be presented to T cells. Immune responses elicited by T-independent antigens are mediated by different mechanisms that bypass the need for T cell help.

Some T-independent antigens, such as bacterial LPS, are mitogenic and can deliver dual signals to B cells, one by occupancy of the antigen-specific receptor (membrane immunoglobulin), and the other through a second, poorly characterized, costimulatory protein. The engagement of these two receptors would be sufficient to stimulate B cells and promote differentiation into antibody-producing cells.

Other T-independent antigens (such as polysaccharides) are not mitogenic, but are composed of multiple sugar molecules, allowing extensive cross-linking of membrane immunoglobulins. Receptor cross-linking delivers strong activating signals that apparently override the need for costimulatory signals.

Special Characteristics of the Immune Response to T-Independent Antigens

The antibody produced in response to stimulation with T-independent antigens is predominantly IgM. The switch to other isotypes, such as IgG and IgA, production requires the presence of cytokines and other signals (e.g., those delivered by CD40 interacting with CD40L) delivered by locally responding T cells. There is, therefore, little (if any) synthesis of IgG and IgA after exposure to T-independent antigens. These antigens also fail to elicit immunological memory, also dependent on the simultaneous activation of T cells, as demonstrated with the hapten–carrier experiments. Finally, the ontogenic development of the T-independent response is slow, and, as a rule, children younger than two years do not respond to polysaccharide immunization.

The use of polysaccharides as immunogens for immunoprophylaxis has always been unsatisfactory. A decade ago it was discovered that polysaccharides induce the same type of immune responses associated with T-dependent immunogens when conjugated to immunogenic proteins. These vaccines act, essentially, as hapten–carrier complexes, in which the polysaccharide plays the role of the hapten and are extremely effective (see Chapter 12).

INDUCTION OF THE IMMUNE RESPONSE
Immune Recognition: Clonal Restriction and Expansion

For the initiation of an immune response an antigen or a peptide associated with a MHC molecule must be recognized as "nonself" by the immunocompetent cells. This phenomenon is designated as immune recognition. The immune system of a normal individual may recognize as many as 10^6 to 10^8 different antigenic specificities. An equal number of different small families (clones) of lymphocytes, bearing receptors for the different antigens, constitute the normal repertoire of the immune system. Each immunocompetent cell expresses on its membrane many identical copies of a receptor for one single antigen. Thus, a major characteristic of the immune response is its clonal restriction, that is, one given epitope will be recognized by a single family of cells with identical antigen receptors, known as a clone. When stimulated by the appropriate specific antigen, each cell will proliferate and the clone of reactive cells will become more numerous (clonal expansion).

Since most immunogens present many different epitopes to the immune system, the normal immune responses are polyclonal, that is, multiple clones of immunocompetent cells, each one of them specific to one unique epitope, are stimulated by any complex immunogen.

Antigen Receptor on T and B Lymphocytes

In B lymphocytes, the antigen receptors are membrane-inserted immunoglobulins, particularly IgD and monomeric IgM molecules (see Chapter 5). In T lymphocytes, the antigen receptors are known as TcR.

As discussed in Chapters 10 and 11, two types of TcR have been identified, depending on the polypeptide chains that constitute them. In differentiated T cells, the TcR most frequently found is constituted by two polypeptide chains, designated as α and β ($\alpha\beta$ TcR), with similar MW (40,000–45,000). A second type of TcR, constituted by two different polypeptide chains known as γ and δ ($\gamma\delta$ TcR) is predominantly found in the submucosal lymphoid tissues.

The two chains of the $\alpha\beta$ TcR have extracellular segments with variable and constant domains, short cytoplasmic domains, and a transmembrane segment (Fig. 5). A disulfide bridge joins them just outside the transmembrane segment. The β chains are highly polymorphic and are encoded by a multigene family that includes genes for regions homologous to the V, C, D, and J regions of human immunoglobulins. The α chains are encoded by a more limited multigene family with genes for regions homologous to the V, C, and J regions of human immunoglobulins (see Chapter 7). Similar polymorphisms have been defined for the $\gamma\delta$ chains. Together, the variable regions of $\alpha\beta$ and $\gamma\delta$ chains define the specific binding sites for peptide epitopes presented in association with MHC molecules. Peptides 7 to 15 amino acids in length are well recognized by CD4 and CD8 TcR, although MHC-II molecules can accommodate larger peptides, up to 30 aminoacids long. There is controversy about the degree of peptide specificity of the TcR. The TcR seems to have a high degree of flexibility, and the configuration of MHC-bound peptides appears to be

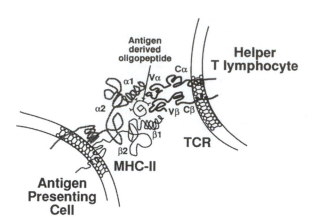

FIGURE 5 Schematic representation of the T lymphocyte receptor and its interaction with a major histocompatibility complex-II-associated peptide. *Abbreviations*: MHC-II, major histocompatibility complex-II; TcR, T-cell receptor. *Source*: Redrawn from Sinha AA, Lopez MT, McDevitt H. Science 1990; 248:1380.

subject to modifications after engagement with the TcR. As suggested by experimental studies, the combination of these two factors increases the number of peptides that can interact with a single TcR, but different studies concerning the degree of cross-reactivity of the TcR have yielded contradictory data, and this issue, critical for vaccine design, remains to be fully resolved.

Antigen Processing and Presentation

Most immune responses to complex, T-dependent antigens involve the participation of several cell types, including T and B lymphocytes that are directly involved in the generation of effector mechanisms, and accessory cells that assist in the inductive stages of the immune response. APCs are accessory cells that express MHC-II molecules on their membrane where antigen fragments can be bound and "presented" to lymphocytes. Additionally, they express ligands for costimulatory molecules and release cytokines that assist the proliferation and/or differentiation of T and B lymphocytes. As described in Chapter 2, several types of cells can function as APCs. The most effective are the dendritic cells found in the paracortical areas of the lymph nodes. The lymph node dendritic cells appear to be largely derived from Langerhans cells and dendritic cells in the dermis and submucosae. The dendritic cells are particularly well suited to initiate the immune response because they express MHC-II molecules constitutively at relatively high levels and because they can ingest microorganisms, dead cells, and proteins by endocytosis or phagocytosis, mediated by interactions with several different constitutively expressed receptors. Once ingested, the infectious agents and soluble antigens are efficiently processed, and the resulting peptides can be presented in association with MHC molecules to resting lymphocytes.

Tissue macrophages are also effective APCs because of their phagocytic and processing properties. However, the phagocytic properties of macrophages are fully expressed only after engagement of Fc and/or the complement receptors by antigen molecules are coated with IgG and/or complement, suggesting that their role maybe more important in the late stages of the primary response and in secondary responses.

The sequence of events leading to antigen processing and presentation in a dendritic cell starts by endocytosis of antigens on membrane patches, transport to an acidic compartment (lysosome) within the cell that allows antigen degradation into small peptides. As antigens are broken down, vesicles coated with newly synthesized human leukocyte antigen (HLA)-II molecules fuse with the lysosome. Some of the peptides generated during processing have high affinity for the binding site located within the MHC-II heterodimer that is initially occupied by an endogenous peptide (class II associated invariant chain peptide, CLIP), displaced by the antigen-derived peptide. The resulting MHC/peptide complexes are then transported to the APC cell membrane where they can interact with and activate CD4$^+$ T cells bearing receptors specific for the peptide (Fig. 6).

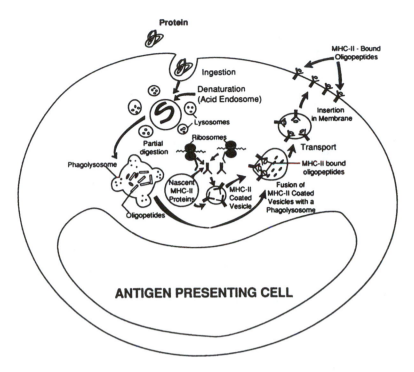

FIGURE 6 Schematic representation of the general steps in antigen processing. The antigen is ingested, partially degraded, and after vesicles coated with nascent major histocompatibility complex (MHC)-II proteins fuse with the phagolysosomes, antigen-derived polypeptides bind to the MHC-II molecule. In this bound form, the oligopeptides seem protected against further denaturation and are transported together with the MHC-II molecule to the cell membrane, where they will be presented to CD4$^+$ T lymphocytes in traffic through the tissue where the antigen-presenting cells are located. *Abbreviation*: MHC-II, major histocompatibility complex-II.

ACTIVATION OF HELPER T LYMPHOCYTES

The activation of resting T helper cells requires a complex and coordinated sequence of signals delivered from the T cell receptor on the cell membrane to the nucleus of the cell. Of all the signals involved, the only antigen-specific interaction is the one that involves the TcR and the peptide/MHC-II complex. The binding of the peptide/MHC complex to the TcR is of low affinity, and other receptor–ligand interactions are required to maintain T lymphocyte adhesion to APC as well as for the delivery of required secondary signals.

The TcR on a helper T lymphocyte interacts with both the antigen-derived peptide and the MHC-II molecule (Fig. 5). This selectivity of the TcR from helper T lymphocytes to interact with MHC-II molecules results from selection in the thymus. During thymic ontogeny, the differentiation of helper and cytotoxic T lymphocytes (CTL) is based on the ability of their TcR to interact with MHC-II molecules (helper T lymphocytes) or with MHC-I molecules (CTL) (see Chapter 10). The interactions between T lymphocytes and MHC-expressing cells are strengthened by cell surface molecules, which also interact with constant (not peptide loaded) regions of MHC molecules: the CD4 molecule on helper T cells interacts with MHC-II molecules, while the CD8 molecule on cytotoxic lymphocytes interacts with MHC-I molecules.

Several other cell adhesion molecules (CAM) can mediate lymphocyte-AC interactions, including lymphocyte function-associated antigen (LFA)-1 interacting with the intercellular adhesion molecules (ICAM)-1, 2, and 3, CD2 interacting with CD58 (LFA-3). Unlike the interactions involving the TcR, these interactions are not antigen-specific. Their role is to promote stable adhesion and signaling between T lymphocytes and APC, essential for proper stimulation through the TcR. Furthermore, T cell activation requires sustained signaling achieved through the establishment of what is known as the immunological synapse, in which

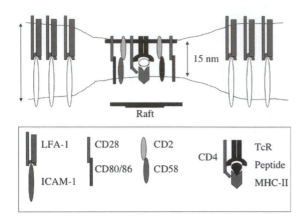

FIGURE 7   Schematic representation of the topography of T cell-antigen-presenting cell (APC) interaction. In the areas where the T cell receptors (TcR) interact with peptide–major histocompatibility complex-II complexes, the cells are in very close aposition. The rafts designate cholesterol-rich membrane domains in the T cell membrane where the TcR, CD4, and other costimulating molecules interact with their respective ligands in the APC. These interactions are primarily responsible for the close aposition of the T cell and APC membranes and for assembling the early signaling complex. Other molecules such as leukocyte function antigen-1 and intercellular adhesion molecules-1 stabilize the interaction between T cells and APCs and are present outside the rafts. *Abbreviations*: ICAM, intercellular adhesion molecules; LFA, lymphocyte function-associated antigen; MHC-II, major histocompatibility complex-II; TcR, T-cell receptor. *Source*: Adapted from Dustin ML, Shaw AS. Science 1999; 283:649–650.

peptide/MHC-II complexes form clusters on the APC membrane allowing aggregation and clustering of multiple TcR molecules on the opposing T cell membrane. In the regions of contact the two cells are separated by a narrow gap surrounded by other interacting molecules such as (CD2/CD58, LFA-1/ICAM-1, etc.). The result is a stable and close apposition between APC and T cell, essential for sustained signaling (Fig. 7).

It is important to stress that accessory cells participate in the activation of helper T lymphocytes through the delivery of signals involving cell–cell contact as well as by the release of soluble factors or cytokines. The cell–cell interaction signals include signals mediated by CD4-MHC-II interactions and signals involving membrane molecules whose expression is increased after initial activation, including:

- CD2 (T cell): CD58 (APC)
- LFA-1 (T cell): ICAM-1, ICAM-2, ICAM-3 (APC)
- CD40 L (T cell): CD40 (APC)
- CD28 (T cells): CD80, CD86 (APC)

Signals mediated by interleukins include those mediated by interleukin-1 (IL-1) and interleukin 12 (IL-12). IL-1 is a cytokine that promotes growth and differentiation of many cell types, including T and B lymphocytes. Both membrane-bound and soluble IL-1 have been shown to be important in activating T lymphocytes in vitro. Membrane-bound IL-1 can only activate T lymphocytes in close contact with the APC. IL-12 promotes Th1 cell differentiation, as discussed later in the chapter.

However, all these costimulatory signals are not specific for any given antigen. The specificity of the immune response is derived from the essential and first activation signal delivered through the antigen-specific TcR.

The sequence of events resulting in T cell proliferation and differentiation involves several major steps. First, the occupancy and cross-linking of the TcR signals cell through a closely associated complex of molecules, known as CD3, which has signal-transducing properties. The TcR heterodimer itself has no recognizable kinase activity. The associated CD3 complex, however, has a 10-intracytoplasmic motifs (ITAMs, for immunoreceptor-tyrosine-based activation motifs) that play a key role in the sequence of cell activation. These ITAMs are associated with the γ, δ, ε, and ζ chains of the CD3 complex. In this very early stages of activation costimulatory signals are delivered by CD4, as a consequence of the interaction with MHC-II, and by CD45, a tyrosine phosphatase, activated as a consequence of TcR occupancy. The activation of CD45 initiates the sequential activation of several protein kinases closely associated with CD3 and CD4. The activation of the kinase cascade has several effects, namely:

1. Calcium influx into the cell through the activation of cell-membrane pumps
2. Phospholipase C activation, leading to the mobilization of Ca^{2+}-dependent second messenger systems, such as inositol triphosphate, that promotes a further increase in intracellular free Ca^{2+} released from intracellular organelles.
3. The increase in intracellular free calcium results in activation of a serine threonine phosphatase known as calcineurin. Diacylglycerol, another product released by phospholipase C, activates another serine/threonine kinase known as protein kinase C. Multiple other enzymes and adapter molecules are activated in the ensuing cascading sequence.

The activation of second messenger systems results in the activation and translocation of transcription factors, such as the nuclear factor-kappa B (NF–κB) and the nuclear factor of activated T cells (NF-AT). Once translocated to the nucleus, these factors induce genes controlling cytokine production and T cell proliferation, such as those encoding IL-2, the IL-2 receptor, and c-myc.

In parallel, there is an increased expression of several proteins on the T cell membrane, such as CD28 and the CD40 ligand (CD40L). These molecules interact, respectively, with CD80/86 and CD40 on the APC membrane. The interactions involving this second set of molecules deliver additional signals that determine the continuing proliferation and differentiation of antigen-stimulated T cells.

ANTIGEN PRESENTATION AND ACTIVATION OF CYTOTOXIC T LYMPHOCYTES

If an APC is infected by an intracellular organism (virus, bacteria, or parasite) the infecting agent will multiply in the cytosol. As described in Chapter 3, peptides derived from microbial proteins are loaded onto MHC-I molecules, transported to the cell surface, and presented to CTL. CTL are a special population of effector T cells capable of killing target cells bearing specific antigen, and are largely CD8$^+$.

The different roles of MHC-I and MHC-II molecules in the immune response and T cell differentiation are summarized in Table 1. It should be noted that the MHC-I molecules, designated as nonclassical, play significant roles in materno-fetal tolerance and in the control of NK activity (see Chapter 10).

The activation of cytotoxic T cells by MHC-I peptide complexes requires peptide loading of MHC-I molecules. The way in which MHC-I molecules and viral peptides become associated involves a complex sequence of events (Fig. 8). Upon infection, intracellular microbes start to produce their own proteins. Some of the nascent microbial proteins diffuse into the cytosolic compartment, where they become associated with degradative enzymes forming a peptide–enzyme complex (proteasome). In these complexes, the protein is partially digested, and the

TABLE 1 Functions of Major Histocompatibility Complex-I and -II Molecules

MHC-I	MHC-II
Classical (HLA-A, B, C): Present intracellular peptide antigens to cytotoxic CD8$^+$ T cells (virus) Involved in intrathymic selection of CD8$^+$ T cells Nonclassical (E, G, F) Inhibit NK cell function Protect fetus from maternal lymphocytes	Present processed peptides derived from extracellular antigens to CD4$^+$ T cells Intrathymic selection of CD4 T cells

Abbreviations: HLA, human leukocyte antigen; MHC, major histocompatibility complex; NK, natural killer.

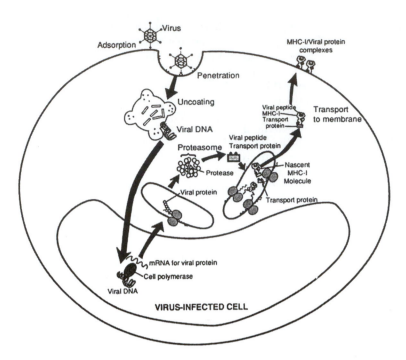

FIGURE 8   Schematic representation of the general steps involved in the presentation of viral-derived peptides on the membrane of virus-infected cells. The virus binds to membrane receptors and is endocytosed, its outer coats are digested, and the viral genome (in this case DNA) is released into the cytoplasm. Once released, the viral DNA diffuses back into the nucleus, where it is initially transcribed into mRNA by the cell's polymerases. The viral mRNA is translated into proteins that diffuse into the cytoplasm, where some will be broken down into oligopeptides. Those small peptides are transported back into the endoplasmic reticulum, where they associate with newly synthesized major histocompatibility complex-I (MHC-I) molecules. The MHC-I/oligopeptide complex becomes associated to a second transport protein and is eventually inserted into the cell membrane. In the cell membrane, it can be presented to CD8$^+$ T lymphocytes in traffic through the tissue, where the viral infected cell is located. A similar mechanism would allow a MHC-II synthesizing cell to present MHC-II/oligopeptide complexes to CD4$^+$ lymphocytes. *Abbreviations*: MHC, major histocompatibility complex; TAP, transporters associated with antigen processing.

resulting peptides bind to specialized proteins (TAP, transporters associated with antigen processing) that deliver them to the endoplasmic reticulum, the site of MHC-I synthesis and assembly. In the endoplasmic reticulum, the viral peptides bind to newly synthesized MHC-class I molecules, and the resulting MHC–viral peptide complex is transported to the membrane of the infected cell.

It has also been demonstrated that MHC-I molecules, particularly in dendritic cells and macrophages, can also be loaded with peptides generated from the processing of ingested exogenous proteins or cells. This phenomenon is known as cross-presentation and involves translocation of internalized antigens to the cytosol, where they are degraded by the proteasomes and the resulting fragments are transported to the endoplasmic reticulum by the TAP system.

The stimulation of cytotoxic T cells requires additional signals and interactions, some of which depend upon cell–cell contact, such as those mediated by the interaction of CD8 with MHC I, CD2 with CD58, LFA-1 with ICAM family members and CD28 with CD80 and CD86. On the other hand, the expansion of antigen-activated CTL requires the secretion of IL-2. In experimental conditions, activated CTL can secrete sufficient quantities of IL-2 to support their proliferation and differentiation, and thus proceed without help from other T cell subpopulations. Physiologically, it seems more likely that activated helper T lymphocytes provide the IL-2 necessary for cytotoxic T-lymphocyte differentiation. The simultaneous expression of immunogenic peptides in association with MHC-I and MHC-II molecules in dendritic cells and macrophages creates the necessary environment for activation of T helper and T cytotoxic lymphocytes in close proximity. In the case of viral infections, macrophages are often infected and, consequently, they express viral peptides associated both with MHC-I (derived from newly synthesized proteins) and with MHC-II (derived from the degradation of endocytosed viral particles) thus becoming able to present viral-derived peptides both to T helper and T cytotoxic lymphocytes.

Mixed Lymphocyte Reaction and Graft Rejection

CTL also differentiate and proliferate when exposed to cells from an individual of the same species but from a different genetic background. In vitro, the degree of allostimulation between cells of two different individuals can be assessed by the mixed leukocyte reaction (see Chapter 15). Two recognition pathways have been proposed (Fig. 9):

1. Direct allorecognition of nonself MHC molecules by lymphocytes expressing alloreactive TcR.
2. Indirect recognition of allogeneic peptides (probably resulting from ingestion and processing of dead donor cells or proteins) associated with MHC-II molecules by Th1 cells expressing receptors for nonself peptides.

This second pathway seems very important in the mixed leukocyte reaction because MHC-II expressing cells must be present for the mixed leukocyte reaction to take place. This requirement suggests that activation of helper T cells by recognition of MHC-II/peptide complexes expressed by APCs is essential for the differentiation of cytotoxic $CD8^+$ cells. The role of helper T cells in the mixed lymphocyte reaction is likely to be very similar to the role of helper T cells that assist B cell responses, that is, to provide cytokines and costimulatory signals essential for cytotoxic T-cell growth and differentiation.

In graft rejection it is also believed that both pathways are involved. Graft rejection is more intense with increasing MHC disparity between donor and host. It seems intuitive that the strength of activation through the direct pathway should be directly related to the degree of structural differences between the nonshared MHC molecules. On the other hand, the transplanted tissues are likely to contain dying cells and activated cells shedding MHC-II molecules. Recipient APCs are likely to express allogeneic MHC-derived peptides either as a consequence of processing of phagocytized dead cells or of endocytosis of soluble donor MHC molecules. Thus, MHC differences are likely to influence the rejection reaction irrespective of which activation pathway is involved. As for what recipient T lymphocytes mediate

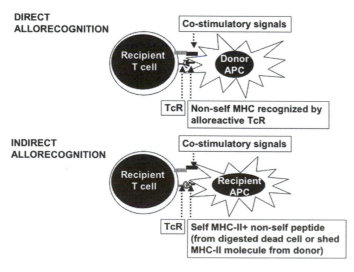

FIGURE 9 Diagrammatic representation of the two pathways involved in allostimulation between cells of two different individuals. *Abbreviations*: MHC, major histocompatibility complex; TcR, T-cell receptor.

the rejection, the indirect pathway can activate both CD4$^+$ and CD8$^+$ lymphocytes, because exogenous peptides can be loaded both to MHC-II and MHC-I molecules (through the cross-presentation pathway discussed earlier in this chapter). Thus, both activated Th1 and CD8 cytotoxic lymphocytes can be activated and become involved in graft rejection.

Alternative Pathways of Antigen Presentation to Cytotoxic T Cells

The best characterized of these pathways involves CD1, a family of nonpolymorphic, MHC-I-related molecules that includes five different isomorphic forms (A to E). APCs, including dendritic cells and B cells express CD1A, B, and C molecules and have been shown to present mycobacterium-derived lipid and lipoglycan antigens to both $\gamma\delta$ and $\alpha\beta$ CD8$^+$ CTL. Both $\gamma\delta$ and CD8$^+$ $\alpha\beta$ T cells stimulated by mycobacterial antigens presented in association with CD1 molecules cause the death of the presenting cells.

STIMULATION OF B LYMPHOCYTE RESPONSES TO T-DEPENDENT ANTIGENS

In contrast to T lymphocytes, B lymphocytes recognize external epitopes of unprocessed antigens, which do not have to be associated to MHC molecules. Some special types of APC, such as the follicular dendritic cells of the germinal centers, appear to adsorb complex antigens onto their membranes, where they are expressed and presented for long periods of time. Accessory cells and helper T lymphocytes provide additional signals necessary for B cell activation, proliferation, and differentiation. A major role is believed to be played by a complex of four proteins associated noncovalently with the membrane immunoglobulin, including CD19, CD21, and CD81. In this complex, the only protein with a known ligand is CD21, a receptor for C3d (a fragment of the complement component 3, C3). It is believed that B cells interacting with bacteria or protein antigens coated with C3 and C3 fragments receive a costimulatory signal through the occupancy of CD21.

Similar to the TcR, membrane immunoglobulins have short intracytoplasmic domains that do not appear to be involved in signal transmission. At least two heterodimers composed of two different polypeptide chains, termed Igα and Igβ, with long intracytoplasmic segments are associated to each membrane immunoglobulin. These heterodimers seem to have a dual function. On one hand, they act as transport proteins, capturing nascent immunoglobulin molecules in the endoplasmic reticulum and transporting them to the cell membrane. On the other, they are believed to be the "docking sites" for a family of protein kinases related to the src gene product, including p56^{lck} and p59^{fyn} that also play a role in T cell activation. In addition, the phosphatase CD45 is essential for p56^{lck} activation, thus initiating a cascade of tyrosine kinase activation. Specific to B cell activation is the involvement of a specific protein kinase, known as Bruton's tyrosine kinase (Btk) in the kinase cascade. The critical role of this kinase was revealed when its deficiency was found to be the cause of infantile agammaglobulinemia (Bruton's disease).

The subsequent sequence of events seems to have remarkable similarities with the activation cascade of T lymphocytes. Activation and translocation of common transcription factors (e.g., NF-AT, NF-κB) induce overlapping but distinct genetic programs. For instance, in B cells NF-κB activates the expression of genes coding for immunoglobulin polypeptide chains. For a B cell to complete its proliferation and differentiation into antibody-producing plasma cell or memory B cell, a variety of additional signals are required.

In the case of the stimulation of a B cell response with a T-dependent antigen, the additional signals are delivered by helper T cells in the form of cytokines and interactions with costimulatory molecules expressed by T cells. A naive B cell is initially stimulated by recognition of an epitope of the immunogen through the membrane immunoglobulin. Two other sets of membrane molecules are involved in this initial activation, the CD45 molecule and the CD19/CD21/CD81 complex. Whether the activation of CD45 involves interaction with a specific ligand on the accessory cell remains to be determined.

In the same microenvironment where B lymphocytes are being activated, helper T lymphocytes are also activated. This could be the result of a dual role of accessory cells, presenting both membrane-absorbed, unprocessed molecules with epitopes reflective of the native

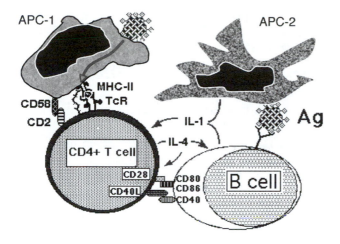

FIGURE 10 Diagrammatic representation of the interactions between antigen-presenting cells (APCs), T cells, and B cells in the early stages of an immune response. In this diagram, two separate APCs are involved in presentation of immunogenic peptides to Th2 cells (APC-1) and adsorbed, unmodified antigen to B cells (APC-2). Costimulatory signals are exchanged between the interacting cells. *Abbreviations*: APC, antigen-presenting cells; MHC, major histocompatibility complex; TcR, T-cell receptor.

configuration of the immunogenic molecule to B lymphocytes as well as MHC-II-associated peptides derived from processed antigen to the helper T lymphocytes (Fig. 10).

The proper progression of the immune response will require complex interactions between accessory cells, helper T lymphocytes, and B lymphocytes (Fig. 10). The helper T cell, as discussed earlier, receives a variety of costimulatory signals from APCs, and the activated helper T cell, in turn, delivers activating signals to APC and B cells. Some of the signals are mediated by interleukins and cytokines, such as IL-2 and IL-4 that stimulate B cell proliferation and differentiation, and interferon-γ that increases the efficiency of APC, particularly macrophages. Other signals are mediated by cell–cell interactions, involving CD40L (on T cells) and CD40 (on B cells). As a consequence of signaling through the CD40 molecule, B cells express CD80 and CD86 that deliver differentiation signals to T cells through the CD28 family of molecules. Additional activation signals are then delivered.

HELPER T LYMPHOCYTE SUBPOPULATIONS

The differentiation of helper T lymphocytes results in specialized functions to assist B cell activation and differentiation (Th2 lymphocytes) and to assist the proliferation and differentiation of CTL and KN cells (Th1 lymphocytes). These two subpopulations cannot be defined on the basis of expression of any specific membrane markers. Their definition is based on the repertoire of cytokines they release: Th1 cells predominantly release IFNγ and TNFβ and Th2 cells predominantly release IL-4 and IL-10 (Table 2).

Several factors appear to control the differentiation of Th1 and Th2. The early stages of proliferation of Th0 cells (as the common precursors are often designated) are IL-2 dependent. IL-2 is the main cytokine releases by activated Th0 cells and has both autocrine and paracrine effects, thus promoting Th0 proliferation. As the cells continue to proliferate, IL-12 promotes Th1 differentiation while IL-4 promotes Th2 differentiation. The cellular source of IL-12 is the APCs, and experimental work suggests that specific antigens or bacterial products with adjuvant properties may induce the release of IL-12 by those cells, thus tilting the immune response toward Th1 differentiation. The cellular source of the IL-4 needed to initiate the differentiation of Th2 cells is not clear. Recent research suggests that the initial drive towards Th2 differentiation may be provided by at least two specialized cell populations. One is a special population of CD4$^+$ T cells expressing a marker known as NK1.1 first defined in IL-2-activated

TABLE 2 Interleukins and Cytokines Released by Th1 and Th2 Helper T Lymphocytes

Th0 interleukins/cytokines	Target cell/effect
Interleukin-2	Th0, Th1, and Th2 cells/expansion; B cells/expansion
Th1 interleukins/cytokines	
Interferon-γ	Macrophages/activation; Th1 cells/differentiation; Th2 cells/downregulation
Lymphotoxin-α (LTα, TNFβ)	Th1 cells/expansion; B cells/homing
Th2 interleukins/cytokines	
Interleukin-4	Th2 cells/expansion; B cells/differentiation; APC/activation
Interleukin-5	Eosinophils/growth and differentiation
Interleukin-6	B cells/differentiation; plasma cells/proliferation; Th1, Th2 cells/activation; CD8$^+$ T cells/differentiation, proliferation
Interleukin-10	Th1, Th2 cells/downregulation; B cells/differentiation
Interleukin-13	Monocytes, macrophages/downregulation; B cells/activation, differentiation; mast cells, basophils/activation
Th1–Th2 interleukins/cytokines	
Interleukin-3	B cells/differentiation; macrophages/activation
TNF	B cells/activation, differentiation
Granulocyte-Monocyte CSF (GM-CSF)	B cells/differentiation

Abbreviations: APC, antigen-presenting cell; Th, helper T lymphocytes 0, 1, and 2; TNF, tumor necrosis factor.

NK cells. These T cells carry a high quantity of preformed IL-4 in their cytoplasm, ready to be released after proper stimulation. What factors control the activation of this specialized population are not known, but once IL-4 is released and Th2 cells start to differentiate, these cells continue to release IL-4 and promote further Th2 differentiation. The other is a subpopulation of dendritic cells known as DC2, which seems to promote Th2 differentiation independently of IL-4 synthesis. The other DC population, DC1, secretes IL-12 and interferon-α and promotes the differentiation of Th1 cells.

Several additional factors playing a role in determining Th1 or Th2 differentiation have been proposed, including the affinity of the interaction of the TcR with the MHC-II–associated peptide, the concentration of MHC-peptide complexes on the cell membrane, and signals dependent on cell–cell interactions (Table 3).

Cell–cell contact also plays a significant role in promoting B cell activation by delivering costimulatory signals to the B cell and/or by allowing direct traffic of unknown factors from helper T lymphocytes to B lymphocytes. Transient conjugation between T and B lymphocytes seems to occur constantly, due to the expression of complementary CAMs on their membranes. For example, T cells express CD2 and CD4, and B cells express the respective ligands, CD58 (LFA-3) and MHC-II; both T and B lymphocytes express ICAM-1 and LFA-1 that can reciprocally interact.

TABLE 3 Signals Involved in the Control of Differentiation of Th1 and Th2 Subpopulations of Helper T-Lymphocytes

Signals favoring Th1 differentiation	Signals favoring Th2 differentiation
Interleukin-12	Interleukin-4[a]
Interferon γ[b]	Interleukin-1
Interferon α[c]	Interleukin-10
CD28/CD80 interaction	CD28/CD86 interaction
High density of MHC-II–peptide complexes on the APC membrane	Low density of MHC-II–peptide complexes on the APC membrane
High affinity interaction between TcR and the MHC-II/peptide complex	Low affinity interaction between TcR and the MHC-II/peptide complex

[a]Released initially by undifferentiated Th cells (also known as Th0) after stimulation in the absence of significant interleukin (IL)12 release from APC; IL-4 becomes involved in an autocrine regulatory circuit, which results in differentiation of Th2 cells (helper T lymphocytes) and in paracrine regulation of B cell differentiation.
[b]Interferon γ does not act directly on Th2 cells, but enhances the release of IL-12 by APC, and as such has an indirect positive effect on Th2 differentiation.
[c]Interferon α is released by dendritic cells and their circulating precursors.
Abbreviations: APC, antigen-presenting cell; MHC, major histocompatibility complex; TcR, T cell receptors.

The continuing proliferation and differentiation of B cells into plasma cells is assisted by several soluble factors, including IL-4, released by Th2 cells; and IL-6 and IL-14, released by T-lymphocytes and accessory cells. At the end of an immune response, the total number of antigen-specific T and B lymphocyte clones will remain the same, but the number of cells in those clones will be increased several-folds. The increased residual population of antigen-specific T cells is long-lived, and is believed to be responsible for the phenomenon known as immunological memory.

BIBLIOGRAPHY

Bottomly K. T cells and dendritic cells get intimate. Science 1999; 283:1124.

Constant S, Pfeiffer C, Woodard A, Pasqualini T, Bottomly K. Extent of T cell receptor ligation can determine functional differentiation of naive CD4$^+$ T cells. J Exp Med 1995; 182:1591.

Duronio V, Scheid M, Ettinger S. Downstream signalling events regulated by phosphatidylinositol 3-kinase activity. Cell Signal 1998; 10:233–239.

Dustin ML, Shaw AS. Costimulation: building an immunological synapse. Science 1999; 283:649.

Farrar M, Doerfler P, Sauer K. Signal transduction pathways regulating the development of $\alpha\beta$ T cells. Biochim Biophys Acta 1998; 1377:F35–F78.

Fruman D, Meyers R, Cantley L. Phosphoinositide kinases. Annu Rev Biochem 1998; 67:481.

Garcia K, Teyton L, Wilson I. Structural basis of T cell recognition. Annu Rev Immunol 1999; 17:369.

Garside P, Ingulli E, Merica RR, Johnson JG, Noelle RJ, Jenkins MK. Visualization of specific B and T lymphocyte interactions in the lymph node. Science 1998; 281:96.

Germain RN, Stefanova I. The dynamics of T cell receptor signaling: complex orchestration and the key roles of tempo and cooperation. Annu Rev Immunol 1999; 17:467.

Heeger PS. T-cell allorecognition and transplant rejection: a summary and update. Am J Transplant 2003; 3:525–533.

June CH, Bluestone JA, Nadler LM, Thompson CB. The B7 and CD28 receptor families. Immunol Today 1994; 15:321.

Justement LB, Brown VK, Lin J. Regulation of B-cell activation by CD45: a question of mechanism. Immunol Today 1994; 15:399.

Krogsgaard M, Davis MM. How T cells "see" antigen. Nat Immunol 2005; 6:239.

Lane P, Flynn S, Walker L, et al. CD4 Cytokine differentiation—who or what decides? In The Immunologist 1998; 6:182.

Lesnchow J, Walunas T, Bluestone J. CD28/B7 system of T cell costimulation. Annu Rev Immunol 1996; 14:233–258.

Moll H. Antigen delivery by dendritic cells. Int J Med Microbiol 2004; 294:337–344.

Noelle RJ. The role of gp39 (CD40L) in immunity. Clin Immunol Immunopath 1995; 76:S203.

Shanafelt M-C, Sondberg C, Allsup A, Adelman D, Peltz G, Lahesmaa R. Costimulatory signals can selectively modulate cytokine production by subsets of CD4$^+$ T cells. J Immunol 1995; 154:1684.

Shen L, Rock KL. Priming of T cells by exogenous antigen cross-presented on MHC class I molecules. Curr Opin Immunol 2006; 18:85–91.

Wilson I, Garcia K. T-cell receptor structure and TcR complexes. Struct Biol 1997; 7:839–848.

5 | Immunoglobulin Structure

Gabriel Virella
Department of Microbiology and Immunology, Medical University of South Carolina, Charleston, South Carolina, U.S.A.

INTRODUCTION

Information concerning the precise structure of the antibody molecule started to accumulate, as technological developments were applied to the study of the general characteristics of antibodies. By the early 1940s, antibodies had been characterized electrophoretically as gamma-globulins (Fig. 1) and also classified into large families by their sedimentation coefficient determined by analytical ultracentrifugation (7S and 19S antibodies), reflective of the molecular weight of monomeric and polymeric immunoglobulins. It was also proven that plasma cells were responsible for immunoglobulin synthesis and that a malignancy known as multiple myeloma was a malignancy of immunoglobulin-producing plasma cells.

As protein fractionation techniques became available, complete immunoglobulins and their fragments were isolated in large amounts, particularly from the serum and urine of patients with multiple myeloma. These proteins were used both for studies of chemical structure and for immunological studies, which allowed to identify antigenic differences between proteins from different patients; this was the basis for the initial identification of the different classes and subclasses of immunoglobulins and the different types of light chains.

STRUCTURE OF IMMUNOGLOBULIN G

IgG is the most abundant immunoglobulin in human serum and in the serum of most mammalian species. It is also the immunoglobulin most frequently detected in large concentrations in multiple myeloma patients. For this reason, it was the first immunoglobulin to be purified in large quantities and to be extensively studied from the structural point of view. The basic knowledge about the structure of the IgG molecule was obtained from two types of experiments.

Proteolytic Digestion

The incubation of purified IgG with papain, a proteolytic enzyme extracted from the latex of *Carica papaya*, results in the splitting of the molecule into two fragments that differ both in charge and antigenicity. These fragments can be easily demonstrated by immunoelectrophoresis (Fig. 2), a technique that separates proteins by charge in a first step, allowing their antigenic characterization in a second step.

Reduction of Disulfide Bonds

If the IgG molecule is incubated with a reducing agent containing free thiol (SH) groups and fractionated by gel filtration (a technique which separates proteins by size) in conditions able to dissociate noncovalent interactions, two fractions are obtained. The first fraction corresponds to polypeptide chains of MW 55,000 (heavy chains); the second corresponds to polypeptide chains of MW 23,000 (light chains) (Fig. 3).

The sum of data obtained by proteolysis and reduction experiments resulted in the conception of a diagrammatic two-dimensional model for the IgG molecule (Fig. 4). The results of proteolytic digestion experiments can be reanalyzed on the basis of this model:

Papain digestion splits the heavy chains in the hinge region (so designated because this region of the molecule appears to be stereoflexible) and results in the separation of two Fab

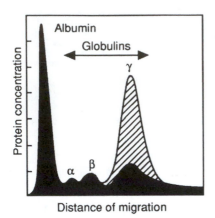

FIGURE 1 Demonstration of the gamma globulin mobility of circulating antibodies. The serum from a rabbit hyperimmunized with ovalbumin showed a very large gamma globulin fraction (*shaded area*), which disappeared when the same serum was electrophoretically separated after removal of antibody molecules by specific precipitation with ovalbumin. In contrast, serum albumin and the remaining globulin fractions were not affected by the precipitation step. *Source*: Adapted from Tiselius A, Kabat EA. J Exp Med 1939; 69:119.

fragments and one Fc fragment per IgG molecule (Fig. 5). The Fab fragments are so designated because they contain the antigen-binding site, whereas the Fc fragment received this designation because it can be easily crystallized.

If the disulfide bond joining heavy and light chains in the Fab fragments is split, one can separate a complete light chain from a fragment that comprises about 50% of one of the heavy chains—half of the NH_2 terminal. This portion of the heavy chain contained in each Fab fragment has been designated as Fd fragment.

Pepsin digestion splits the heavy chains beyond the disulfide bonds that join them at the hinge region, producing a double Fab fragment or F(ab')$_2$ (Fig. 6), whereas the Fc portion of the molecule is digested into peptides. The comparison of Fc, Fab, F(ab')$_2$, and whole IgG molecules shows both important similarities and differences between the whole molecule and its fragments.

1. Both Fab and F(ab')$_2$ contain antibody binding sites, but while the intact IgG molecule and the F(ab')$_2$ are bivalent, the Fab fragment is monovalent. Therefore, a Fab fragment can bind to an antigen, but cannot cross-link two antigen molecules.
2. An antiserum raised against the Fab fragment reacts mostly against light chain determinants; the immunodominant antigenic markers for the heavy chain are located in the Fc fragment.
3. The F(ab')$_2$ fragment is identical to the intact molecule as far as antigen-binding properties are concerned, but lacks most other biological properties of IgG, such as the ability to fix complement, bind to cell membranes, etc., which are determined by the Fc region of the molecule.

STRUCTURAL AND ANTIGENIC HETEROGENEITY OF HEAVY AND LIGHT CHAINS

As larger numbers of purified immunoglobulins were studied in detail, it became obvious that there was a substantial degree of structural heterogeneity, recognizable both by

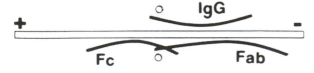

FIGURE 2 Immunoelectrophoretic separation of the fragments resulting from papain digestion of IgG. A papain digest of IgG was first separated by electrophoresis and the two fragments were revealed with an antiserum containing antibodies that react with different portions of the IgG molecule.

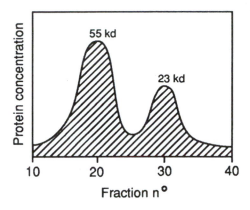

FIGURE 3 Gel filtration of reduced and alkylated IgG (MW 150,000) on a dissociating medium. Two protein peaks are eluted, the first corresponding to a MW 55,000 and the second corresponding to a MW 23,000. The 2:1 ratio of protein content between the high and low molecular weight peaks is compatible with the presence of identical numbers of two polypeptide chains, one of which is about twice as large as the other.

physicochemical methods as well as by antisera able to define different antigenic types of heavy and light chains.

Five classes of immunoglobulins were identified due to antigenic differences of the heavy chains and designated as IgG (the classical 7S immunoglobulin), IgA, IgM (the classical 19S immunoglobulin), IgD, and IgE. IgG, IgA, and IgM together constitute over 95% of the whole immunoglobulin pool in a normal human being and are designated as major immunoglobulin classes. Because they are common to all humans, the immunoglobulin classes can also be designated as isotypes. The major characteristics of the five immunoglobulin classes are summarized in Table 1.

The light chains also proved to be antigenically heterogeneous and two isotypes were defined: Kappa and Lambda. Each immunoglobulin molecule is a homodimer, constituted by a pair of identical heavy chains and a pair of identical light chains; hence, a given immunoglobulin molecule can have either kappa or lambda chains but not both. A normal individual will have a mixture of immunoglobulin molecules in his serum, some with kappa chains (e.g., IgGκ), and others with lambda chains (e.g., IgGλ). Normal serum IgG has a 2:1 ratio of kappa chain over lambda chain, bearing IgG molecules. In contrast, monoclonal immunoglobulins have one single heavy chain isotype and one single light chain

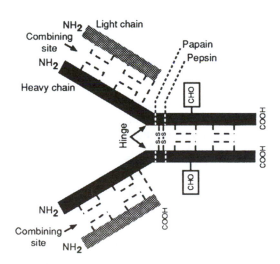

FIGURE 4 Diagrammatic representation of the IgG molecule. *Source*: Modified from Klein J. Immunology. Boston, Oxford: Blackwell Science Publication, 1990.

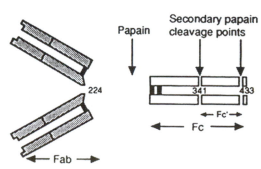

FIGURE 5 The fragments obtained by papain digestion of the IgG molecule. *Source*: Modified from Klein J. Immunology. Boston, Oxford: Blackwell Science Publication, 1990.

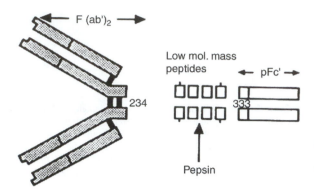

FIGURE 6 The fragments obtained by pepsin digestion of the IgG molecule. *Source*: Modified from Klein J. Immunology. Boston, Oxford: Blackwell Science Publication, 1990.

isotype. This results from the fact that monoclonal proteins are the products of large number of cells all derived from a single mutant, constituting one large clone of identical cells producing identical molecules.

Antigenic differences between the heavy chains of IgG and IgA were later characterized, leading to the definition of IgG and IgA subclasses (Tables 2 and 3). Some interesting biological and structural differences have been demonstrated for IgG and IgA proteins of different subclasses.

In the case of IgG subclasses, IgG1 and IgG3 are more efficient in terms of complement fixation and have greater affinity for monocyte receptors. Those properties can be correlated with a greater degree of biological activity, both in normal antimicrobial responses and in pathological conditions. Physiologically, these properties result in enhanced opsonization and bacterial killing. Pathologically, the assembly or deposition of extravascular immune complexes containing IgG1 and IgG3 antibodies activates pathways that induce tissue inflammation.

From the structural point of view, the IgG3 subclass has the greatest number of structural and biological differences relative to the remaining IgG subclasses. Most differences appear to result from the existence of an extended hinge region (which accounts for the greater MW) and with a large number of disulfide bonds linking the heavy chains together (estimates of their number vary between 5 and 15). This extended hinge region seems to be easily accessible to proteolytic enzymes, and this liability of the molecule is likely to account for its considerably shorter half-life.

Of the two IgA subclasses known, it is interesting to note that a subpopulation of IgA2 molecules carrying the A2m(1) allotype is the only example of a human immunoglobulin molecule, lacking the disulfide bond joining heavy and light chains. The IgA2 A2m(1) molecule is held together through noncovalent interactions between heavy and light chains.

IMMUNOGLOBULIN REGIONS AND DOMAINS
Variable and Constant Regions of the Immunoglobulin Molecule

The light chains of human immunoglobulins are composed of 211 to 217 amino acids. As mentioned earlier, there are two major antigenic types of light chains (κ and λ). When the amino

TABLE 1 Major Characteristics of Human Immunoglobulins

	IgG	IgA	IgM	IgD	IgE
Heavy chain class	γ	α	μ	δ	ε
H-chain subclasses	γ 1,2,3,4	α 1,2	—	—	—
L-chain type	κ and λ	κ and λ	κ and λ	κ and λ	κ and λ
Polymeric forms	No	Dimers, trimers	Pentamers	No	No
Molecular weight	150,000	(160,000)n	900,000	180,000	190,000
Serum concentration (mg/dL)	600–1300	60–300	30–150	3	0.03
Intravascular distribution (%)	45	42	80	75	51

Abbreviations: H, heavy; Ig, immunoglobulin; L, light.

TABLE 2 Immunoglobulin G Subclasses

	IgG1	IgG2	IgG3	IgG4
Percentage of total IgG in normal serum	60	30	7	3
Half-life (days)	21	21	7	21
Complement ixation[a]	++	+	+++	−
Segmental flexibility	+++	+	++++	++
Affinity for monocyte and polymorphonuclear receptors	+++	+	++++	+

[a]By the classical pathway.

TABLE 3 Immunoglobulin A Subclasses

	IgA1	IgA2
Distribution	Predominates in serum	Predominates in secretions
Proportions in serum (%)	85	15
Allotypes	?	A2m(1) and A2m(2)
H-s-s-L	+	− in A2m(1); + in A2m(2)

acid sequences of light chains of the same type were compared, it became evident that two regions could be distinguished in the light chain molecules: a variable region, comprising the portion between end of the amino terminal of the chain and residues 107 to 115; and a constant region, extending from the end of the variable region to the carboxyl terminus (Fig. 7).

The light chain constant regions were found to be almost identical in light chains of the same type, but differ markedly in κ and λ chains. It is assumed that the difference in antigenicity between the two types of light chains is directly correlated with the structural differences in constant regions. In contrast, the amino acid sequence of the light chain variable regions is different even in proteins of the same antigenic type, and early workers thought that this sequence would be totally individual to any single protein. With increasing data, it became evident that some proteins shared similarities in their variable regions, and it has been possible to classify variable regions into three groups, Vκ, Vλ, and VH. Each group has been further subdivided into several subgroups. The light chain V region subgroups (Vκ, Vλ) are "type"-specific; that is, Vκ subgroups are only found in κ proteins, and Vλ subgroups are always associated with λ chains. In contrast, the heavy chain V region subgroups (VH) are not

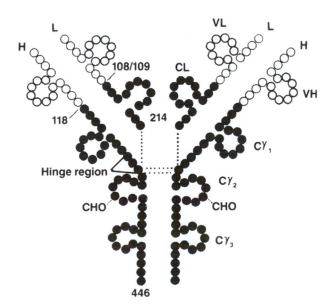

FIGURE 7 Schematic representation of the primary and secondary structure of a human IgG. The light chains are constituted by about 214 amino acids and two regions, a variable (first 108 amino acids, white beads in the diagram) and a constant (remaining amino acids, black beads in the diagram). Each of these regions contains a loop formed by intrachain disulfide bonds and contains about 60 amino acids, which are designated as variable domain and constant domain (VL and CL in the diagram). The heavy chains have slightly longer variable regions (first 118 amino acids, white beads in the diagram), with one domain (VH) and a constant region that contains three loops or domains (Cγ1, Cγ2, and Cγ3), numbered from the NH$_2$ terminus to the COOH terminus.

"class"-specific. Thus, any given VH subgroup can be found in association with the heavy chains of any of the known immunoglobulin classes and subclasses.

The heavy chain of IgG is about twice as large as a light chain; it is constituted by approximately 450 amino acids, and a variable and a constant region can also be identified. The variable region of the IgG heavy chain is constituted by the first 113 to 121 amino acids (counted from end of the amino terminal), and subgroups of these regions can also be identified. The constant region of the IgG heavy chain is almost three times larger than the variable region; for most of the heavy chains, it starts at residue 116 and ends at the carboxyl terminus (Fig. 7). The maximal degree of homology is found between constant regions of IgG proteins of the same subclass.

Immunoglobulin Domains

The immunoglobulin molecule contains several disulfide bonds formed between contiguous residues. Some of them join two different polypeptide chains (interchain disulfide bonds), keeping the molecule together. Others (intrachain bonds) join different areas of the same polypeptide chain, leading to the formation of "loops." These loops and adjacent amino acids constitute the immunoglobulin domains, which are folded in a characteristic β-pleated sheet structure (Fig. 8).

The variable regions of both heavy and light chains have a single domain that is involved in antigen binding. Light chains have one single constant region domain (CL), whereas heavy chains have several constant region domains (three in the case of IgG, IgA, and IgD; four in the case of IgM and IgE). The constant region domains are generically designated as CH1, CH2, CH3, and, if existing, CH4. To be more specific, the constant region domains can be identified as to the class of immunoglobulins to which they belong, by adding the symbol for each heavy chain class ($\gamma,\alpha,\mu,\delta,\epsilon$). For example, the constant region domains of the IgG molecule can be designated as Cγ1, Cγ2, and Cγ3. Different functions have been assigned to the different domains and regions of the heavy chains. For instance, Cγ2 is the domain involved in complement fixation, whereas both Cγ2 and Cγ3 are believed to be involved in the binding to phagocytic cell membranes.

The "hinge region" is located between the CH1 and CH2 domains. This name is derived from the fact that studies by a variety of techniques, including fluorescence polarization, spin-labeling, electron microscopy, and X-ray crystallography, have shown that the Fab fragments can rotate and waggle, coming together or moving apart. As a consequence IgG molecules can change their shape from a "Y" to a "T" and vice versa using the region intercalated between Cγ1 and Cγ2 as a "hinge." The length and primary sequence of the hinge regions play an important role in determining the segmental flexibility of IgG molecules. For example, IgG3 has a 12 amino acid hinge amino terminal segment and has the highest segmental flexibility. The hinge region is also the most frequent point of attack by proteolytic

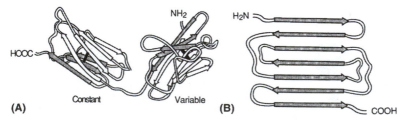

FIGURE 8 Model for the V and C domains of a human immunoglobulin light chain. Each domain has two β-pleated sheets consisting of several anti-parallel β-strands of 5 to 10 amino acids. The interior of each domain is formed between the two β-sheets by in-pointing amino acid residues, which alternate with out-pointing hydrophilic residues, as shown in (**A**). The antiparallelism of the β-strands is diagrammatically illustrated in (**B**). This β-sheet structure is believed to be the hallmark of the extracellular domains of all proteins in the immunoglobulin super-family. *Source*: (A) Modified from Edmundson AB, Ely KR, Abola EE, Schiffer M, Panagiotopoulos N. Biochemistry 1975; 14:3953; (B) Modified from Amzel, Poljak. Ann Rev Biochem 1979; 48:961.

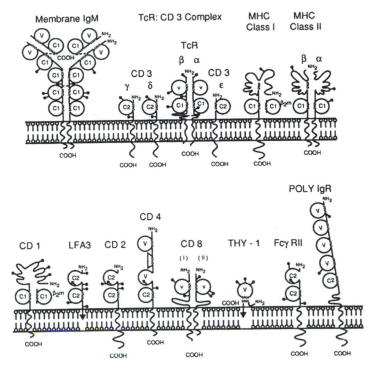

FIGURE 9 Model representations for some proteins included in the immunoglobulin superfamily. *Source*: Modified from Williams AF, Barclay AN. The Immunoglobulin superfamily—domains for cell surface recognition. Ann Rev Immunol 1988: 6:381.

enzymes. In general, the resistance to proteolysis of the different IgG subclasses is inversely related to the length of the hinge amino terminal segments—IgG3 proteins are most easily digestible, whereas IgG2 proteins, with the shortest hinge region, are most resistant to proteolytic enzymes.

IMMUNOGLOBULIN SUPERFAMILY OF PROTEINS

The existence of globular "domains" (Fig. 8) is considered as the structural hallmark of immunoglobulin structure. A variety of other proteins exhibit amino acid sequence homology with immunoglobulins and their molecules also contain Ig-like domains (Fig. 9). Such proteins are considered as members of the immunoglobulin superfamily, based on the assumption that the genes that encode them must have evolved from a common ancestor gene coding for a single domain, much likely the gene coding for the Thy-1 molecule found on murine lymphocytes and brain cells.

The majority of the membrane proteins of the immunoglobulin superfamily seem to be functionally involved in recognition of specific ligands that may determine cell–cell contact phenomena and/or cell activation. The T-cell antigen receptor molecule, the major histocompatibility antigens, the polyimmunoglobulin receptor on mucosal cells (see below), and the CD2 molecule on T lymphocytes (see below) are a few examples of proteins included in the immunoglobulin superfamily.

ANTIBODY-COMBINING SITE

As mentioned earlier, the binding of antigens by antibody molecules takes place in the Fab region, and is basically a noncovalent interaction that requires a good fit between the antigenic

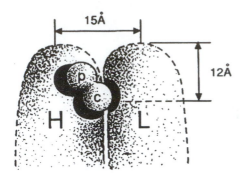

FIGURE 10 Diagrammatic representation of the hypothetical structure of an antigen-binding site. The variable regions of the light and heavy chains of a mouse myeloma protein that binds specifically to the phosphorylcholine hapten form a pouch in which the hapten fits. In this particular example, the specificity of the binding reaction depends mostly on the structure of the heavy chain V region. *Source*: Modified from Padlan E, *et al*. The immune system: genes, receptors, signals. Sercarz A, Williamson C, eds. New York: Academic Press, 1975:7.

determinant and the antigen-binding site on the immunoglobulin molecule. The antigen-binding site appears to be formed by the variable regions of both heavy and light chains, folded in close proximity forming a pouch where an antigenic determinant or epitope will fit (Fig. 10).

Actually, certain sequence stretches of the variable regions vary widely from protein to protein, even among proteins sharing the same type of variable regions. For this reason, these highly variable stretches have been designated as hypervariable regions. The structure of hypervariable regions is believed to play a critical role in determining antibody specificity since these regions are believed to be folded in such a way that they form a "pouch," where a given epitope of an antigen will fit. In other words, the hypervariable regions will interact to create a binding site whose configuration is complementary to that of a given epitope. Thus, these regions can also be designated as complementarity-determining regions.

IMMUNOGLOBULIN M: A POLYMERIC MOLECULE

Serum IgM is basically constituted by five subunits (monomeric subunits, IgMs), each one of them constituted by two light chains (κ or λ) and two heavy chains (μ). The heavy chains are larger than those of IgG by about 20,000 daltons, corresponding to an extra domain on the constant region (Cμ4). A third polypeptide chain, the J chain, can be revealed by adequate methodology in IgM molecules. This is a small polypeptide chain of 15,000 daltons, also found in polymeric IgA molecules. One single J chain is found in any polymeric IgM or IgA molecule, irrespective of how many monomeric subunits are involved in the polymerization. It has been postulated that this chain plays a key role in the polymerization process.

IMMUNOGLOBULIN A: A MOLECULARLY HETEROGENEOUS IMMUNOGLOBULIN
Serum IgA

Serum IgA is molecularly heterogeneous, constituted by a mixture of monomeric, dimeric, and larger polymeric molecules. In a normal individual, over 70% to 90% of serum IgA is monomeric. Monomeric IgA is similar to IgG, constituted by two heavy chains (α) and two light chains ($\kappa or \lambda$). The dimeric and polymeric forms of IgA found in circulation are covalently-bonded synthetic products containing J chains.

Secretory IgA

An IgA is the predominant immunoglobulin in secretions. Secretory IgA molecules are most frequently dimeric, contain J chain as do all polymeric immunoglobulin molecules and, in addition, contain a unique polypeptide chain designated as secretory component (Fig. 11). A single polypeptide chain of approximately 70,000 daltons, with five homologous immunoglobulin-like domains, constitutes this unique protein. It is synthesized by epithelial cells in the mucosa and by hepatocytes, initially as a larger membrane molecule known as

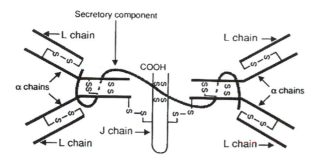

FIGURE 11 Structural model of the secretory IgA molecule. *Source*: Modified from Turner MW. Immunochemistry: an Advanced Textbook. Glynn LE, Steward MW, eds. New York: John Wiley & Sons, 1977.

polyimmunoglobulin receptor, from which the secretory component is derived by proteolytic cleavage that separates it from the intramembrane and cytoplasmic segments of its membrane form (see Chapter 6).

MINOR IMMUNOGLOBULIN CLASSES: IgD AND IgE

IgD and IgE were the last immunoglobulins to be identified due to their low concentrations in serum and low frequency of patients with multiple myeloma producing them. Both are monomeric immunoglobulins, similar to IgG, but their heavy chains are larger than γ chains. IgE has five domains in the heavy chain (one variable and four constant); IgD has four heavy chain domains (as most other monomeric immunoglobulins).

IgD and IgM are the predominant immunoglobulin classes in the B lymphocyte membrane, where they are the antigen-binding molecules in the antigen-receptor complex. Membrane IgD and IgM are monomeric. The heavy chains of membrane IgD and IgM (δm, μm) differ from that of the secreted forms at their carboxyl termini, where the membrane forms have a hydrophobic transmembrane section and a short cytoplasmic tail that are lacking in the secreted forms. In contrast, a hydrophilic section is found at the carboxyl termini of heavy chains of secreted immunoglobulins. The membrane immunoglobulins form a membrane complex with several other membrane proteins, including Igα and Igβ, which have sequence motifs in their cytoplasmic portions that are required for signal transduction. No other biological role is known for IgD besides existing as a membrane immunoglobulin.

IgE has the unique property of binding to Fc$_\epsilon$ receptors on the membranes of mast cells and basophils. The binding of IgE to those receptors has an extremely high affinity (7.7×10^9 L/ M^{-1}), about 100-fold greater than the affinity of IgG binding to monocyte receptors. The high affinity binding of IgE to basophil membrane receptors depends on the configuration of Cϵ3 and Cϵ4 domains. In allergic individuals, if those IgE molecules have a given antibody specificity and react with the antigen while attached to the basophil or mast cell membranes, they will trigger the release of histamine and other substances that cause the symptoms of allergic reactions (see Chapter 21).

BIBLIOGRAPHY

Atassi MA, van Oss CJ, Absolom DR, eds. Molecular Immunology. New York: Marcel Dekker, Inc., 1984.
Ban N, Escobar C, Garcia R, et al. Crystal structure of an idiotype-anti-idiotype Fab complex. Proc Natl Acad Sci USA 1994; 1604.
Day ED. Advanced Immunochemistry. 2nd ed. New York: Wiley-Liss, 1990.
Edmundson AB, Guddat LW, Rosauer RA, Anderson KN, Shan L, Rosauer RA. Three-dimensional aspects of IgG structure and function. In: Zanetti M, Capra DJ, eds. The Antibodies. Vol. 1. Amsterdam: Harwood Acad Pub, 1995:41.
Nezlin R. Internal movements in immunoglobulin molecules. Adv Immunol 1990; 48:1.
Underdown BJ, Schiff JM. Immunoglobulin A: strategic defense initiative at the mucosal surface. Annu Rev Immunol 1986; 4:389.
van Oss CJ, van Regenmortel MHV. Immunochemistry. New York: Marcel Dekker, 1994.

6 | Biosynthesis, Metabolism, and Biological Properties of Immunoglobulins

Gabriel Virella
Department of Microbiology and Immunology, Medical University of South Carolina, Charleston, South Carolina, U.S.A.

IMMUNOGLOBULIN BIOSYNTHESIS

Immunoglobulin synthesis is the defining property of B-lymphocytes and plasma cells. Resting B-lymphocytes synthesize only small amounts of immunoglobulins (Igs) that mainly become inserted into the cell membrane. Plasma cells, considered as end-stage cells arrested at the late G1 phase with very limited mitotic activity, are specialized to produce and secrete large amounts of Igs. The synthetic capacity of the plasma cell is reflected by its abundant cytoplasm, extremely rich in endoplasmic reticulum (Fig. 1).

Normally, heavy and light chains are synthesized in separate polyribosomes of the plasma cell. The amounts of H and L chains synthesized on the polyribosomes are roughly balanced so that both types of chains will be combined into complete IgG molecules, without surpluses of any given chain. The assembly of a complete IgG molecule can be achieved by (*i*) either associating one H and one L chain to form an HL hemimolecule, joining in the next step two HL hemimolecules to form the complete molecule (H_2L_2) or by (*ii*) forming H_2 and L_2 dimers that later associate to form the complete molecule.

The synthesis of light chains is usually slightly unbalanced, so that plasma cells secrete a small amount of excess free light chains, which are eliminated in the urine in very small concentrations. When plasma cells undergo malignant transformation, this unbalanced synthesis of light chains may be grossly aberrant, and this is reflected by the elimination of the excessively produced light chains of a single isotype in the urine (Bence Jones proteinuria, see Chapter 27). In contrast, free heavy chains are generally not secreted. The heavy chains are synthesized and glycosylated in the endoplasmic reticulum, but secretion requires association of light chains to form a complete immunoglobulin molecule. If light chains are not synthesized or heavy chains are synthesized in excess, the free heavy chains associate via their C_H1 domain with a heavy chain binding-protein, which is believed to be responsible for their intracytoplasmic retention. In rare cases, the free heavy chains are structurally abnormal and are secreted. Free heavy chains are usually retained in circulation because of their molecular weight, about twice as large as that of light chains.

Synthesis of Polymeric Immunoglobulins (IgM, IgA)

All polymeric immunogobulins have one additional polypeptide chain, the J chain. This chain is synthesized by all plasma cells including those that produce IgG. However, it is only incorporated to polymeric forms of IgM and IgA. It is thought that the J chain has some role in initiating polymerization. IgM proteins are assembled in two steps. First, the monomeric units are assembled. Then, five monomers and one J chain will be combined via covalent bonds to result in the final pentameric molecule. This assembly seems to coincide with secretion in some cells, in which only monomeric subunits are found intracellularly. However, in other cells the pentameric forms can be found intracellularly and secretion seems linked to glycosylation.

Synthesis of Secretory IgA

Secretory IgA is also assembled in two stages, but each one takes place in a different cell. Dimeric IgA, containing two monomeric subunits and a J chain joined together by disulfide

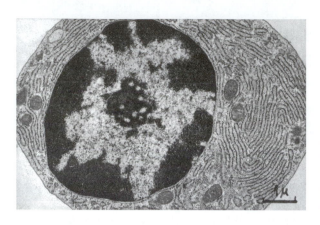

FIGURE 1 Ultrastructure of a mature plasma cell. Note the eccentric nucleus with clumped chromatin, the large cytoplasm containing abundant, distended, and endoplasmic reticulum. *Source*: Electron microphotograph courtesy of Professor P. Groscurth, M.D., Institute of Anatomy, University of Zurich, Switzerland.

bridges, is predominantly synthesized by submucosal plasma cells, although a minor portion may also be synthesized in the bone marrow. Secretory component (SC), on the other hand, is synthesized in the epithelial cells where the final assembly of secretory IgA takes place. Two different biological functions have been postulated for the SC: First, SC is responsible for secretion of IgA by mucosal membranes. The process involves uptake of dimeric IgA, assembly of IgA–SC complexes, and secretion by the mucosal cells. The uptake of dimeric IgA by mucosal cells is mediated by a glycoprotein related to SC, called polyimmunoglobulin receptor (poly-IgR). The poly-IgR is constituted by a single polypeptide chain of approximately 95,000 daltons, composed of an extracellular portion with five immunoglobulin-like domains, a transmembrane domain, and an intracytoplasmic domain. It is expressed on the internal surface of mucosal cells and binds J-chain-containing polymeric immunoglobulins.

The binding of dimeric IgA to poly-IgR seems to be the first step in the final assembly and transport process of secretory IgA. Surface-bound IgA is internalized and poly-IgR is covalently bound to the molecule, probably by means of a disulfide-interchanging enzyme that will break intrachain disulfide bonds in both IgA and poly-IgR and promote their rearrangement to form interchain disulfide bonds joining poly-IgR to an α chain.

After this takes place, the transmembrane and intracytoplasmic domains of the receptor are removed by proteolytic cleavage, and the remaining five domains remain bound to IgA, as SC, and the complete secretory IgA molecule is secreted (Fig. 2).

The same transport mechanisms are believed to operate in the liver at the hepatocyte level. The hepatocytes produce poly-IgR, bind and internalize dimeric IgA reaching the liver through the portal circulation, assemble complete secretory IgA, and secrete it to the bile. Secretory IgA must also flow back to the bloodstream, because small amounts are found in the blood of normal individuals. Higher levels of secretory IgA in blood are found in some forms of liver disease, when the uptake of dimeric IgA backflowing from the gut through the mesenteric lymph vessels takes place, but its secretion into the biliary system is compromised. Under those circumstances, secretory IgA assembled in the hepatocyte backflows into the systemic circulation.

Among all J-chain containing immunoglobulins, the poly-IgR has higher binding affinity for dimeric IgA. In IgA-deficient individuals IgM coupled with SC can be present in external secretions. It is believed that the same basic transport mechanisms are involved, starting by the binding of pentameric IgM to the poly-IgR on a mucosal cell and proceeding along the same lines outlined for the assembly and secretion of dimeric IgA. The fact that secretory IgM with covalently bound SC is detected exclusively in secretions of IgA-deficient individuals is believed to reflect the lower affinity of the interaction between poly-IgR and IgM-associated J chains (perhaps this is a consequence of steric hindrance of the binding sites of the J chain). Therefore, the interaction between IgM and poly-IgR would only take place in the absence of competition from dimeric IgA molecules.

The second function proposed for SC is that of a stabilizer of the IgA molecule. This concept is based on experimental observations showing that secretory IgA or dimeric IgA to

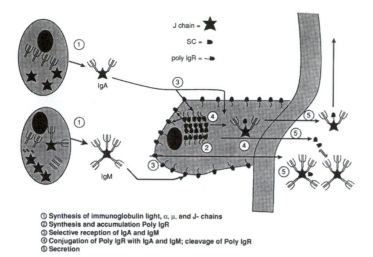

① Synthesis of immunoglobulin light, α, μ, and J- chains
② Synthesis and accumulation Poly IgR
③ Selective reception of IgA and IgM
④ Conjugation of Poly IgR with IgA and IgM; cleavage of Poly IgR
⑤ Secretion

FIGURE 2 Diagrammatic representation of the mechanisms involved in the synthesis and external transfer of dimeric IgA. According to this model, a polyimmunoglobulin receptor is located at the membrane of mucosal cells and binds polymeric immunoglobulins in general and dimeric IgA with the greatest specificity. The poly-IgR–IgA complexes are internalized, and in the presence of a disulfide-interchanging enzyme, covalent bonds are established between the receptor protein and the immunoglobulin. The transmembrane and intracytoplasmic bonds of the poly-IgR are cleaved by proteolytic enzymes, and the extracellular portion remains bound to IgA, constituting the secretory component. The IgA–SC complex is then secreted to the gland lumen. If the individual is IgA deficient, IgM may become involved in a similar process. *Source*: Modified from Brandzaeg P, Baklien K. Intestinal secretion of IgA and IgM: a hypothetical model. In Immunology of the Gut. Ciba Fdtn Symp. 46. North-Holland: Elsevier/ Excerpta, 1977:77.

which SC has been noncovalently associated in vitro are more resistant to the effects of proteolytic enzymes than monomeric or dimeric IgA molecules devoid of SC. One way to explain these observations would be to suggest that the association of SC with dimeric IgA molecules renders the hinge region of the IgA monomeric subunits less accessible to proteolytic enzymes. From a biological point of view, it would be advantageous for antibodies secreted into fluids rich in proteolytic enzymes (both of bacterial and host origin) to be resistant to proteolysis.

IMMUNOGLOBULIN METABOLISM

All proteins produced by an organism will eventually be degraded or lost through the excreta. However, the speed of the metabolic elimination the fractional turnover rate (which is the fraction of the plasma pool catabolized and cleared into urine in a day), and the synthetic rate vary considerably from protein to protein. Within the immunoglobulin group, different immunoglobulin isotypes have different synthetic rates and different catabolic rates.

One of the most commonly used parameters to asses the catabolic rate of immunoglobulins is the half-life (T 1/2) that corresponds to the time elapsed for a reduction to half of the IgG concentration after equilibrium has been reached. This is usually determined by injecting an immunoglobulin labeled with a radio-isotope (^{131}I is preferred for the labeling of proteins to be used for metabolic studies due to its fast decay rate), and follow the plasma activity curve. Figure 3 reproduces an example of a metabolic turnover study. After an initial phase of equilibration, the decay of circulating radioactivity follows a straight line in a semilogarithmic scale. From this graph it is easy to derive the time elapsed between concentration n and n/2, that is, the half-life.

Summary of the Metabolic Properties of Immunoglobulins

1. IgG is the immunoglobulin class with the longest half-life (21 days) and lowest fractional turnover rate (4–10%/12 hrs) with the exception of IgG3, which has a considerably shorter half-life (seven days) close to that of IgA (five to six days) and IgM (five days).

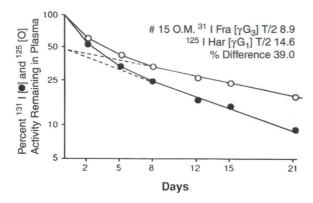

FIGURE 3 Plasma elimination curves of two IgG proteins, one typed as IgG1 (Har) and the other as IgG3 (Fra). The T 1/2 can be determined from the stable part of the curve, and its extrapolation (*dotted line*) as the time necessary for a 50% reduction of the circulating concentration of labelled protein. *Source*: Reproduced from Spiegelberg HL, Fishkin BG, Grey HM. Catabolism of human G immunoglobulins of different heavy chain subclass. J Clin Invest 1968; 47:2323.

2. IgG catabolism is uniquely influenced by its circulating concentration of this immunoglobulin. At high protein concentrations, the catabolism will be faster, and at low IgG concentrations, catabolism will be slowed down. These differences are explained according to Brambell's theory, by the protection of IgG bound to IgG-specific Fc receptors in the internal aspect of endopinocytotic vesicles from proteolytic enzymes. These receptors are structurally different from all other known Fc receptors, and are structurally related to MHC-I molecules (neonatal Fc receptors, FcRn). IgG is constantly pinocytosed by cells able to degrade it, but at low IgG concentrations most molecules are bound to FcRn on the endopinocytotic vesicles and the fraction of total IgG degraded will be small. The undegraded molecules are eventually released back into the extracellular fluids. At high IgG concentrations, the majority of IgG molecules remains unbound in the endopinocytotic vesicle and is degraded resulting in a high catabolic rate (Fig. 4).

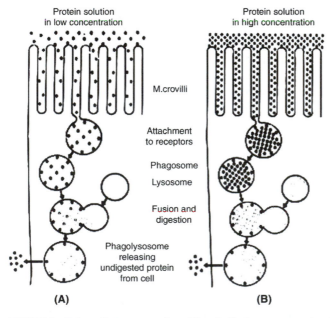

FIGURE 4 Schematic representation of Brambell's theory concerning the placental transfer of IgG and the relationship between concentration and catabolism of IgG. The diagram at the left shows that pinocytotic IgG will be partially bound to phagosome wall receptors and protected from proteolysis, later released undigested. This mechanism would account for transplacental transfer. The diagram on the right side of the figure shows that if the concentration of IgG is very high, the number of IgG molecules bound to phagosome receptors will remain the same as when the concentration is low, while the number of unbound molecules will be much greater, and those will be eventually digested, resulting in a higher catabolic rate. *Source*: Reproduced from Brambell FWR. The transmission of immunity from mother to young and the catabolism of immunoglobulins. Lancet 1966; 2:1089.

3. While most immunoglobulin classes and subclasses are evenly distributed among the intra- and extravascular compartments, IgM, IgD, and to a lesser extent, IgG3, are predominantly concentrated in the intra-vascular space and IgA2 is predominantly concentrated in secretions.
4. The synthetic rate of IgA1 (24 mg/kg/day) is not very different from that of IgG1 (25 mg/kg/day), but the serum concentration of IgA1 is about one-third of the IgG1 concentration. This is explained by a fractional turnover rate three times greater for IgA1 (24%/day).
5. The highest fractional turnover rate and shorter half-life are those of IgE (74%/day and 2.4 days, respectively).
6. The lowest synthetic rate is that of IgE (0.002 mg/kg/day compared to 20–60 mg/kg/day for IgG).

BIOLOGICAL PROPERTIES OF IMMUNOGLOBULINS

The antibody molecules have two major functions: binding to the antigen; a function that basically depends on the variable regions located on the Fab region of the molecule, and several other extremely important functions listed in Table 1, which depend on the Fc region. Of particular physiological interest is the placental transfer, complement fixation, and binding to Fc receptors.

Placental Transfer

In humans, the only major immunoglobulin transferred from mother to fetus across the placenta is IgG. The placental transfer of IgG is an active process; the concentration of IgG in the fetal circulation is often higher than the concentration in matched maternal blood. It is also known that a normal fetus synthesizes only trace amounts of IgG depending on placental transfer for acquisition of passive immunity against common pathogens.

The selectivity of IgG transport has been explained by Brambell's receptor theory for IgG catabolism. The trophoblastic cells on the maternal side of the placenta would endocytose plasma containing all types of proteins, but would have receptors in the endopinocytotic vesicles for the Fc region of IgG and not for any other immunoglobulin. IgG bound to Fcγ receptors would be protected from catabolism, and through active reverse pinocytosis would be released into the fetal circulation. The receptors involved are FcRn, identical to those described earlier, which protect IgG from degradation in endocytic vesicles.

TABLE 1   Biologic Properties of Immunoglobulins

	IgG1	IgG2	IgG3	IgG4	IgA1	IgA2	IgM	IgD	IgE
Serum concentration (mg/dl)[a]	460–1140	80–390	28–194	2.5–16	50–200	0–20	50–200	0–40	0–0.2
Presence in normal secretions	−	−	−	−	+	+ + +	+	−	+
Placental transfer	+	+	+	+	−	−	−	−	−
Complement fixation									
Classic pathway	+ + +	+	+ + +	−	−	−	+ + +	−	−
Alternative pathway[b]	+	+	+	+	+	+	?	+	+
Reaction with Fc receptors on									
Macrophages	+	−	+ +	−	+	+	−	−	−
Neutrophils	+	−	+ +	−	−	−	−	−	−
Basophils/mast cells	−	−	−	−	−	−	−	−	+ + +[c]
Platelets	+	+	+	+	−	−	−	−	−
Lymphocytes	+ +	?	+ +	?	−	−	+	−	−

[a]IgG subclass values after Ref. 5.
[b]After aggregation.
[c]High-affinity receptors.

Complement Activation

The complement system can be activated by three distinct pathways (see Chapter 9). All immunoglobulins have been found able to fix complement by either the classical or the alternative pathway. IgG1, IgG3, and IgM molecules are the most efficient in fixing complement; all of them through the more powerful classical pathway.

Complement activation is an extremely important amplification mechanism, which enhances antibody-dependent neutralization and elimination of infectious agents. These effects depend on two basic mechanisms discussed in greater detail in Chapter 9:

1. Generation of C3b which, when deposited on the membrane of a microorganism, facilitates phagocytosis by cells with C3b receptors. For this reason, C3b is known as opsonin.
2. Disruption of lipid bilayers that depends on the generation of the late complement components (C6–C9). When those components are properly assembled on a cell membrane, they induce the formation of transmembrane channels that result in cell lysis.

Binding to Fc Receptors

Virtually every type of cell involved in the immune response has been found to be able to bind one or more immunoglobulin isotypes through Fc receptors (Table 2). These receptors have been classified according to the isotype of immunoglobulin, which they preferentially bind as FcγR (receptors for IgG), FcαR (receptors for IgA), and FcεR (receptors for IgE). The Fcγ receptors are the most diverse, since they exist in three major types:

1. FcγRI (CD64): a high-affinity receptor, able to bind monomeric IgG, and expressed exclusively by monocytes and macrophages.
2. FcγRII (CD32): a low-affinity receptor for IgG expressed by phagocytic cells, platelets, and B-lymphocytes. Two functionally distinct forms of FcγRII have been identified: FcγRIIa and FcγRIIb.
3. FcγRIII (CD16): a second low-affinity IgG receptor expressed by phagocytic and natural killer (NK) cells.

Fc receptors are constituted by one or several polypeptide chains. The extracellular domains responsible for interaction with the Fc region are located on the α chain, represented in all

TABLE 2   Different Types of Fc Receptors Described in the Cells of the Immune System

Fc receptor	Characteristics	Cellular distribution	Function
FcγRI (I, IIa, and III) (CD64)	Transmembrane and intracytoplasmic domains; high affinity; binds both monomeric and aggregated IgG	Monocytes, macrophages	ADCC (monocytes)
FcγRIIa (CD32) FcγRIIb	Transmembrane and intracytoplasmic domains; low affinity	Monocytes/macrophages; Langerhans cells; granulocytes; platelets; B cells (FcgRIIb)	IC binding; phagocytosis; degranulation; ADCC (monocytes); downregulation (FcgRIIb)
FcγRIII (CD16)	Glycosyl-phosphatidyl inositol anchor in neutrophils; trans-membrane segment in NK cells; low affinity	Macrophages; granulocytes; NK and K cells	IC binding and clearance; "priming signal" for phagocytosis and degranulation; ADCC (NK cells)
FcαR	Transmembrane and intracytoplasmic segments; low affinity	Granulocytes, monocytes/ macrophages, platelets, T and B lymphocytes	Phagocytosis, degranulation
FcεR (I)	High affinity	Basophils, mast cells	Basophil/mast cell degranulation
FcεR (II) (CD23)	Low affinity	T and B lymphocytes; monocytes/macrophages; eosinophils; platelets	Mediate parasite killing by eosinophils

Abbreviations: ADCC, antibody-dependent cellular cytotoxicity; NK, natural killer.

Fc receptors. While FcγRII is constituted exclusively by an α chain, Fcα, FcγRI, and FcγRIII receptors have an additional polypeptide chain (γ), and FcεRI has a third chain ($\bar{\beta}$).

The binding of free or complexed immunoglobulins to their corresponding Fc receptors has significant biological implications. The catabolic rate and the selective placental transfer of IgG depend on the interaction with FcγR on pinocytic vesicles. IgG also mediates phagocytosis by all cells expressing FcγR on their membranes (granulocytes, monocytes, macrophages, and other cells of the same lineage). Thus, IgG is also considered as an opsonin. IgA (particularly its dimeric form) has been shown to mediate phagocytosis but, by itself, it seems to be a weak opsonin, and complement activation by the alternative pathway seems to enhance significantly this activity. In reality, IgG and C3b have synergistic opsonizing effects and their joint binding and deposition on the membrane of an infectious agent is a most effective way to promote its elimination.

A significant property of Fcγ receptors is their ability to transduce activating signals to the cells where they are inserted. Activation is mediated by immunoreceptor tyrosine-based activation motifs (ITAMs) located either in the α polypeptide chain (FcγRIIa) of in one or both of the associated chains (α and β). The activation of ITAMs requires cross-linking of Fc receptors by Ag–Ab complexes containing at least two antibody molecules.

One notable exception to the ability to induce cell activation is the opposite effect mediated by FcγRIIb receptors. These receptors have immunoreceptor tyrosine-based inhibitory motifs (ITIM) in their intracellular portion. As discussed in Chapter 12, these receptors are expressed on B lymphocytes and may play a critical role in the downregulation of humoral immune responses as a consequence of the formation of circulating immune complexes.

Antibody-Dependent Cellular Cytotoxicity

Granulocytes, monocytes/macrophages, and NK cells can destroy target cells coated with IgG antibody [antibody-dependent cellular cytotoxicity (ADCC)]. In this case, the destruction of the target cell does not depend on opsonization but rather on the release of toxic mediators. The specific elimination of target cells by opsonization and ADCC depends on the biding of IgG antibodies to those targets. The antibody molecule tags the target for destruction; phagocytic or NK cells mediate the destruction. Not all antibody molecules are able to react equally with the Fcγ receptors of these cells. The highest binding affinities for any of the three types of Fcγ receptor known to date are observed with IgG1 and IgG3 molecules.

Fcε Receptors

Two types of Fcε receptors specific for IgE have been defined. One is a low-affinity receptor (FcεRII), present in most types of granulocytes. It mediates ADCC reactions directed against helminths, which typically elicit IgE antibody synthesis (see Chapter 14). The other is a high-affinity Fcε receptor (FcεRI) expressed by basophils and mast cells. The basophil/mast cell bound IgE functions as a true cell receptor. When an IgE molecule bound to a high-affinity FcεRI membrane receptor interacts with the specific antigen against which it is directed, the cell is activated, and as a consequence, histamine and other mediators are released from the cell. The release of histamine and a variety of other biologically active compounds is the basis of the immediate hypersensitivity reaction, which is discussed in detail in Chapter 21.

BIBLIOGRAPHY

Brambell FWR. The transmission of immunity from mother to young and the catabolism of immuno globulins. Lancet 1966; 2:1089.
Brandtzaeg P. Molecular and cellular aspects of the secretory immunoglobulin system. APMIS 1995; 103:1.
Brandzaeg P, Baklien K. Intestinal secretion of IgA and IgM: a hypothetical model. In Immunology of the Gut. Ciba Fdtn. Symposium. 46 (new series), Medica/North-Highland, NY: Elsevier/Excerpta 1977:77).
Djistelnloem HM, van de Winkel J, Kellenberg CGM. Inflammation in autoimmunity: receptors for IgG revisited. Trends Immunol 2001; 22:510–516.

Firan M, Bawdon R, Radu C, et al. The MHC class I-related receptor, FcRn, plays an essential role in the maternofetal transfer of g-globulin in humans. Int Immunol 2001; 13:993–1002.

Ghetie V, Ward ES. Multiple roles for the major histocompatibility complex class I-related receptor FcRn. Annu Rev Immunol 2000; 18:739–766.

Janoff EN, Fasching C, Orenstein JM, Rubins JB, Opstad NL, Dalmasso AP. Killing of <i>Streptococcus pneumoniae</i> by capsular polysaccharide-specific polymeric IgA, complement, and phagocytes. J clin Invest 1999; 104:1139.

Nezlin R. Immunoglobulin structure and function. In: van Oss CJ, van Regenmortel MHV, eds. Immunochemistry. New York: Marcel Dekker, 1994:3.

Parkhouse RME. Biosynthesis of immunoglobulins. In: Glynn LE, Steward MW, eds. Immunochemisty: An Advanced Textbook. New York: John Wiley and Sons, 1977.

Ravetch JV, Bolland S. IgG Fc receptors. Annu Rev Immunol 2001; 19:275–290.

Shakib F, Stanworth DR, Drew R, Catty D. A quan study of the distribution of IgG sub-classes in a group of normal human sera. J Immunol Methods 1975; 8:17–28.

Sitia R, Cattaneo A. Synthesis and assembly of antibodies in nature and artificial environments. In: Zanetti M, Capra JD, eds. The Antibodies. Vol. 1. Amsterdam: Harwood Acad Pub, 1995:127.

Spiegelberg HL, Fishkin BG, Grey HM. Catabolism of human G immunoglobulins of different heavy chain subclass: J Clin Invest 1968; 47:2323.

Underdown BJ, Schiff JM. Immunoglobulin A: strategic defense initiative at the mucosal surface. Ann Rev Immunol 1986; 4:389.

Waldmann TA, Strober W. Metabolism of immunoglobulins. Prog Allergy 1969; 13:1.

7 | Genetics of Immunoglobulins

Janardan P. Pandey
Department of Microbiology and Immunology, Medical University of South Carolina, Charleston, South Carolina, U.S.A.

INTRODUCTION

Human immunoglobulin (Ig) molecules are coded by three unlinked gene families: two for light (L) chains located on chromosomes 2 (κ chains) and 22 (λ chains), and one for heavy (H) chains located on chromosome 14. As mentioned in the preceding chapters, each individual is able to produce billions of antibody molecules with different antigenic specificities, and this diversity corresponds to the extreme heterogeneity of the variable (V) regions in those antibody molecules, implying that each individual must possess a large number of structural genes for Ig chains. The allotypic determinants on the constant (C) region (see following discussion), on the other hand, segregate as a single Mendelian trait, suggesting that there may be only one gene for each of the several Ig chain C regions. To reconcile these seemingly contradictory observations, Dreyer and Bennet, in 1965, proposed that two separate genes that are brought together by a translocation event during lymphocyte development encode the V and C regions. Employing recombinant DNA technology, Hozumi and Tonegawa, in 1976, obtained conclusive proof of this hypothesis (for his seminal studies, Tonegawa was awarded the 1987 Nobel prize in Medicine and Physiology).

IMMUNOGLOBULIN GENE REARRANGEMENT

It is well-established that an Ig polypeptide chain is coded by multiple genes scattered along a chromosome of the germ-line genome. These widely separated gene segments are brought together (recombined) during B-lymphocyte differentiation to form a complete Ig gene. The V regions of the Ig-L chains are coded by two gene segments, designated as V and J (J for joining, because it joins V and C region genes). Three gene segments are required for the synthesis of the V region of the H chains: V, J, and D (D for diversity, corresponds to the most diverse region of the H chain). To form a functional L or H chain gene, one or two gene rearrangements are needed. On chromosomes 2 or 22, a V gene moves next to a J gene. On chromosome 14, first the D and J regions are joined, and next one of the V genes is joined to the DJ complex. The VJ segments and one of the L chain C regions (Cκ or Cλ) or VDJ segments and one of the CH-gene complexes (Cμ, Cδ, Cγ3, Cγ1, Cα1, Cγ2, Cγ4, Cε, or Cα2) are then transcribed into nuclear RNA that contains these sequences as well as the interconnecting noncoding sequences. The intervening noncoding sequences are then excised making a contiguous VJC mRNA for an L chain and a contiguous VDJC mRNA for an H chain (Figs. 1 and 2). Gene rearrangements occur in a sequential order: usually H chain genes rearrange first, followed by κ chain genes and lastly by λ genes.

It has been shown that the VDJ joining is regulated by two proteins encoded by two closely linked recombination-activating genes (RAG-1 and RAG-2) localized on the short arm of human chromosome 11. These genes have at least two unusual characteristics not shared by most eukaryotic genes: they are devoid of introns and, although adjacent in location and synergistic in function, they have no sequence homology. The latter implies that, unlike the Ig and major histocompatibility complex (MHC) genes, RAG-1 and RAG-2 did not arise by gene duplication. Recent studies suggest that these genes may be evolutionarily related to transposons, genetic elements that can be transposed in the genome from one location to the other. Conserved recombination signal sequences (RSS) serve as substrate for the enzymes coded by the RAG genes. These enzymes introduce a break between the RSS and the

Kappa Light Chain

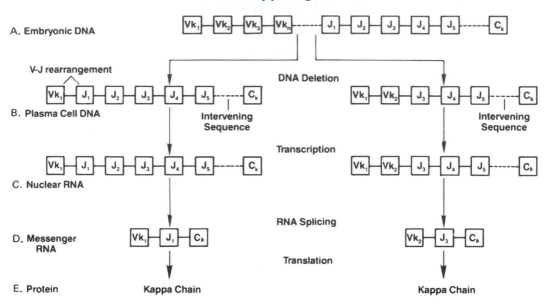

FIGURE 1 The embryonic DNA of chromosome 2 contains over 300 variable (V) genes, five joining (J) genes, and a constant (C) gene (**A**). The V and J gene code for the kappa chain's V region, C for its C region. In the left pathway, differentiation of the embryonic cell to a plasma cell results in deletion of the intervening V genes so that $V_{\kappa 1}$ is joined with the J_1 gene (**B**). The linked $V_{\kappa 1}J_1$ segment codes for one of over 1,500 possible kappa light chain V regions. The plasma cell DNA is transcribed into nuclear RNA (**C**). Splicing of the nuclear RNA produces messenger RNAs with the $V_{\kappa 1}$, J_1, and C genes linked together (**D**), ready for translation of a kappa light chain protein (**E**). The alternate pathway at right (**B–D**) shows another of the many possible pathways leading to a different kappa light chain with a different variable region specificity. *Source*: Modified from David JR. Antibodies: structure and function. Scientific American Medicine. New York: Scientific American Inc., 1980.

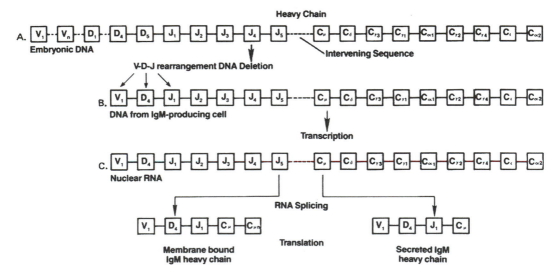

FIGURE 2 A stretch of embryonic DNA in chromosome 14 contains a section coding for the heavy-chain variable region; this DNA is made up of at least 100 variable (V) genes, 50 diversity (D) genes, and four to six joining (J) genes. The section coding for the constant (C) region is formed by nine C genes (**A**). In the pathway shown, when the embryonic cell differentiates into a plasma cell, some V and D genes are deleted so that V_1, D_4, and J_1 are joined to form one of many possible heavy-chain genes (**B**). The plasma cell DNA is then transcribed into nuclear RNA (**C**). RNA splicing selects the C gene and joins it to the V_1, D_4, and J_1 genes (**D**). The resulting messenger RNAs will code for IgM heavy chains (**E**). If RNA splicing removes the $C\mu m$ piece from the $C\mu$ gene, the IgM will be secreted. If the piece remains, the IgM will be membrane-bound. *Source*: Modified from David JR. Antibodies: structure and function. Scientific American Medicine. New York: Scientific American Inc., 1980.

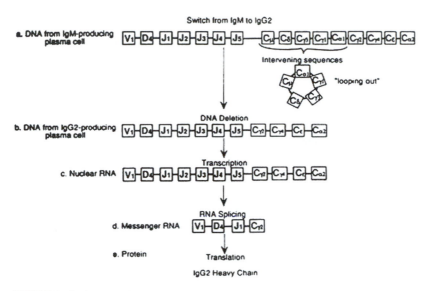

FIGURE 3 In the secondary response, a plasma cell switches from IgM production (**A**) to IgG2 production by deleting a DNA loop containing the constant (C)-region genes $C\mu$, $C\partial$, $C\gamma3$, $C\gamma1$, and $C\mu1$ from the IgM heavy (H)-chain gene (**B**). This DNA is now transcribed into nuclear RNA (**C**). RNA splicing links the $C\gamma2$ gene with the J_1 gene (**D**), and then the mRNA is translated into an IgG2 heavy chain (**E**). *Source*: Modified from David JR. Antibodies: structure and function. Scientific American Medicine. New York: Scientific American Inc., 1980.

coding sequence. Mechanisms involved in subsequent rejoining to form a mature coding segment are not completely understood.

The transcription of Ig genes, like other eukaryotic genes, is regulated by promoters and enhancers. Promoters, located 5′ of the V segment, are necessary for transcription initiation. Enhancers, located in the introns between J and C segments, increase the rate of transcription. For this reason, Ig synthesis (H or L chains) is only detected after the VDJ or VJ rearrangements, which bring the promoter in close proximity to the enhancer.

During ontogeny and functional differentiation, the H chain genes may undergo further gene rearrangements that result in Ig class switching. As the B-lymphocytes differentiate into plasma cells, one H chain C gene segment can be substituted for another without alteration of the VDJ combination (Fig. 3). In other words, a given V region gene can be expressed in association with more than one H chain class or subclass, so that at the cellular level the same antibody specificity can be associated with the synthesis of an IgM Ig (characteristic of the early stages of ontogeny and of the primary response) or with an IgG Ig (characteristic of the mature individual and of the secondary response). Ig class switching is the result of an intrachromosomal recombination between the switch region of $C\mu$ and one of the downstream switch regions. This recombination event leads to looping out deletion of the intervening DNA segment and joins the rearranged V region to a different C region ($C\gamma$, $C\epsilon$, and $C\alpha$).

GENETIC BASIS OF ANTIBODY DIVERSITY

It has been estimated that an individual is capable of producing up to 10^9 different antibody molecules. How this vast diversity is generated from a limited number of germ line elements has long been one of the most intriguing problems in immunology. There are two possible mechanisms for this variability: either the information is transmitted from generation to generation in the germ line, or it is generated somatically during B-lymphocyte differentiation. The following genetic mechanisms have been shown to contribute to the generation of antibody diversity.

V Gene Number

The existence of a large number of V genes and of a smaller set of D and J segments in the germ line DNA, which has probably been generated during evolution as a consequence of environmental pressure. The human VH locus comprises approximately 100 V, 30 D, and 6 J segments.

Combinatorial Association

As mentioned previously, there are at least 100 V region genes for the H chain, and probably this is a conservative estimate. The total number of possible V genes is increased by the fact that any V segment can combine, in principle, with any J and D segments. Imprecise joining of various V gene segments, creating sequence variation at the points of recombination, augments diversity significantly. In the case of the L chain, the number of V region genes is estimated as 300, and they can also recombine with different J region genes. Finally, random association of L and H chains plays an important role in increasing diversity. For example, random association of 1000 H chains and 1000 L chains would produce 10^6 unique antibodies.

Somatic Mutations

Somatic mutations were proposed to be a source of antibody diversity in the 1950s. Experimental support for this hypothesis, however, was only obtained three decades later. Comparison of nucleotide sequences from murine embryonic DNA and DNA obtained from plasmocytomas revealed several base changes, suggesting occurrence of mutations during lymphocyte differentiation. There appear to be some special mutational mechanisms involved in Ig genes since the mutation sites are clustered around the V genes and not around the C genes. In addition to these point mutations, certain enzymes can randomly insert and/or delete DNA bases. Such changes can shift the reading frame for translation (frameshift mutations) so that all codons distal to the mutation are read out of phase and may result in different amino acids, thus adding to the antibody diversity. A large-scale sequencing of H and L chain genes found a much higher proportion of somatically introduced insertions and deletions than previously recognized. These insertions and deletions were clustered around the antigen-binding site, thus constituting a major mechanism of antibody diversity.

Somatic mutations (sometimes termed hypermutations) play a very important role in affinity maturation—production of antibodies with better antigen binding ability. During the initial exposure to an antigen, rearranged antibodies with appropriate specificity bind to the antigen. Late in the response, random somatic mutations in the rearranged V genes result in the production of antibodies of varying affinities. By a process analogous to natural selection, B cells expressing higher-affinity antibodies are selected to proliferate and those with the lower-affinity antibodies are eliminated.

Additionally, gene conversion, a nonreciprocal exchange of genetic information between genes, has also been shown to contribute to the antibody diversity. It is interesting to note that one of the two recombination activating genes described earlier, RAG-2, in addition to its synergistic role with RAG-1, in activating VDJ recombination, appears to be involved in gene conversion events.

Recent discovery of an enzyme—activation-induced cytidine deaminase (AID)—has revolutionized research aimed at delineating the molecular mechanisms underlying various processes that amplify genomic information. AID appears to be an essential catalyst for somatic hypermutation, class switch recombination, and gene conversion, and thus a unifier at the molecular level of three apparently disparate mechanisms of antibody diversity. Its mode of action is under active investigation.

ANTIGENIC DETERMINANTS OF IMMUNOGLOBULIN MOLECULES

Three main categories of antigenic determinants are found on Ig molecules.

Isotypes

These determinants are present on all molecules of each class and subclass of Ig H chains and on each type of L chains; they are defined serologically by antisera directed against the C regions of H and L chains. The antisera are produced in animals, which upon injection of purified human Igs recognize the structural differences between C regions of H and L chains. Isotypic determinants are common to all members of a given species; hence, they cannot be used as genetic markers. Their practical importance results from the fact that they allow the identification of classes and subclasses of Igs through the H chain isotypes and types of L chains (κ, λ). All classes and subclasses of normal Igs share the two L chain isotypes.

Idiotypes

The antigen-combining site in the V region of the Ig molecule, in addition to determining specificity for antigen binding, can also act as an antigen and induce production of antibodies against it. Such antigenic determinants, usually associated with hypervariable regions, are known as idiotypes.

Allotypes

These are hereditary antigenic determinants of Ig polypeptide chains that may differ between individuals of the same species. The loci controlling allotypic determinants are codominant (i.e., both are expressed phenotypically in a heterozygote) autosomal genes, which follow Mendelian laws of heredity. All allotypic markers that have so far been identified on human Ig molecules, with one exception (see later), are present in the C regions of H chains of IgG, IgA, IgE, and on κ-type L chains. Since different individuals of the same species may have different allotypes, these determinants can be used as genetic markers.

The most common technique used for allotype determination is hemagglutination-inhibition. For this purpose, O^+ red cells are coated with IgG immunoglobulins of known allotypes. The coated cells will agglutinate when exposed to specific antibody. The agglutination, however, will be inhibited if the antiserum recognizing the allotype of the Ig coating the red cell is preincubated with soluble IgG carrying the same allotype. Thus, in a first step, the antiallotypic antiserum and an unknown serum to be typed are mixed. In a second step, red cells coated with the relevant allotype are added to dilutions of the mixture. If agglutination is inhibited, it can be concluded that the allotype was present in the unknown serum.

IgG Heavy Chain Allotypes (GM Allotypes)

Allotypes have been found on $\gamma 1$, $\gamma 2$, and $\gamma 3$ H chains, but not as yet on $\gamma 4$ chains. They are denoted as G1M, G2M, and G3M, respectively (G for IgG, the numerals 1, 2, and 3 identify the subclass, the letter M for marker). At present, 18 GM specificities can be defined (Table 1): four associated with IgG1 (G1M), one associated with IgG2 (G2M), and 13 associated with IgG3 (G3M). G1M 3 and G1M 17 are localized in the Fd portion of the IgG molecule while the rest are in the Fc portion. The amino acid/nucleotide substitutions responsible for some allotypes are known. For instance, G1M 3 H chains have arginine at position 214 and G1M 17 H chains have lysine at this position. A single H chain may possess more than one GM determinant; G1M 17 and G1M 1 are frequently present on the Fd and Fc portions of the same H chain in Caucasians.

The four C-region genes on human chromosome 14 that encode the four IgG subclasses are very closely linked. Because of this close linkage, GM allotypes of various subclasses are transmitted as a group called haplotype. Also, because of almost absolute linkage disequilibrium between the alleles of various IgG C-region genes, certain allotypes of one subclass are always associated with certain others of another subclass. For example, the IgG1 gene controls G1M 3, whereas the IgG3 gene controls G3M 5 and G3M 21. We should expect to find G1M 3 associated with G3M 5 as often as with G3M 21; in fact, in Caucasians, a haplotype carrying G1M 3 is almost always associated with G3M 5 and not with G3M 21. Every major ethnic group has a distinct array of GM haplotypes. GM* 3 23 5,10,11,13,14,26 and GM* 1,17 5,10,11,13,14,17,26 are examples of common Caucasian and Negroid

TABLE 1 Currently Testable GM Allotypes

Heavy chain subclass	Numeric	Alphameric
$\gamma 1$	G1M 1	a
	2	x
	3	f
	17	z
$\gamma 2$	G2M 23	n
$\gamma 3$	G3M 5	b1
	6	c3
	10	b5
	11	b0
	13	b3
	14	b4
	15	s
	16	t
	21	gl
	24	c5
	26	u
	27	v
	28	g5

haplotypes, respectively. In accordance with the international system for human gene nomenclature, haplotypes and phenotypes are written by grouping together the markers that belong to each subclass by the numerical order of the marker and of the subclass; markers belonging to different subclasses are separated by a space, while allotypes within a subclass are separated by commas. An asterisk is used to distinguish alleles and haplotypes from phenotypes.

IgA Heavy Chain Allotypes (AM Allotypes)

Two allotypes have been defined on human IgA2 molecules: A2M 1 and A2M 2. They behave as alleles of one another. No allotypes have been found on IgA1 molecules as yet. Individuals lacking IgA (or a particular IgA allotype) have in some instances been found to possess anti-IgA antibodies directed either against one of the allotypic markers or against the isotypic determinant. In some patients, these antibodies can cause severe anaphylactic reactions, following blood transfusion containing incompatible IgA.

IgE Heavy Chain Allotypes (EM Allotypes)

Only one allotype, designated as EM 1, has been described for the IgE molecule. Because of a very low concentration of IgE in the serum, EM 1 cannot be measured by hemagglutination-inhibition, the method most commonly used for typing all other allotypes. This marker is measured by radioimmunoassay using a monoclonal anti-EM 1 antibody.

κ-Type Light Chain Allotypes (KM Allotypes)

Three KM allotypes have been described so far: KM 1, KM 2, and KM 3. (About 98% of the subjects positive for KM 1 are also positive for KM 2.) They are inherited via three alleles, KM* 1, KM* 1,2, and KM* 3 on human chromosome 2. No allotypes have as yet been found on the λ-type L chains.

Heavy Chain V-Region Allotype (HV 1)

So far, HV 1 is the only allotypic determinant described in the V region of human Igs. It is located in the V region of H chains of IgG, IgM, IgA, and possibly also on IgD and IgE.

DNA POLYMORPHISMS: RESTRICTION FRAGMENT LENGTH POLYMORPHISMS

Several new genetic polymorphisms, detected directly at the DNA level, have been described in the Ig region. These are known as restriction fragment length polymorphisms (RFLPs), because they result from variation in DNA base sequences that modify cleavage sites for restriction enzymes. RFLPs have been described in both V and C regions. Their significance is under active investigation.

As mentioned previously, the most widely used method for determining Ig allotypes is hemagglutination-inhibition, using antisera derived from fortuitously immunized human donors. Because of the scarcity of such antisera, investigations to examine the role of allotypes in immune responsiveness and disease susceptibility have been hampered. Recently, molecular methods that allow the detection of allotypes at the genomic level have been developed, thus circumventing the problems arising from the paucity of antisera.

ALLELIC EXCLUSION

One of the most fascinating observations in immunology is that Ig H chain genes from only one of the two homologous chromosomes 14 (one paternal and one maternal) are expressed in a given B lymphocyte. Recombination of VDJC genes described earlier usually takes place on one of the homologues. Only if this rearrangement is unproductive (i.e., it does not result in the secretion of an antibody molecule), the other homologue undergoes rearrangement. Consequently, of the two H chain alleles in a B cell, one is productively rearranged and the other is either in the germ line pattern or is aberrantly rearranged (in other words, excluded). Involvement of the chromosomes is random; in one B cell, the paternal allele may be active, and in another, it may be a maternal allele. (Allelic exclusion is reminiscent of the X-chromosome inactivation in mammals, although it is genetically more complex.)

Two models have been proposed to explain allelic exclusion: stochastic and regulated. The main impetus for proposing the stochastic model was the finding that a high proportion of VDJ or VJ rearrangements are nonproductive, that is, they do not result in transcription of mRNA. Therefore, according to this model, allelic exclusion is achieved because of a very low likelihood of a productive rearrangement on both chromosomes. According to the regulated model, a productive H or L chain gene arrangement signals the cessation of further gene rearrangements (feedback inhibition).

Results from experiments with transgenic mice (mice in which foreign genes have been introduced in the germ line) favor the regulated model. It appears that a correctly rearranged H chain gene not only inhibits further H chain gene rearrangements but also gives a positive signal for the κ chain gene rearrangement. The rearrangement of the λ gene takes place only if both alleles of the κ gene are aberrantly rearranged. (Although in some cases, it appears that the λ gene rearrangement is autonomous, that is, it does not depend on the prior deletion and/or nonproductive rearrangement of both κ alleles.) This mutually exclusive nature of a productive L gene rearrangement results in isotypic exclusion, that is, a given plasma cell contains either κ or λ chains, but not both.

Allelic exclusion is evident at the level of the GM system. A given plasma cell from an individual heterozygous for G1M* 17/G1M* 3 will secrete IgG carrying either G1M 17 or G1M 3, but not both. Since the exclusion is random, serum samples from such an individual will have both G1M 17 and G1M 3 secreted by different Ig-producing cells.

The process of allelic exclusion results in the synthesis of Ig molecules with identical V and C regions in each single plasma cell, because all expressed mRNA will have been derived from a single rearranged chromosome 14 and from a single rearranged chromosome 2 or 22. Therefore, the antibodies produced by each B lymphocyte will be of a single specificity.

GM ALLOTYPES AND IgG SUBCLASS CONCENTRATIONS

Studies from several laboratories have found a correlation between certain GM allotypes or phenotypes and the concentration of the four subclasses of IgG. The results vary; however, virtually all studies report a significant association between the GM 3 5,13 phenotype and a high IgG3 concentration and the G2M 23 allotype and an increased concentration of IgG2. These associations imply that a determination of whether a person's IgG subclass level is in the "normal" range should be made in the context of the individual's GM phenotype.

IMMUNOGLOBULIN ALLOTYPES, IMMUNE RESPONSE, AND DISEASES

Numerous studies have shown that immune responsiveness to certain antigens and susceptibility/resistance to particular diseases are influenced by GM and KM allotypes. How can C-region allotypes influence immune responsiveness thought to be exclusively associated with the V-region genes? The most likely mechanism involves the possible influence of C-region allotypes on antibody affinity. Contrary to the previously held views that the C domains do not play any role in antibody binding affinity, the contribution of CH2 and CH3 domains—where the majority of the GM markers are located—on IgG binding strength is now firmly established. The CH1 domain—where allelic determinants G1M 3 and 17 are located—has also been shown to modulate the kinetic competence of antigen binding sites. A very recent study has conclusively shown that changes in the C region cause changes in the specificity of V-region identical binding sites. Amino acid substitutions associated with various GM/KM allotypic determinants cause structural changes in the C region, and it follows that they could affect the V-region protein conformation, resulting in changes in antibody specificity.

Occasionally, particular alleles of the human leukocyte antigens (HLA), GM, and KM and other genes of the immune system interact to influence immune responsiveness and disease susceptibility. The mechanisms underlying the interaction of these unlinked genetic systems are not understood.

The biological role and reasons for the extensive polymorphism of Ig allotypes remain unknown. The marked differences in the frequencies of Ig allotypes among races, strong linkage disequilibrium within a race, and racially restricted occurrence of GM haplotypes, all suggest that differential selection over many generations may have played an important role in the maintenance of polymorphism at these loci. One mechanism could be the possible association of these markers with immunity to certain lethal infectious pathogens implicated in major epidemics, and different races may have been subjected to different epidemics throughout our evolutionary history. As first suggested by JBS Haldane, high mortality infectious diseases have probably been the principal selective forces of natural selection in humans. After a major epidemic, only individuals with genetic combinations conferring immunity to the pathogen would survive. In this context, it is interesting to note that GM genes have been shown to influence the chance for survival in certain typhoid and yellow fever epidemics, and there is growing evidence of their involvement in immunity to malaria.

BIBLIOGRAPHY

Corcoran AE. Immunoglobulin locus silencing and allelic exclusion. Semin Immunol 2005; 17:141.

Dard P, Lefranc MP, Osipova L, Sanchez–Mazas A. DNA sequence variability of IGHG3 alleles associated to the main G3m haplotypes in human populations. Eur J Hum Genet 2001; 9:765.

Honjo T, Muramatsu M, Fagarasan S. AID: how does it aid antibody diversity? Immunity 2004; 20:659.

Lederberg J. JBS Haldane (1949) on infectious disease and evolution. Genetics 1999; 153:1.

Martomo SA, Gearhart PJ. Somatic hypermutation: subverted DNA repair. Curr Opin Immunol 2006; 18:243.

Muratori P, Sutherland SE, Muratori L, et al. Immunoglobulin GM and KM allotypes and prevalence of anti-LKM1 autoantibodies in patients with hepatitis C virus infection. J Virol 2006; 80:5097.

Pandey JP. Immunoglobulin GM genes and IgG antibodies to cytomegalovirus in patients with systemic sclerosis. Clin Exp Rheumatol 2004; 22:S35.

Pandey JP, Astemborski J, Thomas DL. Epistatic effects of immunoglobulin GM and KM allotypes on outcome of infection with hepatitis C virus. J Virol 2004; 78:4561.

Pandey JP, Prohászka Z, Veres A, Füst G, Hurme M. Epistatic effects of genes encoding immunoglobulin GM allotypes and interleukin-6 on the production of autoantibodies to 60- and 65-kDa heat-shock proteins. Genes Immun 2004; 5:68.

Pandey JP. Genetic polymorphism of Fc. Science 2006; 311:1376.

Pertovaara M, Hurme M, Antonen J, Pasternack A, Pandey JP. Immunoglobulin KM and GM gene polymorphisms modify the clinical presentation of primary Sjögren's syndrome. J Rheumatol 2004; 31:2175.

Selsing E. Ig class switching: targeting the recombinational mechanism. Curr Opin Immunol 2006; 18:249.

Sen R, Oltz E. Genetic and epigenetic regulation of IgH gene assembly. Curr Opin Immunol 2006; 18:237.

Torres M, May R, Scharff MD, Casadevall A. Variable-region-identical antibodies differing in isotype demonstrate differences in fine specificity and idiotype. J Immunol 2005; 174:2132.

8 | Antigen–Antibody Reactions

Gabriel Virella
Department of Microbiology and Immunology, Medical University of South Carolina, Charleston, South Carolina, U.S.A.

GENERAL CHARACTERISTICS OF THE ANTIGEN–ANTIBODY REACTION

The reaction between antigens (Ags) and antibodies (Abs) involves complementary binding sites on the Ab and on the Ag molecules. The sites on the Ag molecule that combine with the binding site of an Ab are known as epitopes. The same way that the binding site is determined by different segments on the variable regions of heavy and light chains that come in close proximity due to the folding of those regions, the epitopes are also formed by discontinuous segments of an Ag molecule. Crystallographic studies have defined protein epitopes as large areas, usually involving 15 to 22 aminoacids located on several surface loops. Some subsets of aminoacids within the epitope are likely to contribute most of the binding energy with the Ab, whereas the surrounding residues provide structural complementary that may play a stabilizing role when Ags and Abs interact. The significance of critical aminoacids in an epitope is illustrated by the fact that Abs can distinguish immunoglobulin allotypes structurally determined by one or two aminoacid substitutions in the constant regions of heavy or light chains (see Chapter 7).

Chemical Bonds Responsible for the Antigen–Antibody Reaction

The interaction between the Ab-binding site and the epitope involves exclusively noncovalent bonds, in a similar manner to that in which proteins bind to their cellular receptors, or enzymes bind to their substrates. The binding is reversible and can be prevented or dissociated by high ionic strength or extreme pH. The following intermolecular forces are involved in Ag–Ab binding:

1. *Electrostatic bonds*. This result from the attraction between oppositely charged ionic groups of two protein side chains; for example, an ionized amino group (NH^{4+}) on a lysine in the Ab, and an ionized carboxyl group (COO^-) on an aspartate residue in the Ag.
2. *Hydrogen bonding*. When the Ag and Ab are in very close proximity, relatively weak hydrogen bonds can be formed between hydrophilic groups (e.g., OH and C=O, NH and C=O, and NH and OH groups).
3. *Hydrophobic interactions*. Hydrophobic groups, such as the side chains of valine, leucine, and phenylalanine, tend to associate due to Van der Waals bonding and coalesce in an aqueous environment, excluding water molecules from their surroundings. As a consequence, the distance between them decreases, enhancing the energies of attraction involved. This type of interaction is estimated to contribute up to 50% of the total strength of the Ag–Ab bond.
4. *van der Waals bonds*. These forces depend upon interactions between the "electron clouds" that surround the Ag and Ab molecules. The interaction has been compared to that which might exist between alternating dipoles in two molecules, alternating in such a way that, at any given moment, oppositely oriented dipoles will be present in closely apposed areas of the Ag and Ab molecules.

All these types of interactions depend on the close proximity of the Ag and Ab molecules. For that reason, the "good fit" between an antigenic determinant and an Ab–combining site determines the stability of the Ag–Ab reaction.

Antibody Specificity

Most of the data concerning this topic was generated in studies of the immune response to closely related haptens. Using a conjugate of *m*-aminobenzene sulfonate (haptenic group) with an immunogenic carrier protein, it was noticed that an animal inoculated with this conjugate would produce Ab that specifically recognized *m*-aminobenzene sulfonate. When the Ab to *m*-aminobenzene sulfonate was tested for its ability to bind to the ortho-, meta-, and para-isomers of aminobenzene sulfonate and to related molecules in which the sulfonate group was substituted by arsonate or carboxylate, it was noted (Table 1) that best reactivity occurred with the hapten used for immunization (m-aminobenzene sulfonate). Of the related haptens, *o*-aminobenzene sulfonate reacted reasonably, whereas *m*-aminobenzene arsonate and *m*-amino-benzene carboxylate reacted very poorly or not at all.

These and other experiments of the same type led to the conclusion that specificity is mainly determined by the overall degree of complementarity between antigenic-determinant and Ab-binding site (Fig. 1). Differences in the degree of complementarity determine the "affinity" of the Ag–Ab reaction.

Antibody Affinity and Avidity

Antibody affinity can be defined as the attractive force between the complementary configurations of the antigenic determinant and the Ab-combining site. Experimentally, the reaction is best studied with antibodies directed against monovalent haptens. The reaction, as we know, is reversible and can be defined by the following equation:

$$\text{Ab} + \text{Hp} \underset{k_2}{\overset{k_1}{\rightleftharpoons}} \text{Ab·Hp} \tag{1}$$

where k_1 is the association constant and k_2 the dissociation constant.

In simple terms, the k_1/k_2 ratio is the intrinsic association constant or equilibrium constant (K). This equilibrium constant represents the intrinsic affinity of the Ab-binding sites for the hapten. High values for K will reflect a predominance of k_1 over k_2 or, in other words, a tendency for the Ag–Ab complex to be stable and not to dissociate. The equilibrium constant (K) can be defined by the equation below:

$$k_1[\text{Ab}][\text{Hp}] = k_2[\text{AbHp}] \tag{2}$$

This can be converted into:

$$K = \frac{k_1}{k_2} = \frac{[\text{Ab} \cdot \text{Hp}]}{[\text{Ab}][\text{Hp}]} \tag{3}$$

where [Ab] corresponds to the concentration of free Ab-binding sites, [Hp] to the concentration of free hapten, and [Ab·Hp] to the concentration of saturated Ab-binding sites.

K, also designated as affinity constant, is usually determined by equilibrium dialysis experiments, in which Ab is enclosed in a semipermeable membrane and dialyzed against a solution containing known amounts of free hapten. Free hapten diffuses across the membrane into the dialysis bag, where it binds to the Abs. Part of the hapten inside the bag will be free, part will be bound, and the ratio of free and bound haptens depends on the Ab affinity. When

TABLE 1 Antigens Tested with Immune Serum for Meta-Aminobenzene Sulfonic Acid (Metanilic Acid)

	Antigens		
	Ortho	Meta	Para
Aminobenzene sulfonic acid	++	+++	+
Aminobenzene arsenic acid	0	+	0
Aminobenzoic acid	0	±	0

Source: Reproduced from Landsteiner K. The Specificity of Serological Reactions. New York: Dover, 1962.

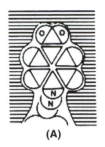

(A)

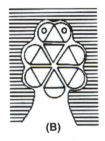

(B)

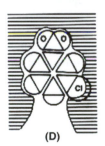

(D)

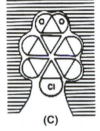

(C)

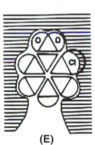

(E)

FIGURE 1 Diagrammatic representation of the "closeness of fit" between antigenic determinants and antibody-binding sites. Antibodies were raised against the *p*-azobenzoate group of a protein-*p*-benzoate conjugate. The resulting anti-*p*-benzoate groups react well with the original protein-*p*-benzoate conjugate (**A**) and with *p*-benzoate itself (**B**). If a chlorine atom (Cl) is substituted for a hydrogen atom at the *p* position, the substituted hapten will react strongly with the original antibody (**C**). However, if chlorine atoms are substituted for hydrogen atoms at the *o* or *m* positions (**D,E**), the reaction with the antibody is disturbed, since the chlorine atoms at those positions cause a significant change in the configuration of the benzoate group. *Source*: Adapted from Van Oss CJ. Principles of Immunology. 2nd Ed. Rose M, Milgram F, Van Oss C, eds. New York: Macmillan, 1979.

equilibrium is reached, the amounts of free hapten will be identical inside and outside the bag. The difference between the amounts of hapten inside the bag minus the concentration of free hapten outside the bag is equal to the amount of bound hapten. If the molar concentration of Ab in the system is known, it becomes possible to determine the values of *r* (number of hapten molecules bound per Ab molecule) and *c* (concentration of free hapten).

Taking Equation (3) as a starting point, if [Ab·Hp] is divided by the total concentration of Ab, the quotient equals the number of hapten molecules bound per Ab molecule [*r*], and the quotient between the number of vacant Ab sites [Ab] divided by the total concentration of Ab equals the difference between the maximum number of Ab molecules that can be bound by Ab molecule [*n* or valency] and the number of hapten molecules bound per Ab molecule [*r*] at a given hapten concentration [*c*]. Equation (3) can be rewritten as:

$$K = \frac{k_1}{k_2} = [Ab·Hp][Ab][Hp] \tag{4}$$

Equation (4), in turn, can be rewritten as the Scatchard equation:

$$\frac{r}{c} = Kn - Kr \tag{5}$$

By determining *r* and *c* concentrations in a series of equilibrium dialysis experiments carried out at different total hapten concentrations, it becomes possible, using Equation 5, to construct what is known as a Scatchard plot, in which *r/c* is plotted versus *r* (Fig. 2). It is also possible to determine the slope of the plot of *r/c* versus *r* values that corresponds to $-K$. The correlation between the slope and the affinity constant is also illustrated in

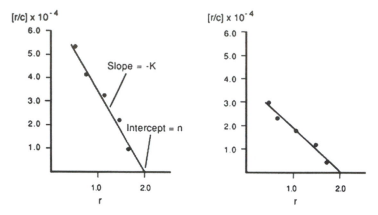

FIGURE 2   Schematic representation of the Scatchard plots correlating the quotient between moles of hapten bound per moles of antibody (*r*) and the concentration of free hapten (*c*), with the concentration of hapten bound per mole of antibody (*r*). The slopes of the plots correspond to the affinity constants, and the intercept with the horizontal axis corresponds to the number of hapten molecules bound per mole of antibody at a theoretically infinite hapten concentration (*n* or valency of the antibody molecule). The plot on the left panel corresponds to a high-affinity antibody, and the slope is very steep; the plot on the right panel corresponds to a low-affinity antibody, and its slope is considerably less steep.

Figure 2. With high-affinity Abs, *r* will reach saturation (*r = n*) at relatively low concentrations of hapten, and the plot will have a steep slope, as shown in the left. With low-affinity Abs, the stable occupancy of the Ab binding sites will require higher concentrations of free hapten, so the r/c quotients will be considerably lower and the slope considerably less steep, as shown on the right. Since the reactants (Abs and haptens) are expressed as moles per liter, the affinity constant is expressed as liters per mole (L/mol).

From the Scatchard plot, it is obvious that at extremely high concentrations of unbound hapten (*c*), *r/c* becomes close to 0, and the plot of *r/c* versus *r* will intercept *r* on the horizontal axis (the interception corresponds to *n*, the Ab *valency*). For an IgG Ab and all other monomeric Abs, the value of *n* is 2; for IgM Abs, the theoretical valency is 10, but the functional valency is usually 5, suggesting that steric hindrance effects prevent simultaneous occupation of the binding sites of each subunit.

In most experimental conditions, an antiserum raised against one given hapten is composed of a restricted number of Ab populations with slightly different affinity constants. Under those conditions, it may be of practical value to calculate an average intrinsic association constant or average affinity (K_0), which is defined as the free hapten concentration required to occupy half of the available Ab binding sites (*r = n/2*). Substitution of *r = n/2* for *r* in Equation (4) leads to the formula $K_0 = 1/c$. In other words, the average affinity constant equals the reciprocal of the free Ag concentration when Ags occupy half of the Ab-binding sites.

High-affinity Abs have K_0 values as high as 10^{10} L/mol. High-affinity binding is believed to result from a very close fit between the Ag-binding sites and the corresponding antigenic determinants that favor the establishment of strong noncovalent interactions between Ag and Ab.

In humans, it has been noted that autoantibodies are usually of low affinity, whereas induced Abs are of high affinity. For example, the affinity of induced antikeyhole limpet hemocyanine (a very strongly immunogenic protein isolated from mollusks -keyhole limpets) IgG antibodies was measured as 7.6 mol/L × E^{-10}, whereas the average affinity of 30 isolated autoantibodies formed spontaneously against oxidized low density lipoprotein (LDL) was 1.02 ± 1.1 mol/L × E^{-8}

Ab avidity can be defined as the strength of the binding of the several different Abs that are produced in response to an immunogen, which presents several different epitopes to the immune system. The strength of the Ag·Ab reaction is enhanced when several different antibodies bind simultaneously to different epitopes on the Ag molecule, cross-linking Ag molecules very tightly. Thus, a more stable bonding between Ag and Ab will be established, due

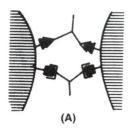 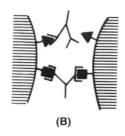

(A)   (B)

FIGURE 3 Diagrammatic representation of the avidity concept. The binding of antigen molecules by several antibodies of different specificities (**A**) stabilizes the immune complex, since it is highly unlikely that all Ag·Ab reactions dissociate simultaneously at any given point in time (**B**). *Source*: Adapted from Roitt I. Essential Immunology. 4th Ed. Oxford: Blackwell, 1980.

to the "bonus-effect" of multiple Ag–Ab bonds (Fig. 3); the increased stability of the overall Ag–Ab reaction corresponds to an increased avidity.

Cross-Reactions

When an animal is immunized with an immunogen, its serum will contain several different Abs directed to the various epitopes presented by the immunizing molecule, reflecting the polyclonal nature of the response. Such serum from an immune animal is known as an anti-serum, directed against the immunogen.

Antisera containing polyclonal Abs can often be found to cross-react with immunogens partially related to that used for immunization, due to the existence of common epitopes or of epitopes with similar configurations. Less frequently, a cross-reaction may be totally unexpected, involving totally unrelated Ags that happen to present epitopes whose whole spatial configuration may be similar enough to allow the cross-reaction.

The avidity of a cross-reaction depends on the degree of structural similarity between the shared epitopes; when the avidity reaches a very low point, the cross-reaction will no longer be detectable (Fig. 4). The differential avidity of given antiserum for the original immunogen and for other immunogens sharing epitopes of similar structure is responsible for the "specificity" of the antiserum; that is, its ability to recognize only one single immunogen or, a few, very closely related immunogens.

SPECIFIC TYPES OF ANTIGEN–ANTIBODY REACTIONS

Ag–Ab reactions may be revealed by a variety of physical expressions, depending on the nature of the Ag and on the conditions surrounding the reaction.

Precipitation

When Ag and Ab are mixed in a test tube in their soluble forms, one of the two things may happen: both components will remain soluble or variable amounts of Ag·Ab precipitate will

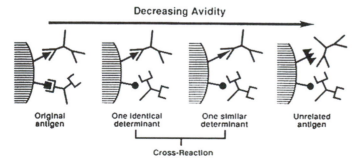

Decreasing Avidity

| Original antigen | One identical determinant | One similar determinant | Unrelated antigen |

Cross-Reaction

FIGURE 4 Diagrammatic representation of the concept of cross-reaction between complex antigens. An antiserum containing several antibody populations to the determinants of a given antigen will react with other antigens sharing common or closely related determinants. The avidity of the reaction will decrease with decreasing structural closeness, until it will no longer be detectable. The reactivity of the same antiserum with several related antigens is designated as cross-reaction. *Source*: Adapted from Roitt I. Essential Immunology. 4th Ed. Oxford: Blackwell, 1980.

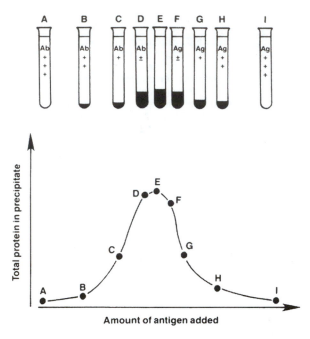

FIGURE 5 The precipitin curve. When increasing amounts of antigen are added to a fixed concentration of antibody, increasing amounts of precipitate appear as a consequence of the antigen–antibody interaction. After a maximum precipitation is reached, the amounts of precipitate begin to decrease. Analysis of the supernatants reveals that at low antigen concentrations, there is free antibody left in solution (antibody excess), and at the point of maximal precipitation, neither antigen nor antibody are detected in the supernatant (equivalence zone); with greater antigen concentrations, antigen becomes detectable in the supernatant (antigen excess).

be formed. If progressively increasing amounts of Ag are mixed with a fixed amount of Ag, a precipitin curve can be constructed (Fig. 5). There are three areas to consider in a precipitin curve:

1. Ab excess—Free Ab remains in solution after centrifugation of Ag·Ab complexes.
2. Equivalence—No free Ag or Ab remains in solution. The amount of precipitated Ag·Ab complexes reaches its peak at this point.
3. Ag excess—Free Ag is detected in the supernatant after centrifugation of Ag·Ab complexes.

    The "lattice theory" was created to explain why different amounts of precipitation are observed at different Ag–Ab ratios. At great Ab excess, each Ag will tend to have its binding sites saturated, with Ab molecules bound to all its exposed determinants. Extensive cross-linking of Ag and Ab is not possible. On the other hand, if one can determine the number of Ab molecules bound to one single Ag molecule, a rough indication of the valency (i.e., number of epitopes) of the Ag will be obtained. At great Ag excess, single Ag molecules will saturate the binding sites of the Ab molecule and not much cross-linking will take place either. If the Ag is very small and has no repeating epitopes, calculation of the number of Ag molecules bound by each Ab molecule will indicate the Ab valency, as discussed earlier in this chapter. When the concentrations of Ag and Ab reach the equivalence point, maximum cross-linking between Ag and Ab will take place, resulting in formation of a large precipitate that contains all Ag and Ab present in the mixture (Fig. 6).

Precipitation in Agar

Semisolid supports, such as agar gel, in which a carbohydrate matrix functions as a container for buffer that fills the interstitial spaces left by the matrix, have been widely used for the study of Ag–Ab reactions. Ag and Ab are placed in wells carved in the semisolid agar and allowed to passively diffuse. The diffusion of Ag and Ab is unrestricted, and in the area that separates Ag from Ab, the two reactants will mix in a gradient of concentrations. When the optimal pro-portions for Ag·Ab binding are reached, a precipitate will be formed, appearing as a sharp, linear opacity (Fig. 7).

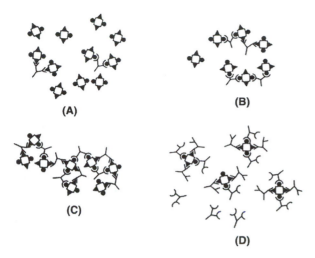

FIGURE 6 The lattice theory explaining precipitation reactions in fluid media: At great antigen excess (**A**), each antibody molecule has all its binding sites occupied. There is free antigen in solution, and the antigen-antibody complexes are very small ($Ag_2 \cdot Ab_1$, $Ag_1 \cdot Ab_1$). The number of epitopes bound per antibody molecule at great antigen excess corresponds to the antibody valency. With increasing amounts of antibody (**B**), larger Ag·Ab complexes are formed ($Ag_3 \cdot Ab_2$, etc.), but there is still incomplete precipitation and free antigen in solution. At equivalence, large Ag·Ab complexes are formed, in which virtually all Ab and Ag molecules in the system are cross-linked (**C**). Precipitation is maximal, and no free antigen or antibody is left in the supernatant. With increasing amounts of antibody (**D**), all antigen-binding sites are saturated, but there is free antibody left without binding sites available for it to react. The Ag·Ab complexes are larger than at antigen excess [$Ag_1 \cdot Ab_{4,5,6 \, (n)}$] but usually remain soluble. The number of antibody molecules bound per antigen molecule at greater antibody excess allows an estimate of the antigen valency.

Agglutination

When bacteria, cells, or large particles in suspension are mixed with antibodies directed to their surface determinants, one will observe the formation of large clumps; this is known as an agglutination reaction.

Agglutination reactions result from the cross-linking of cells and insoluble particles by specific antibodies. Due to the relatively short distance between the two Fab fragments, 7S Abs (such as IgG) are usually unable to bridge the gap between two cells—each of them surrounded by an electronic "cloud" of identical charge that will tend to keep them apart. IgM Abs, on the other hand, are considerably more efficient in inducing cellular agglutination (Fig. 8).

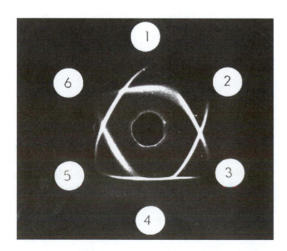

FIGURE 7 Antigen–antibody reactions in agarose gel are often performed in the configuration of a double immunodiffusion test as shown in this photograph. A polyvalent antibody was placed in the middle well, whereas six different antigens were placed in the peripheral wells (1–6). The opaque precipitin lines were visible after overnight incubation, and the complex pattern of interactions between the different lines generated in contiguous wells reflects the degree of structural relationship between the different antigens. For example, the precipitin lines for samples 2 and 3 cross each other completely, indicating lack of identity, whereas the precipitin lines of samples 1 and 2 fuse completely, indicating complete identity.

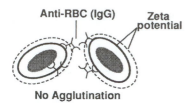

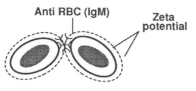

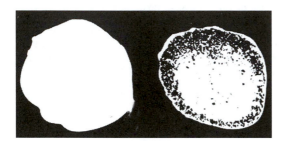

FIGURE 8 IgM antibodies are more efficient in inducing red cell agglutination. Red cells remain at the same distance from each other due to their identical electrical charge (zeta potential). IgG antibodies are not large enough to bridge the space between two red cells, but IgM antibodies, due to their polymeric nature and size, can induce red blood cell agglutination with considerable ease.

FIGURE 9 Latex agglutination assay for rheumatoid factor. Latex particles coated with human IgG were suspended in saline (*left panel*) or in a dilution of the serum of a patient with rheumatoid arthritis positive for rheumatoid factor (*right panel*). Rheumatoid factor is an autoantibody that reacts with human IgG. The reaction of rheumatoid factor with the IgG coated latex particles results in visible clumping (agglutination), whereas no clumping is seen on the particles suspended in saline.

The visualization of agglutination reactions differs according to the techniques used for their study. In slide tests, the nonagglutinated cell or particulate Ag appears as a homogeneous suspension, whereas the agglutinated Ag will appear irregularly clumped (Fig. 9). If Abs and cells are mixed in a test tube, the cross-linking of cells and antibodies will result in the diffuse deposition of cell clumps in the bottom and walls of the test tube, whereas the nonagglutinated red cells will sediment in a very regular fashion, forming a compact red button on the bottom of the tube. In red cell agglutination assays carried out on microtiter plates, agglutinated red cells sediment fast and cover the whole bottom, whereas nonagglutinated red cells roll and sediment in compact buttons at the very bottom of the well (Fig. 10).

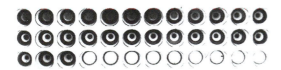

FIGURE 10 Photographic reproduction of a hemagglutination reaction performed in a microtiter plate. In the top row, red blood cells were added to a series of doubling dilutions of a serum sample containing antired cell antibodies. In the second row, red cells were added to an identical series of doubling dilutions of serum obtained from a normal healthy volunteer. The order of dilutions is identical in both rows. On the first well to the left, the sample is diluted 1/20 (1 part serum and 19 parts saline), and on the last well to the right, the sample is diluted 1/81,920 (1 part serum and 81,919 parts saline). The three wells to the left on the third row were filled with red cells added to saline. The purpose of the bottom row wells is to show how red cells sediment as a round button in the absence of antibody. An identical pattern is observed in the red cells mixed with normal serum, indicating that that serum does not contain antibody. On the top row, the sedimentation pattern is different, the bottoms of the wells to the left are diffusely covered by sedimented red cells, and normal sedimentation is only seen on the wells to the extreme right, where the sample has been diluted the most, and the antibody is no longer present in sufficient concentrations to cause visible agglutination.

BIOLOGICAL CONSEQUENCES OF THE ANTIGEN–ANTIBODY REACTION
Opsonization

After binding to particulate Ags or after forming large molecular aggregates, Abs unfold and may interact with Fc receptors on phagocytic cells (see Chapter 6). Such interaction is followed by ingestion by the phagocytic cell (phagocytosis). Substances that promote phagocytosis are known as opsonins.

Fc-Receptor Mediated Cell Activation

The interaction of Ag–Ab complexes containing IgG Abs (especially those of subclasses IgG1 and IgG3) with phagocytic cells through their Fcγ receptors results in the delivery of activating signals to the ingesting cell. The activation is usually associated with enhancement of the phagocyte's microbicidal activity. A less favorable outcome of phagocytic cell activation is an inflammatory reaction, often trigged by spillage of the toxic mediators generated in the activated phagocytic cell. This outcome is more likely when the Ag–Ab complex is immobilized along a basement membrane or a cellular surface (see Chapters 18 and 23).

   Another adverse reaction is the one that results from the engagement of Fc receptor-bound IgE on basophils and mast cells with their corresponding Ag. The result of this reaction is the release of the potent mediators that trigger an allergic reaction (see Chapter 21).

Complement Activation

One of the most important consequences of Ag–Ab interactions is the activation (or "fixation") of the complement system (see Chapter 9).

   The activation sequence induced by Ag–Ab reactions is known as the "classical" pathway. This pathway is initiated by the binding of C1q to the CH2 domain of the Fc region of IgG and equivalent regions of IgM. It must be noted that the complement-binding sequences in IgG and IgM are usually not exposed in free Ab molecules, thus avoiding unnecessary and potentially deleterious activation of the complement system. The Ag–Ab interaction causes configurational changes in the Ab molecule and, therefore, the complement-binding regions become exposed.

   The activation of C1q requires simultaneous interaction with two complement-binding immunoglobulin domains. This means that when IgG Abs are involved, relatively large concentrations are required, so that Ab molecules coat the Ag in very close apposition allowing C1q to be fixed by IgG duplets. On the other hand, IgM molecules, by containing five closely spaced monomeric subunits, can fix complement at much lower concentrations. One IgM molecule bound by two subunits to a given Ag will constitute a complement-binding duplet.

   After binding of C1q, a cascade reaction takes place, resulting in the successive activation of eight additional complement components. Some of the components generated during complement activation are recognized by receptors on phagocytic cells and promote phagocytosis. C3b is the complement fragment with greater opsonizing capacity. Phagocytic cells (see Chapters 9 and 13) take up an Ag coated with opsonizing antibodies and C3b, with maximal efficiency. Others, particularly the terminal complement components, induce cell lysis.

   The activation of the complement system may also have adverse effects, if it results in the destruction of host cells or if it promotes inflammation, which is beneficial with regard to the elimination of infectious organisms, but has always the potential of causing tissue damage and becoming noxious to the host.

Neutralization

The binding of Abs to bacteria, toxins, and viruses has protective effects, because it prevents the interaction of the microbial agents or their products with the receptors that mediate their infectiveness or toxic effects. As a consequence, the infectious agent or the toxin become harmless or, in other words, are neutralized.

BIBLIOGRAPHY

Atassixp M-Z, van Oss CJ, Absolom DR. Molecular Immunology. New York: Marcel Dekker, 1984.

Day ED. Advanced Immunochemistry, 2nd ed. New York: Wiley-Liss, 1990.

Eisen HN. Antibody–antigen reactions. In: Davis BD, Dulbecco R, Eisen HN, Ginsberg HS, eds. Microbiology. Philadelphia: Lippincott, 1990.

Glynn LE, Steward MW, eds. Immunochemistry: An Advanced Textbook. New York: John Wiley & Sons, 1977.

Laver WG, Air GM, Webster RG, Smith-Gill SJ. Epitopes on protein antigens: misconceptions and realities. Cell 1990; 61:663.

van Oss CJ. In: Rose N, Milgram F, van Oss C, eds. Principles of Immunology. 2nd Ed. New York: Macmillan, 1979.

van Oss CJ, van Regenmortel MHV. Immunochemistry. New York: Marcel Dekker, 1994.

Virella G, Lopes-Virella MF. Lipoprotein autoantibodies: measurement and significance. Clin Diagn Lab Immunol 2003; 10:499.

9 | Complement System

Robert J. Boackle
Department of Stomatology and Department of Microbiology and Immunology,
Medical University of South Carolina, Charleston, South Carolina, U.S.A.

INTRODUCTION

As a consequence of antigen-antibody reactions, important changes occur in the physical state of the antibodies. As antigen and antibodies react and form aggregates, the antibody molecules undergo conformational changes. These events are responsible for changes in the spatial orientation and exposure of biologically active domains or segments located on the Fc region of those antibodies. For example, the Fc region of antigen-bound molecules of IgM, IgG3, IgG1, and to a lesser degree IgG2, are able to bind and activate the first component of a series of rapidly acting plasma proteins, known as the complement system.

COMPLEMENT SYSTEM

The complement system includes several components that exist in a nonactive state in the serum. When these complement components are converted to their active form, a sequential, rapid, cascading sequence ensues.

Synthesis and Metabolism of Complement Components

Most of the complement glycoproteins are synthesized predominantly by the liver; but macrophages and many other cell types are also sources of various complement components, especially at sites of infection and/or inflammation. All normal individuals always have complement components in their blood. The synthetic rates for the various complement glycoproteins increase when complement is activated and consumed during an infection. The increased rates appear to be under several regulatory mechanisms, such as the presence of cytokines generated at the site of the infection and the increase of various complement fragments or subcomponents that are released due to complement activation.

Activation of the Complement System

In addition to antigen-antibody complexes, which play a critical role in the activation of the classical complement pathway (see subsequently), several other substances activate the complement system but to lesser degrees. Nonspecific direct activators include proteolytic enzymes, released either from microbes or from host cells (e.g., neutrophils) at the sites of infection, or dying cells at sites of tissue necrosis/damage. In addition, membranes and cell walls of microbial organisms are potential complement activators; they activate the complement system starting at the third complement component (C3) via the alternative pathway, which is to be discussed in the second half of this chapter. A third, mechanism for activating complement is the lectin pathway, which utilizes ficolins and the mannan-binding lectin (MBL) present in human serum. Mannan is a capsular substance present in pathogenic fungi and is one of the several foreign polysaccharide substances to which human MBL binds via Ca^{2+} dependant interactions. Ficolins bind to substances on gram-positive microbes (e.g., peptidoglycans and teichoic acids).

At this point, the following important concepts should be stressed:

1. Complement exists in a stable and nonactivated form.
2. Complement is a biologically potent system. Once it is activated, it may promote local reactions characterized by edema and smooth muscle contraction.
3. Complement is a fast-acting, cascading (amplifying) system, with most effects occurring within a few minutes.
4. Each step in the complement sequence is tightly regulated and controlled to maximize the damage to any foreign substance. Such controls prevent unnecessary consumption of complement components after sufficient complement has deposited on the antigens, and spare the nearby cells of the host from inadvertent complement attack.

Primary Function of the Complement System

The primary function of the complement system is to bind and neutralize any foreign substance that activates it, and then to effectively cause those neutralized complement-coated substances to tightly adhere to phagocytes, thereby enhancing phagocytosis. In this regard, the third complement component (C3) is a major factor due to its position in the classical, alternative, and lectin pathways and because of its relatively high concentration in serum.

CLASSICAL COMPLEMENT PATHWAY
Activation of the Classical Complement Pathway

Immunoglobulins and native complement components are normally found in the serum and in the lymph, but these molecules do not interact with each other until the antibodies interact with their corresponding antigens and undergo the necessary secondary and tertiary conformational changes. These immunoglobulin conformational changes are the basis for specific activation of the very powerful classical complement pathway.

Initiation of the Cascade: C1 Activation
Native, free immunoglobulin does not activate the complement system. A single native IgG molecule cannot bind and activate the first component (C1) in the complement pathway. However, if IgG antibodies form aggregates as a consequence of antigen binding, their Fab arms move about the hinge region in order to bind to the antigenic determinants and therein expose the C_H2_γ region on their Fc, this will result in C1 binding (fixation) and activation.

The IgG subclasses vary with regard to their efficiency in activating C1, which is directly related to the length of the IgG hinge region. A longer hinge region allows movement of the Fab arms further away from the Fc so as to more fully expose the C_H2 region. Thus, IgG3, upon binding the antigen, is by far the most efficient subclass of IgG in activating C1, followed by IgG1 and weakly by IgG2. IgG4 does not effectively activate the classical complement pathway.

For C1 to be activated, it must bind to at least two adjacent IgG antibodies that are bound to antigens. This usually means that the concentration of antibody must be relatively high, and that the specific antigenic determinants recognized by the IgG antibodies must be properly exposed and in close proximity so that for any one IgG antibody molecule each of its Fab regions is able to bind simultaneously to identical antigenic determinants. When sufficient numbers of antigens are in close proximity on a bacterial or viral surface, C1 is very effectively activated, especially when IgG3 or IgG1 antibodies are combined with their respective antigens. For IgM, a pentamer, these logistical problems are less critical. However, IgM antibodies generated during the primary immune response generally have lower affinities for antigens than the IgG antibodies produced during the secondary antibody response. Serum IgA antibodies have relatively weak classical pathway activating properties, but when codeposited with IgG3 or IgG1, the IgA1 antibodies have the ability to accept biologically active complement fragments generated by the IgG-immune complexes, depart from the complement-coated antigenic surface, and transport their bound complement fragments to noncomplement-coated antigenic surfaces. This process is termed complement-coated-antibody transport/transfer (CCAT).

Early Stages: First Complement Component to Third Complement Component

The aggregated Fc regions of the deposited IgG molecules have binding sites, located on the C_H2 domain, for an umbrella-shaped subcomponent of the C1 molecule, known as C1q. Detailed chemical studies have revealed that C1 is actually a complex of three different types of molecules [C1q, dimerized C1r ($C1r_2$), and dimerized C1s ($C1s_2$)] held loosely together through noncovalent bonds and requiring a physiological Ca^{2+} concentration for their proper association.

Under physiological conditions, the subcomponents of C1 (C1q, $C1r_2$, and $C1s_2$) associate, but exist in conformations that partially limit the "tightness" of that association. Physiological levels of calcium ions and ionic strength are essential to maintain these slightly weaker associations within the C1 macromolecular complex. These conditions enable maximal control over C1 to prevent spontaneous C1 activation that would otherwise readily occur upon a tighter association.

C1q contains several distinct portions; there is a collagen-like stalk/stem region that branches into a six-branched umbrella-shape. Within the umbrella portion of the stem, an association with the $C1r_2$ and $C1s_2$ proenzymes occurs. Each of the six collagen-like branches of C1q terminates in a globular head region. It is these globular head regions that have the potential to associate with the exposed Fc regions of the antibodies present on immune complexes (Fig. 1). After the C1q globular head regions interact with the exposed C_H2 of adjacently deposited IgG3 or IgG1 antibodies, C1q undergoes significant conformational changes. This dramatic C1q conformational change spontaneously facilitates a tightened C1q-$C1r_2$-$C1s_2$ association, resulting in the movement and self activation of the $C1r_2$ proenzymes by one another to form activated $C1r_2$enzymes within the macromolecular C1 complex. Each of the activated $C1r_2$ enzymes has a protease activity that cleaves a peptide bond within the adjacent $C1s_2$ molecules, which, in turn, become activated enzymes. Activated $C1s_2$ enzymes (within the C1 macromolecular complex) are then able to cleave and activate the next component in the series, C4.

It is important to realize that at this step, active host $C1s_2$ enzymes are present on the antigenic surface via the association of the immune complexes with activated C1. The deposition of complement enzymes on the antigenic surface is the major reason for the rapid, amplifying effect of the classical complement pathway, because $C1s_2$ enzymes will continue to activate new C4 and C2 until the $C1s_2$ enzymes are inhibited by C1 inhibitor. In fact, the controlling

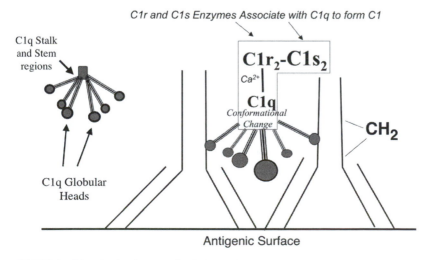

FIGURE 1   C1 activation by an antibody duplet formed by binding to the corresponding antigen.

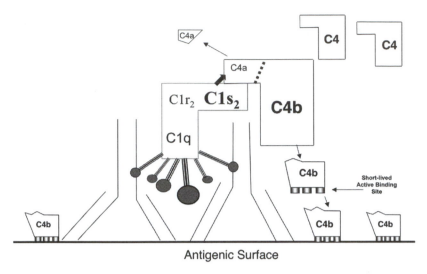

FIGURE 2   Conversion of C4 followed by covalent deposition of C4b on the antigenic surface.

function of C1 inhibitor is the rate-limiting factor in the initiation and progression of the early part of the classical pathway sequence.

As native C4 molecules come into contact with the C1-immune complex, they bind and are cleaved by activated $C1s_2$ into a small fragment, which remains soluble (C4a), and a larger fragment, C4b. As a helpful rule, it is ideal to remember that fragments released into the fluid phase are often designated by the letter "a," while those fragments that remain bound to membranes are designated by the letter "b." However, the nomenclature of C2 fragments is reversed, that is, the bound fragment is designated as C2a, and the soluble fragment as C2b. Each activated C1 is able to cleave and convert many C4 molecules to C4a and C4b. The second fragment derived from C4, C4b, has a very short-lived and highly reactive binding site, an acylating group. This active binding site allows C4b to bind covalently to the nearest hydroxy or amino group, which is usually located on the antigenic surface (Fig. 2). Antibody-coated viral envelopes or antibody-coated bacterial membranes serve as excellent sites for C4b deposition.

Either activated C4b molecules that do not reach the nearby antigenic surface within a few nanoseconds (unable to bind covalently to the antigen) will lose their short-lived active binding site and undergo conformational changes that facilitate binding to a serum factor termed C4-binding protein. Binding of C4b to C4-binding protein causes rapid loss of C4b function and is a very important control mechanism to protect the host's tissues from "bystander attack" by the C4b molecules, being formed in areas of infection.

The activated $C1s_2$ within the bound C1 macromolecular complex is also responsible for the activation of C2—the next complement component to be activated in the classical pathway. In the presence of magnesium ions (Mg^{2+}), C2 interacts with antigen-bound C4b and is, in turn, split by $C1s_2$ into two fragments, termed C2b and C2a. C2b fragments are released into the fluid phase, and C2a binds to C4b (Fig. 3). Thus, proper concentrations of Ca^{2+} ions are needed for optimal $C1q$-$C1r_2$-$C1s_2$ interactions, and Mg^{2+} ions are required for proper C4b-C2a formation. In the absence of Ca^{2+} and/or Mg^{2+} ethylenediaminetetraacetic acid [due to the addition of metal chelators such as ethylenediaminetetraacetic acid (EDTA)], the classical activation pathway is interrupted. An excessive level of Ca^{2+} also tends to disrupt the association of $C1q$-$C1r_2$-$C1s_2$.

The biological role of the soluble C2b is controversial. Some investigators postulate that plasmin-generated fragments of C2b can induce increased capillary permeability, causing leakage of fluid into the interstitial spaces (edema). The relative participation of these fragments in the clinical manifestations of hereditary angioedema (a consequence of C1-inhibitor deficiency, see subsequently) remains unclear because in addition to $C1r_2$ and $C1s_2$, serum C1 inhibitor (C1 INH) regulates kallikrein (bradykinin formation), factor XII, and plasmin.

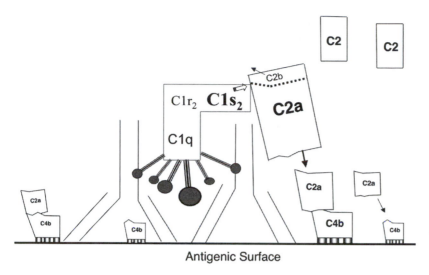

FIGURE 3 Formation of C4b2a complex (C3 convertase) on the antigenic surface. Although activated C1s (within the macromolecular C1 complex) can activate any C2 molecule that it contacts, the cleavage of C2 adjacent to a membrane-bound C4b increases the probability of generating bound-C4b2a complexes on that foreign membrane.

However, the C2 fragment with the best-defined role is C2a, which when bound to C4b, has the active enzyme site necessary for the activation of C3. For C3 to be activated, C2a must remain as a stable complex associated with the membrane-bound C4b molecule. The active C4b2a complex is also known as the classical pathway C3 convertase because it enzymatically converts the next component in the series, C3 to C3b and C3a (Fig. 4). Once active C4b2a complexes are deposited on the antigenic membrane surface surrounding each of the immune complexes, each bound C4b2a complex is capable of rapidly activating many C3 molecules, until the C4b2a complex is disrupted or the enzymatic activity of C2a decays.

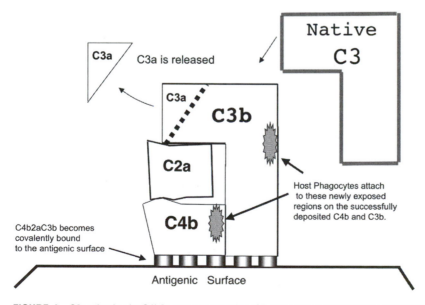

FIGURE 4 C3 activation by C4b2a enzyme complex (C3 convertase) results in the split of C3 into two fragments. While C3b remains associated with C4b2a, C3a is released into the fluid phase. Sites on the deposited C4b and C3b are now exposed and recognized by phagocytic cell receptors.

After at least one deposited C3b molecule associates with the bound C4b2a to form C4b2a3b, the complex acquires the capability of binding to C5 (switches from a C3 convertase to a C5 convertase), wherein C2a (within the C4b2a3b complex) cleaves C5 into C5b and C5a. The newly formed C3b must bind to an amino group or hydroxyl group on the antigen (via its very short-lived active binding site) to remain active. If this fails to happen, the fluid phase C3b associates with Factor H in the serum and is quickly digested by a serum protease, termed Factor I. Some models suggest that an additional C3b molecule may become deposited on top of the C4b within the C4b2a3b complex allowing a stronger interaction with C5.

Thus, a general rule emerges: As each additional component is added to the antigen-antibody-complement complex, the growing complexes acquire the information needed for binding and activating the next component in the series. The activities expressed at each stage of the sequence are regulated by several mechanisms, including the spontaneous decay of C2a activity with time, the short-lived active binding sites on activated complement fragments, the effects of membrane-bound complement inhibitors, and the effects of the normally occurring serum complement inhibitors/regulators. In general, the roles of the serum complement inhibitors are to:

1. Restrict the complement cascade to the surface of the foreign material
2. Prevent bystander damage to the host
3. Limit unnecessary consumption of complement components

Regulatory Mechanisms of the Early Stages

Soon after antigen and antibody react, high levels of C4b and especially C3b accumulate on the antigenic surface, at such high levels that they begin to deposit onto the specific antigenic determinants recognized by the antibody molecules. C4b and especially C3b molecules also bind to the Fab region (C_H1) of the bound antibodies. These phenomena interfere with the ability of antibodies to remain associated with specific epitopes on the antigen. This partial dissolution of the immune complex results in the loosening of the C1 macromolecule from the immune complex. As the antibody molecule recovers its native configuration, the sites on the C_H2 region (that interact with C1q) become less accessible. As C1 begins to separate from the immune complex, the C1q-C1r$_2$-C1s$_2$ macromolecular complex tends to return to its loosely associated form. At that point, the activated C1r$_2$ and C1s$_2$ enzymes are extremely susceptible to irreversible inhibition by a normal serum glycoprotein termed C1-inhibitor, INH. C1 INH forms covalent C1-INH-C1r and C1-INH-C1s complexes, most of which are separated from the bound C1q (Fig. 5) unless the initial attachment of C1 to the immune complexes was weak, in which case C1-INH removes the entire C1q-C1r$_2$-C1s$_2$ macromolecular complex. Activated C1, once having performed its function while bound to the immune

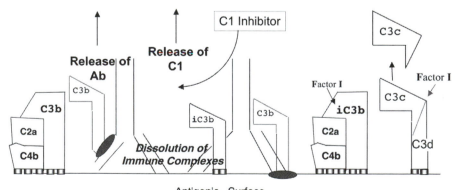

Antigenic   Surface

FIGURE 5 Binding of C4b and C3 fragments to antibody–antigen complexes results in dissolution of those immune complexes. Removal and inactivation of C1 occur as C4b and C3b deposits on the Fab (CH1) of IgG1 and on the antigenic determinants, and thereby disrupt the immune complexes, which in turn cause a loosening of the C1qr$_2$s$_2$ complex, allowing the entrance of C1 Inhibitor.

complex, is then irreversibly inhibited from unnecessary consumption of more native C4 and C2. The proper function of C1-INH represents a very important regulatory mechanism that restricts the range of activated C1 action to the surface of the antigen and prevents useless consumption of C4 and C2. Indeed, the rate-limiting factor in the initiation of the classical complement pathway under normal physiological conditions is not the level of any early complement component but rather the controlling function of C1-INH.

Immune Adherence and Phagocytosis

Prior to its decay or its inactivation, each one of the activated membrane-bound C4b2a enzyme complexes activates C3 molecules, and one or two of the C3b molecules associate with the C4b2a complex. The normal concentration of serum C3 is about 130 mg/dl, which is relatively high and indicates the importance of C3 in the complement activation pathways. C3 is converted through a process that involves its proteolytic cleavage and release of a small biologically active peptide, termed C3a. The larger C3b fragment upon activation behaves very much like the C4b fragment, in that it also has a short-lived, highly reactive binding site, which binds irreversibly to the nearest membrane surface, which is usually the complement-activating antigen.

C3b associates with the bound C4b2a complexes. However, other C3b molecules bind independently to the antigenic membrane. The independently deposited C3b molecules participate in a tremendous amplification of additional C3b deposition via a mechanism termed the amplification loop (to be discussed later in this chapter). It is important to understand that the irreversible (covalent) binding of C4b and of C3b molecules to the antigen actually changes the nature of the antigen. In the case of endotoxin, C4b and C3b deposition abrogates the toxicity of the molecule. Similarly, C4b and C3b contribute to antibody-mediated neutralization of viruses, rendered incapable of properly binding and infecting host cells.

Of great biological significance is the fact that, after C4b and C3b successfully bind to the antigenic surface, they undergo conformational changes that result in the exposure of regions of these two molecules that extend away from the antigenic membrane. These exposed parts of C4b and C3b are biologically important because they contain molecular segments that are able

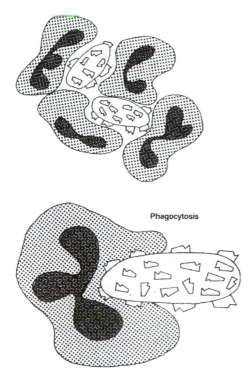

Phagocytosis

FIGURE 6 Opsonization and phagocytosis. The top panel shows immune adherence of phagocytic cells to antigenic cells coated with antibody and complement, and the bottom panel illustrates the ingestion (phagocytosis) of an opsonized cell.

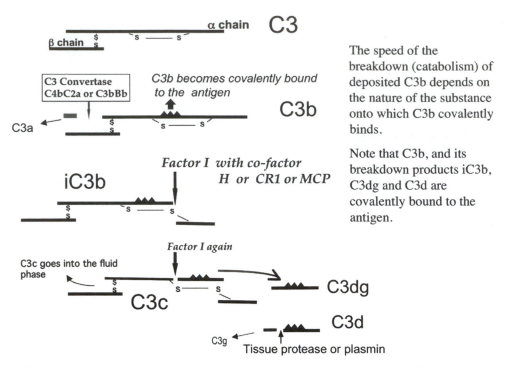

FIGURE 7 Diagrammatic summary of the different steps involved in the breakdown of C3.

to bind to C3b/C4b receptors [currently designated as complement receptor 1 (CR1)] located on host phagocytic cells (Fig. 6). Additional types of receptors for other regions on bound C3b play a significant role in enhancing phagocytosis. Some of those receptors recognize interior (cryptic) regions of C3b exposed, as this component is further catabolized (with time) to form inactivated C3b (iC3b), then C3dg, and finally C3d (Fig. 7).

Polymorphonuclear leukocytes (PMNs), like other phagocytic host cells, have thousands of complement receptors on their membranes allowing them to bind, with high avidity, to particles coated with C3b (and C4b) and/or with breakdown products of bound C3b (i.e., iC3b and C3d). This increased avidity of phagocytic cells for complement-coated particles is known as enhanced immune adherence, and its main consequence is a significant potentiation of the phagocytosis process. In this process, the phagocyte is stimulated to engulf the complement-coated particle because of the interactions with complement receptors on the phagocytic cell membrane. Once engulfed, antigens are digested in phagolysosomes, vesicles that result from the fusion of phagosomes, containing phagocytosed particles, and those lysosomes, which contain a large variety of degradative enzymes. The phagocytic process is one of the most important fundamental defense mechanisms, because it provides a direct way for the host to digest foreign substances (see Chapter 13).

The Late Stages: Fifth Complement Component to Ninth Complement Component

The full effect of the activation of the latter complement components is evident when the activated complement components are deposited on a foreign cell membrane. C5 molecules can be activated by antigen-bound (membrane-associated) C4b2a3b complexes or by alternative pathway/amplification loop enzymes, to be discussed later. As expected, activation of C5 is mediated by the specific proteolytic cleavage of C5 molecules by activated C4b2a3b deposited on the antigen (e.g., foreign cell membrane). Each C5 molecule first binds to an activated C4b2a3b complex and then is split into a small fragment (C5a), which is released into the fluid phase, and a large fragment (C5b). Unlike other complement fragments previously discussed, C5b does not bind immediately to the nearest cell membrane. A complex, consisting

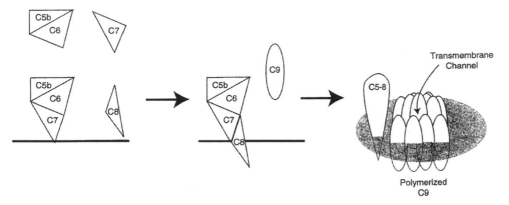

FIGURE 8   Formation of the "membrane attack complex."

of C5b, C6, and C7, is first formed and then the C5b67 complex attaches to the cell membrane through hydrophobic amino acid groups of C7, which become exposed as a consequence of the binding of C7 to the C5b-C6 complex (Figs. 8 and 9). The membrane-bound C5b-6-7 complex acts as a receptor for C8 and then C9. C8, on binding to the complex, will stabilize the attachment of the complex to the foreign cell membrane through the transmembrane insertion of its alpha and beta chains and attracts C9.

The entire C5b-9 complex is also known as the membrane attack complex (MAC). This designation is due to the fact that on binding to C5b-8, C9 molecules undergo polymerization, forming a transmembrane channel of 100 Å diameter, whose external wall is believed to be hydrophobic, while the interior wall is believed to be hydrophilic. This transmembrane channel will allow the free exchange of ions between the cell and the surrounding medium. Due to the rapid influx of ions into the cell and their association with cytoplasmic proteins,

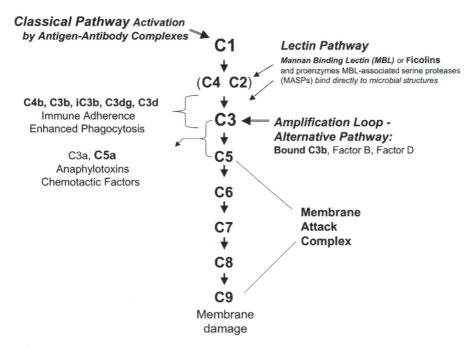

FIGURE 9   The sequence of complement activation pathways.

the osmotic pressure rapidly increases inside the cell. This results in an influx of water, swelling of the cell, and for certain cell types, rupture of the cell membrane, and lysis.

Less than 20 seconds is required for lysis of one million sheep erythrocytes coated with excess IgG antibody when they are mixed with one milliliter of fresh undiluted human serum as a source of complement. In contrast, many Gram-positive bacteria are not susceptible to damage by the MAC, as long as their membrane is covered by an intact cell wall. For these organisms, complement-mediated, enhanced phagocytosis is of prime importance.

Complement Protection Mechanisms in Mamalian Cells

Normal human cells are somewhat resistant to lysis by human complement. Human cells express substances on their membranes that effectively inhibit the human complement sequence (but not the complement of other species). In addition, phagocytes quickly endocytose and destroy inadvertently deposited membrane-bound complement components.

Complement Receptor 1 and Factor I

One of the important inhibitory substances on most types of host cells is the CR1 receptor glycoprotein, which on binding to activated C3b, blocks C3b function in the complement sequence by causing C3b to be rapidly cleaved to iC3b, by a serum enzyme known as Factor I.

Obviously, once the phagocyte actively engulfs the complement-coated particle, there is no reason to continue consuming additional complement or risk inadvertently damaging the phagocyte by depositing C3b and/or MAC complexes on its surface. Therefore, cell surface CR1 molecules after binding to C3b have two independent functions:

1. To enhance phagocytosis of C4b/C3b coated particles by phagocytes
2. Inactivation of C4b/C3b, including those that may become inadvertently deposited on host cells

Decay-Accelerating Factor

Decay-accelerating factor (DAF, CD55) is another important complement-inhibitory substance located on a large variety of host cell membranes. The name of this factor derives from the fact that it can accelerate the dissociation of active C4b2a complexes, turning off their ability to continue activating native C3. In addition, DAF attaches to membrane-bound C4b and C3b and prevents the subsequent interaction of C4b with C2 and of C3b with Factor B, respectively. The role of factor B in the alternative pathway/amplification loop is explained later in this chapter. As a consequence, the two types of C3 convertases, C4b2a and C3bBb, will not be formed or will become dissociated, and the rate of additional C3 activation will be limited. Thus the host cell will be spared from complement-mediated membrane damage. In addition, human hemopoietic cells and various tissues have a C2-binding substance on their membrane, which prevents C4b2a formation on their surfaces.

Several other important complement inhibitory substances are also located on almost all host cell surfaces. These substances are protectin (CD59, which restricts formation of the MAC by binding to C8 and C9) and membrane cofactor protein (CD49, which serves as a cofactor for factor I enzymatic degradation of C3b).

The existence of these multiple protective mechanisms on host cell membranes explains how a phagocyte approaching a complement activating immune complex is itself resistant to bystander damage, initiated by complement inadvertently deposited on its surface. On the other hand, overexpression of complement inhibitors on malignant breast cancer cell membranes and malignant endometrial tissues suggests that avoidance of complement-mediated damage allows better survival of these cancers. In addition, normal human cells and cancer cells have the ability to eliminate the complement MAC from their surface either by endocytosis or by direct emission/release of membrane vesicles (ectocytosis).

Biologically Important Active Fragments: Fifth and Third Complement Component "a" (Anaphylatoxins and Chemotactic factors)

The small complement fragments, C5a and C3a released into the fluid phase are recognized by neutrophils and cause these phagocytes to migrate in the direction from which they originated. The term for this chemical attraction is chemotaxis, and its main biological function is to attract phagocytes into a tissue in which complement-activating antigen-antibody reactions are taking place. Once the PMNs reach the area, by moving toward the highest concentration of freshly generated chemoattractants, the PMNs bind to the C4b and C3b coated antigenic substances via their CR1 receptors (and to iC3b via their CR3 receptors) and proceed to phagocytize the foreign material.

Besides their role as chemokines, C5a and C3a activate the phagocytic cells that carry C5a and C3a receptors. In the case of neutrophils, such activation leads to the expression of cell adhesion molecules (CAMs) and facilitates extravascular migration. In the case of circulating basophils and of mast cells associated with the epithelial and mucosal tissues, C5a and C3a stimulate the release of biologically active mediators such as heparin and vasoactive amines (e.g., histamine). Histamine, when released into the tissues results in increased capillary permeability and in smooth muscle contraction. Fluid is released into the tissue, causing edema and swelling. There is some evidence that the complement fragments C3a and C5a may also act directly on endothelial cells, causing increased vascular permeability. The end result is very similar to the classical anaphylactic reaction that takes place when IgE antibodies bound to the membranes of mast cells and basophils react with the corresponding antigens (see Chapter 21). For this reason, C3a and C5a are known as anaphylatoxins.

ALTERNATIVE COMPLEMENT PATHWAY

Another group of activators of the complement system includes many types of foreign substances, aggregated (hydrophobic) proteins, artificially aggregated immunoglobulins of all classes and subclasses (including IgG4, IgA, and IgE), and microbial membranes and cell walls (Table 1). These activators affect the complement sequence via a mechanism termed the "alternative pathway." The alternative pathway received this designation because its activation does not absolutely require antibody and can proceed in the absence of C1, C4, and C2—all essential for the classical pathway of complement activation.

Once complement is activated by the alternative pathway, it can induce the activation of C5–C9, a property shared with the classical pathway. It must be stressed that activation of the classical pathway is always associated with activation of the alternative pathway which, in that case, functions as an "amplification loop" for the classical pathway, generating more deposited C3b. In fact, the classical pathway is a powerful activator of this pathway/loop.

Some of the most significant activators of the alternative pathway are the bacterial membrane lipopolysaccharides characteristic of gram-negative bacteria and the peptidoglycans and teichoic acids from the cell walls of certain gram-positive bacteria. These substances fix to their surfaces a group of several plasma glycoproteins, including C3b, factor B, factor D,

TABLE 1 Activators of the Alternative Pathway

Bacterial membranes (endotoxic lipopolysaccharides) and viral envelopes
Bacterial and yeast cell walls
Classical pathway (via C3b generation)
Proteases (i.e., via enhanced C3b generation), released by:
  Polymorphonuclear leukocytes
  Bacteria
  Organ failure (pancreatitis)
  Damaged tissue (burns, necrosis, trauma)
  Fibrinolytic system (plasmin)
Aggregated immunoglobulins (including IgA, IgG4, and IgE)
Virus-transformed host cells (limited effects)

Abbreviations: C, complement component; Ig, immunoglobulin.

TABLE 2 Alternative Pathway Sequence

C3 fragmentation (C3 cleavage via classical pathway or via natural turnover, tissue proteases, or bacterial proteases)
Deposition of C3b (via its labile binding site) on a surface, which retards its rapid inactivation by
   Factor I and its cofactors (factor H or CR1)
Binding of Factor B to C3b leading to C3bB
Activation of the bound B by D leading to C3bBb
C3bBb activation of more C3, leading to formation of C3bnBb (and liberation of more C3a)
Binding of properdin to C3b and stabilization of the association of Bb on C3b
C3bnBb activation of C5 (with liberation of C5a); activation of the terminal sequence
   (i.e., membrane attack complex)

Abbreviations: C3, third complement component; C5, fifth complement component.

and properdin, which constitute the initial portion of the alternative pathway sequence. The generation of a "protected" (i.e., nondegraded and stable) bound form of C3b must first occur for the alternative complement pathway/amplification loop to be initiated. So, the alternative pathway begins with at least one stable C3b covalently bound to the activator/antigen, and proceeds with the cleavage of many additional C3 molecules to form more bound C3b and fluid phase C3a. It is important to understand that as a part of the classical pathway, the amplification loop rapidly utilizes the abundant levels of C3 to completely coat the foreign surface and change its very nature due to the covalent binding of C3b molecules, which continue to bind covalently even as C3b is degraded to iC3b, C3dg, and C3d.

Sequence of Activation of the Alternative Pathway/Amplification Loop

C3b fragments are formed slowly during normal C3 turnover in blood, but faster whenever complement is activated by any of the known pathways. Once formed, C3b has an opportunity to bind via its short-lived labile binding site to the nearest surface. By definition, if the surface is an activator of the alternative pathway, then C3b upon binding to the substance will not be rapidly inactivated by natural inhibitory systems and will survive on the activating surface long enough to bind to serum factor B, forming a C3bB complex.

The interaction between deposited C3b and factor B is stabilized by Mg^{2+}, which is the only ion required for functional activation of the alternative pathway. Therefore, tests to discriminate between the two complement activation pathways are often based on the use of a particular chelator (EGTA) that selectively chelates Ca^{2+} (to disrupt C1q, C1r$_2$, and C1s$_2$) with the addition of sufficient Mg^{2+} to allow activation of the alternative pathway.

Factor B, within the C3bB complex, is specifically activated by a circulating active plasma enzyme, Factor D, to yield activated C3bBb. C3bBb is an important C3 convertase, which (like C4b2a) activates C3, leading to the formation C3bBb, which in turn is capable of activating more C3 as well as C5 and the MAC. C3b$_n$Bb may contain one or two C3b molecules (enabling a stronger interaction with C5) and is stabilized by properdin, a plasma glycoprotein that binds to C3b. Since factor D has never been isolated in its proenzyme form, it is generally believed to

TABLE 3 Third Component Receptors

Complement receptor	Most notably expressed on	Primary binding specificity
CR1 (CD35)	Phagocytes—all types Erythrocytes Almost All Human Cell Types	C3b and C4b
CR2 (CD21)	B lymphocytes, Follicular Dendritic Cells	C3d, C3dg, and iC3b
CR3 (CD11b/CD18) (Mac-1)	Neutrophils, Macrophages—all types Monocytes, Follicular Dendritic Cells	iC3b
CR4 (CD11c/CD18) (p150,95)	Neutrophils, Monocytes, Macrophages—all types B lymphocytes—Activated Natural Killer Cells	iC3b

be activated immediately upon leaving the adipose tissues, where it is synthesized. The most important point is the tremendous C3 amplification step that occurs in regard to C3b deposition and C3a formation. Every time a new C3b is deposited on the activating substance there is a chance to form a new C3bBb enzyme, which is capable of activating more C3, causing more C3b deposition. Likewise, amplified C3a and C5a production leads to an enhanced neutrophil chemotaxis and to edema.

It must be kept in mind that the nature of the surface (to which the C3b binds) regulates to a great extent C3b survival time. It is the absence of a C3b degradation system on the surface to which C3b is bound that "allows" bound C3b to remain intact and, consequently, the alternative pathway/amplification loop to be activated. If C3b binds to a surface or a molecule that does not support activation of the alternative pathway, then C3b is rapidly inactivated by Factor I, acting in concert with several cofactors, such as CR1 and membrane cofactor protein (CD46), or Factor H in plasma.

As CR1 and/or membrane cofactor protein are found on the surface of most host cells, these cofactors are most effective in binding and regulating C3b that inadvertently binds to bystander host cells. Factor H appears to be primarily responsible for inactivating fluid phase C3b. However, Factor H binds to C3b molecules accidentally deposited on host (sialic acid-rich tissue) surfaces and therein serves as a cofactor for Factor I. Several pathogens acquire serum Factor H onto their surfaces enabling a circumvention of the neutralizing effects of the complement amplification loop.

Biological Significance of the Alternative Complement Pathway

The biological significance of the alternative pathway can be understood if we consider, as an example, an infection with a hypothetical bacterium. Since all normal individuals have low levels of antibody to most bacteria, some limited classical pathway activation occurs. Theoretically, in the presence of large numbers of bacteria, the relatively low levels of specific antibody may be effectively absorbed by antigens present on the proliferating bacteria, allowing uncoated bacteria to escape destruction by the more effective classical pathway.

While optimal classical pathway function is awaiting production of large amounts of specific antibody, C3b molecules (produced via normal C3 turnover) are slowly (inadvertently) deposited on the bacteria, initiating the alternative complement sequence. Most bacteria, fungi, and viruses activate the alternative pathway, but with varying efficiencies. That is, there is a large variability in the avidity and degree of the interaction with this pathway, depending on the species and strain of microorganism. Perhaps aiding the activation of the alternative pathway are the proteolytic enzymes being produced by microorganisms, which directly activate components like C3. If a higher rate of C3 conversion to C3b and C3a occurs near the membrane of the organism, C3b molecules will more rapidly deposit on the foreign surface via their highly reactive C3b-binding site, and the alternative complement pathway will be more effectively initiated. On the other hand, large levels of powerful broad-spectrum proteases, located on bacterial surfaces could protect the bacteria from the effects of complement by simply degrading the complement components as they deposit.

In summary, the alternative pathway of complement activation is important especially during the early phase of the infection, when the concentrations of specific antibody are very low. After the antibody response is fully developed, the classical and alternative pathways work synergistically, with the alternative pathway functioning as an amplification loop of the classical pathway.

Activation and Inactivation of Third Complement Component

When C3b is inadvertently deposited on host cells containing cofactors for Factor I, C3b is rapidly cleaved into small products, which will not activate additional complement components. On the other hand, C3b molecules deposited on antigens are slowly degraded by Factor I, allowing time for activation of the amplification loop and the MAC. As a result, a more prolonged presence of iC3b is observed on antigens. While iC3b has irreversibly lost the ability to participate in the complement activation sequence, it remains bound to the foreign substance and enhances its phagocytosis.

Therefore, very important reactive sites become exposed when Factor I cleaves bound-C3b molecules. The newly exposed regions react with other cell receptors, CR2 and CR3. CR3, which avidly binds to iC3b, is not a ubiquitous complement receptor (like CR1), rather it is expressed on phagocytes and is very important in enhancing phagocytosis. However, even the site that reacts with CR3 is eventually lost as iC3b continues to be degraded by Factor I, which causes the iC3b to break into two major fragments: C3dg and soluble C3c. The C3dg fragments remain covalently bound to the antigen and retain the site that interacts with CR2 (a complement receptor expressed by B cells and follicular dendritic cells). With time, C3dg is further degraded into C3d by the continued action of plasma or tissue proteases; this fragment remains bound to the antigen, and like C3dg, continues to express the site for interaction with CR2.

OTHER COMPLEMENT ACTIVATION PATHWAYS
Proteolytic Enzymes as Nonspecific Activators of Individual Complement Components

A variety of proteolytic enzymes, some released by microbes at the site of an infection, and others released from host cells in areas of inflammation or necrosis, are capable of activating the complement system. For example, PMNs leak oxidative products and lysosomal proteolytic enzymes into the extracellular fluids during the phagocytosis process. Oxidation of native C5 increases its susceptibility to the process of conversion by proteases, and increases C5a formation. Also, within inflamed or traumatized tissue, damaged host cells release lysosomal proteases during their degeneration. These bacterial and/or host proteases are able to directly cleave C1, C3, and C5. As a consequence of direct cleavage of C3 and C5, biologically active peptides (C3a and C5a) are generated, contributing to a local inflammatory reaction by their direct action, and by attracting and activating additional PMNs to the area of tissue damage.

Lectin Pathway of Complement Activation

The newest discovered pathway for activating the second, fourth, and third complement components is the lectin complement pathway, which involves a serum MBL and other serum lectins called ficolins. Mannan, a constituent of the polysaccharide capsules of many pathogenic fungi and yeasts (e.g., *Cryptococcus neoformans* and *Candida albicans*), is one of the several polysaccharide substances to which human MBL binds via Ca^{2+}-dependant interactions, while bacterial lipoteichoic acid and peptidoglycan associate with serum ficolins. In addition to carbohydrate motifs of microorganisms, MBL can bind to glycoproteins on the envelope of several types of viruses.

The activation of the lectin pathway does not involve antigen-antibody interactions. Like the alternative complement pathway, the lectin pathway is a primitive backup system to activate complement, before substantial levels of specific IgG antibodies are produced. Both MBL and ficolins are acute phase reactants, that is, their concentration increases during infection and inflammation. Structurally, MBL and ficolins are members of the collectin family (C-type lectin) characterized by having a collagen-like sequence that resembles the structure of C1q, and several Ca^{2+}-dependent carbohydrate recognition domains. Both types of lectins stay associated with serum serine proteases and upon binding to microbial structures the proteases in the complexes become activated, and, in turn, activate the early complement components (C4, C2). The activation of C4 and C2 generates deposition of C4b2a and subsequent C3b deposition and terminal component activation. Thus, the initiation of the lectin pathway has several features that somewhat parallel the classical complement pathway. It is important to realize that under normal conditions, the classical pathway activation by immune complexes is a much more efficient and powerful activation than the activation by the lectin pathway.

COMPLEMENT RECEPTORS IN HUMAN CELL MEMBRANES
Complement Receptor 1

CR1 is a common membrane glycoprotein that can be detected on almost all types of human cells including erythrocytes and cells from various tissues and organs. CR1 reacts with C3b until C3b becomes cleaved by factor I. In phagocytic cell membranes, the main biological role of CR1 is to enhance the phagocytosis of those antigenic substances to which C3b is covalently bound. Also, cell surface CR1 molecules protect the cells on which they are expressed from complement-mediated bystander damage. CR1 molecules move on the cell surface to quickly bind any nearby C3b inadvertently deposited on host cells and act as a cofactor for the serum factor-I enzyme, which cleaves C3b to form iC3b and thereby prevent further activation of the complement sequence.

CR1 on erythrocytes effectively removes inflammatory complement-coated particles from the fluid phase of the blood. These particles (antigens) are the ones that are actually becoming freshly coated with newly deposited C4b and/or C3b molecules (with the local release of C3a and C5a). Their removal from the plasma reduces the probability that those complement-coated immune complexes will freely circulate in the serum and be able to enter and inadvertently damage (via their inadvertent inflammatory potential) vital organs and tissues. Likewise, the ubiquitous presence of CR1 on almost all host cell membranes not only protects those host cells from inadvertent complement-mediated membrane attack, but also sequesters any residual fluid phase complement-coated antigens, preventing deeper penetration of these inflammatory complexes into those tissues and vital organs while awaiting the arrival of phagocytes. It is important to understand that the site on C3b, which binds to the CR1 receptor on erythrocytes and other host cells, is lost as iC3b is formed. Therefore, a preferred binding to phagocytes increases. The most important point is that erythrocytes provide a protective function by carrying inflammatory complement-coated immune complexes to the various host phagocytic systems (e.g., spleen and liver).

Complement Receptor 2

Complement Receptor 2 is another important cell surface glycoprotein that has primary binding specificity for a molecular site on the alpha chain of C3, exposed on C3d, C3dg, and on iC3b. B-lymphocytes have both CR2 and CR1 molecules on their surface. Follicular dendritic cells (important in antigen presentation) have CR2, CR3, and CR1 on their surface. Antibody production is greatly enhanced by complement-coated antigens, which stimulate B cells via their CR2 and CR1. In animal models, when C3d was chemically linked to an antigen, and added to specific B cells in vivo, a thousand-fold enhancement of antibody production occurred. The CR2 not only stimulates the B cell directly but also associates with CD19 (another B cell membrane protein that is known to greatly stimulate antibody production). Of course, this complement-mediated synergistic effect on B cells occurs only in the presence of specific antigen (and with helper T cells).

Complement Receptor 3

Complement Receptor 3 is a cell surface glycoprotein that, via Ca^{2+} dependant interactions, binds to site(s) exposed predominantly on iC3b; this CR3 receptor is expressed on neutrophils, monocytes/macrophages, certain natural killer cells, and on a low proportion of B and T lymphocytes.

Complement Receptor 4

Complement Receptor 4 is expressed mainly in neutrophils, monocytes, and tissue macrophages. Like CR3, it binds to iC3b that remains irreversibly bound to the antigenic surface.

In addition to the CR1, CR2, CR3, and CR4 glycoproteins, certain host cells also have receptors for C3a and C5a. For example, neutrophils, mast cells, basophils, and certain lymphocyte populations have receptors for C3a and C5a. The binding of C3a and/or C5a to these receptors stimulates several cellular functions, such as release of active mediators, upregulation of complement receptors, leading to enhanced phagocytosis and upregulation of cell-adhesion molecules that contributes to their extravascular migration.

Besides the role in B cell activation mentioned earlier, complement receptors mediate the stimulation of many cell types that express them. Antigens coated with antibody and complement (i.e., C4b, C3b, iC3b, and C3dg) adhere strongly to macrophages, neutrophils, and lymphocytes (B lymphocytes and activated T lymphocytes) and cause them to release many biologically active factors, including a variety of soluble mediators (such as cytokines, interleukins, prostaglandins, and/or leukotrienes) that influence immune responses and cause inflammation.

PATHOLOGICAL SITUATIONS ASSOCIATED WITH EXAGGERATED COMPLEMENT ACTIVATION

Once the complement cascade is activated, the complement components are under very tight regulation and control. An important aspect of this regulation is the constant presence of plasma inhibitors for the activated complement components. For each type of activated fragment there is at least one inhibitor or inhibitory mechanism. The tight regulation and rapid neutralization of the active fragments limit their range of action.

In the case of C3a and C5a, there are several serum inhibitors, one of which is believed to be a serum protease that removes the carboxy-terminal arginine residue of the peptides and limits their ability to stimulate PMNs, leukocytes, basophils, and mast cells.

The inhibitor for C3b, as described in detail in previous sections of this chapter, is factor I, which only works in conjunction with appropriate cofactors [factor H, CR1, or MCP (CD46)]. C4b is also inhibited by Factor I, and a cofactor termed C4 Binding Protein (C4BP). Factor I cleaves C4b and C3b and prevents their capacity to be involved in activating downstream components of complement pathways.

The serum inhibitor for C1 is a serum protein termed C1-INH that tends to stabilize the nonactivated C1 macromolecular complex, preventing spontaneous activation. More importantly, C1-INH has the ability to bind irreversibly to the activated form of $C1r_2$ and $C1s_2$, at or near their active site. If a deficiency of any of these complement inhibitors or cofactors exists within an individual, an imbalance in complement regulation occurs, and disease may ensue.

Hereditary Angioedema

This is a rare genetic disorder due to a genetically inherited C1-INH deficiency, of which two main variants are known. In the most common, the genetic inheritance of a silent gene results in a significantly lower level of C1-INH. The second variant is characterized by normal levels of C1-INH protein, but 75% of the molecules are dysfunctional, that is, will not inhibit activated $C1r_2$ or $C1s_2$ because of an aberrant amino acid substitution. While the lack of C1-INH can be easily detected by a quantitative assay, the synthesis of dysfunctional C1-INH can only be revealed by a combination of quantitative and functional tests. An acquired form of C1-INH deficiency can be detected in certain malignant diseases. Individuals with congenital C1-INH deficiency may present clinically with a disease known as hereditary angioedema, characterized by spontaneous swelling of the face, neck, genitalia and extremities, often associated with abdominal cramps and vomiting. The disease can be life threatening if the airway is compromised by laryngeal edema; and tracheotomy maybe a lifesaving measure. This anaphylactoid reaction is due not to IgE-mediated reactions, but rather to spontaneous uncontrolled activation of the complement system by C1 and other systems controlled by C1-INH. The complement reaction is usually self-limiting and will cease after all C4 and C2 have been consumed. However, in vivo there is no substantial consumption of the remaining complement sequence (C3–C9) due to the action of several other regulatory mechanisms, which are especially effective against the unbound (free) forms of C4b and C3b (i.e., C4b and C3b that are not bound to any antigen).

Attacks in patients with C1-INH deficiency occur after surgical trauma, particularly after dental surgery or after severe stress. It is notable that activated Hageman factor, kallikrein, and plasmin are also controlled (in part) by binding to C1-INH. After surgical trauma, binding to each of the enzymes mentioned earlier further depletes the available C1-INH in deficient patients. In the absence of sufficient C1-INH, spontaneous activation of a limited number of C1 molecules and the other substances controlled by C1-INH will gradually accentuate the depletion of C1-INH to the point that unbound activated C1 and other activated enzymes controlled by C1-INH are present in the circulation. These blood enzymes controlled by C1-INH become much less restricted. For example, the continued presence of activated, uninhibited fluid phase C1s will cause spontaneous and continuous activation of the next two components in the sequence, C4 and C2 until their complete consumption. Low C4 levels are considered diagnostic of C1-INH deficiency, and they remain low even when the patients are not experiencing an attack, probably due to a continuously exaggerated C4 catabolism by activated C1. Loss of control over unbound (fluid-phase) activated C1 results in total depletion of C4 and C2 and a further rapid depletion of any residual C1-INH. At the same time, there is a reduction in control by C1-INH over any activated kallikrein. Plasma prekallikrein circulates complexed with high molecular weight kininogen, and uncontrolled activated kallikrein cleaves kininogen to release bradykinin. There is mounting evidence to suggest that the major angioedema-producing substance is bradykinin, although earlier reports suggest a role for a fragment of C2 (C2a) liberated by the action of C1 on C2 followed by the cleavage of C2 by unrestricted plasmin. While it is generally accepted that serum C3 levels are not significantly altered during attacks of angioedema, in vitro evidence has shown that if appropriate levels of antibody to human C1-INH are added to whole human serum, 100% C3 conversion occurs. This complete C3 conversion can only be achieved when the function of C1-INH is blocked. Thus, minor participation of low levels of C3a in angioedema cannot be ruled out when localized C1-INH levels approach zero. As mentioned earlier in this chapter, C1-INH helps to control several other blood system enzymes. During attacks of hereditary angioneurotic edema, when C1-INH is being consumed, the activation of the kallikrein-kinin system occurs and the released bradykinin is considered a key contributor to the edema scenario.

Paroxysmal Nocturnal Hemoglobinuria

Paroxysmal nocturnal hemoglobinuria (PNH) is an acquired disorder on the surface of selected hemopoietic stem-cell lines and their erythrocyte progeny. The patients develop hemolytic anemia associated with the intermittent passage of dark urine (due to hemoglobinuria), which usually is more accentuated at night. The spontaneous hemolysis is due to an increased susceptibility of the abnormal population of erythrocytes to complement-mediated lysis. The erythrocytes are not responsible for the activation of the complement system; rather, they are lysed as innocent bystanders when complement is activated.

Detailed studies of the circulating erythrocytes in PNH patients have demonstrated the existence of three erythrocyte subpopulations with varying degrees of sensitivity to complement. The reason for the existence of these subpopulations was elucidated when the molecular basis of PNH was established. Several membrane proteins are attached to cell membranes through phosphatidylinositol "anchors." The red cell membrane contains two such proteins: DAF (CD55) which prevents or disrupts the formation of C4b2a and C3bBb and protectin (CD59), which prevents the proper assembly of the MAC by binding to C8 and C9. These two proteins (together with CR1 and MCP) have an important protective role for "bystander" erythrocytes by controlling the rate of complement activation on the erythrocyte membrane. The deficiency of the phosphatidylinositol anchoring system is reflected by deficiencies of DAF and protectin. Type I PNH red cells have normal or slightly lowered levels of these two proteins and usually show normal resistance to complement-mediated hemolysis; type III PNH red cells lack both proteins and are very sensitive to hemolysis; type II PNH red cells lack DAF and have intermediate sensitivity to hemolysis.

Phosphatidylinositol is involved in the membrane binding of other proteins, such as the predominant type of Fc receptor in the neutrophil (Fc RIII). Therefore, in these patients, neutrophils, platelets, and other cells are deficient both in DAF and in Fc receptors. These deficiencies seem to be the basis of other abnormalities seen in PNH patients: thrombotic complications, attributed to increased complement-induced platelet aggregation; bacterial infections, and persistence of immune complexes in the circulation, both attributed to a lack of Fc-mediated phagocytosis.

Pulmonary Vascular Leukostasis as a Side Effect of Hemodialysis

Passage of heparinized blood over a variety of filter materials (i.e., artificial hemodialysis membranes and nylon fiber substances used in the heart-lung machine) causes varying degrees of complement activation. The classical pathway may be activated by interfacially (solid-liquid or air-liquid) aggregated immunoglobulins or by direct binding of C1q. Also, membrane (filter)-bound C3b (via C3 turnover and C3b deposition) mediates activation of the alternative pathway. Rapid generation of C5a causes a transient leukopenia with a short-term, reversible accumulation and aggregation of granulocytes in the blood capillaries of the lungs, where they release superoxide that damages the tissues surrounding the areas of PMN accumulation. As a result, repeated hemodialyses may lead to chronic fibrosis of the lung.

Pancreatitis, Severe Trauma, and Pulmonary Distress Syndrome

Any pathologic process that causes a rapid release of high levels of C5a into the blood may cause massive PMN aggregation and consequent pulmonary distress syndrome. For example, when large amounts of proteases are released into the blood (i.e., pancreatitis or severe tissue trauma), pulmonary distress syndrome and, sometimes, temporary blindness occur due to blockage of small blood vessels with aggregated granulocytes. Similarly, in myocardial infarction, blockage of critical heart capillaries with leukocyte aggregates may extend cardiac damage. Steroids that prevent and reverse leukocyte aggregation have been used to retard such damage in experimental animals. Cardiolipin released from within the damaged heart tissues onto cell surfaces may directly activate C1 and therein exaggerate the complement activation being induced by the tissue proteases.

Septic Shock and First Complement Component-Inhibiter Depletion

The classical complement pathway, the contact activation system, and the coagulation cascade are activated during severe sepsis and septic shock. Activation of these cascades in severe sepsis contributes to the development of multiple organ failure (which may or may not be reversible), associated with high mortality rates. A depletion of C1-INH occurs due to the activation of these host enzyme systems. Depletion of C1-INH to less than about 10% of its normal serum level allows many bacterial substances and charged host cellular substances to directly activate C1 (which otherwise would be prevented from activating complement). In experimental animals, C1-INH substitution reduces mortality by severe sepsis or septic shock.

COMPLEMENT LEVELS IN DISEASE

The complement proteins have some of the highest turnover rates of any of the plasma components. At any one time, the level of a complement component is a direct function of its catabolic and synthetic rates. There are many factors that cause the increased production of complement components by the liver and from cells present at local sites of inflammation. In tissue culture models, the addition of cytokines, such as interleukin-1α, interferon-γ, and especially tumor necrosis factor (TNF), upregulate C3 synthesis. Interleukin-1α, interleukin-6, and especially interferon-γ upregulate factor B synthesis. Interestingly, TNF and interferon-γ concomitantly increase DAF expression on host cells (e.g., vascular endothelial cells) in order to protect the host from bystander complement attack, especially in areas where the MAC is inadvertently being deposited (e.g., on the vascular endothelium) during localized inflammation.

The catabolic rates of the complement system are primarily a function of the extent of complement activation by all the pathways involved. Therefore, the levels of complement proteins are influenced by the levels of complement activators (i.e., immune complexes), the class and subclass of immunoglobulin within the immune complexes, the release of direct complement-activating bacterial products, and, in certain chronic inflammatory diseases, the presence of auto-antibody to complement components (immunoconglutinins).

   The synthetic rates of complement glycoproteins vary widely in disease states and during the course of a given disease. In the end, the level of a complement component is a function of its metabolic rate (synthesis vs. catabolism) and the type and, course of, the inflammatory reaction. Elevated levels of a given complement component in a disease state probably means that there is both a rapid synthetic and catabolic rate. Lower overall complement levels indicate that consumption is greater than synthesis at that particular time, usually in association with acute inflammation or an exacerbation of a chronic inflammatory process. Severe complement depletion, on the other hand, is usually associated with impaired hepatic synthesis (e.g., as in liver failure).

Hypocomplementemia and Clearance of Immune Complexes

The development of immune complex diseases is believed to be a consequence of the inability to properly eliminate immune complexes from the kidney and/or from the basement membrane of dermal tissues. As previously mentioned in our discussion of the classical pathway, activation of a normal complement system by immune complexes will eventually lead to partial dissolution of the immune complex. This phenomenon is due to the deposition of large complement fragments such as C4b and C3b on the antigen and on the Fab region of the antibody, which interferes with the antigen-antibody binding reaction. If a deficiency in the early complement components exists, there will likely be a corresponding defect in the production and binding of C4b and C3b to the immune complex. As a result, the rate of formation of new immune complexes surpasses the inefficient rate of immune complex dissolution and/or phagocytic clearance, and the generation of pro-inflammatory complement fragments will be possible for a longer period of time. The reasons for the lower levels of early complement components (i.e., C1q, C4, and/or C2) are multiple and include not only genetic factors but also a variety of metabolic control mechanisms mentioned earlier in the chapter.

   In patients with systemic lupus erythematosus (SLE), a reduction in the levels of CR1 on erythrocyte has been reported. As previously discussed, the binding of complement-coated immune complexes to erythrocytes is an important physiological mechanism of immune complex removal from the circulation. Small to medium-sized immune complexes are not taken up as efficiently by CR1 and tend to persist longer in circulation. However, when the number of CR1 receptors on erythrocyte membranes is decreased, even large-sized (complement coated) immune complexes may persist for longer periods in circulation and may have a greater opportunity to be deposited in organs and tissues thereby causing inflammation. The depleted number CR1 per erythrocyte may be partly due to the overwhelming utilization of the erythrocyte CR1 in SLE and subsequent CR1 catabolism as the complement-coated immune complexes are presented to phagocytic cells in the liver and spleen.

Complement Deficiencies

Deficiencies of several of the components of the complement system are associated with two types of clinical situations: chronic bacterial infections, caused by capsulated organisms such as *Neisseria* species, and autoimmune disease, mimicking SLE (see Chapter 29).

MICROBIAL ANTICOMPLEMENTARY MECHANISMS

In general, complement-mediated phagocytosis is the most effective mechanism for elimination of infectious microorganisms. However, pathogenic organisms have evolved several mechanisms to circumvent either effective complement activation or effective complement deposition on their outer surface. These evasion strategies are most efficient during the early stages of an infection, when the levels of specific antibodies are low.

   In some cases, the microorganisms (e.g., *Candida*) have on their surface a structural protein that mimics the protective effect of DAF or other complement regulators. *Streptococcus pyogenes*, *Neisseria gonorrhoeae*, and *Candida albicans* have surface structures that attract host serum factor H and promote host serum factor I mediated cleavage of any deposited C3b to form iC3b. iC3b does not participate in the amplification loop. As a result, less C3b is deposited on these organisms. Interestingly, HIV acquires membrane DAF (CD55) upon leaving the infected host cell, and during the infection process appears to adsorb Factor H from serum. In these situations, if insufficient levels of high affinity antibody fail to deposit on the pathogen, a reduced deposition of complement components leads to a less effective neutralization/ elimination.

Other less sophisticated complement-restrictive mechanisms that different micro-organisms have acquired include the shedding of MAC-coated pili, destruction of C3b by proteases on the bacterial surface, and protection of the cytoplasmic membrane from the dis-solving effect of the MAC by slime layers, peptidoglycan layers, polysaccharide capsules, etc. With the deposition of sufficient levels of high affinity antibodies, these protective mechan-isms are usually overridden, and the microorganisms are properly phagocytosed, although some bacteria have acquired anti-phagocytic capsules that further complicate the job of the immune system (see Chapter 14).

BIBLIOGRAPHY

Banki Z, Kacani L, Rusert P, et al. Complement dependent trapping of infectious HIV in human lymphoid tissues. AIDS 2005; 19:481–486.

Boackle RJ, Nguyen QL, Leite RS, Yang X, Vesely J. Complement-coated antibody-transfer (CCAT); serum IgA1 antibodies intercept and transport C4 and C3 fragments and preserve IgG1 deployment (PGD). Mol Immunol 2006; 43:236–245.

Bracho FA. Hereditary angioedema. Curr Opin Hematol 2005; 12:493–498.

Cai S, Dole VS, Bergmeier W, et al. A direct role for C1 inhibitor in regulation of leukocyte adhesion. J Immunol 2005; 174:6462–6466.

Davis AE III. The pathophysiology of hereditary angioedema. Clin Immunol 2005; 114:3–9. Review.

Kemper C, Atkinson JP. T-cell regulation: with complements from innate immunity. Nat Rev Immunol 2007; 7:9–18. Review.

Mason JC, Yarwood H, Sugars K, et al. Induction of decay-accelerating factor by cytokines or the mem-brane-attack complex protects vascular endothelial cells against complement deposition. Blood 1999; 94:1673.

Nielsen EW, Waage C, Fure H, et al. Effect of upraphysiologic levels of C1-inhibitor on the classical, lectin and alternative pathways of complement. Mol Immunol 2007; 44:1829–1836.

Rawal N, Pangburn MK. Formation of high affinity C5 convertase of the classical pathway of complement. J Biol Chem 2003; 278:38476–38483.

Rooijakkers SH, Ruyken M, Roos A, et al. Immune evasion by a staphylococcal complement inhibitor that acts on C3 convertases. Nat Immunol 2005; 6:920–927.

Shichishima T, Noji H. A new aspect of the molecular pathogenesis of paroxysmal nocturnal hemoglobi-nuria. Hematology 2002; 7:211–227. Review.

Sjoholm AG, Jonsson G, Braconier JH, Sturfelt G, Truedsson L. Complement deficiency and disease: an update. Mol Immunol 2006; 43:78–85.

Thangam EB, Venkatesha RT, Zaidi AK, et al. Airway smooth muscle cells enhance C3a-induced mast cell degranulation following cell-cell contact. FASEB J 2005; 19:798–800.

van Doorn MB, Burggraaf J, van Dam T, et al. A phase I study of recombinant human C1 inhibitor in asymptomatic patients with hereditary angioedema. J Allergy Clin Immunol 2005; 116:876–883.

Wallis R, Dodds AW, Mitchell DA, Sim RB, Reid KB, Schwaeble WJ. Molecular interactions between MASP-2, C4 and C2 and their activation fragments leading to complement activation via the lectin pathway. J Biol Chem 2007 Jan 3.

Watson NF, Durrant LG, Madjd Z, Ellis IO, Scholefield JH, Spendlove I. Expression of the membrane comp-lement regulatory protein CD59 (protectin) is associated with reduced survival in colorectal cancer patients. Cancer Immunol Immunother 2005; 3:1–8.

Ziller F, Macor P, Bulla R, Sblattero D, Marzari R, Tedesco F. Controlling complement resistance in cancer by using human monoclonal antibodies that neutralize complement-regulatory proteins CD55 and CD59. Eur J Immunol 2005; 35:2175–2183.

Zipfel PF, Skerka C, Hellwage J, et al. Factor H family proteins: on complement, microbes and human dis-eases. Biochem Soc Trans 2002; 30:971–978. Review.

10 | Lymphocyte Ontogeny and Membrane Markers

Virginia M. Litwin
MDS Pharma Services, Central Lab, North Brunswick, New Jersey, U.S.A.

INTRODUCTION

This chapter describes the differentiation process of the main lymphocyte subsets and the membrane markers expressed on the mature cells. A brief introduction to the key technological approaches used in the study of lymphopoiesis and membrane markers will be useful before broaching this intricate and intriguing topic. Identification of expression patterns of surface and intracellular marker have made it possible to define, purify, and characterize lymphocytes with regard to type, maturation stage and activation state. Standardized nomenclature has been adopted for many cellular markers, the letters "CD" (for cluster of differentiation) followed by a number. Cellular markers are most often identified using fluorescence-tagged monoclonal antibodies and detected by flow cytometry or immunofluorescence microscopy (see Chapter 15).

Sophisticated and complicated in vivo experimental systems, such as genetically engineered animals and animals in which cells have been adoptively transferred, have been critical tools for the immunology research community. Elucidation of the role of various cellular receptors, transcription factors, and cytokines in the development of an immune response or lymphocyte ontogeny has been facilitated by these experimental systems. Transgenic animals express the genes of another species or strain (e.g., human genes can be inserted into the germline of mice); whereas, "knock-out" mice have a specific gene disrupted or deleted. The crossbreeding of transgenic and knockout mice has generated animals that express only the human form of a given gene. The use of multiparameter flow cytometry and cell sorting has allowed the isolation of highly purified cell populations, and even single cells, for use in subsequent in vitro cultures. Purified populations of stem cells or progenitor populations can be adoptively transferred into knock-out or normal animals and be analyzed for their ability to differentiate or home to a given organ in the environmental conditions present in each particular recipient animal or in vitro culture. These genetic and cellular manipulations are only possible, for experimental purposes, in animal models; most of our understanding of lymphocyte ontogeny is based on the study of mice. Given that regulatory components and critical factors, involved in hematopoiesis and lymphopoiesis, are thought to be broadly conserved, most of the information garnered in the murine system is believed to be relevant to the human system.

STEM CELL DIFFERENTIATION

All blood cell types, including lymphocytes, are derived from pluripotent precursors known as hematopoietic stem cells (HSC). HSC are found primarily in the fetal liver and bone marrow and persist throughout adult life. By definition a stem cell must be capable of both self-renewal and differentiation. Self-renewal is the ability to give rise to at least two daughter cells at the same stage of development as the parent and is dependent on growth factors such as, granulocyte-monocyte colony simulating factor (GM-CSF), granulocyte-colony stimulating factor (G-CSF), interleukin (IL-3), and 5. Differentiation of HSC along the various hematopoietic lineages is progressive, in that cells develop first into multipotent progenitors and then into precursors with decreasing pluripotency and increasing commitment to a single differentiation pathway. This progression was once thought to be an orderly sequence of events; however, this view may be oversimplified. As research in this field continues, new questions emerge. For example, it is not clear whether lymphoid progenitors are discrete, homogeneous populations, or overlapping populations. Nor is it clear whether lineage commitment occurs via a continuum of differentiation with a progressive loss of lineage options or via abrupt events resulting in the acquisition of certain properties. Whatever the precise mechanism, HSC give rise to progeny with progressively more restricted myeloid, erythroid, or lymphoid developmental potential. This differentiation is accompanied by the silencing of some genes and the activation of others. Changes in the expression levels of cytokine receptors, signal transduction molecules, and transcription factors are key components in lymphoid differentiation.

Hematopoietic Stem Cells Markers

HSC are characteristically described as lacking FMS-like tyrosine kinase3 (Flt3) and the markers specific to discrete lymphoid lineages (Lin), but expressing high levels of Sca1 and c-kit. HSC also express CD44, low levels of Thy1.1 (CD90), but no IL-7Rα or CD27. Thus the phenotype of HSC can be expressed as Lin$^-$, Sca1^{high}, c-kit^{high}, CD44$^+$, Thy1.1^{low}, CD27$^-$, and IL-7Rα^-. Progression of HSC differentiation and lineage commitment is indicated by changes in this phenotype as described subsequently and summarized in Figure 1.

   Flt3 is a cytokine tyrosine kinase receptor thought to be important in early lymphoid development. In addition, Flt3 plays a major role in maintaining B lymphoid progenitors. CD27 plays a role in lymphoid proliferation, differentiation, and apoptosis. The acquisition of CD27 and Flt3 by the HSC coincides with the loss of long-term repopulating potential. At this stage the cells retain both lymphoid and myeloid potential and are referred to as multipotent progenitors.

Stem Cell Growth Factor Receptor

The level of expression of the stem cell growth factor receptor or c-kit (CD117), a cytokine tyrosine kinase receptor, is thought to progressively decline with lineage commitment, and thus can

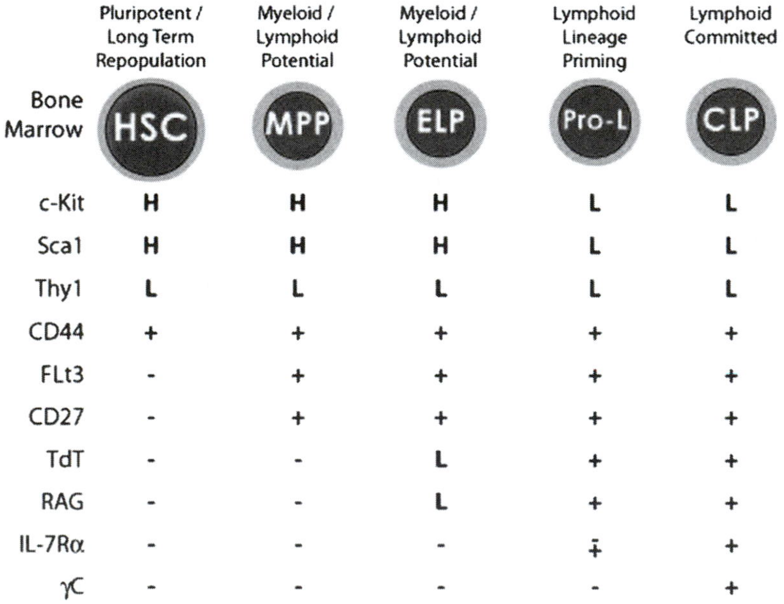

	Pluripotent / Long Term Repopulation	Myeloid / Lymphoid Potential	Myeloid / Lymphoid Potential	Lymphoid Lineage Priming	Lymphoid Committed
Bone Marrow	HSC	MPP	ELP	Pro-L	CLP
c-Kit	H	H	H	L	L
Sca1	H	H	H	L	L
Thy1	L	L	L	L	L
CD44	+	+	+	+	+
FLt3	-	+	+	+	+
CD27	-	+	+	+	+
TdT	-	-	L	+	+
RAG	-	-	L	+	+
IL-7Rα	-	-	-	∓	+
γC	-	-	-	-	+

FIGURE 1   Hypothetical model of lymphopoiesis. The differentiation of the pluripotent, self-renewing, hematopoietic stem cells in the bone marrow is progressive. First, cells develop into multipotent progenitors and then into early lymphoid progenitors, prolymphocytes, and finally to the common lymphoid progenitor that is fully committed to the lymphoid lineage. Changes in the expression of the hallmark surface markers and intracellular proteins that typify each stage of differentiation are shown. *Abbreviations*: CLP, common lymphoid progenitors; ELP, early lymphoid progenitors; HSC, hematopoietic stem cell; MPP, multipotent progenitors; RAG, recombinase activation gene.

be used to distinguish general categories of lymphoid progenitors. In the bone marrow, HSC and early lymphoid progenitors are c-kit^{high}, as are the early thymocyte progenitors, the most primitive cells in the thymus. The early lymphoid progenitors are primarily restricted (but not fully committed) to the lymphoid lineage. This intermediate step in the differentiation pathway may also be described as "lineage priming." A population of c-kit^{low} cells in the bone marrow called pro-lymphocytes has limited self-renewal capacity and has lymphoid but not myeloid potential.

Recombinase-Activation Genes 1 and 2 and Terminal Deoxynucleotidyl Transferase

Recombinase-activation genes 1 and 2 (RAG-1, RAG-2) are transposases. Terminal deoxynucleotidyl transferase (Tdt) is a template-independent DNA polymerase believed to play an important role in the generation of antigen receptor diversity both in B cells and T cells. The expression of this enzyme is restricted to lymphoid precursors and transformed cells in patients with acute lymphoblastic leukemia. The absence of the RAG affects both T and B cells differentiation and results in severe combined immunodeficiency (see Chapter 29).

Common γ Chain, Interleukin 7 Receptor α

The common γ chain (γc) (CD132) is a subunit shared by the membrane bound receptors for IL-2, IL-4, IL-7, IL-9, IL-13, IL-15, and IL-21 (see Chapter 11). A common lymphoid progenitor cell exists within the Pro-L population and is defined on the basis of upregulation of the interleukin-7 receptor alpha (IL-7Rα), CD127, and γc. This progenitor cells have the ability to give rise to all lymphoid lineages -T cells, B cells, Natural Killer (NK) cells, and Dendritic cells (DC), but not myeloid cells. Patients with γc chain gene deficiency (see Chapters 11 and 29) display defects in T, B, and NK cell development, and suffer from X-linked severe combined immunodeficiency.

LYMPHOPOIESIS

Lymphocytes start to differentiate into separate lineages early in fetal life. In humans, the embryonic yolk sac of the developing embryo is the first hematopoietic structure, which forms stem cells that develop into leukocytes, erythrocytes, and thrombocytes. Hematopoietic activity begins when the fetal liver receives stem cells from the yolk sac at the sixth week of gestation. NK cells are probably the first functionally active lymphocytes in the developing fetus and can be isolated from the fetal liver, prior to formation of the thymic rudiment. There is also evidence of extrathymic T cell development in the fetal liver, early in the development of the fetus. In the 12th week, a minor contribution is made to the production of blood cells by the spleen. At 20 weeks of gestation, thymus, lymph node, and bone marrow begin hematopoietic activity. The bone marrow becomes the sole hematopoietic center after 38 weeks. At that time, differentiated T and B lymphocytes appear in the circulation. In adults, T cells represent 55% to 84% of the circulating peripheral blood lymphocytes; B cells 6% to 25%, NK cells 5% to 27% and DC less than 1%.

Antigen-Specific T Cell and B Cell Receptors

A critical step in T lymphopoiesis and B lymphopoiesis is the complex process of forming functional, but not autoreactive, antigen-specific receptors. The tremendous diversity and specificity of the immune system is mediated by the T cell receptor (TcR) and the surface immunoglobulins (Igs) that constitute the B cell receptor (BcR) (Figs. 2 and 3). These receptors are somewhat similar in structure and are formed by a similar process. They are comprised of highly diverse, antigen-specific variable regions and more conserved constant regions. A nearly limitless array of diverse receptors is generated from a limited number of germline gene segments by V(D)J (V, variable; D, diversity; J, joining) recombination. (Figs. 1 and 2 in Chapter 7 and Fig. 4 in this chapter). Initiation of the V(D)J recombination requires the expression of RAG genes. V(D)J recombination proceeds via precise DNA cleavage initiated by the RAG proteins at short conserved signal sequences (see Chapter 7). Disruption or

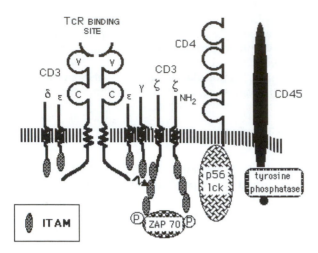

FIGURE 2 Diagrammatic representation of the T cell receptor (TcR) and its coreceptors on a mature CD4$^+$ T lymphocyte. The $\alpha\beta$ heterodimer is associated with the CD3$\gamma\delta\varepsilon\zeta$ complex, which contains tyrosine-based activation motifs. It is believed that activating signals are transmitted by the ζ chain. Coreceptors also contribute to the initial T cell activation. CD45 has intrinsic phosphatase activity and CD4 is associated to a p56lck tyrosine kinase. At least two more tyrosine kinases—p59fyn and zeta-associated p70 appear to play a role in the initial signaling cascade (see Chapter 11). *Abbreviations*: TcR, T cell receptor; ZAP, zeta-associated protein kinase.

deletion of RAG genes results in the absence of mature T and B lymphocytes, which are arrested at the progenitor stage prior to TcR and BcR gene rearrangement.

V(D)J recombination is tightly controlled by regulatory mechanisms that prevent TcR and BcR gene rearrangement in nonlymphoid tissues. For example, RAG expression is restricted to lymphocyte progenitors and developing lymphocytes. In addition, lineage-specific, *cis* elements control the accessibility of DNA regions to RAG-1 and RAG-2. This and other control processes ensures that TcR genes are only rearranged to completion in T lymphocytes and BcR genes are only rearranged to completion in B lymphocytes.

Due to the random nature of gene rearrangement, a productive V(D)J rearrangement occurs only about a third of the time. If rearrangement of one allele is nonproductive, the process will proceed on the second allele. However, by a mechanism called allelic exclusion, the generation of a functional protein will result in RAG inactivation and thus gene rearrangement on the second allele will not occur. Consequently, only one functional antigen-specific receptor will be expressed per developing T or B lymphocyte.

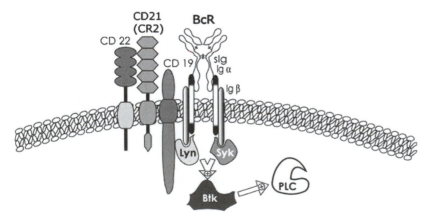

FIGURE 3 Diagrammatic representation of the B cell receptor (BcR) constituted by a membrane immunoglobulin molecule closely associated with Igα and Igβ molecules. Three additional molecules, CD19, CD21, and CD22 are associated with the BcR complex and play a role in B cell signaling. *Abbreviations*: BcR, B cell receptor; PLC, Phospholipase C.

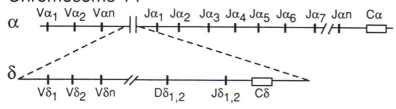

Chromosome 7

Chromosome 14

FIGURE 4 Genomic organization of the T cell receptor (TcR) genes. The genes for the β and γ chains rearrange independently at their own end of chromosome 7. The δ genes are in the middle of the α gene locus on chromosome 14. Rearrangement of the α genes leads to removal of the δ genes that are found as extrachromosomal DNA in cells that have productive rearrangements of the α and β genes yielding a $TcR2^+$ T cell. In $TcR1^+$ ($\gamma\delta$) T lymphocytes, the α and β genes are deleted.

The polypeptides comprising the TcR and BcR are members of the Ig gene superfamily, display similar macromolecular structures, and associate with homologous coreceptors. The short intracytoplasmic regions of these antigen-recognition receptors are not capable of signal transduction. The TcR and BcR associate in the cytoplasm with other molecules, forming receptor complexes, which are then transported to the cell membrane. The coreceptor molecules lend signal transduction capacity to the mature receptor complex. The selection process for the TcR and BcR provides a mechanism of deleting nonfunctional receptors or receptors that are autoreactive (see Chapter16).

A major difference between TcR and BcR is that once the rearrangements are completed in the thymus, the TcR will not change, whereas, the BcR will undergo additional gene modifications such as class switching and affinity maturation in the secondary lymphoid organs. The estimated diversity of $TcR\alpha\beta$ and $TcR\gamma\delta$ TcR (10^{15} to 10^{18}) exceeds the potential diversity of Igs (10^9 to 10^{11}) by several orders of magnitude.

Transcription Factors

Although this chapter focuses mainly on membrane markers, the critical role of transcription factors during lymphocyte ontogeny cannot be overlooked. Some transcription factors act at multiple stages of hematopoiesis and lymphopoiesis, whereas others play determinant roles and have the ability to drive an uncommitted precursor to a distinct lineage. Examples of such "commitment factors" are Pax-5 for B cell lineage commitment and Notch-1 for T cell lineage commitment.

Ikaros, part of a family of zinc finger transcription factors, is expressed in hematopoietic lineages including stem cells and myeloid pluripotent precursors. Ikaros is essential in activating c-kit and flt3 genes in those cell populations. Ikaros and related family members are also required for the development of all lymphocytes and act at multiple stages of differentiation from stem cells to mature lymphocytes. Ikaros is believed to drive cells toward lymphoid commitment by repressing expression of factors that lead to myeloid development.

T Lymphopoiesis

Unlike other bone-marrow derived lymphoid lineages, T cell development occurs almost exclusively in the thymus (Fig. 5). T-lymphopoiesis does not occur autonomously, but requires signals generated from the thymic stromal cells. A complex set of regulatory and growth factors acting in various combinations drives the T cell developmental choice points. Several stages at which specific regulators are required for T cell development to proceed have been defined. Interestingly, later in T cell development and its maturation these same regulatory factors influence T cell specialization. T cells are unique among the lymphocyte populations in their ability to further specialize as mature cells. In recent years, many sublineages of T cells have been described: the conventional TcR$\alpha\beta$ T cells; the so-called unconventional TcR$\gamma\delta$ T cells; NKT cells; and T regulatory cells (Treg). Details regarding the lineage commitment and developmental progression of the unconventional T cells are less well-described compared to the conventional T cells.

Stage One: Thymic Migration

Multipotent precursors enter the T cell pathway as they immigrate to the thymus. The most primitive cells in the thymus are the early thymocyte progenitors, which retain all lymphoid and myeloid potential but exist only transiently, rapidly differentiating into T and NK lineages, with a possible intermediate stage—the common lymphoid recursor.

Stage Two: Proliferative Expansion and T Lineage Commitment

Final commitment to the T cell lineage occurs within the thymic microenvironment. The c-Kit$^+$, IL-7R$^+$ T lymphocyte precursor cells proliferate rapidly once they reach the thymus, where IL-7 and c-kit ligand are plentiful. As ontogenic development proceeds, thymocytes express several enzymes of the purine salvage pathway, such as ADA and PNP, as well as Tdt.

Notch1, a member of a highly conserved Notch Family of signaling receptors, is upregulated on the early thymocytes and is essential for T cell lineage commitment. Features of Notch receptor proteins include an extracellular domain containing epidermal growth-factor like repeats and an intracellular signaling domain. When thymoctyes expressing Notch1 engage thymic stromal cells expressing Notch1 ligands, they become restricted to the T-cell lineage. Higher levels of Notch1 signaling are thought to favor T lymphocytes expressing TcR$\alpha\beta$ lineage over T lymphocytes expressing TcR$\gamma\delta$.

Early thymocytes do not express CD4 or CD8 and are known as double negative thymocytes (Fig. 5). Within the thymic cortex, the most primitive double negative T cells, which are CD44$^+$ and CD25$^-$, retain multipotential ability and can differentiate into cells of the myeloid or lymphoid lineages (B cells, DC, T cells, or NK cells). More differentiated double negative T cells (DN2 cells) are CD44$^+$ and CD25$^+$ and have more limited potentiality but are not yet fully restricted to the T cell lineage (they can still develop into DC, T cells, or NK cells). Later on, as the cells cease to express CD44 but remain CD25$^+$, they are fully committed to the T cell lineage. With the commitment to the T cell lineage, comes the simultaneous induction of T-cell specific gene expression and initiation of TcR gene rearrangement. At this point the cells become CD25$^-$ and the TcRβ rearrangement is initiated.

Productive rearrangement of the TcRα, β, γ, and δ genes can result in the generation of either of two types of receptors TcR1 ($\gamma\delta$ TcR) or TcR2 ($\alpha\beta$ TcR). TcR gene rearrangement, or V(D)J recombination, involves the transposition of noncontiguous segments of DNA and the deletion of intervening and noncoding sequences (Fig. 4). Transposition is mediated by the RAG. The β and γ chain genes are located in distant regions of chromosome 7, whereas the α and δ chain genes are located on chromosome 14. The generation of the extensive diversity needed for a complete TcR repertoire relies almost exclusively on the D regions, where extensive of random nucleotide addition occurs, particularly at the DJ junction. Of the four genes available for TcR synthesis, only the β and δ genes contain D regions. As such β and δ chains display hypervariability as compared to the less polymorphic α and γ chains.

TcR gene rearrangement occurs in an ordered and sequential fashion. Due to the chromosomal organization of the TcR genes, the TcRγ and TcRδ genes are rearranged before the TcRα and TcRβ genes. The δ gene is located in the middle of the α chain gene, between Vα and Jα regions. When RAG transposes the elements of the δ genes to form a VδJδ complex, it eliminates the V and J regions of the α gene. The rearranged δ chain pairs with the γ chain. T cells expressing TcR1 ($\gamma\delta$ TcR) leaves the thymus to migrate to the skin and mucosae.

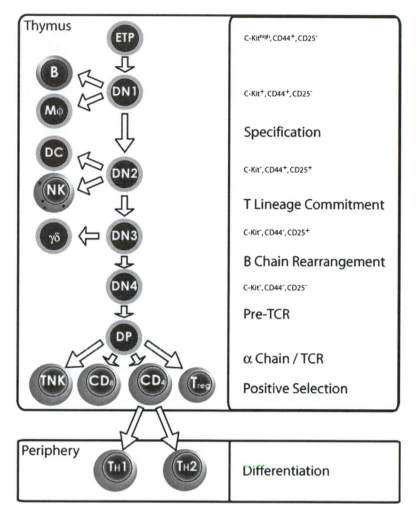

FIGURE 5 Schematic representation of intra-thymic T lymphopoiesis. Early thymocyte progenitors give rise to double negative (DN) thymocytes, which become increasingly committed to the T-cell lineage in thymic cortex. DN1 retain myeloid and B-cell potential. DN2 retain dendritic cell and natural killer cell potential. DN3 are T-cell lineage committed. DN4 give rise to double positive (DP) thymocytes expressing the $\alpha\beta$ T cell receptor cells and both CD4 and CD8. In the thymic medulla, mature single positive CD4 and CD8 T cells emerge, as well as natural killer T cells and regulatory T cells emerge from the DP population. Further differentiation into T helper (Th)1 and Th2 occurs in the periphery. *Abbreviations*: DC, dendritic cells; ETP, early T cell progenitors; NK, natural killer cell; TCR, T-cell receptor.

Stage Three: β-Selection

The rearrangement of the TcRβ gene occurs in two steps. First, Dβ-to-Jβ rearrangement, followed by the Vβ-to-DβJβ rearrangement. Finally, the Cβ region gene is added to the VβDβJβ. The productively rearranged β chain triggers the inactivation of the RAG genes, so that rearrangements on the second allele do not take place. The phenomenon of allelic exclusion, originally described for Ig synthesis (see Chapter 7), also exists for TcR synthesis.

The productively rearranged β chain will be present in the cytoplasm for several days prior to TcRα gene rearrangement. During that period, β chain will associate with a protective polypeptide, known as the pre-Tα. When the β chain/pre-Tα associates with CD3 molecules and is transported to the cell membrane the pre-TcR is formed. CD3 is a complex of 5 unique subunits designated γ, δ, ε, ζ and η (note that the γ and δ chains of the CD3 unit are distinct from the $\gamma\delta$ chains of the TcR1). The CD3$\gamma\delta\varepsilon$ trimolecular complex is synthesized first and remains intracytoplasmic, where it becomes associated with pre-Tα molecules.

Soon thereafter, the CD3ζ chains are synthesized and become associated to the CD3 complex. Once the ζ chain has been added to the CD3 molecule, the whole CD3-pre-Tα complex is transported from the Golgi apparatus to the cell membrane. A critical characteristic of the ζ chain is its long intracytoplasmic tail, which has affinity for the zeta-associated protein kinase (ZAP70). The association of ZAP70 to the ζ chain is critical for further differentiation of the T cell. The congenital absence of ZAP70 is associated with a block at the DN stage of T cell development.

Signaling through the pre-TcR generates activation signals, which lead to a cascade of proliferation and differentiation, such as the coexpression of CD4 and CD8—characteristic of the double-positive thymocyte population. These cells re-express their RAG genes and undergo TcRα gene rearrangement. Rearrangement of the TcRα gene results in the deletion of the δ gene, which will appear as extrachromosomal circular DNA in germline configuration. Upon successful rearrangement of the VαJαCα chain, the pre-Tα chain of the pre-TcR is replaced by the newly synthesized α chain and the TcR2, ($\alpha\delta$ with a full complement of CD3 molecules, is inserted in the T cell membrane (Fig. 2).

Stage Four: T Cell Receptors Selection

TcR selection occurs in the thymic medulla where the double-positive thymocytes encounter epithelial cells expressing major histocompatibility complex (MHC) class I and II molecules. Only 2% to 3% of the differentiating thymocytes, those that express TcR capable of interaction with MHC molecules, but tolerant to self-peptides, survive the selection process. Many newly formed thymocytes are subject to negative selection, probably as a consequence of several different sets of circumstances. Some are eliminated because the TcR is abnormal (the recombination process resulted in out-of-frame rearrangements), or because the resulting TcR is unable to interact with MHC molecules. A small percentage of double-positive thymocytes are thought to die from apoptosis because their interaction with the MHC-peptide complexes is too strong (they would be activated by self-peptides). The recognition of self-peptides in the thymus is likely to involve both thymic-derived peptides and peptides of extra-thymic origin. During the time T cells are differentiating, extensive development of most other tissues is taking place, hence, large numbers of cells are undergoing apoptotic death. This results in the extensive release of self-antigens, which are eventually captured by the thymic epithelial cells, and presented to the pre-T cells in the context of self-MHC. The thymocytes whose TcR interact strongly with MHC-peptide complexes receive apoptotic signals and are eliminated. This negative selection process is critical to the development of self-tolerance during embryonic differentiation (see Chapter 16).

Positive selection results in the selection of thymocytes that express a TcR capable of interaction with MHC molecules but fails to recognize the self-peptides associated to the MHC molecules. If the TcR is MHC class I-restricted, CD8 must also associate with MHC class I. The CD8-TcR-MHC class I interaction results in the activation of repressor genes that turn off CD4 expression. Conversely, double positive T cells that have MHC class II-restricted TcR engage CD4, and the expression of CD8 is turned off. The single positive CD4 or CD8 T cells emerging from the medulla leave the thymus and colonize the peripheral lymphoid organs.

The positive signal delivered to the double positive thymocytes through these TcR-MHC interactions involves CD45 and the lymphocyte-specific tyrosine kinase, p56lck. These molecules are utilized by both CD4 and CD8 T cells. As the TcR interacts with MHC, the phosphatase activity of CD45 is upregulated and ZAP70 is activated. Both activities contribute to the dephosphorylation of p56lck, which becomes activated. The activation of p56lck is critical for further differentiation of T cell, because mice deficient in either CD45 or p56lck cannot proceed beyond the double positive stage. Also critical is the proper expression of MHC molecules. MHC class-I deficient mice do not develop normal numbers of CD8$^+$ T cells, while class-II deficient mice or humans do not develop normal numbers of CD4$^+$ T cells.

Stage Five: Continuing Differentiation in the Periphery

It was previously believed that the human thymus remained active as the site of T cell differentiation only until early adulthood and that later in adult life the thymus became atrophic. However, several recent reports indicate that the human thymus is active throughout adult life. Thus several factors may contribute to the supply of T cells in adult life, generation in the thymus, extrathymic differentiation, and the fact that memory T cells are long-lived and survive for decades.

Transcription Factors Controlling T Cell Development

The key components that drive precursor cell toward the T lineage are the levels of NOTCH, E proteins, and GATA-enhancer binding protein 3 (GATA-3). The Notch pathway is involved in embryonic viability, HSC self-renewal, and plays an established role in T lineage commitment. Notch1 is essential for T cell commitment and early thymocyte development. When activated, the intracellular domain of Notch1 is cleaved off and translocates to the nucleus where it activates T cell-specific gene expression. The transcription factor GATA-3 is expressed in a T cell-specific manner and is required for T cell development. During T cell development, GATA-3 is important in the β selection and positive selections stages by regulating the expression of RAG-2, TcR gene enhancers, and CD4. E proteins, such as E2A, are important in the regulation of CD4, RAG-1/RAG-2, and GATA.

Unconventional T Cells

The thymus also gives rise to the so-called unconventional T cells such at $\gamma\delta$ T cells, Natural Killer T cells (NKT) and regulatory T cells (Treg).

$\gamma\delta$ T Cells

$\gamma\delta$ T cells expressing TcR1 represent only 1% to 5% of the circulating T cells, but are abundant in the mucosal immune system and the skin, where they represent the dominant T cell population. These non-MHC restricted T cells are involved in specific primary immune responses, tumor surveillance, immune regulation and wound healing. Factors that drive a thymocyte to the $\alpha\beta$ or $\gamma\delta$ TcR lineage are not well-understood.

Several differences between $\alpha\beta$ and $\gamma\delta$ T cell development have been described. $\gamma\delta$ T cells do not pass through the critical CD4/CD8 double positive stage of the $\alpha\beta$ T cells, they are positively, rather than negatively, selected on cognate self-antigen and they emigrate the thymus in "waves" of clonal populations, which are home to discrete tissues. For example, Vγ9Vδ2 TcR cells are found in the peripheral blood while Vδ2 predominate in the intestinal tract.

Natural Killer T Cells

Human NK T cells are a unique population, which express a semi-invariant form of the TcR2 (Vα24Jα18/Vβ11) and NK cell markers such as CD56 and KIR. They recognize glycolipid antigens presented in association with CD1d, an MHC molecule that associates with β2 microglobulin. NKT cells are thought to play an important role in tumor immunity and immunoregulation.

T Regulatory Cells

CD4$^+$, CD25$^+$ regulatory T cells, are also referred to as naturally occurring regulatory T cells. Tregs comprised about 5% of the circulating CD4$^+$ T cells. These cells are thought to possess important autoimmunity property by regulating autoreactive T cells in the periphery. The transcription factor foxp3 appears to correlate with the Treg activity.

Natural Killer Cell Ontogeny

Although considered part of the innate immune system, NK cells are more closely related to T cells than to other cells of the innate immune system. NK cells not only share many surface markers and functional activities in common with T lymphocytes, they also arise from a common bipotential progenitor (the T/NK precursor). The T/NK precursor population is also believed to be the source of a subpopulation of DC, which expresses lymphoid phenotypic markers, in contrast with the predominant population of DC that are of myeloid lineage.

Phenotypically mature NK cells are defined as CD3$^-$, CD16$^\pm$, CD56$^+$ lymphocytes. Although committed NK progenitors can be found in the thymus, NK cells can develop in athymic nude mice; therefore, the thymus is not required for NK development. It is believed that NK cells can develop in a variety of organs; however, the major site of NK cell development has yet to be identified.

A multi-stage model of NK cell development indicates that IL-15, c-kit ligand and Flt3 ligand are required for both the differentiation (IL-15) and expansion (c-kit ligand and Flt3 ligand) of functionally active NK cells. The expression of γc seems critical for NK cell development; γc knock-out mice lack NK cells. NK cell maturation also requires the T cell-derived cytokine, IL-21.

In humans, the majority (85–90%) of the NK cells are CD56$^+$, CD16$^+$, CD3$^-$ and have a high cytolytic capacity. A smaller subset (10–15%) express high levels of CD56 (CD56^{bright}), little or no CD16, and in addition they express IL-2Rα (CD25) and c-kit (CD117). The CD56^{bright} NK cell subset is chiefly responsible for cytokine production and has an enhanced survival capacity. In the periphery, the CD56^{bright} NK cells also express the lymph node homing receptors. At the lymph nodes, they differentiate into functionally mature CD56$^+$, CD16$^+$, CD3$^-$ NK cells which express killer cell immunoglobulin-like receptors (KIR), natural cytotoxicity receptors (NCR), and critical adhesion molecules.

Dendritic Cell Ontogeny

DC are highly specialized, highly efficient, antigen-presenting cells. Although, these cells were originally thought be of the myeloid lineage (referred to as myeloid dendritic cells), it is now recognized that a subset of DC of the lymphoid lineage also exists (referred to as plasmacytoid dendritic cells). The development and regulation of DC is not well-characterized. DC may represent a unique hematopoietic lineage with a more plastic developmental pathway than that followed by the conventional myeloid and lymphoid lineages. Several models of DC ontogeny have been proposed including a common precursor and lineage conversion. Some studies have shown that both the common lymphocytic and the common myeloid progenitors can give rise to either plasmacytoid or myeloid DC. While the DC precursors have been identified in the human fetal liver, thymus, and bone marrow, during adult life DC are thought to be produced from the bone marrow and released into the periphery.

B Lymphopoiesis

B-lymphopoiesis occurs exclusively in the bone marrow (Fig. 6). B lymphocytes are made continuously throughout life in the human bone marrow. The microenvironment in the bone marrow is composed of stromal cells, extracellular matrix, cytokines, and growth factors, which are critical for proliferation, differentiation, and survival of early lymphocyte and B-lineage precursors. The relative proportion of precursor B cells in the bone marrow remains constant throughout the life span of the organism. Pre-B-I cells comprise about 5% to 10% of the total. Pre-B-II cells represent 60% to 70% while the remaining 20% to 25% are immature B cells. Immature B cells then migrate to the spleen where they go through transitional stages before final maturation.

B lymphocytes are identified by the presence of sIg. After antigenic stimulation, B cells differentiate into plasma cells that secrete large quantities of Igs. Within a single cell or a clone of identical cells, the antibody-binding sites of sIg and that expressed on the cell membrane are identical. B-lymphopoiesis can be divided into distinct stages based on the sequential expression, or loss, of cell surface or intracellular proteins, and Ig gene rearrangement. Deregulation of B-lymphopoiesis can lead to autoimmunity, leukemia, or lymphoma. The most critical aspects in B-lymphopoiesis are the Ig gene rearrangement and expression of the pre-BcR and the BcR. Pre-BcR and BcR receptors signaling play a crucial role at the developmental checkpoints such as negative selection, anergy, receptor editing, and positive selection.

Progenitor B Cells

In the bone marrow, the earliest cells in B lymphopoiesis are referred to as the progenitor B cells (pro-B cells), which express c-kit, Flt3, Tdt, RAG, CD34, and CD45RA, but no lineage-specific markers. Coinciding with the onset of RAG expression, μIg heavy (μIgH) gene rearrangements

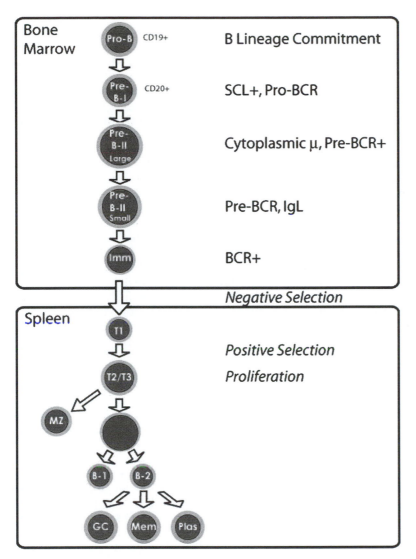

FIGURE 6 Schematic representation of B lymphopoiesis in the bone marrow and spleen. The completion of the immunoglobulin heavy (IgH) D to J rearrangement marks the transition from progenitor B cells (pro-B cells) to B cell precursors (Pre-B). Pre-BI expresses a pro-B cell receptor (pro-BcR) while pre-BII expresses cytoplasmic IgHμ and the pre-BcR. After light (IgL) chain rearrangement, the complete BcR is expressed on the immature B cells, which migrate to the spleen. Selection and maturation of immature B cells occurs through a series of transitional B cells, (T1, T2/T3). Mature B cells are classified into two to three lineages B-1, B-2, and marginal zone B cells. The B-2 lineage, or follicular B cells, is composed of conventional B cells—memory, germinal center, and plasma cells. *Abbreviations*: BcR, B cell receptor; GC, germinal center; Imm, immature; Mem, memory; MZ, marginal zone; Plas, plasma cells.

begin. The D to J gene segment rearrangement on both alleles is initiated, but not completed, at the pro-B cell stage. At this stage the pro-B cell is not fully committed to the B cell lineage.

Like TcR gene rearrangement, Ig genes rearrangement occurs in an ordered fashion. μIgH genes are the first to be rearranged, followed by Igκ, and, finally, byIgλ. μIgH variable region exons are assembled from component V, D, and J gene segments; Igκ and Igλ light chain variable regions are assembled from component V and J gene segments. Most B cells express the functional product of only one IgH allele and one IgL allele as a consequence of allelic exclusion (see Chapter 7). Cells in which the first V(D)J rearrangement at the μIgH, Igκ, or Igλ locus that was nonproductive, will proceed with V to (D)J rearrangement of the second allele.

B Cell Precursors

B cell precursors (pre-B cells) exist in two distinct stages, pre-BI and pre-BII. The pre-BI cells still express c-kit and have a unique capacity for self-renewal (extended proliferation at the same stage of differentiation). During the pre-BI stage, the μIgH D to J gene segment rearrangement on both alleles is completed. Rearrangement of the V region gene segments has been initiated, but the μIgH chain is not yet expressed in the cytoplasm. Pre-BI cells have down regulated Tdt and CD34. They express genes specific to the B-lineage (CD19, CD20, Igα, Igβ) and are committed to the B-lineage. A surrogate light chain associates with other proteins to form the pro-BcR that is expressed on the surface or the pre-B-I cells.

Pre-BII cells downregulate c-kit and upregulate CD2, CD25, and CD72. In addition, μIgH rearrangement is completed during the pre-BII stage. The resultant VDJ variable region exon is then linked to the μ constant region exon via RNA splicing to form a cytoplasmic μIgH chain. The product of a functionally rearranged μIgH chain from the first allele prevents initiation of V to DJ gene rearrangement on the second allele, and the RAG expression is terminated. The expression of the μIgH chain on the cell membrane is required for allelic exclusion to occur.

Successful VDJ rearrangements of the μIgH chain gene result in the high levels of cytoplasmic μIgH chain expression. The μIgH chain associates with surrogate light chains and the signaling components Igα and Igβ (CD79a and CD79b) to form the pre-BcR, which is expressed on the membrane of the pre-BII cells. The physiological role of surrogate light chains seems to be that of a stabilizer, protecting nascent μIgH chains from degradation, until light chain synthesis is turned on. The expression of surrogate light chains is critical to normal B cell development. Patients defective in the genes coding for surrogate light chains have a severe form of B cell deficiency.

Although the pre-BcR is only transiently expressed on the pre-B cell, signaling through the pre-BcR is essential for the selection, proliferation, and differentiation of pre-B cells. Pre-BcR expression serves as a checkpoint that monitors for functional μIgH chain rearrangement, triggers clonal expansion and developmental progression of surface IgM$^+$ pre-B cells. The pre-BcR is not activated in an antigen-specific manner, but via interaction with stromal cells. Pre-BcR signaling regulates the pre-B cell proliferative phase by a negative feedback mechanism. The interaction of the surrogate light chains with complementary proteins induces internalization of the pre-BcR and subsequent suppression of surrogate light chain synthesis, followed by re-expression of the RAG genes. During the second wave of RAG expression, further arrangement of the μIgH loci are prevented, as the chromatin is no longer accessible to RAG. Because these pre-BII cells are cycling, they are also referred to as large pre-B cells. After cellular proliferation subsides, the pre-BII cells are also referred to as small pre-B cells. These cells no longer express the pre-BcR and μIgH chain accumulates in the cytoplasm. The small pre-BII cells express CD2, CD22, CD45RA, and MHC class II. The second wave of RAG expression occurs in the small pre-BII cells and promotes the rearrangement of the Ig light (IgL) chain (V$_L$J$_L$), resulting synthesis of IgL chains. By a process known as IgL isotype exclusion, an individual B cells will produce only one type of light chain (Igκ or Igλ). In pre-B cells, the Igκ locus is rearranged first. Only cells that fail to generate a productive Igκ chain will go on to rearrange the Igλ locus. Once a productive IgL is formed, it will pair with the previously rearranged μIgH chain to create a mature BcR. In the bone marrow the majority of the cells are CD19$^+$, membrane IgM$^+$, characteristics shared by pre-BII cells and immature B cells. Cell fate decisions at specific antigen-independent checkpoints are controlled by the pre-BcR and BcR. There are many similarities as well as significant differences in the signaling by the pre-BcR and the BcR. Notably the pre-BcR is able to stimulate proliferative expansion in a cell-autonomous fashion. Activation signals from the pre-BcR and BcR involves the phosphorylation of tyrosine-based activation motifs (ITAMs) present in Igα and Igβ. This complex contains three classes of activated protein tyrosine kinases (PTKs)—Src family kinase, Lyn (Syk/Zap70 kinase), and the Tec-family kinase (Btk); as well as other proteins including the adapter molecule, phosphoinositide 3-kinase (PI3K), and phospholipase C-γ2.

B Cell Maturation

Immature B cells are characterized as resting cells (not cycling) that express CD19, sIgM, Igα, and Igβ, but are sIgD$^-$. Like the small pre-B-II cells, RAG-2 expression is high in the immature

B cells, indicating that additional IgL gene rearrangement can still occur. Final differentiation occurs when RAG expression is terminated.

Immature B cells leave the bone marrow and emigrate to the spleen where they advance through several developmental stages before final maturation. Signaling through the BcR plays a key role in inducing the elimination of self-reactive B cells during the final stages of differentiation. Immature and transitional B cells expressing BcR reactive with self-antigens are either eliminated by selective death or become anergic and thus fail to progress through subsequent developmental stages. Cell fate—death (by apoptosis) or anergy—is determined by the strength of the BcR signal, ligand density, as well as other factors. Negative selection in the immature B cells may occur in the bone marrow or in the periphery (spleen); positive selection occurs in the periphery. Positive selection, the survival and subsequent development of transitional B cells, requires that a subthreshold survival signal be generated through the BcR. Failure to receive such antiapoptotic signals will result in cell death.

The immature B cells are $CD19^+$, $sIgM^{high}$, $sIgD^{low}$, $CD21^-$, $CD23^-$. Most of immature T cells entering the spleen are negatively selected. They most likely undergo clonal deletion or anergy as evident by their lack of expression of survival factor, Bcl-2 and high expression of the pro-apoptotic molecule, FAS (CD95). The surviving cells display a phenotype close to that of a mature B cell, $CD19^+$, $sIgM^{high}$, $sIgD^{high}$, $CD21^{high}$, and $CD23^{high}$. BcR signaling of these cells results in extensive proliferation.

Mature B cells express phenotype CD19, sIgM, and sIgD. About 80% of adult B cells are found in the lymph node follicle (follicular B cells), and this population include memory B cells, germinal center B cells, and plasma cells (terminally differentiated). Differentiation of the mature B cells into germinal center B cells, memory B cells, or Ig-secreting plasma cells can occur in the spleen, lymph nodes, or mucosa associated lymphoid tissue. Recirculating peripheral B cells express CD23 and CD24. Human memory B cells are characterized by CD27 expression. Most plasma cells are home in the bone marrow, and, to a lesser extent, in the spleen, and peripheral tissues. A small percentage of B cells will differentiate into the marginal zone (MZ) pool, which is uniquely located in the MZ of the spleen. These cells exist in a pre-activated state, enabling them to rapidly respond. They are key players in T-independent responses and are responsible for early antibody production in primary T-dependent responses. Typically this population displays a phenotype of $sIgM^{high}$, $sIgD^{lo}$, $CD19^+$, $CD21^+$, and $CD23^-$. Because of their role in rapid antibody production and the fact that they express Toll-like receptors, MZ B cells are thought to be cells that bridge the innate and the adaptive immune systems.

Isotype Switching

Around birth, mature, resting B cells coexpress sIgM and sIgD on their membranes. The sIgM and sIgD expressed on individual B cell clones have the same antigenic specificity. These mature, naïve B lymphocytes home to secondary lymphoid organs where, upon antigenic challenge, they downmodulate sIgD and, less constantly, sIgM. Activated B cells undergo subsequent heavy chain constant region gene rearrangements or isotype switching by a process called class switch recombination (Fig. 3 in Chapter 7). Hence the same variable region can be associated with a different heavy chain isotype (IgG, IgE, or IgA). The resultant sIg of different isotypes are expressed on nonoverlapping B cell subsets, sometimes in association with sIgM.

In addition to isotype switching, activated B cells undergo antibody affinity maturation by a process called somatic hypermutation, which results in the emergence and selection of B cell clones producing antibodies of similar specificity but higher affinity (see Chapter 7).

Ontogenic Development of Immunoglobulin Synthesis

A normal newborn infant, though having differentiated B lymphocytes, produces very small amounts of Igs for the first two to three months of life. During that period of time, the newborn is protected by placentally-transferred maternal IgG, which starts to cross the placenta at the 12th week of gestation. By the 3rd month of age, IgM antibodies produced by the newborn are usually detectable. The concentration of circulating IgM reaches adult levels by one year. In cases of intra-uterine infection, IgM antibodies are synthesized in relatively large amounts by the fetus and detected in cord blood by conventional assays. The onset of the synthesis of IgG and IgA occurs later and the concentration of these reaches adult levels at six to seven years.

Transcription Factors Essential for B Cell Differentiation

B lymphopoiesis requires three transcription factors, E proteins (E2A and EBF), and Pax5. E2A and EBF act in concert to drive the differentiation of common lymphocyte precursors toward the B-lineage pathway by activating B cell-restricted gene expression and μIgH chain gene rearrangements. Commitment to the B-cell lineage is orchestrated by Pax5, which simultaneously represses the transcription of B-cell lineage-inappropriate and activates the expression of B-cell lineage-specific genes. Terminal differentiation of B cells to memory cells and plasma cells depends on the transcriptional repressor Blimp-1.

Regulation of Lymphopoiesis and Immune Responses by Opposing Signaling Events

The immune system is controlled by balance of stimulatory and inhibitory signals mediated by lymphocyte membrane markers. While the presence of inhibitory receptors was first recognized in NK cells and subsets of T cells, inhibitory receptors are also found on B cells, monocytes, macrophages, and DC. Engagement of activation receptors on lymphocytes can induce cellular migration, proliferation, differentiation, anergy, or apoptosis. Several factors that influence the outcome include: antigen concentration; binding avidity; duration of antigen recognition; association with costimulatory molecules; cytokines; and the developmental stage of the lymphocyte. Engagement of cellular inhibitory receptors will inhibit functional responses. In most cases conserved sequences within the cytoplasmic domains of the receptors and/or association with intracellular adapter proteins mediates the activation or inhibitory cascade.

Most inhibitory receptors contain one or more copies of the conserved tyrosine-based inhibitory motif (ITIM), Ile/Val/Leu/Ser-x-Tyr-x-x-Leu/Val, within the cytoplasmic domain. Upon receptor ligation, inhibitory signaling is mediated by tyrosine phosphorylation within this region and the subsequent recruitment of the tyrosine-specific phosphatases, SHP-1 and SHP-2 or the phospholipid-specific phosphatases, SHIP. In general, these phosphatases work by degrading phosphatidylinositol triphosphate or decreasing the phosphorylation of intracellular signaling proteins such as ZAP70, Syk, and pospholipase Cγ

In a similar fashion, activation receptors share common signaling pathways mediated by the transmembrane association with adapter proteins containing the conserved tyrosine-based activation motif (ITAM), Asp/Glu/-x-x-Tyr-x-xLeu/Ile-x_{6-8}-Tyr-x-x/Leu/Ile. Upon tyrosine-phosphorylation of ITAM, the tyrosine kinases Syk and ZAP70 are recruited via their SH2 domains and stimulate the activation of intracellular signaling proteins. ITAM-containing adapter proteins include FcϵRIγ and CD3ζ.

LYMPHOCYTE MEMBRANE MARKERS

The list of lymphocyte membrane markers and transcription factors continues to grow. Membrane markers include a wide variety of functional proteins, such as antigen-specific receptors, costimulatory molecules, adhesion molecules, inhibitory receptors, growth factor receptors, cytokine receptors, chemokine receptors, and receptors that mediate cell death. Membrane markers can be shared as various hematopoietic and nonhematopoietic cell types, be pan-lineage specific, or lineage subset specific. Pan-lineage specific markers are common to all cells of a given lineage, whereas, subset-specific markers are present on only a subpopulation of cells of a given lineage. For example, all leucocytes express CD45 albeit at different levels—lymphocytes express the highest level of CD45, monocytes express intermediate levels, and neutrophils, low levels; CD3 and CD19 are pan-T cell and pan-B cell-specific markers, respectively; and CD4 and CD8 represent subset-specific T cell markers.

Most of the membrane markers on leukocytes are members of the Ig gene superfamily. The notable feature of these proteins is the presence of one or more Ig-like domains (see Chapter 5). These domains—approximately 100 amino acids in length—are characterized by a common fold formed between two antiparallel β-sheets stabilized by a disulfide bond. The result is a conserved structural platform that allows for the display of unique determinants required for specific ligand binding.

T Lymphocyte Markers

T cells are often referred to as "directors" of the adaptive-immune response and are discussed in detail in Chapters 2 and 4. Upon antigen-specific activation, they can provide help to B cells, influence the type of immune response via their cytokine secretion profile, or engage in cytolytic activity. Approximately three-quarters of peripheral blood mononuclear cells are T lymphocytes, and among T lymphocytes, $CD4^+$ cells often referred to as T helper cells predominate over $CD8^+$ cells, or cytotoxic T lymphocytes (CTL) by a 2:1 ratio.

CD4 is expressed on most thymocytes, two-thirds of T cells and monocytes. CD4 defines the T helper cell population and binds to MHC Class II antigens during antigen-specific TcR binding. CD4 is also the binding receptor for HIV-1.

CD8 is expressed on most thymocytes, one-third of T cells, and some NK cells. CD8, which binds to MHC Class I antigens during antigen-specific TcR binding, can be expressed as a $CD8\alpha\beta$ heterodimer or $CD8\alpha\alpha$ homodimer. $CD8\alpha\beta$ is only found on $TcR\alpha\beta$ T cells, the CTL. $CD8\alpha\alpha$ can be found on NK cells, $\gamma\delta$ T cells or $\alpha\beta$ T cells.

Markers Associated with T Cell Signaling and Activation
T Cell Receptor
Although the structure of the $\alpha\beta$TcR has been more extensively characterized than the structure of the $\gamma\delta$TcR both heterodimers are believed to have a similar structure. The comparison of the general characteristics of TcR and BcR reveals many similarities, as well as notable differences. The α (acidic) chain is about 40 to 50 Kd, whereas, the β (basic) chain is slightly smaller, 40 to 45 Kd. Each chain is composed of an extracellular, a transmembrane, and an intracytoplasmic domain. Like the BcR, the TcR has a small intracytoplasmic region. In the extracellular domain, the constant region is about 120 to 140 amino acids and the variable domains 100 to 120 amino acids. The variable regions are located on the amino-terminal end of each chain. Their length is similar to that of the Ig variable regions. The hypervariable regions within the variable domain form the antigen-binding site, unique for each TcR. Monoclonal antibodies generated against the antigen-binding site of the TcR detect idiotypic specificity unique to that particular TcR or T cell clone. The surface area of the antigen-binding site on the TcR is similar to that of the BcR, yet the degree of genetic diversity for TcR is more extensive.

CD3
CD3 is first expressed during thymic differentiation and continues to be expressed in all mature T cells in the periphery. CD3 is a complex of five unique, invariant chains [$\gamma\delta\varepsilon\zeta\eta$ (Fig. 2)]. The cytoplasmic domains of the CD3ζ chain contain ITAM motifs and are responsible for signaling. The ζ chain also associates with CD16 and functions as the signaling domain of that receptor expressed on NK cells. Phosphorylated ITAM motifs of the CD3ζ chain bind to SH2 domains of the intracellular signaling molecules, for example, ZAP70.

CD28
CD28 is the dominant costimulatory pathway in T cell activation resulting from the interaction of CD28 with the B lymphocyte antigens CD80 and CD86 (see Chapter 11).

TNF Receptor Family
Several members of the tumor necrosis factor receptor (TNFR) family (CD27, CD30, CD137, CD154) have costimulatory effects on T cells. Their expression is regulated and transiently expressed, and they are key mediators of generating survival signals, sustaining responses, and generating effector/memory populations. Members of the TNF family are involved in cancer, infectious diseases, autoimmunity, and transplantation and thus are attractive therapeutic targets.

CD40 Ligand (CD40L, CD154)

CD40 ligand is one of the first activation-induced cell surface molecules expressed on T cells. It is expressed on all activated $CD4^+$ cells and a small population of $CD8^+$ cells and $\gamma\delta$ T cells. CD154 interacts with CD40, expressed on B cells. This interaction is required for the development and maturation of T-dependent B lymphocyte responses. As discussed in Chapter 29, the lack of expression of the CD154 is the molecular basis of most cases of a unique immunodeficiency disease known as hyper-IgM syndrome.

CD27

CD27 has recently been identified as a costimulatory molecule expressed on most T and NK cells and is induced on primed B cells. Its activity is regulated by the transiently expressed TNF-like ligand CD70 expressed on T cells, B cells, and DC. The CD27–CD70 system acts by increase cell survival and is important in effector and memory cell formation.

4-1BB (CD137)

4-1BB (CD137) is transiently expressed on activated T cells. 4-1BB ligand is expressed on DC, B cells, and macrophages. Signaling through 4-1BB can activate T cells, but the major effect is to prolong survival in activated cells. Interest in 4-1BB as a cancer therapeutic comes from the fact that antibodies to 4-1BB have been found to enhance CD8 expansion and interferon γ production.

CD30 and CD30 Ligand

CD30 is expressed on activate TcR1 and TcR2 T cells. CD30 ligand (CD153) is expressed on resting B cells and activated cells. Like other members of the TNFR family, CD30 activation results in enhanced proliferation and cytokine secretion.

CD25

CD25 is the α chain of the IL-2 receptor, or the low-affinity IL-2R. CD25 is expressed at low levels by about 30% of resting lymphocytes and is upregulated upon activation. Thus, CD25 expression can be used as an indicator of the number of activated lymphocytes. As mentioned earlier, $CD4^+$ T cells expressing high levels of CD25 represent a unique unconventional T cell population, regulatory T cell population (Treg).

CD2 and LFA-3 (CD58)

CD2 is expressed on all thymocytes, T cells, and NK cells. The heterotypic interaction between CD2 and its major ligand leukocyte function antigen-3 (LFA-3, CD58) enhances T cell antigen recognition. CD2 engagement by LFA-3 expressed on an APC stimulates T cell proliferation and differentiation (see Chapter 11).

CD45: Isoforms

CD45, expressed by all leukocytes, is a major cell surface component occupying up to 10% of the surface. CD45 plays an important role in T lymphocyte activation, due to the fact that its intracytoplasmic domain has tyrosine phosphatase activity. Three isoforms (CD45RA, CD45RB, CD45RO), generated by alternate splicing of nuclear RNA, have been identified. These isoforms share the intracellular domains, but vary in their extracellular domains. The ontogenic development of the CD45 isoforms is not clear, but in mature lymphocytes their expression becomes restricted. CD45RA is expressed both by naive and memory $CD4^+$ T cells. In the case of naive populations, CD45 is coexpressed with CD62L, while memory T cells either express CD45RA only, or switch from CD45RA to CD45RO. $CD45RO^+$ T cells are considered either as primed T lymphocytes or as memory T lymphocytes (the expression of this marker seems to be maintained long after the primary response has waned).

CD71

CD71, the transferrin receptor, is a type II membrane glycoprotein that is upregulated during leukocyte activation. The CD71 homodimer associates with $CD3\zeta$ suggesting a role in signal transduction. The CD71-controlled supply of iron to the cell is important during proliferative responses.

CD69

CD69 is a lectin receptor encoded in a region of chromosome 12 known as the "NK gene complex." CD69 is expressed on a variety of hematopoietic cells. CD69 is absent on resting lymphocytes but rapidly upregulated during activation of T, B, and NK cells. Because monoclonal antibodies directed against CD69 can activate lymphocytes, a role for CD69 in signal transduction has been suggested.

ICAM-1, -2, -3, and LFA-1 (CD11a/18)

Intercellular cell adhesion molecule (ICAM)-I (CD54), is expressed by both hematopoietic and nonhematopoietic cell types. The expression on leukocytes is upregulated during activation. Similarly, the expression on the endothelium is upregulated during inflammation. ICAM-1, ICAM-2 (CD102), and ICAM-3 (CD53) are all coreceptors for the integrin LFA-1. LFA-1 is a heterodimer composed of CD11a and CD18, which is expressed on APC and other leukocytes. ICAM-1 also binds to other related integrins such as those that share CD18 but express unique CD11 chains—(MAC-1) (CD11b/CD18) and p150, 95 (CD11c/CD18). LFA-1 and ICAM are expressed by T, B, and NK cells and are responsible for homotypic adhesion. An LFA-1 expressing cell will bind with the counter receptor on another cell type and vice versa.

Markers Associated with T Cell Downregulation

Inhibitory receptors first identified on NK cells are also found on subsets of T cells and are discussed subsequently.

CTLA-4 (CD152)

Cytotoxic T cell Late Antigen (CTLA)-4, CD152 binds the same ligands as CD28 (CD80 and CD86), but with a much higher affinity. Unlike CD28, which is constitutively expressed, CTLA4 is upregulated on activated T cells. CTLA4 engagement results in downregulation of T cell responses induced by CD28 signaling. CTLA4 is thought to be important in establishing peripheral T cell tolerance.

NATURAL KILLER CELLS

NK cells, part of the innate immune system, are considered one of the first lines of defense against infection. NK cells, active in the naive, or nonimmunized host, do not require prior antigen exposure, or priming, nor do they express the exquisitely specific antigen receptors found on T and B cells. They possess potent cytolytic activity and produce an array of immunoregulatory cytokines and chemokines (IFN-γ TNF-α, GM-CSF, MIP-1α, MIP-1β, RANTES). Given that, NK produced cytokines are important regulators of the adaptive immune system, NK cells provide a bridge between adaptive and innate immunity.

NK cells distinguish normal and abnormal cells through a sophisticated repertoire of stimulatory and inhibitory receptors, which are invariant and constitutively expressed. NK cell activation, proliferation, and effector functions are controlled by: the competition between signals resulting from stimulatory and inhibitory receptors; the affinity of the receptor for the ligand; as well as, the level of ligand expression on the target cell. Positive stimuli are required to activate NK cell effector function, while cytokines and inhibitory receptors control specificity and regulation. In essence, NK cells are activated by cells lacking the ligands for the inhibitory receptors or overexpressing the ligands for the activation receptors as described subsequently, diagrammatically represented in Figure 7.

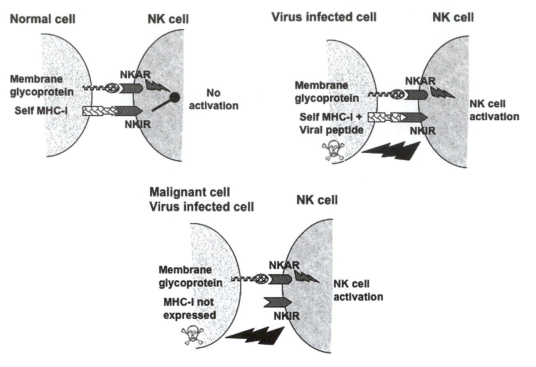

FIGURE 7 Diagrammatic representation of the mechanism of target cell recognition by natural killer cells. The activation or lack of activation of cytotoxic pathways depends on the balance between activating receptors (NKAR, such as NKR-P1, which interacts with cellular glycoproteins) and inhibitory receptors [NKIR, such as KIR, which interacts with self-major histocompatibility complex (MHC)-I molecules]. If the inhibitory receptor is not triggered (due to either lack of interaction of the inhibitory receptor with MHC-I−peptide complex or downregulation of expression of MHC-I molecules on the cell membrane), stimulatory activity prevails and the target cell is killed. Overexpression of modified cellular glycoproteins (in malignant cells of viral-infected cells) can cause a very strong activating signal, able to override the downregulating signal mediated by MHC-I recognition.

Markers Associated with Natural Killer Cell Stimulation and Activation
CD16
CD16 was the first activation molecule described on NK cells and remains the best characterized. CD16 is a low affinity IgG Fc receptor (FcγRIII) expressed on most NK cells, activated monocytes, and a subset of T cells. CD16 engagement on NK results in antibody dependent cellular cytotoxicity and cytokine secretion. The transmembrane-anchored CD16 isoform is complexed with the CD3ζ chain or the FcεRγ chain. Receptor ligation results in the phosphorylation of tyrosine residues within the ITAM motif in the cytoplasmic domains of the CD3ζ chain or the FcεRγ chain.

CD2
CD2 is expressed on NK and T cells. CD2 activation by monoclonal antibody LFA-3 induces NK cell-mediated cytotoxicity. CD2 ligation induces similar cascade of intracellular signaling events as CD16. CD2 is not thought to be a primary activation receptor on NK cells, rather a costimulatory receptor, which augments NK cell activation.

Natural Cytotoxicity Receptors
Natural cytotoxicity receptors (NKp46, NKp3, NKp44) are selectively expressed on NK cells and varying surface densities. They associate with different ITAMs such as CD3ζ FcεRIγ, or DAP-12 and play a major role in activating lysis of tumor and virally infected targets, although their cellular ligands have not yet been identified.

NKG2D is a lectin-like, homodimer activation receptor, which is constitutively expressed on NK and CD8$^+$ T cells. It forms a transmembrane association with the ITAM-bearing adapter protein DAP-10. NKG2D is involved in tumor and viral immunity and recognizes two families of stress-induced, MHC class I-like molecules.

DNAM-1 (CD226) activation results in enhanced NK cell activity (lysis and cytokine production). Ligands for DNAM-1 include 2 members of the nectin family, the polio virus receptor (CD112) and nectin-2 (CD155), highly expressed on many tumor cell lines and normal tissues.

The human NKR-P1 (CD161) receptor is a member of the C-type lectin superfamily, which is expressed on a subset of NK cells, $\gamma\delta$TcR$^+$ T cells, and about 25% of CD4$^+$ and CD8$^+$ T cells, primarily of the effector/memory phenotype. These receptors interact with glycoproteins, such as those expressed in mammalian cells, and are believed to deliver activating signals to the NK cells.

2B4 (CD244) is present on all NK cells, most $\gamma\delta$TcR$^+$ T cells, and CD8$^+$ T cells. Both 2B4 and its ligand CD48 are members of the CD2/CD150 family, which is characterized by the four Thr-x-Tyr-x-xLeu/Ile motifs in the cytoplasmic tail.

Markers Associated with Natural Killer Cell Downregulation

For many years, NK cells were defined as mediators of MHC nonrestricted cytolysis because of their ability to lyse allogeneic as well as autologous virally-infected or transformed targets. However, the observation that NK cells preferentially lysed target cells which expressed low levels or no MHC class I antigens, precipitated the study of MHC class I receptors on NK cells. Two distinct MHC class I receptor families have been described in humans: KIR and CD94/NKG2A. Although structurally distinct, each of these receptor families relies on ITIM sequences in the cytoplasmic domains to meditate inhibitory signaling. NK cell proliferation, cytotoxicity, and cytokine production are all downregulated as a consequence of MHC class I—NK receptor interaction.

Killer Cell Immunoglobulin-Like Receptors

In humans, the killer cell Ig-like receptors (KIR) family members recognize classical MHC class I antigens and are expressed on overlapping subsets of human NK cells, $\gamma\delta$TcR$^+$ T cells, and memory/effector $\alpha\beta$TcR$^+$ T cells. There are 15 genes in the KIR family coding for Type I transmembrane glycoproteins containing two or three Ig-like domains. Variability also exists within the cytoplasmic domains. The KIR with the longer cytoplasmic tails contain one to two ITIM sequences. The KIR with the shorter cytoplasmic region do not contain ITIM and form a transmembrane association with ITAM-bearing DAP-12 adapter protein, resulting in an activation rather than an inhibitory receptor.

CD94 and NKG2

CD94 and NKG2 are type II membrane proteins of the C-type lectin-like family, which form disulfide-linked heterodimers. They recognize the nonclassical MHC [human leukocyte antigen E(HLA-E)]. CD94 associates with human NKG2 proteins (NKG2A or NKG2C) and is expressed on most NK cells, and $\gamma\delta$TcR$^+$ T cells, and a subset memory/effector CD8$^+$ $\alpha\beta$TcR$^+$ T cells. CD94/NKG2A contains an ITIM in the cytoplasmic domain and functions as an inhibitory receptor; whereas, CD94/NKG2C functions as an activation receptor when associated with DAP-12. CD94/NKG2 expression is modulated by cytokines. IL-15, Il-2, and TGF-β will induce CD94/NKG2.

DENDRITIC CELLS

DC represent a complex and heterogeneous population involved in the initiation of innate and adaptive immune responses. These cells were initially defined by their antigen-presenting properties and their capacity to prime naïve T cells. More recently, their important role in Type 1 interferon (α and β) production and in the maintenance of immunological tolerance has been highlighted.

DC express HLA-DR, but not the markers specific to lymphoid and myeloid lineages. Plasmacytoid DC express blood dendritic cell antigen 2 (BDCA2), and high levels of CD123; whereas, myeloid-derived DC are CD11c$^+$.

The subpopulation of DC known as interferon-producing cells produces up to 1000 times more type 1 interferon (α, β) upon viral infection than other hematopoietic cells. This type 1 interferon not only directly inhibits viral replication, but also contributes to activation of T, B, and NK cells. The activated interferon producing cells subsequently differentiate into mature DC that directly regulates T cell functions by consequence of antigen presentation and cytokine secretion. In summary, this population of DC is not only one of the most important effector cells of the innate immune system, it is also a critical link between the innate and adaptive immunity. There is considerable interest in the use of DC in cancer immunotherapy. Preliminary clinical trials in which DC were isolated, loaded with tumor antigen, and reinfused into patients have been successful with B cell lymphoma and prostate cancer.

B LYMPHOCYTES

As the producers of Ig, B lymphocytes are the principal cellular mediators of humoral immune responses. B lymphocytes are identified by the presence of sIg. After antigenic stimulation, B cells differentiate into plasma cells that secrete large quantities of Igs. Within a single cell or a clone of identical cells, the antibody-binding sites of membrane and secreted Igs are identical. Molecules expressed on B cells involved in cell-to-cell interactions may deliver activating signal or inhibitory signals.

Markers Associated with B Cell Signaling and Activation
B Cell Receptor
The BcR complex is constituted by sIg associated with Igα (CD79a) and Igβ (CD79b) (Fig. 3). Antigen recognition occurs though the sIg, whereas Igα and Igβ mediate signal transduction. After antigen binding, the recruitment of tyrosine kinase to the cytoplasmic domains of Igα and Igβ initiates the activation cascade. The major kinase that is recruited to the BcR complex is known as Bruton's tyrosine kinase (Btk). Congenital Btk deficiency is associated with a block in B cell differentiation, demonstrating that signals delivered through the fully assembled BcR and associated kinases are necessary for B cell development during ontogeny.

Receptors for Activation and Proliferation Factors
TNF Receptor Family
Three cellular receptors of the TNFR family are involved in proliferation and maturation of B cells: the B cell maturation antigen (BCMA), the transmembrane activator and calcium modulator, and cyclophilin ligand interactor, and the BLyS receptor 3 (BR3). B cell activating factor (BAFF) and a proliferation inducing ligand (APRIL) are soluble ligands belonging to a TNF subfamily that interact with those receptors.

BAFF has a costimulatory effect in B cell activation but is not sufficient to induce B cell activation independently. Costimulation through BAFF allows a greater proportion of cells to be activated and induces antiapoptotic members of the Bcl-2 gene family, which allows for longer postactivation survival.

CD19, CD20, and CD21
CD19 is expressed on all B lineage cells with the exception of plasma cells. It is also found on most malignancies of B lymphocyte origin (see Chapter 27). CD19 contains potential phosphorylation sites in the cytoplasmic domain and associates with CD21 and other molecules. The formation of this molecular complex lowers the activation threshold for the BcR and results in early activation events such as modulates Ca^{2+} influx.

CD21 is expressed at high levels on mature, resting B cells but is lost upon activation. The cytoplasmic domain of CD21 contains potential phosphorylation sites. CD21 is also known as CR2, because this molecule functions as a receptor for the iC3b and C3d fragments of complement. The interaction between antigen-bound C3d and CD21 can deliver a costimulating signal to the B cell that results in amplification of humoral immune responses. Moreover, CD21 and CD23 (FcεRII) interact on the cell surface, and this interaction may play a regulatory role in IgE production. CD21 is also the receptor used by Epstein-Barr virus to infect B lymphocytes.

CD20 is an antigenic cluster associated with the first membrane marker to be found on a developing B lymphocyte. It is detectable on pre-B lymphocytes expressing cytoplasmic μ chains and remains expressed during maturation on the mature B lymphocyte, but is not expressed on plasma cells. It is a highly unusual molecule in that it crosses the membrane several times, and both the N-terminal and the C-terminal residues are intracellular. The extracellular domain contains only 42 amino acids. The carboxyl terminal end has 15 serine and threonine residues, the hallmark of a protein susceptible to phosphorylation by protein kinases, which occurs after mitogenic stimulation. This suggests that CD20 may play an important role in the activation and proliferation of mature B lymphocytes (see Chapter 11).

CD45

CD45 exists in several isoforms. B lymphocytes express only the highest molecular weight isoform of CD45. The most remarkable feature of CD45 is its cytoplasmic domain that comprises 705 amino acids and is the largest intracytoplasmic domain of all known membrane proteins. This intracytoplasmic domain has intrinsic tyrosine phosphatase activity and plays an essential role in lymphocyte activation.

CD38

CD38 is a type II transmembrane glycoprotein, which is expressed on immature B and T cells, but not on most mature, resting peripheral lymphocytes. CD38 is present on activated T cells and NK cells. CD38 disappears from the membrane of memory B cells differentiated in the mantle zone of the lymph nodes, which subsequently leaves the nodes as CD20$^+$, CD38$^-$ memory B cells and migrate to different lymphoid organs. Antibodies to CD38 induce T and B cell proliferation.

LFA-3 (CD58)

LFA-3 (CD58) is expressed on about half of the circulating T and B cells. When LFA-3 on antigen-presenting cells (APC) engages CD2 on T cells, intercellular adhesion is increased and costimulatory signals are delivered to the T cell.

CD80/86

CD80 (B7.1) and CD86 (B7.2), expressed at low levels on resting B cells and other APC, are upregulated upon activation. They bind CD28 and CTLA-4, expressed on T lymphocytes (see Chapter 11).

CD40

CD40 interacts with the CD40 ligand (CD40L, CD154). CD40 is expressed on all mature B cells, but is absent from plasma cells. It is also present on some epithelial, endothelial, DC, and activated monocytes. The interaction of CD40 and its coreceptor expressed on helper T cells is required for B lymphocyte maturation and isotype switching. The interaction of CD40:CD154 results in signaling, which leads to the upregulation of anti-apoptotic members of the Bcl-2 family's increasing cell survival.

Markers Associated with B Cell Downregulation
CD22

CD22, an integral part of the BcR complex, is first detected in the cytoplasm of pre-BII cells containing cytoplasmic μ chains. Later, it is found on the surface of 75% of sIgM$^+$ immature B cells, and, on 90% of sIgM$^+$, sIgD$^+$ mature, resting cells. In the adult, CD22 is expressed at relatively high levels in tissue B cells (e.g., in the tonsils and lymph nodes), but not in circulating B cells. CD22 is upregulated during activation, but is lost in the terminally differentiated plasma cells. CD22 binds to sialylated carbohydrate ligands (e.g., CD45RO) and plays an important regulatory role in B cell activation by raising the B cell activation threshold. CD22-deficient mice produce excessive antibody responses to antigen stimulation, as well as increased levels of auto-antibodies. In contrast, cross-linking of CD22 suppresses the response of B cells to antigenic stimulation because the intracytoplasmic segment has numerous ITIM motifs that function as docking sites for SHP-1. The binding of SHP-1 to CD22 prevents phosphorylation of the kinases needed for further B cell activation. In this way, CD19 and CD22 cross-regulate each other because activation through CD22 inhibits the CD19 pathway.

CD32

CD32 (FcγRII) is expressed on a range of leukocytes including, monocytes, macrophages, Langerhans cells, granulocytes, B cells, and platelets. CD32 is one of two low-affinity IgG Fc receptors, which only binds aggregated IgG. The cytoplasmic domains are associated with SHP-1 and other downregulatory kinases. Coligation of CD32 with membrane Ig (a situation that emerges during the immune response, due to the formation of antigen–antibody complexes in antigen excess, as described in Chapter 12) leads to the biding and activation of SH2-containing inositol phosphatase (SHIP). This is followed by inhibition of inositol 1,4,5 triphosphate (IP3), thus blocking the activation pathways activated after BcR occupation.

CD72 and CD100

CD72 is a type II transmembrane protein of the C-type lectin family. CD72 is expressed on B cells, dendritic cells, and on a subpopulation of T cells and macrophages. CD72 contains intracellular ITIMs and is known to have an inhibitory role in B cell signaling. CD100 has recently been identified as a ligand for CD72. CD100 is expressed at high levels on T cells and at low levels on B cells and dendritic cells, but is upregulated upon activation.

Other B Cell Membrane Markers

CD10 is expressed on precursor and immature B cells, pre-T cells, neutrophils, bone marrow stromal cells. CD10 is a commonly used marker for pre-B acute lymphocytic leukemias and some lymphomas. This molecule is a member of the type II membrane metalloproteinases and has neutral endopeptidase activity. CD10 knockout mice exhibit enhanced lethality to endotoxin, suggesting a role for CD10 in septic shock modulation. CD10 on bone marrow stromal cells appears to regulate B cell development, since inhibition of CD10 in vivo enhances B cell maturation.

CD5 is expressed on most T lymphocytes and on a small subpopulation of B lymphocytes. CD5 is found on most chronic lymphocytic leukemias. In nonleukemic individuals, B lymphocytes expressing CD5 appear to be activated and committed to the synthesis of IgM auto-antibodies. However, there is no apparent correlation between disease activity and the numbers of circulating CD5$^+$ cells. Thus, the precise role of these cells remains speculative. The cytoplasmic domain of CD5 contains ITAM motifs and is phosphorylated during T cell activation. CD5 is thought to be involved in thymic selection and in T-B cell recognition. MHC antigens, both HLA-I and II, are expressed at high levels by B lymphocytes. The presence of HLA class II enables B lymphocytes to serve as antigen-presenting cells. B lymphocytes are unique in that they express antigen-specific receptors and have the potential to act as antigen-presenting cells.

BIBLIOGRAPHY

Cancro MP. Peripheral B-cell maturation: the intersection of selection and homeostasis. Immunol Rev 2004; 197:89.

Hendriks RW, Middendorp S. The pre-BcR checkpoint as a cell-autonomous proliferation switch. Trends Immunol 2004; 25:249.

Lanier LL. NK cell recognition. Annu Rev Immunol 2005; 23:225.

Pelayo R, Wlener R, Perry SS, et al. Lymphoid progenitors and primary routes to becoming cells of the immune system. Curr Opin Immunol 2005; 17:100–107.

Rothenberg EV, Taghon T. Molecular genetics of T cell development. Annu Rev Immunol 2005; 23:601.

Star TK, Jameson SC, Hogquist KA. Positive and negative selection of T cells. Annu Rev Immunol 2003; 21:139.

http://mpr.nci.nih.gov/prow/

11 | Cell-Mediated Immunity

Donna L. Farber
Department of Surgery, Division of Transplantation, University of Maryland School of Medicine, Baltimore, Maryland, U.S.A.

Gabriel Virella
Department of Microbiology and Immunology, Medical University of South Carolina, Charleston, South Carolina, U.S.A.

INTRODUCTION

Adaptive immune responses have been traditionally subdivided into humoral (antibody-mediated) and cellular (cell-mediated) immune responses. As a rule, humoral (B cell-mediated) immune responses function predominantly in the elimination of soluble antigens and the destruction of extracellular microorganisms, whereas cell-mediated (T cell) immunity is more important for the elimination of intracellular organisms (such as viruses). Both humoral and cellular immunity are coordinated by T lymphocytes, and there is significant interplay between these two arms of the immune response. The humoral response to proteins depends on "help" provided by T lymphocytes in the form of cytokines and other ancillary signals, and cell-mediated immunity involves T-cell directed recruitment and activation of multiple types of immune cells for antigen clearance. In this chapter, we discuss how T lymphocytes become activated after encountering antigen, how they differentiate into effector cells, and the multiple consequences of this effector response in coordinating antigen clearance. We also discuss how T cell activation can culminate in a memory immune response that can persist for the lifetime of an individual, and how T-cell subsets also play central roles in immunoregulation.

T-CELL ACTIVATION
Initial Recognition of Antigen-Derived Peptides by T-Cell Receptors

A major distinction between antigen-recognition by T versus B lymphocytes is the inability of T cells to recognize free, soluble antigen through the T-cell receptor (TcR), whereas B cells recognize free antigen via surface immunoglobulin. T cells recognize antigen-derived peptides associated to self-major histocompatibility complex (MHC) molecules (see Chapters 3 and 4), and the tertiary structure of the oligopeptides generated as a consequence of processing by antigen-presenting cells (APCs) often has no resemblance to its structure within native antigen. As a result, T and B lymphocytes bind structurally distinct antigenic determinants.

The antigen-derived oligopeptides that fit into the binding sites of MHC-I or MHC-II molecules interact with TcR of different T-cell subpopulations. MHC-II/peptide complexes expressed on the surface of APC are recognized by the TcR of CD4$^+$ lymphocytes, whereas MHC-I/peptide complexes expressed by a variety of cells are recognized by the TcR of CD8$^+$ lymphocytes. This dichotomy of recognition of CD4 and CD8 T cells is due to specific interaction of the CD4 and CD8 coreceptor with MHC class II and class I, respectively. This trimolecular complex of the TcR/MHC-peptide and CD4 or CD8 coreceptor form a focal point of contact between the T cell and the APC. The CD4 molecule on the lymphocyte membrane interacts with nonpolymorphic areas of the class II MHC molecules on the APC, and CD8 interacts with analogous nonpolymorphic regions of MHC class I. This interaction helps stabilize the contact between MHC-II and TcR, but is also involved in signal transduction in the early stages of T lymphocyte activation, as discussed later in this chapter.

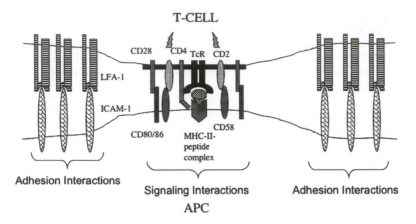

FIGURE 1   The immunological synapse. T cells recognizing a major histocompatibility complex–peptide complex presented by an antigen-presenting cell interact through a variety of membrane proteins, some primarily involved in promoting attachment of the two cells, and others delivering activating signals to the T cell.

In addition to the TcR-coreceptor/MHC interaction, other interactions between T cells and APC are necessary for proper interaction and are required for full T-cell activation and differentiation into effector T cells, for mediating antigen clearance. These additional interactions comprise both adhesive interactions that strengthen the interaction between T cells and APC, and costimulatory signals that are required both for activation of naive T cells and to regulate T-cell activation and prevent unchecked propagation of the immune response. Both of these interactions are graphically illustrated in Figure 1 and described in detail next.

Adhesive Interactions Between T Cells and Antigen-Presenting Cell

Activation of a T lymphocyte requires the close and prolonged interaction between T cells and APC. In order for two cells to come together in intimate association, the natural electrostatic repulsions on the membrane must be overcome. The interaction between the TcR and APC is a low-affinity one, and not sufficient to keep the T cell and APC together, so other molecular interactions between these cells are required. A class of molecules called adhesion molecules fulfills this requirement.

Two sets of adhesion molecules of the integrin family [CD2/CD58 and leukocyte function antigen-1 (LFA-1)/intercellular adhesion molecule 1 (ICAM-1)] play a primary role in T lymphocyte–APC adhesion. CD2 molecules expressed by essentially all T lymphocytes bind to CD58 (LFA-3) molecules expressed by most nucleated cells as well as by erythrocytes. The initial interaction between the MHC/peptide complex and the TcR causes a conformational change on the CD2 molecule that increases the affinity of CD2 for the CD58 molecule expressed by the APC. In addition to its role in stabilizing cell–cell contact, the interaction between CD2 and CD58 delivers an activating signal to the T lymphocyte.

The LFA-1 molecule that interacts with the ICAM-1 also undergoes conformational changes in the early stages of T-cell activation. Both APC and T cells express LFA-1 and ICAM-1, and the heterotypic interaction between pairs of these molecules results in the formation of strong intercellular bonds. The strengthening of the adhesive interaction via CD2 and LFA-1 occurs due to contact of the TcR with MHC-peptide complexes and is referred to as "outside-in signaling."

The establishment of APC-T lymphocyte interactions brings the membranes of the two cells into close proximity (immunological synapse, see Chapter 4). Such close contact is critical for the delivery of additional activating signals to the T cell and allows for high local concentrations and maximal effects of the interleukins (ILs) and cytokines released by APC and T lymphocytes.

Costimulatory Interactions Between T Cells and Antigen-Presenting Cell

The interaction of a T cell and APC via adhesive interactions and TcR/MHC-peptide contacts is not sufficient to fully activate the T cell and promote differentiation to effector cells that are essential for the recruitment and activation of additional immune cells for antigen clearance. An additional signal is required for T-cell activation, which is called the costimulatory signal. The costimulatory signal was initially proposed by Bretscher and Cohn in the 1970s in their "two signal hypothesis," as a mechanism whereby the immune system could monitor whether a pathogen was present, and represented a checkpoint against self-reactivity. In the absence of costimulatory signals, TcR occupancy, by itself, induces T-cell unresponsiveness or anergy (see Chapter 16).

The identity of the costimulatory signal for T-cell activation was reported in 1990 as an interaction between a cell surface glycoprotein receptor on T cells, CD28, which binds two related ligands on the surface of APCs—B7-1 (CD80) and B7-2 (CD86). CD28 is expressed by all T cells, and CD28/B7 engagement is required for activation of naive CD4 T cells and for IL-2 production. The ligands for CD28, and CD80/CD86 are expressed only by activated APC, such as activated macrophages and B cells, and by mature dendritic cells (DC). Induction of these costimulatory ligands on the surface of APC is triggered via toll-like receptors (TLR) (see Chapter 14) that bind pathogen-associated molecules such as lipopolysaccharides, components of bacterial cell walls (peptidoglycans and lipotechoic acids), and bacterial DNA (CpG motifs). In addition, the engagement of TLR triggers upregulation of B7 costimulatory ligands. This pathogen-mediated control of costimulation ensures that T cells only see their second signal in the presence of a foreign invader and not from the endogenous self.

Although the CD28/CD80/CD86 interaction is the most important costimulatory pathway for activation of naive T cells, these molecules are but a few in the growing family of costimulatory proteins that function to both positively and negatively regulate T-cell activation (Table 1). Although CD28 is the main costimulatory molecule on resting T cells, activation induces upregulation of additional members of the costimulatory family, such as inducible costimulator (ICOS) for positive regulation of effector function and CD154 (also called CD40 ligand) for promoting interaction with other APC and for promoting T-B cell cooperation. Importantly, there are additional regulatory molecules that are upregulated following activation, which play critical roles in turning off T-cell activation and cytokine production. The cytotoxic T cell late antigen (CTLA)-4 molecule is rapidly upregulated on T cells upon activation, and also binds the B7-1/B7-2 (CD80/86) ligands similar to CD28, but with higher affinity. A negative regulatory role for CTLA-4 was established from the findings that mice deficient in this molecule displayed severe lymphoproliferation early in life with profound lymphocytic infiltration into peripheral organs. These CTLA-4$^{-/-}$ deficient mice die at 4 weeks of age of severe autoimmunity (normal lab mouse lifespan is one to two years). Two mechanisms have been proposed to explain the effect of CTLA-4 expression. One is a direct downregulation of effector T cells as a consequence of the CD28/CTLA-4 interaction. The second mechanism would be the activation of CTLA-4$^+$, CD4$^+$, and CD25$^+$ regulatory

TABLE 1 Costimulatory Receptor–Ligand Interactions Between T Cells and Antigen-Presenting Cells

Costimulatory receptor	Expression	Ligand	Function
CD28	Resting and activated T cells	CD80/CD86	Promote IL-2 production, required for naive T-cell activation
CD154 (CD40L)	Activated T cells	CD40	Promote T–B cell collaboration and activation of APC
ICOS	Activated T cells	ICOS-L	Promote effector function
CTLA-4	Activated T cells	CD80/CD86	Downregulate T-cell activation
BTLA-4	Th1 effector cells	Unknown	Negative regulator
PD-1	Activated T cells	PD-L1	Negatively regulate T-cell activation/effector function

Abbreviations: APC, antigen-presenting cells; CTLA, cytotoxic T cell late antigen; BTLA, B and T lymphocyte attenuator; ICOS, inducible costimulator; PD, programmed death.

T cells (Tregs). Thus, CTLA-4 plays critical roles early after activation in dampening the T-cell response and preventing prolonged, unchecked activation that can lead to immunopathology.

Additional negative costimulatory regulators of T-cell activation have recently been identified and are designated programmed death-1 (PD-1) and BTLA-4 (Table 1). Less is known about these newer molecules, although they likewise bind ligands expressed by the APC. Both positive and negative costimulatory regulators can serve as potential therapeutic targets for enhancing immune responses in vaccines and abrogating T-cell activation in auto-immunity. For example, a fusion molecule, CTLA-4Ig that binds the B7-1/B7-2 (CD80/86) ligands with high affinity shows efficacy as a treatment for rheumatoid arthritis, and recently became an approved drug for this condition. Moreover, direct blockade of CTLA-4 is now in clinical trials for enhancement of antitumor immunity. Thus, identification of T cell-specific control molecules has real therapeutic applications.

Intracellular Events Associated with CD4 T-Cell Activation

When the adequate complement of activating signals is delivered to a $CD4^+$ T lymphocyte, a cascade of intracellular signals is triggered. As discussed in Chapters 4 and 10, the TcR hetero-dimer itself has a very short intracytoplasmic portion with no recognizable kinase activity. The signal transduction functions of the TcR are mediated by the CD3 complex, consisting of four different protein subunits (CD3γ,ε,δ and the CD3ζ homodimer) that are noncovalently associated to the TcR and contain short extracellular domains, and long intracytoplasmic portion. Within the cytoplasmic portion of each CD3 subunit are immunoreceptor tyrosine-based activation motifs (ITAMs) containing tyrosine residues (2 per ITAM) that are substrates for tyrosine kinases that initiate the TcR-mediated signaling cascade.

Signal transduction events following TcR engagement by antigen/MHC class II com-plexes serve to transmit activating signals from the cell surface through the cytoplasm, culmi-nating in the nucleus, where transcription factors for genes promoting T-cell growth and differentiation are activated. For activation of naive T cells, these signals start with phosphoryl-ation of CD3 molecules and activation of tyrosine kinases, proceed via a cascade of phosphoryl-ation and recruitment of additional signaling molecules, and ultimately lead to IL-2 gene transcription in the nucleus.

While signal transduction is a dynamic process, TcR-coupled signaling can be divided into three distinct phases: proximal, linker/adapter, and distal (Fig. 2). In the proximal phase, initial TcR engagement triggers phosphorylation of the CD3 subunits on ITAMs by the src-related tyrosine kinase $p56^{lck}$, which is noncovalently associated with the cyto-plasmic domains of CD4 and of CD8. The src-related kinase p59fyn has also been shown to phosphorylate CD3 components. Both the lck and fyn kinases are themselves regulated by phosphorylation and dephosphorylation events. The cell surface molecule CD45 is expressed by all leukocytes and contains an intracytoplasmic phosphatase that, in T cells, can serve to regulate the activity of src family kinases by dephosphorylation. Phosphorylation of the CD3ζ subunit is particularly important for the activation and coupling of downstream signaling processes. CD3ζ phosphorylation results in the recruitment and activation of a third tyrosine kinase, called zeta-associated protein of 70 kdal (ZAP-70). In resting peripheral CD4 T cells, a proportion of CD3ζ is already ZAP-70 associated, but this increases greatly fol-lowing activation, causing phosphorylation and concomitant activation of ZAP-70 kinase activity. Thus, the activation and mobilization of src family kinases, phosphorylation of CD3 subunits, and recruitment and activation of ZAP-70 comprise the major proximal events in T-cell signaling.

The second temporal cluster of signaling events involves the mobilization of linker-adapter molecules that form a scaffold on which multiple signaling intermediates are com-plexed, to couple proximal signaling to downstream events. The role of linker-adapter molecules in signaling is a general feature in multiple immune and nonimmune cell types. In T cells, two molecules, linker of activation T cells (LAT) and SLP-76 (SH2-containing Leuko-cyte Protein of 76 kdal), both serve as substrates of ZAP-70 and form the linker/adapter bridge coupling ZAP-70 activation to downstream events such as MAP kinase activation and Ca release. LAT and SLP-76 are linked to each other via additional molecular adaptor molecules,

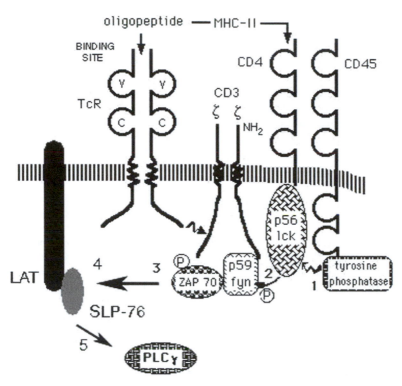

FIGURE 2 Sequence of events during the initial stages of T-cell activation. Antigen occupancy of the T-cell receptor (TcR) induces modifications of the CD45 transmembrane protein. These modifications result in activation of its tyrosine phosphatase activity; one of the substrates of CD45 is a p56^{lck} tyrosine kinase. Dephosphorylation of p56^{lck} results in its enzymatic activation. Activated p56^{lck} initiates a cascade involving the src-related kinase p59^{fyn} as well as the activated immunoreceptor tyrosine-based activation motifs of the ζ chain of the TcR complex, leading to the phosphorylation of ZAP70. This is followed by phosphorylation of the linker of activator T cells (LAT) and the associated SH2-containing leukocyte protein of 76 kdal (SLP-76), which in turn will activate phospholipase C and other substrates involved in cell activation.

and both also complex with phospholipase C (PLC)-γ, which gets phosphorylated and promotes the release of intracellular calcium stores via hydrolysis of inositol phosphates. LAT and SLP-76 also serve distinct roles in signaling. LAT is coupled to the Ras signaling pathway, and SLP-76 is involved in pathways related to cytoskeletal reorganization, integrin activation, and to additional kinases that promote downstream events. Thus, LAT and SLP-76 play central roles in the overall coordination of TcR-mediated signaling events. Their critical roles have been further established in vivo, as mice deficient in either LAT or SLP-76 are profoundly impaired in T-cell development (that requires TcR-mediated signaling, see Chapter 10) and lack peripheral T cells.

The distal events in TcR signaling are directly coupled to transcription factor mobilization in the nucleus. One important distal event is the activation of mitogen-activated protein (MAP) kinases, including p38, Erk1/2, and Jnk kinases in T cells, which control activation of transcription factors for IL-2 and effector cytokine production. Another important distal event is the activation and release of calcium from intracellular stores via second messengers. One of these messengers is inositol 1,4,5-triphosphate (IP3), responsible for an additional rise in intracellular ionized calcium concentration by mobilizing Ca^{2+} from intracytoplasmic stores. The activation of the calcium and calmodulin-dependent serine/threonine phosphatase calcineurin follows this second cytosolic calcium peak. The second critical messenger is diacylglycerol (DAG), responsible for the activation of protein kinase C (PKC). Together, calcium flux and MAP kinase activation coordinate and lead to mobilization of transcription factors such as nuclear factor of activated T cells (NFAT), nuclear factor-kappa B (NF-κB), and AP-1 that all control transcription of the IL-2 gene (see subsequently).

The sequence of signaling events described earlier refer to those directly coupled to the TcR; however, full T-cell activation requires engagement of the CD28 costimulatory receptor. While less is known concerning the precise signaling pathways coupled to CD28, two important processes have been found to be coupled to CD28 ligation. The first process is activation of a phosphoinositol (PI)-3 kinase that leads to PI hydrolysis for mobilization of intracellular calcium stores. The second CD28-mediated signal target is the serine/threonine kinase Akt that is associated with cell survival and metabolic control. CD28 has also been shown to have quantitative effects on TcR signaling, facilitating the biochemical processes from TcR ligation to IL-2 production.

Transcription Factors for T-Cell Activation

The signaling cascades emanating from TcR and CD28 ligation culminate in transcription factor activation in the nucleus. Transcription factors need to be activated in order to induce the expression of a large number of molecules that control T-cell proliferation and differentiation. These molecules are not expressed by resting T cells, and their genes must be transcribed de novo. Multiple genes are expressed in a defined sequence starting minutes after activation of a helper cell and continuing for the next several days. Those genes encode critical transcription factors, enzymes, and substrates involved in proliferation, differentiation, and effector function.

Among the well-characterized transcription factors involved in T-cell activation NFκB, NF-AT and AP-1 are particularly important in IL-2 production and in coordinating the initial functional events in T-cell activation. NFκB is a DNA-binding protein found complexed with a specific inhibitor (IκB) in the cytoplasm of resting T lymphocytes. After phosphorylation by an IκB kinase, IκB is destroyed and the untethered NFκB moves into the nucleus, where it binds to the promoters of many genes, including the IL-2 receptor (IL-2R) gene and the c-myc gene, mediating their transcriptional activation (Fig. 3). Additionally, NFκB activation is essential for the prevention of apoptotic cell death. NF-AT1 is almost exclusively found in hematopoietic cells. NF-AT1, along with AP-1, binds to regions of specific DNA sequences found in the 5′ promoter region of most cytokine genes. An inactive phosphorylated form of NF-AT is located in the cytoplasm of resting T cells. This form is activated by dephosphorylation catalyzed by a calcium-dependent serine/threonine phosphatase known as calcineurin. AP-1 is a nuclear protein induced when T cells are stimulated via the TcR plus ancillary signals mediated by CD28 cross-linking. It is formed by the association of two proto-oncogene products, c-Fos and c-Jun, whose synthesis is activated by PKC. The full expression of cytokine and cytokine receptor genes is controlled by promoter sequences recognized by NFκB and/or by the complex of NFAT-1 and AP-1. Their occupancy by these transcription factors is essential for control of their expression during T-cell activation.

Interleukin-2 Synthesis and T Lymphocyte Proliferation

Two critical early events in T-cell activation are the appearance of transcripts for IL-2 and for the IL-2R in the cytoplasm. The upregulation of the IL-2 gene, an essential step for T-cell proliferation at the onset of the immune response, requires occupancy of the promoter region by NF-AT/AP-1/NFκB complexes. The expression of the IL-2R, on the other hand, seems to be primarily controlled by NFκB. The release of IL-2 into the cellular environment of activated T cells expressing IL-2Rs has significant biological consequences.

Autocrine and Paracrine Effects of IL-2

IL-2 stimulates lymphocyte proliferation both in autocrine and paracrine loops. Autocrine stimulation involves release of IL-2 from an activated T cell and binding and activation of IL-2Rs expressed by the same T cell. Paracrine stimulation is likely a consequence of IL-2 overproduction after persistent stimulation of CD4$^+$ T cells. The released IL-2 exceeds the binding capacity of the IL-2Rs expressed by the producing cell and can stimulate other nearby cells expressing those receptors. The targets of the paracrine effects of IL-2 are helper T lymphocytes,

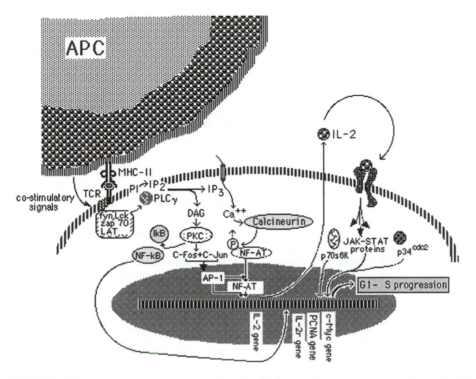

FIGURE 3 Diagrammatic representation of a simplified second messenger cascade involved in T-lymphocyte activation. After the sequence of events illustrated in Figure 2 takes place, two important enzymes are activated. Calcineurin, a serine/threonine phosphatase, dephosphorylates and activates the cytoplasmic component of the nuclear factor of activated T cells (NF-AT). A complex of NF-AT and calcineurin translocates to the nucleus where it forms a complex with AP-1, and this complex activates the expression of the IL-2 gene. Protein kinase C (PKC) is also activated, and the active form has at least two critical effects: (*i*) It promotes the association of c-Fos and c-Jun into AP-1, which translocates to the nucleus. In the nucleus AP-1 binds directly to the IL-2 gene enhancer region and combines with NF-AT to form the active form of NF-AT that synergizes with AP-1, enhancing the expression of the IL-2 gene. (*ii*) PKC activates a kinase that causes the dissociation of the complex formed between the nuclear factor κ B (NFκB) and its inhibitory protein (IkB). The activated NFκB then translocates to the nucleus where it enhances the expression of several genes, including the one encoding the IL-2 receptor. The phosphorylated adaptor protein linker of activator T cells (LAT) triggers additional signaling pathways, including the Ras pathway, which results in Raf, Mek, and ERK activation. The activation of these pathways results in transcriptional activation of cytokine and other genes, and other activation genes leading to progression from G0 to G1. Additional signals are required for progression to S1. Synthesis and release of IL-2 associated with increased expression of the IL-2R creates the conditions necessary for such progression. The occupancy of the IL-2R is followed by activation of protein kinases and diacylglycerol kinase, followed by the activation of several transcription factors of the JAK-STAT (signal transducers and activators of transcription) family, and increased transcription of proteins controlling cell proliferation, such as the proliferating-cell nuclear antigen (PCNA), an obligate cofactor of DNA polymerase delta, an enzyme that itself plays a significant role in DNA replication, and c-myc, which controls cell proliferation.

cytotoxic T lymphocytes (CTL), B lymphocytes, and natural killer (NK) cells, all of which express IL-2Rs of varying affinities.

IL-2 Receptor

The IL-2R expressed by T and B lymphocytes is composed of three different polypeptide chains.

1. CD25, a 55 kD polypeptide chain (IL-2Rα chain), is expressed at very low levels in about 10% of the circulating (nonactivated) T cells, but is sharply upregulated a few hours after activation. CD25 binds IL-2 with low affinity and has a short intracytoplasmic domain unable to transduce growth signals upon binding to its ligand.

2. The IL-2Rβ chain (also called CD122) is a 70 to 75 kD polypeptide chain expressed by resting T lymphocytes. The IL-2R$\alpha\beta$ heterodimer has an increased affinity for IL-2. The β chain appears capable of signal transduction, as its intracytoplasmic domain is 286 amino acids long. In addition, engagement of $\alpha\beta$ dimers results in the recruitment of γ chains, forming the high affinity IL-2R.
3. The IL-2R γ chain or γ c is the third polypeptide chain that comprises the trimeric IL-2R expressed after T-cell activation. The γ chain has a long intracytoplasmic segment for intracellular transmission. This protein subunit is shared by a number of cytokine receptors in addition to the IL-2R, including those for IL-4, IL-7, IL-9, and IL-15.

Consequences of IL-2 Binding to the IL-2 Receptor

The binding of IL-2 to the trimeric high affinity IL-2R induces the association of the IL-2R to the src-related p56lck tyrosine kinase and to other specific tyrosine kinases of the janus tyrosine kinase (JAK) family. These proximal events lead to phosphorylation of transcription factors of the signal transducers and activators of transcription (STAT) family, which dimerize after phosphorylation and then translocate to the nucleus. In the nucleus, activated STAT factors upregulate the expression of genes coding for cytokine receptors and induce the appearance of cyclins that drive the cell into cell cycle (Fig. 3). In addition, signals transduced via the CD28/B7 interaction stabilize IL-2 production, via triggering the synthesis of DNA-binding proteins that appear to block the rapid decay of the IL-2 mRNA, and induce members of the antiapoptotic Bcl-2 gene family. If the CD28/B7 interaction is blocked, T cells will be unable to stabilize IL-2 production, and this results in an anergic state. T cells experiencing anergy are rendered unresponsive to subsequent stimulation.

T-Lymphocyte Proliferation and Differentiation

The production of IL-2 and upregulation of IL-2R promote entry of the T cell into the cell cycle to initiate its proliferation and expansion. The purpose of this proliferation step is to expand out the antigen-specific T cells to effect antigen clearance. Since a given T cell clone specific for a particular antigen is expected to be present in relatively low frequencies, this expansion step is necessary to fortify the immune response against a particular antigen or pathogen when it is encountered.

It is estimated that the initial helper T lymphocyte population is capable of expanding 100-fold in six days, reaching more than 1000-fold its starting number by day 10—the time that it takes to elicit a detectable primary immune response to most infectious agents. This expansion results in the differentiation not only of the short-lived effector cells needed for the ongoing immune response but also of long-lived memory cells. Following such rapid and robust T-cell expansion, many of the activated effector cells will undergo apoptosis. However, when the immune response subsides, an expanded population of memory T cells will remain and will be able to assist the onset of subsequent responses to the same antigen with greater efficiency and speed, which is characteristic of an anamnestic (memory) response.

Soluble Factors Involved in T-Cell Responses

A variety of soluble factors, cytokines and interleukins (ILs) (cytokines responsible for cross-signaling between different lymphocyte subpopulations), play significant roles in T-cell differentiation, activation, and effector functions. The critical role of IL-2 has been discussed earlier. For the sake of organization, we discuss cytokines and lymphokines by their predominant function, well-aware that most have multiple sources and functions, and that the same functions can be shared by multiple cytokines (Table 2).

Interleukins Involved in T-Cell Differentiation

IL-1, IL-4, IL-7, and IL-12 are the three main ILs with this type of function. IL-1, released by a variety of cell types, including APCs, acts as a growth factor on the bone marrow. It is a major factor leading to the general mobilization of leukocytes, objectively reflected by peripheral

TABLE 2 Major Interleukins and Cytokines

Interleukin/cytokine	Predominant source	Main targets	Biological activity
IL-1α,β	Monocytes, macrophages, and other cell types	T and B lymphocytes, dendritic cells, granulocytes, monocytes	Activates a variety of cell types through the NFκB pathway; IL-1 activated T cells are induced to secrete IL-2; cytotoxic for β cells of the pancreatic islets; proinflammatory.
IL-2	Activated T lymphocytes	T and B lymphocytes, NK cells	Promotes T- and NK-cell proliferation; cofactor for the proliferation of activated B cells; activates NK cells
IL-3	Activated T lymphocytes; also mast cells and others	Hematopoietic stem cells; basophils	Hematopoietic growth factor; chemotactic for eosinophils
IL-4	Th2 lymphocytes; also mast cells, basophils, and macrophages	Th1 lymphocytes, macrophages, B lymphocytes	Growth and differentiation factor for B lymphocytes; causes the expansion of Th1 lymphocytes (autocrine loop); promotes IgE synthesis
IL-5	Th2 lymphocytes, mast cells, eosinophilss	Eosinophils, B lymphocytes	Promotes the growth and differentiation of eosinophils; chemotactic for eosinophils; B cell differentiation
IL-6	Monocytes, fibroblasts, endothelial cells; also B and Th2 lymphocytes, plasma cells, macrophages	B and T lymphocytes, others	B cell differentiation factor; polyclonal B lymphocyte activator; cofactor for T lymphocyte differentiation; proinflammatory mediator; pyrogen
IL-7	Bone marrow, thymic stromal cells	Pro-B lymphocytes; activated T lymphocytes, thymocytes	Stimulates proliferation of pro-B lymphocytes and activated T lymphocytes; promotes thymic differentiation of T lymphocytes
IL-8 (CXCL8)	Macrophages, activated monocytes, fibroblasts, endothelial cells	Neutrophils, monocytes, T lymphocytes	Neutrophil and T-lymphocyte chemotactic factor
IL-9	Thymocytes, CD4$^+$T lymphocytes	Mast cells, B lymphocytes, thymocytes	Growth factor
IL-10	Th2 lymphocytes, Tregs, CD8$^+$ T cells	B lymphocytes, Th1 lymphocytes, macrophages, granulocytes	Inhibits cytokine synthesis predominantly in Th1 T lymphocytes and activated APCs; thymocyte growth factor; cytotoxic T cell and B cell differentiation factor; chemotactic factor for CD8$^+$ T lymphocytes; mast cell costimulator
IL-11	Bone marrow stromal cells and mesenchymal cells	Hematopoietic stem cells	B-cell differentiation factor; stimulates proliferation and differentiation of hematopoietic stem cells, particularly megakaryocytes
IL-12	Monocytes, macrophages, dendritic cells	Th1 lymphocytes, NK cells	Natural killer cell stimulating factor; Th1 lymphocyte activation and proliferation; enhances the activity of cytotoxic cells; induces interferon-γ production

(Continued)

TABLE 2 Major Interleukins and Cytokines (*Continued*)

Interleukin/ cytokine	Predominant source	Main targets	Biological activity
IL-13	Activated Th2 and CD8$^+$ T lymphocytes, Nk cells	B lymphocytes, monocytes, macrophages	Promotes immunoglobulin synthesis; induces the release of mediators from basophils and mast cells; suppresses monocyte/macrophage functions
IL-14	T lymphocytes	B lymphocytes	B lymphocyte growth factor
IL-15	Monocytes/macrophages, microglia	T lymphocytes, monocytes, NK cells	Lymphocyte, mast cell, and NK cell growth factor; maturation factor for NK cells; chemoattractant for T lymphocytes
IL-16	CD8$^+$ T lymphocytes, fibroblasts, eosinophils, mast cells	CD4$^+$T lymphocytes	Chemotactic and activating factor for CD4$^+$ T lymphocytes; macrophages and eosinophils
IL-17	Activated CD4$^+$T lymphocytes and CD4$^+$T memory cells	Multiple	Proinflammatory; promotes osteoclast activation; promotes angiogenesis; chemoattractant for PMN leukocytes; promotes neutrophil maturation
IL-18	Dendritic cells, monocytes, macrophages, etc.	T cells and others	Proinflammatory; induces interferon-γ; promotes angiogenesis
IL-21	CD4$^+$T lymphocytes	NK, T and B lymphocytes	B lymphocyte proliferation; T- and NK-cell costimulation
IL-23	Activated macrophages	T lymphocytes	Induces interferon-γ synthesis; induces T lymphocyte proliferation
IL-27	Activated APCs and mature dendritic cells	Naive CD4$^+$T lymphocytes, NK cells	Promotes proliferation of naive CD4$^+$ T lymphocytes; activates Th1 responses (induces T-bet and downregulates GATA-3); induces interferon-γ synthesis
IL-32	Activated T and NK lymphocytes	Macrophages	Proinflammatory; induces the production of TNF; IL-8 and MIP-2
GM-CSF	Activated Th2 lymphocytes, macrophages, and endothelial cells; malignant plasma cells	Hematopoietic stem cells	Promotes proliferation and maturation of granulocytes and monocytes; proinflammatory; chemoattractant for neutrophils and eosinophils; activates neutrophils and basophils
IFN α/β	Leukocytees, fibroblasts	Lymphocytes	NK activator; proinflammatory
IFNγ	Th1 lymphocytes	Multiple	Macrophage and NK activator
TGFβ	Macrophages, lymphocytes (Tregs), endothelial cells	Multiple	Inhibits T-, B-, and NK-cell proliferation; deactivates macrophages; anti-inflammatory and immunosuppressive
TNF (TNF-α, cachectin)	Activated APCs, CD4$^+$T lymphocytes, NK cells	Multiple	Cytotoxic for tumor cells; induces cachexia; septic shock mediator; B lymphocyte activator; proinflammatory
LT-α (lymphotoxin, TNFβ)	T and B lymphocytes, leukocytes in general	Multiple	Activates B-lymphocytes, PMN leukocytes, and NK cells; promotes fibroblast proliferation

Abbreviations: APC, antigen-presenting cells; GM-CSF, granulocyte, monocyte-colony stimulating factor; IFN, interferon; IL, interleukin; MIP, macrophage inflammatory protein; NFκB, nuclear factor-kappa B; NK, natural killer; PMN, polymorphonuclear; TGF, tumor growth factor; TNF, tumor necrosis factor; Tregs, regulatory T cells.

blood leukocytosis, characteristic of bacterial infections. It is also, along with IL-12, one of the cytokines that seems to favor T-helper 1 (Th1) differentiation.

IL-4, primarily released by Th2 lymphocytes, is both a B cell growth and differentiation factor, as well as major determinant, through an autocrine loop, of the proliferation and differentiation of Th2 lymphocytes, whereas it has downregulatory effects on the Th1 population.

IL-7 is produced in the bone marrow, thymus, and spleen. Its main role seems to be to induce the proliferation of B- and T-lymphocyte precursors. In the thymus, IL-7 drives pre-T cell differentiation into double positive $CD4/CD8^+$ T-cell precursors. In the periphery, IL-7 seems to play a key role promoting the expansion of antigen-stimulated T cells. The molecular mechanism for this effect on activated T-cell expansion seems linked to the upregulation of the expression of bcl-2 and related genes, whose products protect the cell against apoptotic death IL-12, primarily released by APCs, has significant role in promoting Th1 cell differentiation (see below).

Interleukins Involved in B-Cell Differentiation

IL-4, 5, 6, 7, 10, 13, 14, 21, TNF, and lymphotoxin-α (LT-α) have been implicated as mediating different steps of B-cell proliferation and differentiation. They also have other significant characteristics, and some will be discussed in greater detail in other chapters of this book (see Chapters 14, 19, and 20).

IL-4 has been discussed earlier. Of note is the fact that its effect in B-cell differentiation seems associated with a predominant switch to IgE synthesis. High levels of IL-4 are often measured in patients with type I (IgE-mediated) hypersensitivity.

IL-6 promotes the differentiation of B-lymphocyte precursors, as well as the differentiation of T-lymphocyte precursors into CTL. It has also proinflammatory properties (see Chapter 14).

IL-10 promotes B-cell differentiation and has important regulatory functions, turning off Th1 (and to a lesser degree Th2) activity as well as inhibiting cytokine synthesis from activated lymphocytes and macrophages.

IL-13 promotes the synthesis of IgE by activated B cells. In addition, it has direct effects on basophils and mast cells. The important role this pathogenic cytokine has in bronchial asthma is discussed elsewhere (see Chapter 21).

IL-14 and 21 have also been reported to promote B-cell proliferation.

Interleukins with Regulatory Functions

Several cytokines have been reported to have regulatory functions.

IL-10, released by activated Th2 cells and $CD4^+$ regulatory T lymphocytes (Tregs), suppress the activities of Th1 cells and Th2 cells.

Tumor growth factor-β (TGF-β), released by macrophages, Tregs, and endothelial cells, inhibits T-, B-, and NK-cell proliferation. It also deactivates macrophages. Thus, this cytokine has a combination of anti-inflammatory and immunosuppressive effects.

Interferon-γ (IFN-γ), produced by $CD4^+$ cells and NK cells has a wide range of effects, the most important of which being monocyte/macrophage activation. After exposure to IFN-γ, monocytes undergo a series of changes, typical of their differentiation into phagocytic effector cells. First, the cell membrane becomes ruffled; the number of cytoplasmic microvilli increases by a factor of ten. This change reflects a considerable increase in phagocytic capacities. Second, the expression of MHC class II antigens and Fcγ receptors increases. The increase in the expression of MHC-II enhances the efficiency of monocytes as APC, and the increased expression of Fc receptors further enhances their efficiency as phagocytic cells. Third, the production of cytokines (TNF, IL-12), chemokines (CXCL9, CXCL10, and CXCL11), and of several antimicrobial proteins and compounds (including defensins, cathepsins, collagenases, superoxide radicals nitric oxide) is upregulated. As a consequence, a variety of cell types is attracted, engulfed organisms are rapidly killed, and ingested proteins are efficiently digested in the phagolysosomes. Some of these effects result in cell-mediated inflammation (see Chapter 14).

Cytokine Genes and Structure

The precise role of individual cytokines in the immune and inflammatory responses is difficult to determine, because the same cells produce so many cytokines, and each cytokine can exert different and overlapping effects on multiple targets. Shared biological effects cannot be explained by structural similarities between molecules. On the one hand, many cytokine receptors activate different but overlapping sets of protein kinases and other signaling molecules. On the other, several IL genes appear to be regulated by the same set of nuclear binding proteins, and several IL receptors are structurally similar. These may be keys to understanding the plurality of IL responses and apparent redundancy of effects among structurally different ILs.

While IL genes differ from each other in their coding sequence, they have greater than 70% homology in their untranslated 5′ region, suggesting the use of common transcription factors such as NF-AT. In addition, the mRNA transcripts have many AUUUA repeats near the 3′ end, which, in part, determine the rapid rate of mRNA decay. The expression of IL genes, therefore, is generally very transient, but may be more prolonged, depending on the activating signals received by the cell. Increased stability of IL mRNAs is observed after calcineurin phosphorylation and after CD28 engagement.

In spite of the diversity of IL genes, all monomeric ILs have similar tertiary structure: at least four α helices arranged in pairs of parallel symmetry, each pair being antiparallel relative to the other. The α helices are joined by connecting loops that contain β helical sheets of variable length. The helix located near the aminoterminal end is the one that interacts with the cytokine receptor.

Cytokine Receptors

Cytokine receptors can be grouped into several families depending on structural characteristics (Fig. 4). Upregulation of a given subunit of these receptors is often a consequence of cellular activation, and usually results in the expression of a high affinity receptor able to transduce activation signals. The activation pathways triggered after receptor occupancy tend to be similar for receptors of the same family but differ for receptors of different families. The fact that several cytokines may share a given receptor explains why some biological properties are common to several ILs.

Interleukin Receptor Family

The IL receptor family is the most common type of receptor. The receptors of this family are heterodimers or heterotrimers and always include an α and a β chain, the latter with a longer intracytoplasmic segment and signaling functions. The receptors for IL-2, 3, 4, 5, 6, 7, 9, and 15, and granulocyte, monocyte-colony stimulating factor (GM-CSF) are included in this family. The receptors for IL-2, 4, 7, 9, and 15 share a third chain (γ_c), which plays a significant

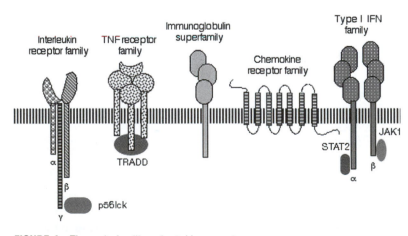

FIGURE 4   The main families of cytokine receptors.

role in signal transduction. One of the forms of severe combined immunodeficiency is secondary to abnormalities in the γ chain gene (see Chapter 30). Receptors for IL-3, IL-5, and GM-CSF share a common β chain. A different β chain is shared by the receptors for IL-6 and IL-11.

Tumor Necrosis Factor Receptor Family

Other receptor families include the tumor necrosis factor receptor family, including receptors for TNF, lymphotoxin-a (LT-α, TNFβ), CD40, and Fas. There are two types of TNF receptors, the TNFR-1 and TNFR-2. TNFR-1 and CD40 both have "death domains" in their intracytoplasmic tails [TNF receptor-associated death domains (TRADD)], whose activation induces apoptosis (see later in the chapter). Engagement of TNFR-1, however, does not necessarily trigger cell death, because an antiapoptotic pathway leading to NFκB synthesis is simultaneously triggered; the balance between proapoptotic and antiapoptotic signals dictates the choice between proliferation and apoptosis. In contrast, the engagement of TNFR-2 usually results in cell activation.

Immunoglobulin Superfamily Receptors

The immunoglobulin superfamily receptors that include the IL-1 (α and β) and IL-18 receptors, a receptor for colony-stimulating factor 1, and, as a special subfamily, the interferon receptors.

Interferon Receptors

The interferon receptors are constituted by two different chains. In the resting state, the two chains are loosely associated with kinases, including members of the JAK family. After occupancy with interferon, one or two members of the STAT family of transcription factors undergo phosphorylation and translocation into the nucleus. The JAK–STAT system is polymorphic. There are three known JAK kinases and seven STAT transcription factors. The STAT-1 transcription factor is predominantly involved in signaling after occupancy of interferon receptors. Its biological significance is underlined by the results of inactivating the encoding gene in mice. The STAT-1 deficient mice do not respond to interferons and are highly susceptible to bacterial and viral infections.

Chemokine Receptor Family

The chemokine receptor family, whose common feature is seven transmembrane domains and include receptors for IL-8, platelet factor-4, Regulated on Activation, Normal T-Cell Expressed and Secreted (RANTES), and macrophage chemotactic and activating proteins (see Chapter 14).

EFFECTOR T-CELL DIFFERENTIATION

T-cell differentiation into effector cells is a critical step in adaptive immunity, as it is the job of the effector lymphocytes to clear the antigen, either by the recruitment and activation of additional immune effectors, as for CD4 effector T cells, or via direct effector function and cytotoxicity, as for CD8 effector T cells. Both types of effector cells secrete soluble mediators called cytokines, and it is the specific cytokine and target that governs the type of immune response elicited by each effector cell type. We will next discuss the different types of effector T cells, mechanisms for their generation, and their specific role in adaptive immunity.

CD4 Effector T Cells

CD4 T cells differentiate to effector T cells, designated as such due to the effector cytokines they produce. It takes several days from the initial activation for a naïve CD4 T cells to differentiate into an effector-cytokine producing cell, and the time point for differentiation depends on the type of cytokine produced. In addition to effector cytokine production, effector CD4 T cells also undergo additional phenotypic and functional alterations. Effector CD4 T cells are larger, blast-like cells, contrasting the small resting phenotype of naive T cells. They also show increased expression of activation and differentiation markers, including adhesion molecules such as the integrin LFA-1 and CD44, reflecting the increased ability of effector T cells to interact with APC. Effector CD4 T cells also loose the requirement for CD28/B7-derived costimulation

TABLE 3   Types of Differentiated CD4 T Cells and Their Properties

Effector cell type	Cytokines produced	Transcription factors	Cellular targets
T-helper 1 (Th1)	IL-2, IFN-γ, TNF-α, IL-3, GM-CSF	T-bet	Macrophages, CD8 T cells
T-helper 2 (Th2)	IL-4, IL-5, IL-6, IL-10, IL-3, TGF-β	GATA-3, c-maf	B cells, mast cells, eosinophils
Cytotoxic T lymphocyte (CTL)	IFN-γ, TNF-α, perforin	T-bet, Eomes	MHC class I$^+$ Infected or tumor targets
Regulatory T cells (Treg)	IL-10, TGF-β	FoxP3	T cells, dendritic cells

Abbreviations: IFN, interferon; IL, interleukin; MHC, major histocompatibility complex; TGF, tumor growth factor; TNF, tumor necrosis factor.

to reactivate. Importantly, effector T cells also change their homing and recirculation patterns in vivo. Although naive lymphocytes primarily traffic through lymphoid tissue and blood, effector T cells have downregulated expression of the lymph node homing receptor CD62L, or L-selectin, and are able to migrate to peripheral tissue sites. In this way, effector T cells can readily traffic to peripheral sites of antigen encounter for efficacious clearance.

In addition to profound changes in the cellular phenotype and function, effector T cells are relatively short-lived, lasting only days to weeks in vivo. The brief lifespan of effector T cells probably accounts for the lack of circulating effector T cells in healthy individuals. It is only in situations of chronic activation, such as chronic infection or autoimmunity, where effector T cells can be detected. However, effector CD4 T cells can be propagated in vitro through repeated stimulation, and it is through the study of these in vitro-stimulated T cell lines and clones that important findings regarding the control of effector cytokine function have emerged. From these studies, Mosmann et al. defined two main types of CD4 effector T cells, Th1 and Th2 cells (Table 3). Th1 cells were found to produce primarily proinflammatory cytokines such as IFN-γ and TNF-α for macrophage recruitment and activation in addition to IL-2, whereas Th2 cells produced primarily cytokines involved in B cell help and immunoregulation, including IL-4, IL-5, and IL-10. Effector CD4 T cells whose cytokine profile can be delineated according to Th1/Th2 definitions are referred to as "polarized" (Fig. 5). In addition to their functional profile, Th1 and Th2 effector cells can also be distinguished by their expression

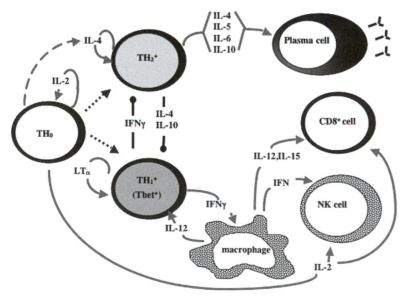

FIGURE 5   Diagrammatic representation of the cytokine repertoire of Th1 and Th2 helper lymphocyte subpopulations and their autocrine and exocrine interactions with CD8$^+$ T cells, natural killer cells, and antigen-presenting cells.

of transcription factors. Th1 cells express the transcription factor T-bet, which is both necessary and sufficient for driving Th1 differentiation. By contrast, Th2 effector cells express the other transcription factors that have dominant roles, in promoting IL-4 production and Th2 differentiation.

Because it has been difficult to isolate Th1 and Th2 effector cells among human CD4 T cells, the Th1/Th2 dichotomy remains somewhat controversial. However, it is well-recognized that response to certain pathogens, autoimmune diseases, and allergies are associated with a predominant Th1 (Type 1) or Th2 (Type 2) cytokine profile. For example, the immune response to parasitic worm infections is predominantly Th2, consistent with the presence of IL-5, important in promoting recruitment of eosinophils that play a key role in the elimination of parasites. Responses to intracellular pathogens tend to be biased toward Th1, due to the requirement for a vigorous cellular response for pathogen clearance. Autoimmune diseases such as rheumatoid arthritis and diabetes are characterized by a Th1 cytokine profile that is associated with a pathogenic proinflammatory T-cell response. In mouse models of these autoimmune diseases, protection from pathogenic T-cell destruction is associated with a switch in overall cytokine profile from a Th1 to a Th2 profile. Finally, allergic responses are primarily of the Th2 type, and atopic individuals tend to be more Th2-inclined. Thus, the balance of Type 1 versus Type 2 cytokines produced in an immune response appears critical in regulating the balance between productive and pathogenic immunity.

It is due to the important role of effector cytokine profile in immune responses that determining mechanisms for the control of Th1 versus Th2 generation has been at the forefront of immunology research for the past 15 years. One important factor determining effector cell differentiation is the cytokine environment the T cells encounter during their initial activation. IL-12, produced by APCs such as activated DC, promotes the differentiation and activation of Th1 effector cells. Activated Th1 cells release IFN-γ that activates macrophages, inducing additional release of IL-12 and a more efficient antimicrobial response, particularly against intracellular organisms. On the other hand, IL-4 promotes the differentiation and activation of Th2 lymphocytes. IL-4 can be provided by mast cells, a certain subset of "innate-type" T cells, or by the T cell themselves. Other factors that may drive Th1 versus Th2 polarization are the antigen dose, APC type, and cellular environment. In addition, there is reciprocal counter-regulation of Th1 and Th2 effector cells, with sustained production of IFN-γ suppressing IL-4 production, and high levels of IL-4 and IL-10 inhibiting the release of FN-γ and IL-12 (Fig. 5).

T-Helper Cells in Cell-Mediated Immunity

Th1 effector cells are central orchestrators of cell-mediated immunity and also promote inflammation. IFN-γ and TNF-α produced by Th1 effector cells act directly on monocytes and macrophages, promoting maturation, activation, phagocytic, and bactericidal functions of these cells. Th1 cells also promote inflammation through the actions of these cytokines on vascular permeability, and mediate delayed-type hypersensitivity seen with response to poison oak and to *Mycobacterium tuberculosis*. This hypersensitivity response is manifested in the skin with a cellular infiltrate comprised of CD4 T lymphocytes and monocytes, reflecting Th1-mediated recruitment of monocytes to the antigen site. Finally, IL-2 produced by Th1 effectors can act on CD8 T cells to promote their differentiation to cytotoxic effector cells for direct target cell lysis (see later). Thus, by inflammation and activation of additional immune cells, Th1 effector cells direct antigen clearance.

Although Th1-mediated responses can be beneficial in clearing intracellular pathogens, unchecked or chronic persistence of Th1 effector cells can lead to pathological consequences. One prime example of an unchecked Th1 response is granulomatous reactions that are observed when certain intracellular pathogens have developed mechanisms of resistance to antimicrobial defenses or present with chronic infection. The granulomas contain T lymphocytes, macrophages, histiocytes, and other cell types, often forming a barrier circumscribing a focus of infection. The formation of granulomas is due to the release of cytokines that attract and immobilize other mononuclear cells. The activation of these cells in situ results in the release of enzymes that cause tissue destruction, and cytokines, which attract and activate additional inflammatory cells.

T-Helper Cells in Humoral Immunity

As discussed in Chapter 4, antigens can be broadly subdivided into T-dependent and T-independent according to the need for T cell help in the induction of a humoral immune response. Most complex proteins are T-dependent antigens, whereas most polysaccharides can elicit antibody synthesis without T cell help.

It is also clear that T and B lymphocytes cooperating in the inductive stages of an immune response do not recognize the same epitopes in a complex immunogen. The membrane immunoglobulin of the B cell reacts with surface epitopes expressed on the native antigen, whereas the cooperating T cell recognizes MHC-II-associated peptides derived from the processing of the antigen by accessory cells (Fig. 6).

Activated Th2 cells play a key role in B-cell activation. B cells recognize epitopes on cell-adsorbed antigens that maintain their tertiary structure, but require additional costimulatory signals to further proliferate and differentiate. There is a need for high lymphocyte density and intense recirculation to fulfill the optimal conditions for T–B-cell cooperation, and those are most likely achieved in lymphoid tissues, such as the lymph nodes. The cooperative interaction between T- and B-lymphocytes is believed to start outside of the primary follicles, in the paracortical area.

At the very early stages of the immune response, T and B cells are not tightly adherent. The initial contact involves molecules used by T cells in their nonspecific interactions with APC, such as CD2, CD4, LFA-1, and ICAM-1. In addition, CD5 molecules on the T cell that bind CD72 molecules on the B cell may also be involved at that stage. Some time after this initial interaction, T and B cells become firmly attached due to the upregulation of several sets of membrane molecules. Some molecules play a predominant role in promoting the stable interaction between the cooperating cells, while others deliver activating signals. The CD40–CD40L interaction is critical for T–B interaction and for the ability of Th2 cells to help B cells. Activated CD4$^+$ lymphocytes express increased levels of CD40L (CD154) able to interact with CD40 expressed by B cells. The interaction of CD40 with CD40L induces two

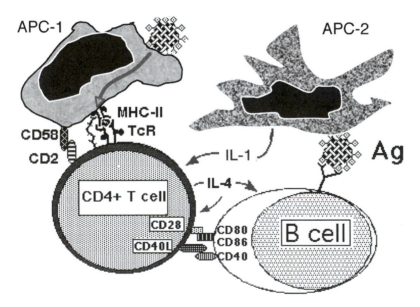

FIGURE 6 Diagrammatic representation of the sequence of signals and interactions between Th2 cells and B cells taking place at the onset of an immune response. The B lymphocyte receives activating signals from the occupancy of the binding sites of membrane immunoglobulin by unprocessed antigen and costimulatory signals (cytokines and cell membrane interactions involving CD40 and CD40L, as well as CD28 and CD80/86) from activated Th2 cells. The Th2 cells recognize antigen-derived peptides associated with MHC-II molecules and receive costimulatory signals from the antigen-presenting cell (cytokines and cell membrane interactions involving CD2 and CD58). Additional costimulatory signals result from the interaction with activated B cells, involving CD40L interacting with CD40 and CD28 interacting with CD80/86.

protein kinase pathways on B lymphocytes. One of the pathways involves JAK kinases and STAT transcription factors while the other pathway involves the MAP kinase and results in the activation of NFκB. Once activated, B cells increase their expression of CD80 (B7-1), expressed at low or undetectable levels on B lymphocytes, and CD86 (B7-2), constitutively expressed at low levels on B cells (Fig. 6).

Requirement for T-Helper Cells for B-Cell Proliferation and Differentiation

Following activation, B cells enter mitosis, proliferate and differentiate into antibody-producing plasma cells. This evolution is associated with migration through different areas of the lymph node. First, the activated B cells separate from the helper T cell and migrate to the denser areas of the follicle, around the germinal centers, where they proliferate with a rapid cycling time of about seven hours. In five days, the antigen-stimulated B-lymphocyte population in a given germinal center increases by about 1000-fold. Most resting B cells express IgM and IgD on the cell membrane, and in the initial stages of cell proliferation and differentiation many cells will produce and secrete IgM antibody, characteristic of the early stages of the primary immune response.

As B cells continue to proliferate and differentiate, recombination genes will be activated (apparently as a consequence of cytokine-mediated signaling) and class switch takes place. The constant region genes for μ and δ chains are looped out and one of the constant region genes for IgG, IgA, or IgE moves into the proximity of the rearranged V-D-J genes (see Chapter 7). Subsequently, the synthesis of IgM antibody declines, replaced by antibody of the other classes, predominantly IgG. The isotype class switch seems to depend on signals delivered both by cytokines (e.g., IL-4) and by cell–cell interactions involving CD40 and CD40L. The signaling pathways that lead to the activation of the recombination genes and, subsequently, to isotype switch have yet to be defined.

The functional differentiation of B lymphocytes coincides with migration of the differentiating B cells and plasmablasts to different territories. First, the dividing B cells migrate into the clear areas of the germinal centers and into the mantle zone. Those areas are rich in $CD4^+$, $CD40L^+$ T cells that apparently deliver a critical signal to B cells, mediated by CD40–CD40L interaction. Once committed to differentiation into antibody production, the activated B cells differentiate into plasmablasts that exit the lymph nodes through the medullary cords and migrate to the bone marrow, where they become fully differentiated, antibody-secreting plasma cells.

In murine models, activated B cells receiving a CD40-mediated signal differentiate either into memory B cells or antibody-producing plasma cells. What determines that B cells differentiate into antibody-producing plasma cells or memory cells is not known. It has been suggested that costimulatory signals delivered by IL-2 and IL-10 promote the differentiation of B memory cells, but this remains to be confirmed. In humans, CD40-mediated activating signals must be involved both in the differentiation of IgG-producing plasma cells and of memory B cells. Children born with a defective CD40L gene suffer from an immunodeficiency known as the Hyper-IgM syndrome, in which B cells cannot switch from IgM to IgG production and no immunological memory is generated (see Chapter 30).

Activation and Differentiation of CD8 Effector T Cells

An essential function of cell-mediated immunity is the defense against intracellular infectious agents, particularly viruses. For example, circulating T lymphocytes isolated from individuals who are recovering from measles infection destroy MHC-identical fibroblasts infected with this virus in two to three hours. A number of experimental models have provided insights into the mechanisms of lymphocyte-mediated cytotoxicity against virus-infected cells.

The first signal leading to the differentiation of CTL involves recognition of a viral peptide associated with an MHC-I molecule. As pointed out in Chapters 3 and 4, such recognition is only possible if the TcR and MHC-I molecules are able to interact weakly in the absence of the viral-derived oligopeptide, and this is only possible when the two interacting cells are MHC-identical, because only T lymphocytes able to interact with self-MHC molecules are selected during differentiation (see Chapter 10).

Like CD4 effector cells, CD8 T cells when activated by antigen and APC undergo prolif-erative expansion coincident with their differentiation. The resultant differentiated effector CD8 T cells adopt distinct functional characteristics (Table 3). They produce high levels of IFN-γ and TNF-α, similar to Th1 effector cells. Like Th1 effectors, the transcription factor T-bet controls IFN-γ production, although an additional transcription factor, Eomesodermin, also plays integral roles in controlling effector cytokine production by CD8 effector cells. Most effector CD8 T cells, unlike Th1 cells, however, exhibit cytotoxic capacity, with the ability to lyse MHC Class I-expressing target cells harboring specific antigen. This cytotoxic capability is mediated by the presence of perforins and esterases in cytoplasmic granules and have increased expression of the membrane-associated Fas ligand.

Target Cell Killing

The cytotoxic reaction takes place in a series of successive steps (Fig. 7). The first step in the cytotoxic reaction involves the conjugation of cytotoxic T cells with their respective targets. This conjugation involves, in the first place, the recognition by the TcR of a peptide-MHC-I complex. However, additional interactions are required to achieve the strong adhesion of the T cell to the target cell required for effective killing:

1. The CD8$^+$ molecule itself interacts with the nonpolymorphic domain of the MHC class I molecule, specifically with its $\alpha3$ domain. The avidity of this interaction increases after TcR occupancy.
2. The CD2 molecule, present on all T cells, interacts with the CD58 molecules expressed by the target cells. Any resting T cell can interact with CD58$^+$ cells, but this interaction by itself is weak and does not lead to cell activation. The modification of the CD2 molecule after TcR engagement increases the affinity of the interaction between CD2 and CD58.
3. In addition, the interaction between LFA-1 and ICAM-1 provides additional stabilizing bonds between the interacting cells. LFA-1 avidity for its ligand(s) is also upregulated by T-cell activation.

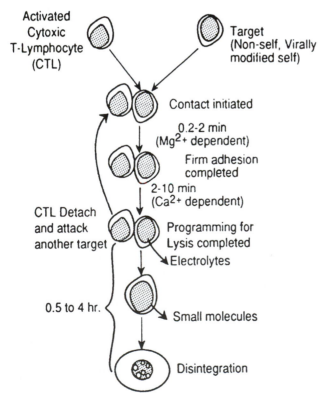

FIGURE 7 Diagrammatic representation of the sequence of events in a cytotoxic reaction. Notice that an activated cytotoxic (CD8$^+$) T cell is able to kill several targets.

The conjugation of CD8$^+$ T cell to its target cell is firm but transient and, after about 30 minutes, the affinity of ICAM-1 for LFA-1 and of CD58 for CD2 reverts to resting levels. The cytotoxic T cell can then move on to another antigen-bearing target with which it will develop the same interaction. In this way, CTL can be serial killers.

During the short period of intimate contact with its target, a series of reactions takes place, eventually resulting in the killing of the target cell. First, the cytoskeleton of the cytotoxic cell reorganizes. The microtubule-organizing center and the Golgi apparatus reorganize in the direction of the area of contact with the target cell. This is associated with transport of cytoplasmic granules toward the target. When the cytoplasmic granules reach the membrane, their contents are emptied into the virtual space that separates the cytotoxic T cells and target cells. These granules contain a mixture of proteins, including perforins and granzymes.

Perforins polymerize as soon as they are released, forming "polyperforins." These polyperforins are inserted in the target cell membrane where they form transmembrane channels. The formation of these channels may lead to influx of water into the cell and may cause cell death in a manner analogous to the effects of the assembly of the terminal complement components on a cell membrane. On the other hand, the perforin channels are believed to facilitate the penetration of granzymes A and B into the target cell. Once in the cytoplasm of the target cell, granzymes activate proteolytic enzymes that initiate a cascade of events leading to apoptotic death of the target.

Apoptosis or programmed cell death is characterized by nuclear and cytoplasmic changes. At the nuclear level, DNA is degraded and fragmented. The cytoplasm shows condensation and there is an abnormal increase of membrane permeability, especially significant at the mitochondrial level.

The nuclear alterations involve the activation of a series of caspases, cysteineproteases that cleave after aspartic acid residues, which includes 13 different enzymes. Of those, some are considered as initiators of the sequence that leads to apoptosis (e.g., caspase 8 and 9), and others are considered as effector caspases, involved in the final steps of the cycle (e.g., caspase 3 and 7). All caspases exist as inactive proenzymes that need to be cleaved by proteases, and granzymes appear to be able to activate the effector caspases, either directly or through a pathway mediated by increased mitochondrial membrane permeability and release of cytochrome c and other caspase activators. This leads to the activation of initiator caspases, particularly caspase 9. Once activated, the effector caspases, such as caspase 3, cleave an endonuclease-inactivating protein that forms an inactive complex with a cytoplasmic DNAs. As that protein is digested, the endonuclease becomes active, translocates to the nucleus, causing the DNA breakdown that is characteristic of apoptotic cell death (Fig. 8).

A second pathway to apoptosis is primarily mediated by Fas (CD95)–FasL interactions that induce a death-inducing signaling complex in the Fas-bearing cell. The activation of this pathway is associated with activation of caspase 8, which in turn will trigger the cascade that leads to activation of effector caspases and apoptosis. However, the two pathways are not mutually exclusive, and Fas–FasL interactions often result in direct activation of caspase 8 as well as in increased mitochondrial permeability, release of cytochrome c, and activation of caspase 9.

Experiments carried out with animals transgenic for the hepatitis B virus (HBV) suggest that activation of both pathways seems to be a requirement for efficient cytotoxicity in vivo. Two groups of knockout mice were injected with cytotoxic T cell clones. One group was FasL deficient, and the second group lacked the perforin genes. Normal mice expressing both FasL and perforins were used as control. Although the clones from all animals could kill HBV-infected cells in vitro, in vivo cytotoxicity was only observed in normal mice that expressed both the FasL and the perforin genes.

Because the expression of Fas and FasL is very widespread, even in resting cells, there are negative control mechanisms to avoid unnecessary triggering of the pathway. Two proteins seem to play major roles blocking the caspase 8 apoptosis pathway induced by Fas–FasL interactions (cFLIP and CrmA, the product of a cytokine response modifier gene). On the other hand, a protein encoded by the proto-oncogene Bcl-2 blocks the mitochondrial pathway to apoptosis.

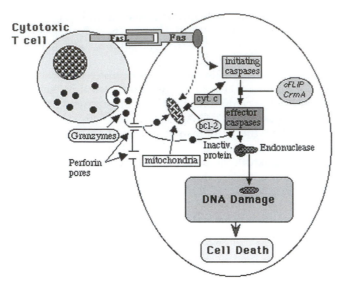

FIGURE 8   Diagrammatic representation of the sequence of events leading to apoptosis of a target cell after interaction with an activated cytotoxic T lymphocyte. Two pathways leading to activation of a critical initiator caspases have been described: one involves the interaction between Fas and FasL, an interaction that activates caspase 8. The other involves granzymes, released by the T lymphocyte and diffused into the cytoplasm through polyperforin clusters. Granzymes can trigger apoptosis either by activating directly terminal caspases or by inducing increased mitochondrial permeability, followed by release of cytochrome c and other caspase activators. The activation of terminal caspases is followed by denaturation of an inactivating protein complexed with a cytoplasmic endonuclease. The activated endonuclease translocates to the nucleus, where it causes DNA breakdown, the hallmark of apoptosis. Two levels of control appear to exist: One, controlling mitochondrial permeability, is regulated by a member of the Bcl-2 proto-oncogene family. The other, blocking the pathway between initiator and effector caspases, involves CrmA, the product of a cytokine response modifier gene, and cFLIP.

IMMUNE MEMORY

Effector CD4 and CD8 T cells as discussed earlier play critical roles in coordinating multiple aspects of the immune response to clear the antigen. These effector cells, however, are relatively short-lived, lasting only days to weeks in vivo. Once antigen is removed, the majority of these effector cells die during the contraction of the immune response. Indeed, without this contraction phase, whereby the expanded population of effector T cells is killed off, there would be risk of immunopathology and potential infiltration into peripheral organs. For many antigen encounters, however, this contraction phase does not result in elimination of all the T cells that have been activated by antigen. A small proportion of previously activated or effector T cells enters a resting state and persists as a long-lived memory T cell. Memory T cells, like naive T cells, are small and resting with low level expression of CD25; however, memory T cells exhibit other striking functional and phenotypic differences when compared to naive T cell counterparts (Table 4).

       In terms of cell surface phenotype, memory T cells maintain upregulated expression of adhesion molecules, such as LFA-1 and CD44, and also exhibit specific expression of the CD45RO isoform for human memory T cells. Functionally, memory T cells are capable of rapid recall effector function when recalled with antigen and can produce high levels of effector cytokines, such as IFN-γ, within hours after restimulation. For CD8 memory T cells, they are also capable of rapid target cell killing. This rapid recall function is a hallmark of memory immune responses and is the underlying basis for protective immunity mediated by the memory response. Memory T cells are also more easily activated than naive T cells, and have reduced requirements for CD28/B7 costimulation, respond to lower antigen doses, and can be activated by a broader range of APC types, such as resting B cells and endothelial cells that fail to stimulate naïve T cells. Memory T cells are also heterogeneous and exist in multiple

TABLE 4 Distinguishing Features of Naive and Memory T Cells

Property	Naive T cell	Memory T cell
Phenotype	CD45RBhi (mo)/CD45RA(hu)	CD45RBlo(mo)/CD45RO(hu)
	CD44lo	CD44hi
	CD11alo	CD11ahi
	CD62Lhi	CD62Llo/hi
	CCR7hi (hu)	CCR7lo/hi
Activation requirements		
Costimulation CD28/B7	Mandatory	Dispensable
Antigen-presenting cells	DC	Many types: DC, resting B cells, macrophages, endothelial cells
Responses to low antigen dose	Weak	Strong
Effector function	None (produce IL-2)	Effector cytokines, cytolysis (CD8)
Kinetics	Slow (days)	Rapid (hours)
Homing	Lymphoid tissue	Lymphoid and nonlymphoid tissue
Heterogeneity	Unknown, homogenous	Multiple subsets

Abbreviation: DC, dendritic cells.

subsets in both lymphoid and nonlymphoid peripheral tissues such as lung, liver, and gut, contrasting the phenotypic homogeneity of naïve T cells and exclusive residence in lymphoid tissue. At least two subsets of memory T cells have been defined, based on expression of the lymph node homing receptors CD62L (L-selectin) and the chemokine receptor CCR7 that likewise mediate homing to lymphoid tissue. The $CD62L^+/CCR7^+$ subset has been designated a "central memory" subset and is primarily found in lymphoid tissue. The $CD62L^-/CCR7^-$ subset is referred to as the "effector-memory" subset. These memory subsets have different trafficking patterns throughout the body. Although the precise function and regulation of memory subsets in anamnestic immune responses are not known, they may play distinct roles in protective immunity and in memory maintenance, and their characterization is an active area of research.

Memory T cells can be maintained by continual cellular turnover for the lifetime of an individual. Although the maintenance requirements for memory T cells are not all defined, memory CD4 T cells seem to require an interaction with self MHC class II/peptide complexes and also require the cytokine IL-7 for survival. IL-7 is a stromal-derived cytokine that likewise is required for survival of naïve T cells. Memory CD8 T cells also are maintained by cellular turnover, but do not require self MHC molecules. Memory CD8 T cells also require IL-7 for survival and regulate their proliferative turnover via responses to IL-15. IL-15 is produced by many somatic cell types and binds to the IL-2β receptor (CD122). Interestingly, memory CD8 T cells require CD4 T cells for their generation and functional maintenance, underscoring the central role of CD4 T cells in both primary and memory immune response. The long-term maintenance of memory T cells is therefore due to their responses to endogenous cells and cellular factors.

While the generation of memory T cells is a goal for vaccines particularly for intracellular viral pathogens, currently all efficacious vaccines work by generating neutralizing antibodies (that also require CD4 T cell help). It remains a challenge for future research in this area to elucidate how memory T cells are generated and begin to design vaccines that promote their development.

REGULATION OF THE IMMUNE RESPONSE

Normal immune responses are tightly regulated. As antigen is removed from the host, downregulatory systems become operative and turn off the response. There are several mechanisms by which the immune system self-regulates. One mechanism is via upregulation of inhibitory molecules for endogenous downregulation of T-cell activation. Earlier in this chapter, we saw how members of the costimulatory receptor family such as CTLA-4 and PD-1 are upregulated after activation and play critical roles in turning off T-cell activation. These molecules are important therapeutic targets for enhancing immunity in cancer and vaccines. Another mechanism for downregulation of the immune response is via induction of apoptosis, as seen earlier. It is well-known that continuous exposure to antigen results in activation-induced cell death of effector T cells via apoptosis. A third mechanism functions via regulatory cytokines. The cytokines IL-10 and TGF-β both have regulatory function and can downregulate an existing effector response. These cytokines are produced either by activated T cells, or both subpopulations of regulatory lymphocytes. While once controversial, there is now compelling evidence for existence of regulatory T-cell populations, the most predominant being the CD4$^+$CD25$^+$ T-cell subset (see next). Thus, by a combination of intrinsic and extrinsic factors, the immune system self-regulates inappropriate and prolonged responses.

Regulatory Lymphocytes

Over two decades ago, Gershon et al. identified a regulatory T-cell population among CD8 T cells. The population could be generated during an immune response and could suppress immune responses in both antigen-specific and nonspecific manners. However, studies on these CD8 suppressor T cells abruptly halted when a particular molecule associated with this cell was found to be an artifact. Nevertheless, the concept of a T-suppressor cell never completely left the field of immunology and, in recent years, there has been a strikingly dramatic resurgence in research on Tregs.

There are at least three different cell populations that have been shown to contain regulatory function, and whose presence is associated with downregulation of immune responses in autoimmune disease models. These three types include a subset of CD4 T cells, a subset of CD8 T cells, and a subset of invariant T cells, termed NKT cells. Because most of the research and direct evidence for regulation is attributed to the CD4 subset, we focus on that population here. For the other subsets, there is still controversy on their roles in vivo in regulation of immune responses.

The CD4$^+$ regulatory T lymphocytes are referred to as Tregs. They are characterized by certain phenotypic, functional, and molecular attributes (Table 3). Phenotypically, they are in the resting state, yet exhibit upregulation of the IL-2α chain, CD25. When stimulated through the TcR, Tregs fail to undergo proliferation, or produce IL-2, but they can respond to exogenous IL-2. Tregs have been shown to produce regulatory cytokines IL-10, IL-4, and/ or TGF-β, although the pattern of cytokine production by Tregs appears to differ in distinct antigen systems and disease models. On the molecular level, Tregs are marked by expression of the FoxP3 transcription factor, a member of the forkhead transcription factor family. Mice lacking FoxP3 exhibit profound lymphoproliferation and autoimmunity and lack the Treg subset. Importantly, individuals born with a defect in the human FoxP3 gene develop a severe syndrome called IPEX, for immunodysregulation, polyendocrinopathy, enteropathy, X-linked syndrome. Individuals with IPEX present during infancy with profound lymphocyte proliferation and lymphocytic infiltration into peripheral organs, leading to death after several months. The only viable treatment for IPEX is bone marrow transplantation, although this treatment fails to be effective long-term, and the malignant-type of lymphoproliferation eventually prevails. Thankfully, IPEX is an extremely rare disorder, as it has proved fatal in all but two known cases.

There are several mechanisms by which Treg cells exert their regulatory function. One mechanism is via the production of immunoregulatory cytokines, as stated earlier. However, production of these cytokines is not unique to Treg cells, as effector T cells and other immune cells such as DC and macrophages can produce IL-10, and many immune and nonimmune cell types produce TGF-β. Moreover, the role of particular cytokines in immunoregulation differs according to the system being studied, so there is no unifying role for these cytokines in Treg-mediated immunoregulation. Another mechanism by which Treg have been shown to act is through modulation of APC. For example, Tregs can modulate certain types of DC to render them tolerogenic rather than activating. This interplay between Treg and APC is an active area of investigation. Finally, another way Treg have been proposed to function is via direct effects on T cells, either by sequestration of IL-2 or other nonspecific effects. As the potential for harnessing Tregs has great therapeutic value for treating autoimmunity and inducing tolerance in transplantation, these mechanistic issues are likely to be at the forefront of research in this field for many years to come.

CONCLUDING REMARKS

We have shown in this chapter how T cells become activated when they encounter antigen, including the molecular and cellular requirements and events involved in this process. We have detailed how differentiation to effector T cells provides the key players for coordinating immune responses and removing foreign antigens. Finally, we have discussed how immune memory is generated as a result of this process, and the different mechanisms the immune system uses to regulate immunity that could result in immunopathology. These cellular and molecular processes that form the basis of cellular immunity are important candidates for immunotherapies for modulating these responses in vaccines, autoimmunity, allergy, and transplantation.

BIBLIOGRAPHY

Bradley LM, Haynes L, Swain SL. IL-7: maintaining T-cell memory and achieving homeostasis. Trends Immunol 2005; 26:172.

Bretscher P, Cohn M. A theory of self-nonself discrimination. Science 1970; 169:1042.

Calderhead DM, et al. CD40-CD154 interactions in B-cell signaling. Curr Top Microbiol Immunol 2000; 245:73.

Constant SL, Bottomly K. Induction of Th1 and Th2 CD4$^+$ T cell responses: the alternative approaches. Annu Rev Immunol 1997; 15:297.

Dutton RW, Bradley LM, Swain SL. T cell memory. Annu Rev Immunol 1998; 16:201.

Farber DL. Commentary: Differential TcR signaling and the generation of memory T cells. J Immunol 1998; 160:535.

Farber DL, Ahmadzadeh M. Dissecting the complexity of the memory T cell response. Immunol Res 2002; 25:247.

Fontenot JD, Rasmussen JP, Williams LM, Dooley JL, Farr AG, Rudensky AY. Regulatory T cell lineage specification by the forkhead transcription factor Foxp3. Immunity 2005; 22:329.

Gershon RK, Cohen P, Hencin R, Liebhaber SA. Suppressor T cells. J Immunol 1972; 108:586.

Hori S, Nomura T, Sakaguchi S. Control of regulatory T cell development by the transcription factor Foxp3. Science 2003; 299:1057.

Intlekofer AM, Takemoto N, Wherry EJ, Quezada SA, Jarvinen LZ, Lind EF, Noelie R. Effector and memory CD8$^+$ T cell fate coupled by T-bet and eomesodermin. Nat Immunol 2005; 6:1236.

Jiang H, Chess L. An integrated view of suppressor T cell subsets in immunoregulation. J Clin Invest 2004; 114:1198.

Jordan MS, Singer AL, Koretzky GA. Adaptors as central mediators of signal transduction in immune cells. Nat Immunol 2003; 4:110.

Kaech SM, Wherry EJ, Ahmed R. Effector and memory T-cell differentiation: implications for vaccine development. Nat Rev Immunol 2002; 2:251.

Kuo CT, Leiden JM. Transcriptional regulation of T lymphocyte development and function. Annu Rev Immunol 1999; 17:149.

Mosmann TR, Coffman RL. TH1 and TH2 cells: different patterns of lymphokine secretion lead to different functional properties. Annu Rev Immunol 1989; 7:145.

Quezada SA, Jarvinen LZ, Lind EF, Noelle RJ. CD40/CD154 interactions at the interface of tolerance and immunity. Annu Rev Immunol 2004; 22:307.

Riley JL, June CH. The CD28 family: a T-cell rheostat for therapeutic control of T-cell activation. Blood 2005; 105:13.

Rudd CE, Schneider H. Unifying concepts in CD28, ICOS and CTLA-4 coreceptor signalling. Nature Rev Immunol 2003; 3:544.

Sakaguchi S, Sakaguchi N, Asono M, Itoh M, Toda M. Immunologic self-tolerance maintained by activated T cells expressing IL-2 receptor alpha-chains (CD25). Breakdown of a single mechanism of self-tolerance causes various autoimmune diseases. J Immunol 1995; 155:1151.

Sprent J, Surh CD. T cell memory. Annu Rev Immunol 2002; 20:551.

Szabo SJ, Jacobson NG, Dighe AS, Gubler U, Murphy KM. Developmental commitment to the Th2 lineage by extinction of IL-12 signaling. Immunity 1995; 2:665.

Szabo SJ, Kim ST, Costa GL, Zhang X, Fathman CG, Glimcher LH. A novel transcription factor, T-bet, directs Th1 lineage commitment. Cell 2000; 100:655.

von Herrath MG, Harrison LC. Antigen-induced regulatory T cells in autoimmunity. Nature Rev Immunol 2003; 3:223.

Wherry EJ, Teichgraber V, Becker TC, Masopust D, Kaech SM, Antia R, von Andrian UH, Ahmed R. Lineage relationship and protective immunity of memory CD8 T cell subsets. Nature Immunol 2003; 4:225.

Zhang DH, Cohn L, Ray P, Bottomly K, Ray A. Transcription factor GATA-3 is differentially expressed in murine Th1 and Th2 cells and controls Th2-specific expression of the interleukin-5 gene. J Biol Chem 1997; 272:21597.

12 | Humoral Immune Response and Its Induction by Active Immunization

Gabriel Virella
Department of Microbiology and Immunology, Medical University of South Carolina, Charleston, South Carolina, U.S.A.

INTRODUCTION

The recognition of a foreign cell or substance triggers a complex set of events that result in the acquisition of specific immunity against the corresponding antigen(s). The elimination of "nonself" depends on effector mechanisms able to neutralize or eliminate the source of antigenic stimulation. While the inductive stages of most immune responses require T and B cell cooperation, the effector mechanisms can be clearly subdivided into cell-dependent and antibody-dependent (or humoral). The sequence of events that culminates in the production of antibodies specifically directed against exogenous antigen(s) constitutes the humoral immune response.

OVERVIEW OF THE INDUCTION OF A HUMORAL IMMUNE RESPONSE
Exposure to Natural Immunogens

Infectious agents penetrate the organism generally via the skin, upper respiratory mucosa, and intestinal mucosa. In most cases, the immune system is stimulated in the absence of clinical symptoms suggestive of infection (subclinical infection). The constant exposure to immunogenic materials penetrating the organism through those routes is responsible for continuous stimulation of the immune system and explains why relatively large concentrations of immunoglobulins can be measured in the serum of normal animals. In contrast, animals reared in germ-free conditions synthesize very limited amounts of antibodies, and their sera have very low immunoglobulin concentrations.

Active Immunization

Many infectious diseases can be prevented through active immunization. When live, attenuated organisms are used for immunization, they are usually delivered to the natural portal of entry of the organism. For example, a vaccine against the common cold using attenuated rhinoviruses would be most effective if applied as a nasal aerosol. On the other hand, if inert compounds (such as inactivated infectious agents, polysaccharides, or toxoids) are used as immunogens, they have to be introduced in the organism by injection, usually intramuscularly, subcutaneously, or intradermally.

In humans, immunization is usually carried out by injecting the antigen intradermally, subcutaneously or intramuscularly, or by administering it by the oral route (e.g., attenuated viruses, such as poliovirus). As a rule, injected immunogens are mixed or emulsified with adjuvants—compounds that enhance the immune response.

Adjuvants
The most potent adjuvant is complete Freund's adjuvant (CFA)—a water-in-oil emulsion containing killed mycobacteria. This adjuvant is widely used for the production of antisera in laboratory animals, but it tends to cause an intense inflammatory reaction in humans and for that reason is not used in human vaccines. In humans, the most commonly used adjuvants are inorganic gels such as alum and aluminum hydroxide.

The mechanism of action of the adjuvants is similar for all and involves two important factors:

1. Adjuvants slow down the diffusion of the immunogen from the injected spot, so that antigenic stimulation will persist over a longer period of time.
2. Adjuvants induce a state of activation of antigen-presenting cells in the site of inoculation. This activation can be more or less specific—CFA causes a very intense local inflammation, while some bacterial compounds with adjuvant properties have a more targeted effect on macrophages and other antibody producing cell (APC), and have strong adjuvant properties without causing a very intense inflammatory reaction. Alum and aluminum hydroxide share both types of effects, but they do not induce an inflammatory reaction as intense as CFA and this is the reason for their use in human immunization.

B Cell Activation

As discussed in greater detail in Chapters 4 and 11, B cell activation requires multiple signals. The only specific signal is the one provided by the interaction between the antigen-binding sites of membrane immunoglobulins with a given epitope of an immunogen. The additional signals, provided by Th2 helper cells and APC, are nonspecific with regard to the antigen.

The recognition of an antigen by a resting B cell seems to be optimal when the immunogen is adsorbed to a follicular dendritic cell or to a macrophage. B lymphocytes recognize either unprocessed antigen or antigen fragments, which conserve the configuration of the native antigen. All techniques used for measurement of specific antibodies use antigens in their original configuration as their basis, and succeed in detecting antibodies reacting with them. Whether some B cells may have membrane immunoglobulins reactive with immunogen-derived peptides associated with major histocompatibility complex (MHC-II) molecules is not known.

Helper Th2 lymphocytes provide other signals essential for B cell proliferation and differentiation. The activation of this CD4 subpopulation is favored by a low-affinity interaction between an immunogen-derived oligopeptide associated with an MHC-II molecule and the T cell receptor, as well as by additional signals, some derived from cell-cell interactions, such as the CD28/CD86 interaction, and others from cytokines, such as IL-4. Activated Th2 cells, in turn, provide several costimulatory signals that promote B cell proliferation and differentiation. Some of these signals derive from the interaction between cell membrane molecules upregulated during the early stages of Th2 and B cell activation, for example, CD40L (CD159) on T cells and CD40 (on B cells), while others are mediated by cytokines, such as IL-4, IL-5, IL-6, and IL-10 (Fig. 1).

When the proper sum of specific signals and costimulatory signals is received by the B cell, clonal proliferation and differentiation ensues. Since each immunogen presents a

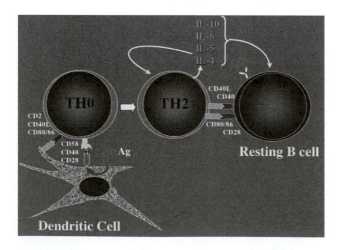

FIGURE 1 Induction of a humoral response. The activation of a resting B cell requires recognition of unprocessed antigen and costimulatory signals, provided by activated Th2 cells through the release of cytokines and the increased expression of membrane proteins able to deliver activating signals to B cells, expressing the corresponding ligand molecules.

multitude of epitopes, a normal immune response is polyclonal, that is, involves many different clones recognizing different epitopes of an immunogen. The induction of an immune response requires some time for activation of all the relevant cells and for proliferation and differentiation of B cells into plasma cells. Thus, there is always a lag phase between the time of immunization and the time when antibodies become detectable. It must be noted that while most activated B cells will become antibody-producing plasma cells, some will become memory cells (see subsequently).

Experimental animals immunized with a given immunogen (e.g., tobacco mosaic virus) often show marked postimmunization hypergammaglobulinemia, but only a very small fraction of the circulating immunoglobulins react with the immunogen. In humans, the initial burst of IgE production, after first exposure to an allergen, seems to be mainly constituted by nonspecific antibodies. This apparent lack of specificity of the immune response is more obvious in the primary immune response after the first exposure to an immunogen. Most likely, it is a consequence of the fact that the antibodies produced early in the immune response are of low affinity, and may not be detectable in assays that favor the detection of high affinity antibodies. It is also possible that the costimulatory signals provided by Th2 cells may enhance the immune response of neighboring B cells engaged in unrelated immune responses. This may result in the enhanced synthesis of antibodies reacting with other immunogens that the immune system is simultaneously recognizing. While the synthesis of unrelated antibodies is usually beneficial or inconsequential (see Chapter 14), it can also be the basis for at least some autoimmune reactions if strong help is provided to autoreactive B cells, which otherwise would remain quiescent (see Chapter 16).

THE PRIMARY IMMUNE RESPONSE

The first contact with an antigen evokes a primary response, which has the following characteristics:

1. A relatively long lag between the stimulus and the detection of antibodies by current methods (varying between 3 to 4 days after the injection of heterologous erythrocytes and 10 to 14 days after the injection of killed bacterial cells). Part of this variation depends on the sensitivity of antibody detection methods, but it is also a reflection of the potency of the immunogen.
2. The first antibody class to be synthesized is usually IgM. Later in the response, IgG antibodies will predominate over IgM antibodies. This phenomenon, known as IgM-IgG switch, is controlled by different interleukins released by activated helper T lymphocytes and by specific costimulatory signals mediated by CD28/CD80, CD40/CD40L, and CD21/CD23.
3. After rising exponentially for some time, antibody levels reach a steady state and then decline (Fig. 2). Adjuvant administration will keep the antibody levels high for months.

Downregulation of the Humoral Immune Response

Several regulatory mechanisms will operate in order to turn off antibody production after the infectious agent (or any other type of immunogen) has been eliminated.

Antigen Elimination
The most obvious downregulatory mechanism is the elimination of the antigen, which was the primary stimulus of the immune response.

T reg Activation
As immune response progresses, the activity of T cells with suppressor activity, such as T regs, starts to predominate. IL-10, the major immunosuppressive cytokine relased by activated $CD4^+$, $CD25^+$, $FoxP3^+$ T regs, downregulates both Th1 and Th2 cells, thus reducing the

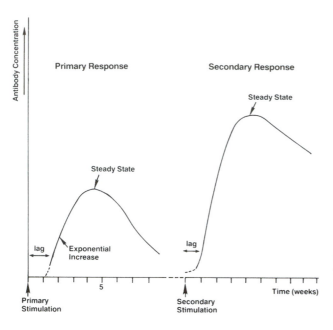

FIGURE 2 Diagrammatic representation of the sequence of events during a primary and a secondary immune response. *Source*: Modified from Eisen, HN. Immunology. 2nd Ed. Cambridge: Harper & Row, 1980.

delivery of costimulatory signals to B cells. T cells with suppressor activity persist after the antigen is eliminated, either as a consequence of their late activation or of a longer life span.

Immunoregulatory Effects of Soluble Antigen–Antibody Complexes and Anti-idiotypic Antibodies

As the immune response proceeds and IgG antibodies are synthesized, IgG-containing antigen–antibody complexes are formed in circulation and in the extravascular compartments. The appearance of soluble antigen–antibody complexes is apparently perceived by the immune system as evidence for having reached the main goal—elimination of the antigen. B cells express the FcγRIIb on their membranes, and experimental evidence shows that the ligation of B cell FcγRIIb with antigen–antibody complexes has a downregulating effect (Fig. 3).

Also during the immune response, as levels of antibodies keep increasing, anti-idiotypic antibodies reacting with variable region epitopes or idiotypes presented by the antibodies produced against the antigen, which elicited the immune response start being synthesized. The easiest way to understand this response is to accept that the normal state of tolerance to the millions of idiotypes that are presented by antigen receptors is broken when one or a few specific antibodies are produced in large concentrations, suddenly exposing the immune system to large concentrations of molecules with unique idiotypes.

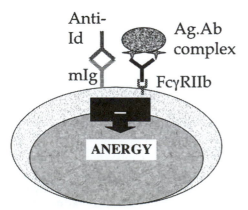

FIGURE 3 Downregulation of activated B cells. The diagram depicts two mechanisms proposed to downregulate the humoral immune response. Anti-idiotypic antibodies specific for the binding site of a given antibody emerge during the humoral response. The anti-idiotypic antibodies bind to binding site of the surface immunoglobulins from the clone producing the antibody that triggered the anti-idiotype. In doing so, the anti-idiotype delivers an incomplete signal and prevents further interactions with unprocessed antigen. On the other hand, immune complexes formed by soluble, unprocessed, antigen and antibody interact with the down-regulatory FcγRIIb expressed by B cells. Both mechanisms can turn off activated B cells and are not mutually exclusive.

Anti-idiotypic antibodies are believed to participate in negative regulation of the immune response by binding to membrane immunoglobulins from antigen-specific B cells, expressing variable regions of the same specificity as the antibody molecules that triggered the anti-idiotypic antibody. The binding of an antibody to a membrane immunoglobulin induces B lymphocyte proliferation, but the proliferating B cells fail to differentiate into antibody-producing cells for lack of costimulatory signals. At the same time, the occupancy of the membrane immunoglobulin binding sites by the anti-idiotypic antibodies prevents the proper antigenic stimulation of the B lymphocyte (Fig. 3).

SECONDARY OR ANAMNESTIC RESPONSE

Re-exposure of an immune animal or human being to an immunizing antigen to which they have been previously exposed induces a secondary recall or anamnestic response. The capacity to mount a secondary immune response can persist for many years, providing long-lasting protection against reinfection.

The secondary response has some important characteristics, some dependent on the existence of an expanded population of memory cells, ready to be stimulated, and others dependent on the prolonged retention of antigen in the lymph nodes with continuous stimulation of B cells over long periods of time.

Differentiation of B Memory Cells

During the peak of a primary response, there is a duality in the fate of activated B cells: while most will evolve into antibody-producing plasma cells, others will differentiate into memory B cells.

The differentiation of memory cells is believed to take place in the germinal centers of secondary lymphoid tissues. As a prememory B cell enters a follicle, it migrates into the germinal center, where it undergoes active proliferation. At this stage, the "switch" from IgM to IgG or other isotype synthesis is taking place and the variable (V) region genes undergo somatic hypermutation. After completing this round of proliferation, the resulting memory B cells need additional signals for full differentiation.

1. Clones with high affinity mIg in the membrane will be able to interact with antigen molecules immobilized by follicular dendritic cells. As a consequence, these clones will receive strong activation and differentiation signals. In contrast, clones with low affinity mIg will not be able to compete with preformed antibody for binding to the immobilized antigen epitopes, will not receive adequate signals, and will undergo apoptosis.
2. The evolution of this antigen-stimulated memory B cell precursor into a memory B cell requires a second signal provided by a helper T cell, in the form of the CD40/CD40 ligand interaction. Other signals, such as the one delivered by the CD21/CD23 interaction, may result into direct evolution of the prememory B cell into an antibody producing plasma cell.

As discussed in Chapter 4, immunological memory is largely a T cell function, but the expansion of the responding population of B cells will certainly contribute to the ability to respond more rapidly and effectively to a second exposure to the same antigen.

Consequences of the Existence of Expanded Populations of Memory Cells

Four major features of a secondary immune response (Fig. 2) result from the existence of expanded populations of memory cells, both T and B:

1. Lower threshold dose of immunogen, that is, the dose of antigen necessary to induce a secondary response is lower than the dose required to induce a primary response.
2. Shorter lag phase, that is, it takes a shorter time for an antibody to be detected in circulation after immunization.

3. Faster increase in antibody concentrations and higher titers of antibody at the peak of the response.
4. Predominance of IgG antibody is characteristic of the secondary immune response, probably a consequence of the fact that memory B cells express IgG on their membranes and will produce IgG after stimulation.

Consequences of Prolonged Retention of Antigen and Persistent B Cell Stimulation

We have previously discussed the downregulating effects of the interaction of soluble antigen–antibody complexes with B cells. However, antigen–antibody complexes formed early in a secondary immune response have a totally opposite effect when taken up by follicular dendritic cells that express Fcγ receptors on their membrane. They remain associated to these cells for a long period of time with the following consequences:

1. Longer persistence of antibody synthesis, slowing down the decay of antibody levels caused by the downregulatory mechanisms discussed earlier.
2. Affinity maturation: It is known that the affinity of antibodies increases during the primary immune response and even more so in the secondary and subsequent responses. This maturation is a result of the selection of memory B cells with progressively higher affinity mIg antibodies during a persistent immune response. This selection is a direct consequence of the retention of antigen–antibody complexes by the follicular dendritic cells. The antigen moieties of the retained immune complexes are effectively presented to the immune system for as long as the complexes remain associated to the dendritic cells. As free antibodies and mIg compete for binding to the immobilized antigen, only B cells with mIg of higher affinity than the previously synthesized antibodies will be able to compete effectively and receive activation signals. Consequently, the affinity of the synthesized antibodies will show a steady increase.
3. Increased avidity and increased cross-reactivity: During a long-lasting secondary response to a complex immunogen, clones responding to minor determinants emerge. Cryptic epitopes that are not recognized in the primary immune response may also be recognized as a consequence of repeated stimulation. Therefore, a wider range of antibodies is produced in the secondary immune response. This results in increased avidity (as discussed in Chapter 8, avidity is the sum of binding forces mediated by different antibody molecules binding simultaneously to the same antigen). On the other hand, as the repertoire of antibodies recognizing different epitopes of a given immunogen increases, so do increase the probabilities for the emergence of cross-reactive antibodies recognizing antigenic determinants common to other immunogens.

FATE OF ANTIGENS ON THE PRIMARY AND SECONDARY RESPONSES

Following intravenous injection of a soluble antigen, its concentration in serum tends to decrease in three phases (Fig. 4):

1. Equilibration phase: This phase is characterized by a sharp decrease of brief duration corresponding to the equilibration of the antigen between intra-and extravascular spaces.
2. Metabolic decay: During this phase the antigen slowly decays, due to its catabolic processing by the host.
3. Immune elimination: When antibodies start to be formed, there will be a phase of rapid immune elimination, in which soluble antigen–antibody complexes will be formed and taken up by macrophages. The onset of this phase of immune elimination is shorter in the secondary immune response and virtually immediate if circulating antibody exists previously to the introduction of the antigen.

A similar sequence of events, with less distinct equilibration and metabolic decay phases, occurs in the case of particulate antigens. If the antigen is a live, multiplying, organism, there might be an initial increase in the number of circulating or tissue-colonizing organisms, until

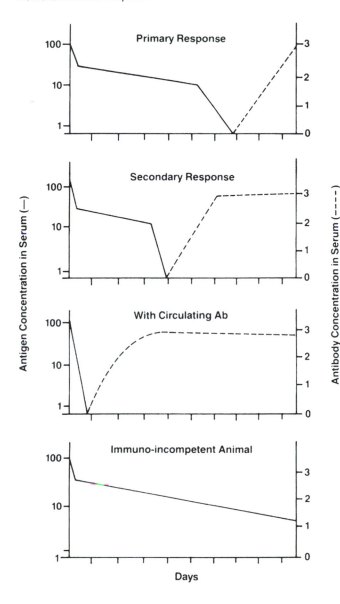

FIGURE 4 Diagrammatic representation of the fate of injected antigen in a nonimmune animal, which will undergo primary immune response; an immune animal, which will show an accelerated, secondary response; an animal with circulating antibodies, which will very rapidly eliminate the corresponding antigen from circulation; and an immunoincompetent animal, which will slowly metabolize the antigen. *Source:* Modified from Talmage DF, Dixon FJ, Bukantz SC, Damin GJ. J Immunol 1951; 67:243.

the immune response promotes the elimination of the antigen by a variety of mechanisms (see Chapters 13 and 14).

MUCOSAL HUMORAL IMMUNE RESPONSE

The gastrointestinal and respiratory mucosae are among the most common portals of entry used by infectious agents. Since this constant exposure only rarely results in clinical disease, it seems obvious that strongly protective mechanisms must exist at the mucosal level. Some of those protective mechanisms are nonspecific and of a physicochemical nature, including the integrity of mucosal surfaces, gastric pH, gastrointestinal traffic, proteases and bile present in the intestinal lumen, as well as the flow of bronchial secretions, glucosidases, and bactericidal enzymes (e.g., lysozyme) found in respiratory secretions. At the same time, cell-mediated and humoral immune mechanisms are also operative in mucosal membranes.

Cell-Mediated Immune Mechanisms at the Mucosal Levels

Most evidence suggests that innate cell-mediated mechanisms predominate, including phagocytic cells and γ/δ T lymphocytes.

1. Phagocytic cells (particularly macrophages) abound in the submucosa and represent an important mechanism for nonspecific elimination of particulate matter and microbial agents of limited virulence.
2. γ/δ T lymphocytes are also present in large numbers in the submucosal tissues. It has been proposed that these cells seem to be able to cause the lysis of infected cells by MHC-independent recognition of altered glycosylation patterns of cell membrane glycoproteins or by recognition of cell-associated microbial superantigens.

Humoral Immunity at the Mucosal Level

A large volume of data has been compiled concerning the induction and physiological significance of humoral immunity at the mucosal level. A major established fact, supported by several lines of experimental work, is that the induction of secretory antibodies requires direct mucosal stimulation. Ogra and coworkers demonstrated that the systemic administration of an attenuated vaccine results in a systemic humoral response while no secretory antibodies are detected. In contrast, topical immunization with live, attenuated poliovirus results in both a secretory IgA response and a systemic IgM-IgG response (Fig. 5).

In addition, it has been demonstrated that the stimulation of a given sector of the mucosal system (GI tract) may result in detectable responses on nonstimulated areas (upper respiratory tract). This protection of distant areas is compatible with the unitarian concept of a mucosal immunological network with constant traffic of immune cells from one sector to another (Fig. 6). For example, antigen-sensitized cells from the gut-associated lymphoid tissue (GALT), or from the peribronchial lymphoid tissues, enter the general circulation via the draining lymphatic vessels. Their systemic recirculation results in their migration towards the remaining secretory-associated lymphoid tissues including the gastro-intestinal tract, the airways, the urinary tract, and the mammary glands, the salivary glands, and the cervical glands of the uterus.

Passive Transfer of Mucosal Immunity

In some mammalian species, milk-secreted antibodies are actively absorbed in the newborn's gut and constitute the main source of adoptive immunity in the neonate. This is usually observed in species in which there is limited or no placental transfer of antibodies. In mammalians in which placental transfer of immunoglobulins is very effective (such as humans), the antibodies ingested with maternal milk are not absorbed. However, milk antibodies seem to provide passive immunity at the gastro-intestinal level, which may be a very important factor in preventing infectious gastroenteritis in the newborn whose mucosal immune system is not fully developed.

Physiological Significance of Mucosal Immunity

The main immunological function of secretory IgA is believed to be to prevent microbial adherence to the mucosal epithelia, which usually precedes colonization and systemic invasion. However, in several experimental models it has been demonstrated that disease can be prevented without interference with infection, so there are unresolved questions concerning the anti-infectious mechanism(s) of secretory antibodies.

The relative importance of cellular versus humoral mucosal defense mechanism has not been properly established. However, many IgA deficient individuals, with very low or absent circulating and secretory IgA, are totally asymptomatic suggesting that cell-mediated mechanisms may play a significant protective role.

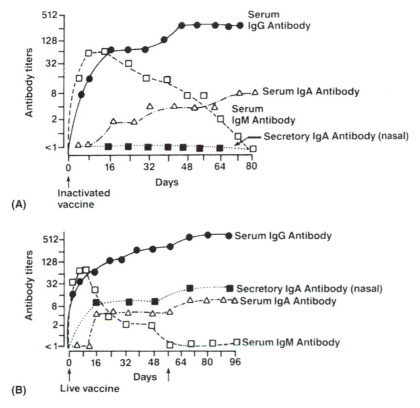

FIGURE 5 Comparison of the systemic and mucosal immune responses in human volunteers given killed polio vaccine (**A**) and live attenuated polio vaccine (**B**). Note that secretory antibody was only detected in children immunized with live, attenuated vaccine. *Source*: Modified from Ogra PL, Karzon DT, Roghthand F, MacGillivray M. N Engl J Med 1968; 279:893.

PASSIVE IMMUNIZATION

The parallel development of microbiology and immunology resulted in the discovery of the protective role of antibodies against a variety of infectious agents. This lead Roux and other eminent bacteriologists to develop serotherapy, that is, the use of antibodies raised in animals to treat infectious diseases caused by bacteria they had just identified as the causative agents. The approach was successful, particularly for diseases caused by exotoxins, such as diphtheria and tetanus, but it was also verified that the administration of horse serum was not without problems, leading to serum sickness as a consequence of the deposition of complexes made of horse proteins and antibodies produced by the patient who received them in different tissues and organs (see Chapter 23).

However, the advantages of immediate protection for the treatment and prevention of diseases in exposed patients remained obvious and eventually human immunoglobulins, purified from patients with high antibody titers, were used for passive immunization without the risk of developing serum sickness. Other than antisnake venom antibodies, still produced in horses, passive immunization is currently carried out with human antibodies.

IMMUNOPROPHYLAXIS
Introduction

The concept of active immunization as a way to prevent infectious diseases is about two centuries old, if we consider the introduction of cowpox vaccination by Jenner in 1796 as the starting point. Jenner observed that milkmaids that had contracted cowpox were protected from smallpox and developed an immunization procedure based on the intradermal scarification

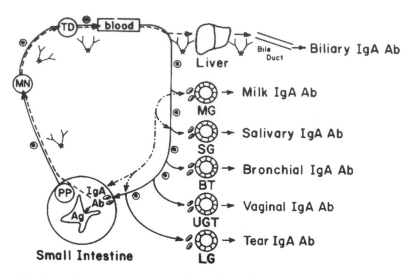

FIGURE 6 Diagrammatic representation of the pathways leading to the expression of IgA antibodies after antigenic stimulation of the gut-associated lymphoid tissue. IgA immunocytes (•) originating in Peyer's patches (PP) migrate to mesenteric lymph nodes (MN). Cells leave MN via the thoracic duct (TD) and enter circulation with subsequent homing to the mammary gland (MG), salivary gland (SG), lacrimal gland (LG), and the lamina propria of the bronchial tree (BT), intestinal or urogenital tract (UGT) (•). The IgA antibodies are then expressed in milk, saliva, tears, and other secretions. IgA antibodies ($\curlyvee$) entering circulation (- - -) are selectively removed by the liver and subsequently expressed in bile. Cell traffic between peripheral mucosal sites (- • - MG to SG, LG, and small intestine) is included in this scheme. *Source*: Reproduced from Montgomery PC, Standera CA, Majumdar AS. Evidence for migration of IgA bearing lymphocytes between peripheral mucosal sites. Protides of the Biological Fluids. Peeters H, Ed. New York: Pergamon, 1985:43.

of material from cowpox lesions. Empirically, he had discovered the principle of vaccine with live, attenuated microbes, which was later picked up by Louis Pasteur when he developed several of his vaccines. As infectious agents became better characterized, new vaccines were developed, some with inactivated organisms, others with microbial components, others still with attenuated infectious agents. Mass vaccination has had some remarkable successes, such as the eradication of smallpox and the significant declines in some of the most common or most serious infectious diseases of childhood, such as diphtheria, measles, and polio. However, at the global scale infectious diseases are still a major cause of mortality, and the development of new and more effective vaccines remains a high priority.

Traditionally, vaccines are administered with the ultimate goal of inducing the synthesis of protective antibodies. However, most induce cell-mediated immunity as well. In some cases (e.g., tetanus toxoid), the cell-mediated immune reaction is inconsequential. But in the case of viral vaccines, it may be as important or more than humoral immunity. This seems to be particularly the case in HIV vaccines, because the elicited antibodies are not very effective in neutralizing the virus. However, this raises significant difficulties because the evaluation of protective cell-mediated immunity is technically difficult.

Types of Vaccines

A wide variety of immunizing agents has been developed. The following are examples of the types of immunizing agents that are most widely used for immunoprophylaxis in humans.

Killed Vaccines
Killed vaccines are generally safe, but not as effective as attenuated vaccines.

1. Killed bacteria, such as the cholera vaccine, prepared with killed *Vibrio cholerae*, are still in use, but not as widely as some decades ago.

2. Inactivated viruses, such as the influenza vaccine, the hepatitis A vaccine, and Salk's polio vaccine, are still widely used. While the efficiency of the influenza vaccine is relatively poor (average of 60% protection), the hepatitis A and polio vaccines are very efficient. The inactivated polio vaccine contains a mixture of the three known types of poliovirus after inactivation with formalin. This vaccine has been as successful in the eradication of poliomyelitis as Sabin's attenuated oral vaccine. Its main advantage is safety, but it is not as effective or amenable to mass immunizations as the oral vaccine (see subsequently). However, the safety concerns have resulted in its exclusive use in the United States and other countries where poliomyelitis has been virtually eradicated, and there is greater risk of contracting polio from the attenuated vaccine than from a wild virus strain.

Component Vaccines

Component vaccines are safe and their use has increased in the last decade. The original component vaccines were mostly made of bacterial toxoids and polysaccharides. Other modalities such as conjugate vaccines and recombinant component vaccines have been introduced with considerable success.

1. Bacterial polysaccharide vaccines are widely used for *Streptococcus pneumoniae* and *Neisseria meningitidis*. A typhoid fever vaccine made of the Vi capsular polysaccharide is also available. Because of their T-independent nature, polysaccharide vaccines are not very potent (especially in young children) and do not elicit long-lasting memory. While conjugate vaccines (see subsequently) have replaced some polysaccharide vaccines, such as the old *Haemophilus influenzae* type B vaccine, the *S. pneumoniae* 23 serotype vaccine (Pneumovax 23) continues to be widely used in the adult population.
2. Inactivated toxins (toxoids), such as tetanus and diphtheria toxoids, are basically formalin-inactivated toxins that have lost their active site, but maintained their immunogenic determinants. Toxoids are strongly immunogenic proteins and induce antibodies able to neutralize the toxins. Immunization with toxoids also results in long-lasting memory. Chemically inactivated pertussis toxin is a key component of the acellular pertussis vaccine currently used.
3. Recombinant bacterial antigens have been shown to be potent immunogens. A Rocky Mountain spotted fever vaccine using a recombinant *Rickettsia rickettsi* antigen produced in *Escherichia coli* is currently being evaluated. A recombinant inactive variant of the diphtheria toxin is used as a "carrier" in some conjugate vaccines (see subsequently).
4. Viral component vaccines are based on the immunogenicity of isolated viral constituents. The best example is the hepatitis B vaccine, produced by recombinant yeast cells. The gene coding for the hepatitis B surface antigen (HBsAg) was isolated from the hepatitis B virus and inserted into a vector flanked by promoter and terminator sequences. That vector was used to transform yeast cells from which HBsAg was purified. All the available hepatitis B vaccines are obtained by this procedure.

Mixed Component Vaccines

The interest in developing safer vaccines for whooping cough led to the introduction of mixed component acellular vaccines. The acellular pertussis vaccine is constituted by a mixture of inactivated pertussis toxin, a major determinant of the clinical disease, and one or several additional bacterial proteins, including adhesins (filamentous hemagglutinin) and outer membrane proteins (pertactin). These vaccines have replaced the old vaccine prepared with killed *Bordetella pertussis*.

Conjugate Vaccines

Most polysaccharide vaccines have shown poor immunogenicity, particularly in infants. This lack of effectiveness is a consequence of the fact that polysaccharides induce mostly T-independent responses with little immunological memory. This problem appears to be eliminated if the polysaccharide is conjugated to an immunogenic protein, very much like a hapten-carrier conjugate.

1. The Hib conjugate vaccine: The first conjugate vaccines to be developed involved the poly-ribositolribophosphate (PRP) of *H. influenzae* type b (Hib). Four conjugate vaccines are available based on Hib-polysaccharide conjugated to different protein carriers, such as diphtheria toxoid (PRP-D), a diphtheria toxoid-like protein (PRP-HbOC), tetanus toxoid (PRP-T), or meningococcal outer membrane protein (PRP-OMP). All are equally efficient, but in order not to lose the carrier effect, the same vaccine should be used for the primary immunization and boosters.
2. The introduction of these vaccines was followed by a 95% decrease in the incidence of *H. influenzae* type b infections affecting children of less than 5 years of age.
3. The pneumococcal polysaccharide vaccine (Prevnar): This vaccine contains the capsular polysaccharides of seven *S. pneumoniae* serotypes (4, 6B, 9V, 14, 18C, 19F, and 23F) conjugated to an inactive recombinant version of the diphtheira toxin. This vaccine has markedly reduced the incidence of severe pneumococal infections but is not effective against all strains that cause otitis media in infants and young children.
4. The meningococcal conjugate vaccine (MCV4 or MenactraT): This can prevent four types of meningococcal disease (serogroups A, C, Y, and W-135), which include two of the three types most common in the United States. However, serogoup B polysaccharide is nonimmunogenic and is not included in the conjugate vaccine. New formulations including serogroup B outer membrane protein are being evaluated.

DNA Vaccines

The observation that intramuscular injection of nonreplicating plasmid DNA encoding the hemagglutinin (HA) or nucleoprotein (NP) of influenza virus elicited humoral and cellular protective reactions attracted enormous interest from the scientific community. The recombinant DNA is taken up by APCs at the site of injection and is presented to T helper cells in a way that both humoral and cell-mediated immune responses are elicited. The safety and easy storage of candidate DNA vaccines are extremely appealing and several different trials are ongoing. However, the initial impression from human trials is that DNA vaccines are far less potent in humans that they appear to be in experimental animals.

Attenuated Vaccines

Attenuated vaccines are generally very efficient, but in rare cases can cause the very disease they are designed to prevent, particularly in immunocompromised individuals.

1. Attenuated viral vaccines: Most anti-viral vaccines are made of viral strains attenuated in the laboratory, including the classical smallpox vaccine, the yellow fever vaccine, the oral polio vaccine (a mixture of attenuated strains of the three known types of poliovirus), the mumps-rubella-measles vaccine, and the Varicella-Zoster vaccine.
    Attenuated viral vaccines tend to be very potent, probably because of the infective nature of the immunizing agent. In the case of polio vaccines, the attenuated virus can be transmitted by the fecal-oral route to nonimmunized individuals, thus increasing the proportion of immunized individuals in any given population. Another advantage of attenuated vaccines administered topically (by mouth or aerosol) is the simplicity of the immunization procedure. However, their use in the field is made difficult by the need for refrigeration.
2. Attenuated bacterial vaccines: The Bacillus of Calmette–Guérin (BCG), an attenuated strain of *Mycobacterium bovis*, has been used for decades as a vaccine for tuberculosis. Unfortunately, the rates of protection obtained with this vaccine are rather variable, from 80% to 0%. The trials conducted in the United States were particularly disappointing and resulted in the lack of interest in BCG as an immunoprophylactic agent. Current research with this agent is centered on creating recombinant strains of increased immunogenicity.
3. Recombinant attenuated bacteria have also been approved for immunoprophylaxis. The best example is the oral vaccine prepared with the attenuated Ty21, a strain of *Salmonella typhi*, that grows poorly and is virtually nonpathogenic, but induces protective immunity in 90% of the individuals and is the recommended vaccine for typhoid fever.

Immunization with Recombinant Organisms

Recombinant technology has also been used to create genetically attenuated strains in which genes critical for replication of virulence are deleted and replaced with genetic information encoding immunogenic components of other organisms. Vaccinia virus, because of its large genome, appears to be an ideal candidate to create multivalent vaccines, for example carrying the genes for the HBsAg, glycoprotein D for Herpes virus, and influenza virus hemagglutinin. The potential value of these constructs is obvious, since they could induce protection against multiple diseases after a single immunization. However, attenuated viruses have the potential of causing severe infections in the immunocompromised, and this is well-substanbtiated in the case of vaccinia virus. Other candidate viruses are animal poxviruses, such as the canarypox virus, which has been tried for the development of HIV vaccines, and adenovirus. None of those vaccines has been approved for human use.

Recommended Immunizations

At the present time, a wide variety of vaccines are available for protection of the general population or of individuals at risk for a specific disease due to their occupation or other factors. Table 1 summarizes the recommended schedule for active immunization of normal infants and children. In many cases, several vaccines are combined in a single preparation to reduce the number of injections in children.

Additional information concerning recommended immunizations for adults, travelers, special professions, and so on, can be obtained in a variety of specialized publications, including the Report of the Committee on Infectious Diseases, published annually by the American Academy of Pediatrics, the booklet Health Information of International Travel, also published annually by the United States Public Health Service, and the Morbidity and Mortality Weekly Report published by the Centers for Disease Control in Atlanta.

TABLE 1 Recommended Immunization Schedule for Persons Aged 0–6 Year—United States, 2007[a]

Vaccine ▼ / Age ▶	Birth	1 month	2 months	4 months	6 months	12 months	15 months	18 months	19–23 months	2–3 years	4–6 years	
Hepatitis B[1]	HepB	HepB		See footnote 1		HepB			HepB Series			Range of recommended ages
Rotavirus[2]			Rota	Rota	Rota							
Diphtheria, Tetanus, Pertussis[3]			DTaP	DTaP	DTaP		DTaP				DTaP	
Haemophilus influenzae type b[4]			Hib	Hib	Hib[4]	Hib			Hib			
Pneumococcal[5]			PCV	PCV	PCV	PCV				PCV / PPV		
Inactivated Poliovirus			IPV	IPV		IPV					IPV	Catch-up immunization
Influenza[6]						Influenza (Yearly)						
Measles, Mumps, Rubella[7]						MMR					MMR	
Varicella[8]						Varicella					Varicella	Certain high-risk groups
Hepatitis A[9]						HepA (2 doses)				HepA Series		
Meningococcal[10]									MPSV4			

Note: Light-shaded boxes represent ranges of recommended ages; dark shaded boxes represent recommended schedules for catch-up vaccination of nonimmune or improperly immunized individuals; the dark shaded column at 11 to 12 years of age indicated the recommended age for Tdap and MCV4 boosting in the age groups covered by these recommendations; boosters at later ages are also recommended for Tdap.

[a]Recommendations approved by the Advisory Committee on Immunization Practices, the American Academy of Pediatrics, and the American Academy of Family Physicians.

Abbreviations: DtaP, diphtheria, tetanus, and acellular pertussis; HepA, hepatitis A; HepB, hepatitis B; Hib, *Haemophilus influenzae* type b; IPV, inactivated polio vaccine; MCV4, tetravalent meningococcal polysaccharide conjugate vaccine; MMR, measles, mumps, rubella; MPSV4, tetravalent meningococcal polysaccharide vaccine; PCV, pneumococcal polysaccharide conjugate vaccine; PPV, pneumococcal polysaccharide vaccine; Tdap, tetanus, reduced diphtheria toxoid, acellular pertussis.

Vaccines as Immunotherapeutic Agents

The use of vaccines to stimulate the immune system as therapy for chronic or latent infections is receiving considerable interest. Initial enthusiasm in HIV-positive patients failed to materialize. Recent observations suggest that the papilloma virus vaccines not only prevent cervical carcinoma, but also cause regression of early lesions. This issue is being actively investigated. The use of vaccines for tumor treatment is discussed in greater detail in Chapter 26.

BIBLIOGRAPHY

Ahmed R, Gray D. Immunological memory and protective immunity: understanding their relation. Science 1996; 272:54.

Churchill Rb, Pickering LK. The pros (many) and cons (few) of breastfeeding. Contemp Pediatr 1998; 15:108.

Cui Z. DNA vaccine. Adv Genet 2005; 54:257–289.

Dennehy M, Williamson AL. Factors influencing the immune response to foreign antigen expressed in recombinant BCG vaccines. Vaccine 2005; 26:1209–1223.

Dunman PM, Nesin M. Passive immunization as prophylaxis: when and where will this work? Curr Opin Pharmacol 2003; 35:486–496.

Hammarlund E, Lewis MW, Hansen SG, et al. Duration of antiviral immunity after smallpox vaccination. Nat Med 2003; 9:1131–1137.

Källberg E, Jainandunsing S, Gray D, Leanderson T. Somatic mutation of immunoglobulin V genes in vitro. Science 1996; 271:1285.

Klaus GGB, Humphrey JH, Kunkel A, Dongworth DW. The follicular dendritic cell: its role in antigen presentation in the generation of immunological memory. Immunol Rev 1980; 53:3.

Kniskern PJ, Marburg S, Ellis RW. *Haemophilus influenzae* type b conjugate vaccines. Pharm Biotechnol 1995; 6:673.

Levine MM, Woodrow GC, Kaper JB, Cobon GS. New Generation Vaccines. 2nd ed. New York: Marcel Dekker, 1997.

McCullough KC, Summerfield A. Basic concepts of immune response and defense development. ILAR J 2005; 46:230–240.

Mestecky J, Lue C, Russell MW. Selective transport of IgA. Cellular and molecular aspects. Gastroenterol Clin North Am 1991; 20:441.

Noelle RJ, Erickson LD. Determinations of B cell fate in immunity and autoimmunity. Curr Dir Autoimmun 2005; 8:1–24.

Sabin AB. Oral poliovirus vaccine: history of its development and use and current challenge to eliminate poliomyelitis from the world. J Infect Dis 1985; 151:420.

13 | Phagocytosis

Gabriel Virella
Department of Microbiology and Immunology, Medical University of South Carolina,
Charleston, South Carolina, U.S.A.

INTRODUCTION

The failure or success of an antibody response directed against an infectious agent depends entirely on their ability to trigger the complement system and/or to induce phagocytosis. Most mammals, including humans, have developed two well-defined systems of phagocytic cells: the polymorphonuclear (PMN) leukocyte system (particularly the neutrophil population) and the monocyte/macrophage system. Both types of cells can engulf microorganisms and cause their intracellular death through a variety of enzymatic systems, but the two-cell systems differ considerably in their biological characteristics.

PHYSIOLOGY OF THE POLYMORPHONUCLEAR LEUKOCYTES

Neutrophils and other PMN leukocytes are "wandering" cells, constantly circulating around the vascular network, able to recognize foreign matter by a wide variety of immunological and nonimmunological mechanisms. Their main biological characteristics are summarized on Table 1. Their effective participation in an anti-infectious response depends on the ability to respond to chemotactic signals, ingest the pathogenic agent, and kill the ingested microbes.

Chemotaxis and Migration to the Extravascular Compartment

In normal conditions, the interaction between leukocytes and endothelial cells is rather loose and involves a family of molecules known as selectins, which are constitutively expressed on endothelial cells and glycoproteins, expressed on the leukocyte cell membrane. Their interactions cause the slowing down ("rolling") of leukocytes along the vessel wall, but do not lead to firm adhesion of leukocytes to endothelial cells.

A variety of chemotactic stimuli can be involved in the recruitment of leukocytes to the extravascular space. In most cases, those chemotactic factors can be of bacterial origin, but can also be released as a consequence of tissue necrosis, as a result of monocyte and lymphocyte activation, or as a by-product of complement activation.

Among bacterial products, formyl-methionyl peptides, such as f-methionine-leucine-phenylalanine (f-met-leu-phe), are extremely potent chemotactic agents. Complement-derived chemotactic factors (such as C5a) can be generated in several ways. Tissue damage may result in the activation of the plasmin system that may, in turn, initiate complement activation with generation of C5a. After the inflammatory process has been established, proteases released by activated neutrophils and macrophages can also split C5, and the same cells may release leukotriene B4, another potent chemotactic factor, attracting more neutrophils to the site. On the other hand, many microorganisms can generate C5a by activation of the complement system through the alternative pathway.

Finally, activated T cells and monocytes can also release chemokines such as IL-8, monocyte chemotactic protein-1, and Regulated on Activation, Normal T cell Expressed and Secreted (RANTES) that have neutrophils and/or monocytes as targets.

After receiving a chemotactic stimulus, the neutrophil undergoes changes in the cell membrane, which is smooth in the resting cell, and becomes "ruffled" after the cell receives the chemotactic signal. The activated PMN has a marked increase in cell adhesiveness,

TABLE 1 Comparison of the Characteristics of Polymorphonuclear Leukocytes and Monocytes/Macrophages

Characteristic	PMN leukocytes	Monocyte/macrophage
Numbers in peripheral blood	$3 - 6 \times 10^3/\mu L$	$285-500/\mu L$
Resident forms in tissues (macrophage)	−	+
Nonimmunological phagocytosis	++	+
Fc receptors	FcγRII,III	FcγRI,II,III
C3b receptors	++	++
Enzymatic granules	++	++
Bactericidal enzymes	++	++
Ability to generate superoxide and H_2O_2	+++	++
Synthesis and release of leukotrienes	+ (B4)	++ (B4, C4, D4)
Synthesis and release of prostaglandins	−	++
PAF release/response	++	±
Response to nonimmunologic chemotactic factors	+	−
Response to C5a/C3a	+	−
Response to cytokines	+ (IL-8)	++ (IFN-γ)
Release of cytokines	+	++
Antigen processing	−	++
Expression of HLA class II antigens	−	++
Phagocytosis-independent enzyme release	++	−

Abbreviations: HLA, human leukocyte antigens; IFN, interferon; PMN, polymorphonuclear.

associated with increased expression of adherence molecules, namely integrins of the CD11/CD18 complex, which includes:

1. CD11a [the α chain of leukocyte function antigen (LFA)-1],
2. CD11b (the C3bi receptor or CR3, also known as Mac-1) molecule,
3. CD11c (also known as protein p150, 95), and
4. CD18 (the β chain of LFA-1).

These cell adhesion molecules (CAMs) are common to the majority of leukocytes, but their individual density and frequency may vary in the two main groups of phagocytic cells. While CD11a and CD18 are expressed virtually by all monocytes and granulocytes, CD11b is more prevalent among granulocytes, and CD11c is more frequent among monocytes.

The expression of these CAMs mediates a variety of cell–cell interactions such as those that lead to neutrophil aggregation, and, most importantly, those that mediate firm adhesion of neutrophils to endothelial cells. For example, CD11a (LFA-1) and CD11b interact with molecules of the immunoglobulin gene family, such as ICAM-1, ICAM-2, and VCAM-1, expressed on the endothelial cell membrane. The expression of VCAM-1, and to a lesser degree, of ICAM-1, and -2 are also upregulated by cytokines released by activated monocytes and lymphocytes, such as IL-1 and tumor necrosis factor (TNF). Consequently, the adhesion of leukocytes to endothelial cells is further enhanced.

After adhering to endothelial cells, leukocytes migrate to the extravascular compartment. The transmigration involves interaction with a fourth member of the immunoglobulin gene family—platelet endothelial CAM 1 (PECAM-1)—which is expressed at the intercellular junctions between endothelial cells. The interaction of leukocytes with PECAM-1 mediates the process of diapedesis, by which leukocytes squeeze through the endothelial cell junctions into the extravascular compartment.

The diapedesis process involves the locomotor apparatus of the neutrophils, a contractile actin–myosin system stabilized by polymerized microtubules. Its activation is essential for the neutrophil to move to the extravascular space and an intact CD11b protein seems essential for the proper modulation of microtubule assembly, which will not take place in CD11b–deficient patients.

Phagocytosis

At the area of infection, PMN leukocytes recognize the infectious agents, which are ingested and killed intracellularly. The sequence of events leading to opsonization and intracellular killing is summarized in Figure 1.

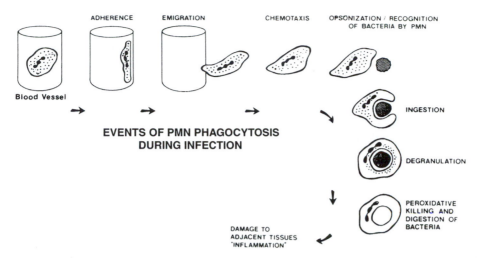

FIGURE 1 Diagrammatic representation of the sequence of events that take place during polymorphonuclear leukocyte phagocytosis. *Source*: Reproduced from Wolach B, Baehner RL, Boxer LA. Israel J Med Sci 1982; 18:897.

Several recognition systems appear to be involved in the phagocytosis step. The most important recognition systems are those that mediate the ingestion of opsonized particles. Two major types of receptors expressed by phagocytic cells are involved in this process:

1. $Fc\gamma$ receptors are predominantly involved in promoting ingestion of antibody-coated particles. Neutrophils express two types of $Fc\gamma$ receptors, $Fc\gamma RII$ and $Fc\gamma RIII$, both of which are involved in phagocytosis. In experimental conditions, $Fc\alpha$ receptors may also be involved in phagocytosis, but their efficiency seems to be much lower than that of $Fc\gamma$ receptors.
2. The CR1 (C3b) receptor is also able to mediate phagocytosis with high efficiency. This receptor is expressed by all phagocytic cells, including PMN leukocytes, monocytes, and macrophages. The binding and ingestion of microorganisms through this receptor has been well-established.

Opsonization with both immunoglobulin G (IgG) antibodies and C3b seems to be associated with maximal efficiency in ingestion.

Opsonization is not an absolute requirement for ingestion by phagocytic cells. A variety of receptors may be involved in nonimmune phagocytosis, as described in greater detail in Chapter 14. These nonimmune mechanisms are particularly effective in promoting the ingestion of microorganisms with polysaccharide-rich outer layers. In addition, neutrophils are able to ingest a variety of particulate matter, such as latex beads, silicone, asbestos fibers, and so on, in the absence of opsonizing antibodies or complement.

Intracellular Killing

Irrespective of the nature of the receptors that may mediate it, ingestion is achieved through formation of pseudopodia that surround the particle or bacteria, and eventually fuse at the distal pole forming a phagosome. The cytoplasmic granules of the neutrophil (lysosomes) then fuse with the phagosomes, and their contents empty inside the phagosomes (degranulation). This degranulation process is very rapid and delivers a variety of antimicrobial substances to the phagosome:

1. The azurophilic or primary granules contain, among other substances, myeloperoxidase, lysozyme, acid hydrolases (such as β-glucuronidase), cationic proteins, defensins, metalloproteinases (including proteases and collagenases), elastase, and cathepsin (C2).

2. The secondary granules or lysosomes contain lysozyme and lactoferrin.
   Killing of ingested organisms depends on the effects of cationic proteins from the primary granules, lysosomal enzymes, such as lysozyme and lactoferrin, defensins, nitric oxide (NO), and, most significantly, of by-products of the respiratory burst, activated as a consequence of phagocytosis.
3. Cationic proteins bind to negatively charged cell surfaces (such as the bacterial outer membrane) and interfere with microbial growth.
4. Lactoferrin has antimicrobial activity by chelating iron and preventing its use by bacteria that need it as an essential nutrient.
5. Lysozyme splits the β-1,4 linkage between the N-acetylmuramic acid peptide and N-acetylglucosamine on the bacterial peptidoglycan. Some bacteria are exquisitely sensitive to the effects of this enzyme that causes almost immediate lysis. However, the importance of this enzyme as a primary killing mechanism has been questioned due to the relative inaccessibility of the peptidoglycan layer in many microorganisms, which may be surrounded by capsules or by the lipopolysaccharide-rich outer membrane (Gram-negative bacteria).
6. Defensins are antimicrobial peptides released by almost all eukaryotic species, including plants, invertebrate animals, and vertebrate animals. Structurally, defensins are cationic molecules with spatially separated hydrophobic and charges regions, which insert themselves into phospholipid membranes, causing their disruption. In mammalians, defensins are produced by specialized mucosal cells (i.e., the Paneth cells in the gut) and by phagocytic cells. The mucosal defensins are believed to play an important role protecting mucosal cells from pathogenic bacteria. The neutrophil defensins are packaged on the azurophilic granules, and are delivered to the phagosomes and also spilled into the extracellular environment.

Respiratory Burst

From the bactericidal point of view, the activation of the superoxide generating system (respiratory burst) is the most significant killing mechanism of phagocytic cells. This system is activated primarily by opsonization, but also by a variety of PMN activating stimuli, ranging from f-met-leu-phe to C5a. The activating stimuli are responsible for the induction of a key enzymatic activity [the reduced from of nicotinamide adenine dinucleotide phosphate (NADPH), a molecular complex located on the cell membrane, responsible for the transfer of a single electron from NADPH to oxygen, generating superoxide (O_2^-)].

The molecules responsible for NADPH oxidase activity are:

1. Cytochrome b588, which is an heterodimer formed by two polypeptide chains, alpha, of high molecular weight (91 Kd, gp91phox) and beta, of low molecular weight (22 Kd, p22phox), believed to play the key role in the reduction of oxygen to superoxide, possibly by being the terminal electron donor.
2. Two cytosolic proteins (neutrophil cytosolic factors 1 and 2, termed p47phox and p67phox, respectively). p47phox is a substrate for protein kinase C.
3. $p21^{rac}$, an ubiquitous ras-related GTPase.

In a resting cell, the complex is inactive and its components are not associated. After the cell is activated, p47phox is phosphorylated, and becomes associated with p67phox and with $p21^{rac}$. The phosphorylated complex binds to cytochrome b588 in the lysosomal membranes, forming what is considered to be the active oxidase.

The electron transfer from NAPDH to oxygen is believed to involve through at least three steps:

1. Reduction of a flavin adenine dinucleotide (FAD), bound to the alpha chain of cytochrome b
2. Transfer of an electron from FADH2 to ferric iron in a heme molecule associated to the beta chain of cytochrome b
3. Transfer of an electron from reduced iron to oxygen, generating superoxide

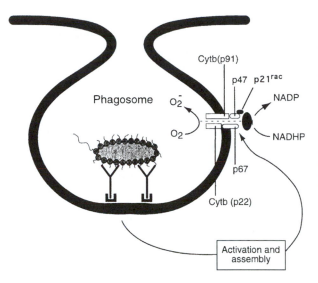

FIGURE 2 Schematic representation of the major events involved in the respiratory burst of phagocytic cells. The occupancy of Fc and/or CR1 receptors triggers the activation sequence, which involves protein kinase activation, enzyme activation, and phosphorylation of at least one cytosolic protein (p47). As a result, a molecular complex, constituted by cytochrome b (Cyt b), p47, and p67, is assembled on the cell membrane, which folds to constitute a phagosome. This complex has NADPH oxidase activity, oxidizes NADPH and transfers the resulting electron to an oxygen molecule, resulting in the formation of superoxide (O_2^-). *Abbreviations*: Cytb, cytochrome b; NADP, nicotinamide adenosine diphosphate; NADHP, nicotinamide adenine dinucleotide phosphate.

The formation of the active molecular complex with oxidase activity coincides with phagolysosome fusion. Thus, the brunt of the active oxygen radicals generated by this system is delivered to the phagolysosome (Fig. 2).

The respiratory burst generates two toxic compounds, essential for intracellular killing of bacteria—superoxide and H_2O_2. Through myeloperoxidase, H_2O_2 can be peroxidated and led to form hypochlorite and other halide ion derivatives, which are also potent bactericidal agents. These compounds are also toxic to the cell, particularly superoxide, which can diffuse into the cytoplasm. The cell has several detoxifying systems, including superoxide dismutase, which converts superoxide into H_2O_2, and in turn, H_2O_2 is detoxified by catalase and by the oxidation of reduced glutathione, which requires activation of the hexose monophosphate shunt.

Activated phagocytic cells also express an inducible form on NO synthase (iNOS), which generates NO from arginine and molecular oxygen, using a variety of cofactors that include NADPH. NO is a short-lived, highly cytotoxic free radical gas, which is believed to contribute significantly to intracellular killing. It can also participate in the induction of inflammatory reactions when spilled to the extracellular space.

PHYSIOLOGY OF THE MONOCYTE/MACROPHAGE
Comparison of Polymorphonuclear Leukocytes and Monocyte/ Macrophages

The two populations of phagocytic cells share many common characteristics, such as:

1. Presence of Fcγ and C3b receptors on their membranes
2. Ability to engulf bacteria and particles
3. Metabolic and enzymatic killing mechanisms and pathways

In contrast, other functions and metabolic pathways differ considerably between these two types of cells (Table 1). One important distinguishing feature is the involvement of the monocyte/macrophage series of cells in the inductive stages of the immune response, due to their ability to process antigens and present antigen-derived peptides to the immune system. The monocyte/macrophage is also involved in immunoregulatory signals, providing both activating signals (in the form of IL-1, IL-6, and IL-12) and downregulating signals (mainly in the form of PGE_2) to T lymphocytes.

These two types of phagocytic cells have different preferences as far as phagocytosis is concerned. For example, PMN leukocytes are able to ingest inert particles such as latex, but have very little ability to engulf antibody-coded homologous erythrocytes, while the reverse is true for the monocyte/macrophage. On the other hand, while neutrophils seem to be constitutively ready to ingest particulate matter, the circulating monocytes and the tissue-fixed (resident) macrophages are usually resting cells that need to be activated by several types of stimuli before they can fully express their phagocytic and killing potential. The activating factors include microorganisms or their products and cytokines. The main activating cytokine is interferon-γ, released by activated Th1 cells.

Activated Macrophage

The Activated Macrophage has unique morphologic and functional characteristics. Morphologically, the activated macrophage is larger, and its cytoplasm tends to spread and attach to surfaces. The composition of the plasma membrane is changed, and the rates of pinocytosis and engulfment are increased (phagocytosis through C3b receptors is only seen after activation). Intracellularly, there is a marked increase in enzymatic contents, particularly of plasminogen activator, collagenase, and elastase, and the oxidative metabolism (leading to generation of superoxide and H_2O_2) as well as the activity of iNOS are greatly enhanced.

Role of Macrophages in the Phagocytosis of Dead Cells

As cells die, either by apoptosis or by necrosis, they express cell membrane markers that allow ingestion by macrophages, dendritic cells, and related cells. This results in the presentation of peptides derived from the dead cells on major histocompatibility complex (MHC)-I molecules. In physiological conditions the ingestion of dead cells by tissue macrophages is associated with the release of anti-inflammatory cytokines such as TGFβ1 and IL-10 and the immune system remains ignorant of the presented self-peptides. However, presentation of peptides derived from ingested dead cells cross-loaded to MHC-I molecules by dendritic cells may elicit a CD8$^+$ immune response against those peptides. It can be theorized that if the dead cells are ingested in nonphysiological conditions, for example, as a consequence of the reaction against an infective agent, the likelihood for uptake and presentation in conditions favorable to the induction of an immune response increases. Such immune responses have been postulated to play a significant role in the emergence of autoimmune diseases (see Chapter 16).

LABORATORIAL EVALUATION OF PHAGOCYTIC FUNCTION

The evaluation of phagocytic function is usually centered on the study of neutrophils that are considerably easier to isolate than monocytes or macrophages. Phagocytosis by neutrophils can be depressed as a result of reduction in cell numbers or as a result of a functional defect. Functional defects affecting every single stage of the phagocytic response have been reported and have to be evaluated by different tests. The following is a summary of the most important tests used to evaluate phagocytic function.

Neutrophil Count

This is the simplest and one of the most important tests to perform since phagocytic defects due to neutropenia are, by far, more common than the primary, congenital, defects of phagocytic function. As a rule, it is believed that a neutrophil count below 1000/μL represents an increased risk of infection, and when neutrophil counts are lower than 200/μL, the patient will invariably be infected.

Adherence

The increased adherence of activated phagocytic cells to endothelial cells is critical for the migration of these cells to infectious foci. Although there are specialized tests to measure aggregation and adherence of neutrophils in response to stimuli such as C5a$_{desarg}$ (a nonchemotactic derivative of C5a), presently this property is evaluated indirectly, by determining the expression of the different components of CD11/CD18 complex that mediate adhesion by flow cytometry.

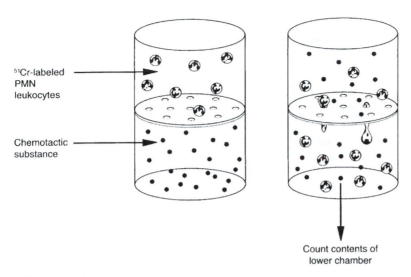

51Cr-labeled
PMN
leukocytes

Chemotactic
substance

Count contents of
lower chamber

FIGURE 3 Schematic representation of the principle of chemotaxis assays using the Boyden chamber and ^{51}Cr-labeled polymorphonuclear leukocytes.

Chemotaxis and Migration

The migration of phagocytes in response to chemotactic stimuli can be studied in vitro, using the Boyden chamber. The basic principle of all versions of the Boyden chamber is to have two compartments separated by a membrane whose pores are too tight to allow PMN leukocytes to passively diffuse from one chamber to the other, but large enough to allow the active movement of these cells from the upper chamber, where they are placed, to the lower chamber.

The movement of the cells is stimulated by adding to the lower chamber a chemotactic factor such as C5a, the bacterial tetrapeptide f-met-leu-phe, IL-8, leukotriene B4, or platelet-activating factor (PAF). The results are usually based on either counting the number of cells that reached the bottom side of the membrane, or on the indirect determination of the number of cells reaching the bottom chamber using ^{51}Cr-labeled PMN (Fig. 3).

It must be noted that all versions of this technique are difficult to reproduce and standardize and are not used in routine laboratory diagnosis.

Ingestion

Ingestion tests are relatively simple to perform and reproduce. They are usually based on incubating PMN with opsonized particles, and after an adequate incubation, determining either the number of ingested particles or a phagocytic index:

$$\text{Phagocytic index} = \frac{\text{No. of cells with ingested particles}}{\text{Total no. of cells}} \times 100$$

Several types of particles have been used, including latex, zymosan (fragments of fungal capsular polysaccharidic material), killed *Candida albicans* and IgG-coated beads (Immunobeads). All these particles activate complement by either one of the pathways and become coated with C3, although opsonization with complement is not the major determinant of phagocytosis. The easiest particles to visualize once ingested are fluorescent latex beads; their use considerably simplifies the assay (Fig. 4), particularly if performed in a flow cytometer. Fluorescein-labeled killed *C. albicans* and killed *Staphyloccocus aureus* can also be used in flow cytometry-based ingestion assays.

Ingestion tests are also not used routinely because other tests are available that test both for ingestion and for the ability to mount a respiratory burst (see later).

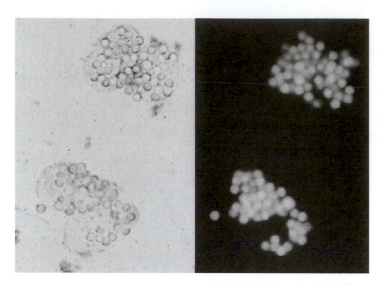

FIGURE 4 Use of fluorescent latex beads for evaluation of phagocytosis. The panel on the left reproduces a photograph of microscopic field showing the phagocytic cells that have ingested latex beads under visible light. The panel on the right shows the same field under UV light.

Degranulation

When the contents of cytoplasmic granules are released into a phagosome, there is always some leakage of their contents into the extracellular fluid. The tests to study degranulation involve ingestion of particulate matter as mentioned earlier, but in this case, the supernatants are analyzed for their contents of substances released by the PMN granules such as myeloperoxidase, lysozyme, β-glucuronidase, and lactoferrin.

Oxidative Burst

Most diganostic laboratories that test for neutrophil function run one variant or another of a test to measure the oxidative burst. Several different assays are available, using different parameters and methodologies. Tests based on the reduction of nitroblue tetrazolium (NBT reduction tests) were the first successfully used for the evaluation of the oxidative burst, but have been largely replaced by flow cytometry tests based on the reduction of fluorescent substrates.

The principle of the NBT assays is relatively simple. Oxidized NBT, colorless to pale yellow in solution, is transformed by reduction into blue formazan. The test usually involves incubation of purified neutrophils, NBT, and a stimulus known to activate the respiratory burst. Two types of stimuli can be used:

1. Opsonized particles, which need to be ingested to stimulate the burst. In this way, the test examines both the ability to ingest and the ability to produce a respiratory burst.
2. Diffusible activators, such as phorbol esters. Those compounds diffuse into the cell and activate protein kinase C, which, in turn, activates the NADPH-cytochrome b system and induce the respiratory burst directly, bypassing the ingestion step. A patient whose neutrophils respond to stimulation with phorbol ester but not to stimulation with opsonized beads is likely to have an ingestion defect. In contrast, neutrophils from a patient with a primary defect in the ability to generate the respiratory burst will not respond to any kind of stimulus.

The first generation of reduction assays relied on conventional microscopy to count the number of PMN with blue-stained cytoplasm after incubation with opsonized particles. However, the microscopic assay is difficult to standardize, and its interpretation can be affected by subjectivity.

Colorimetric assays proved to be more amenable to standardization. The classical quantitative technique involves the extraction of intracellular NBT with pyrimidine and measure its absorbance at 515°nm (which corresponds to the absorbance peak of reduced NBT). This modality of the NBT test is extremely sensitive and accurate, but is difficult to perform because the reagents used to extract the dye from the cells are highly toxic. An alternative are tests in which the PMN are simultaneously exposed to opsonized particles and NBT, and the change of color of the supernatant from pale yellow to gray or purple (as a result of the spillage of oxidizing products during phagocytosis) is measured. This assay was rendered practical and convenient by the introduction of kinetic colorimeters. Using this type of equipment, the color change of NBT can be measured without the need to extract the dye from the cells or to separate the cells from the supernatant (Fig. 5).

The techniques more widely used in diagnostic laboratories utilize fluorescent dyes, which allow the use of flow cytometry to measure the oxidative burst. One of the best studies techniques is based on the oxidation of 2′,7′-dichlorofluorescein diacetate (nonfluorescent) that results in the formation of 2′,7′-dichlorofluorescein (highly fluorescent). The numbers of fluorescent cells and fluorescence intensity of activated and nonactivated PMN suspensions from patients and suitable controls can be determined by flow cytometry. In patients with primary defects of the enzymes responsible for the respiratory burst, both the mean fluorescence intensity and the numbers of fluorescent cells after stimulation with phorbols are considerably lower than those determined in normal, healthy volunteers. This particular assay seems to depend primarily on the production of H_2O_2, and secondarily, on NO generation. Other fluorescent substrates that can be used include hydorethydine, which seems to be more specific for superoxide, and dihydrorhodamine.

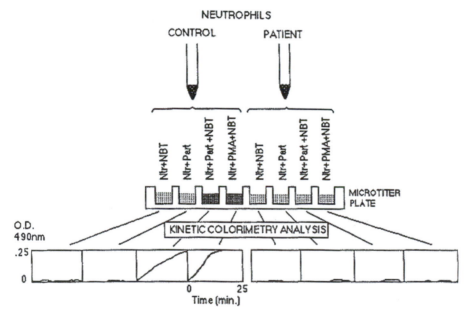

FIGURE 5 Diagrammatic representation of a quantitative NBT assay carried out by kinetic colorimetry. Neutrophils are isolated from a patient under a normal control, and incubated separately in a microtiter plate with NBT (to check for spontaneous activation of neutrophils), with opsonized particles (to check for interference of cells and particles with the colorimetric assay), and with opsonized particles and phorbol myristate acetate in the presence of NBT (to check for the induction of the respiratory burst). A kinetic colorimeter is used to monitor changes in OD due to the reduction of NBT over a 25-minute period, and the results are expressed diagrammatically and as an average of the variation of the OD/unit of time. The graphic depiction of the results obtained with neutrophils from a normal control and from a patient with chronic granulomatous disease are reproduced in the lower part of the diagram. *Abbreviations*: NBT, nitroblue tetrazolium; OD, optical density.

Killing Assays

The main protective function of the neutrophil is the ingestion and killing of microorganisms. This ability can be tested using a variety of bacteria and fungi that are mixed with PMN in the presence of normal human plasma (a source of opsonins) and after a given time, the cells are harvested, lysed, and the number of intracytoplasmic viable bacteria is determined.

Killing assays are difficult and cumbersome, and require close support from a microbiology laboratory, and for this reason have been less used than the indirect killing assays based on detection of the oxidative burst of the PMN, mentioned in the previous section. Alternative and simpler approaches to the evaluation of intracellular killing are based on the differential uptake of dyes (such as acridine orange) between live and dead bacteria.

BIBLIOGRAPHY

Aderem A, Unerhill DM. Mechanisms of phagocytosis in macrophages. Annu Rev Immunol 1999; 17:593.

Boxer LA, Blackwood RA. Leukocyte disoreders: quanrtitative an qualitative disorders of the neutrophil. Pediatr Rev 1996; 17:19 (Pt 1), 47 (Pt 2).

Ottonello L, Dapino P, Pastorino G, et al. Neutrophil dysfunction and increased susceptibility to infection. Eur J Clin Invest 1995; 25:687.

Pallister CJ, Hancock JT. Phagocytic NADPH oxidase and its role in chronic granulomatous disease. Br J Biomed Sci 1995; 52:149.

Robinson JP, Carter WO, Narayanan P. Functional assays by flow cytometry. In: Rose NR, de Macario EC, Folds JD, Lane HC, Nakamura RM, eds. Manual of Clinical Laboratory Immunology. 5th ed. Washington, DC: ASM Press, 1997:245–254.

Umeki S. Mechanisms for the activation/electron transfer of neutrophil NADPH-oxidase complex and molecular pathology of chronic granulomatous disease. Ann Hematol 1994; 68:267.

Virella G, Thompson T, Haskill-Stroud R. A new quantitative NBT reduction assay based on kinetic colorimetry. J Clin Lab Anal 1990; 4:86–89.

Virella G. Diagnostic evaluation of neutrophil function. In: Gabrilovich DI, ed. The Neutrophils: New Outlook for Old Cells. London: Imperial College Press, 1999:275.

Vuorte J, Jansson SE, Repo H. Standardization of a flow cytometric assay for phagocyte respiratory burst activity. Scand J Immunol 1996; 43:329–334.

14 | Infections and Immunity

Gabriel Virella and Stephen Tomlinson
Department of Microbiology and Immunology, Medical University of South Carolina, Charleston, South Carolina, U.S.A.

INTRODUCTION

During evolution, an extremely complex system of anti-infectious defenses has emerged. However, as vertebrates and mammals developed their defenses, so microbes continued to evolve and many became adept at avoiding the consequences of anti-infectious defense mechanisms. The interplay between host defenses, microbial virulence, and microbial evasion mechanisms determines the outcome of the constant encounters between humans and pathogenic organisms.

NONSPECIFIC ANTI-INFECTIOUS DEFENSE MECHANISMS
Constitutive Nonspecific Defense Mechanisms

Constitutive nonspecific defense mechanisms play an important role as a first line of defense by preventing penetration of microorganisms beyond the outer exposed surfaces of the body. As summarized in Table 1, some of these nonspecific defense mechanisms are local, while others are systemic. The local mechanisms consist of physical and chemical barriers that protect the organism from infectious agents, and their importance is apparent from the prevalence of infections when their integrity is compromised. The systemic mechanisms can be activated directly by infectious agents, and are designated as innate immunity. This term was designed to contrast with the active or adaptive immune response (adaptive immunity) that takes several days to develop. A summary of the characteristics that differentiate some of the best-defined components of innate immunity from adaptive immunity is presented in Table 2.

Innate Immunity Mechanisms

Several anti-infectious systems can be included in the broad category of innate immunity, ranging from antibacterial compounds to phagocytic cells.

Antimicrobial Peptides: Defensins and Cathelicidins

Defensins are antimicrobial peptides released by specialized mucosal cells (i.e., the Paneth cells in the gut) and by phagocytic cells. The mucosal defensins are believed to play an important role in protecting mucosal cells from pathogenic bacteria. The neutrophil defensins are packaged in the azurophilic granules and are delivered to the phagosomes as well as being spilled into the extracellular environment. Mammalian defensins are grouped into two families: α and β. β defensins have been shown to have chemotactic properties for immature dendritic cells and T lymphocytes, and because of this activity may play a significant role in promoting the onset of the immune response.

Cathelicidins are expressed by lymphocytes, phagocytic cells, and epithelial cells of the gastrointestinal and respiratory tracts. Their antibacterial activity affects both gram-positive and gram-negative bacteria. In addition, engagement of toll-like receptors (TLRs) 1 and 2 (see subsequently) by mycobacterial lipopeptides triggers a vitamin D-dependent antimycobacterial response mediated by increased synthesis of cathelicidin.

TABLE 1   Nonspecific Anti-infectious Defense Mechanisms

Local	Systemic
Physical integrity of skin and mucosae	Fever
Lysozyme in tears, saliva, sweat, and other secretions	Defensins
Gastric acidity	Production of interferons
Flow of mucosal secretions in the respiratory tract	Nonimmune opsonization; phagocytosis
Intestinal transit	Nonimmune killing; NK cells
Urinary flow	

Abbreviation: NK, natural killer.

Activation of the Complement System via the Alternative Pathway

A variety of microorganisms (bacteria, fungi, viruses, and parasites, Table 3) can activate complement directly in the nonimmune host via all three activation pathways. Certain microbial structures can directly bind C1q (initiates classical pathway), mannose-binding protein (MBP) (lectin pathway), and can accept spontaneously deposited C3 (alternative pathway). The subsequent generation of chemotactic complement activation products (C3a and C5a) and the opsonization of microbes by C3b and iC3b promote leukocyte recruitment and microbe phagocytosis.

γ/δ T Lymphocytes

This T cell subpopulation is predominantly localized to the mucosal epithelia, and appears to recognize and eliminate infected epithelial cells by a nonimmunological mechanism (i.e., not involving the T cell receptors).

Phagocytosis

As a microbe penetrates beyond the skin or mucosal surface, it will encounter cells able to ingest it. Two types of cells are particularly adept at nonimmune phagocytosis: granulocytes (particularly neutrophils) and tissue macrophages. This nonimmune phagocytosis involves a variety of recognition systems (Fig. 1).

CR1 and CR3 Receptors

CR1 and CR3 receptors able to interact with complement opsonins C3b and iC3b on the microbial surface that are deposited as a consequence of complement activation.

Mannose Receptors

Mannose receptors able to mediate ingestion of organisms such as *Candida albicans* that have mannose-rich polysaccharides. Mannose-mediated phagocytosis is amplified by a MBP that

TABLE 2   Features of Innate and Adaptive Immunity

Innate immunity	Adaptive immunity
Pathogen recognized by receptors encoded in the germline	Pathogen recognized by receptors generated randomly during differentiation
Receptors have broad specificity, that is, recognize many related molecular structures called PAMPs.	Receptors have very narrow specificity; that is, recognize a unique epitope
PAMPs are essential polysaccharides and polynucleotides that differ little from one pathogen to another but are not found in the host.	Most epitopes are derived from polypeptides (proteins) or polysaccharides and reflect the individuality of the pathogen.
Receptors are PRRs	Receptors are BCR and TcR for antigen
Immediate response	Slow (3–8 days) response (because of the need for clones of responding cells to develop)
No memory of prior exposure	Memory of prior exposure

Abbreviations: BCR, B-cell receptor; PAMPs, pathogen-associated molecular patterns; PRRs, pattern-recognition receptors; TcR, T-cell receptor.

TABLE 3 Examples of Infectious Agents Able to Activate the Alternative Pathway of Complement Without Apparent Participation of Specific Antibody

Bacteria
Haemophilus influenzae Type b
Streptococcus pneumoniae
Staphylococcus aureus
S. epidermidis
Fungi
Candida albicans
Parasites
Trypanosoma cyclops
Schistosoma mansoni
Babesia rodhaini
Vesicular stomatitis virus

promotes phagocytosis through complement activation and direct interaction with C1q receptors on phagocytic cells.

C-Reactive Protein
C-reactive protein binds to certain bacterial polysaccharides and has very similar effects to the MBP, activating complement, and promoting phagocytosis, both through CR1 and CR3, as well as by other receptors including the FcγRI and C1q receptors.

Toll-Like Receptors
TLRs, structurally similar to the Toll receptors of insects, recognize pathogen-associated molecular patterns (PAMPS) or, in other words, are pattern-recognition receptors. There are 10 types of TLR, most of them present in phagocytic cells and antigen-presenting cells (APCs), and six of which recognize microbial products:

1. TLR-1 and 2 recognize glucan, peptidoglycan, lipopeptides, and some lipopolysacharides.
2. TLR-3 recognizes viral dsRNA.
3. TLR-4 recognizes most types of lipopolysaccharide.
4. TLR-5 recognizes flagellin.

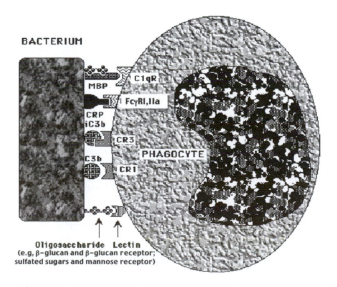

FIGURE 1 Diagrammatic representation of the different receptors that may mediate nonimmune phagocytosis. *Abbreviations*: CRP, C-reactive protein; MBP, mannose-binding protein.

5. TLR-7 recongnizes viral ssRNA.
6. TLR-9 recognizes bacterial DNA.

Binding of these products to TLRs induces phagocytosis, activation of signaling cascades involving nuclear factor-kappa B (NFkB) and, in some cases (TLR-1/2), synthesis of antimicrobial peptides, such as cethelicidin. It is now clear that these processes are also of significance in bridging innate and adaptive immune responses, such by activating APCs. A special case seems to be that of TLR-7, expressed in endosomal vesicles, where it can interact with viral ssRNA released as engulfed viral particles are denatured. The stimulation of TLR-7 by viral ssRNA induces the release of interferon-α (IFN)-α and proinflammatory cytokines, which may play an important role in the innate response to viruses.

Proinflammatory Cytokines and Chemokines

One of the most remarkable consequences of the activation of CD4$^+$ T cells is the synthesis of cytokines, soluble molecules that deliver activating or inhibitory signals to other leukocyte populations. A special subset of cytokines is the interleukins (ILs), of which 18 different ones have been well-characterized. Although activated CD8$^+$ cells may produce some cytokines, and APCs themselves produce others, CD4$^+$ T cells are their major source. The biological effects of cytokines and chemokines are extremely diverse; they influence not only the immune response, but also inflammatory processes and hematopoiesis (see Chapter 11).

The group of soluble factors that influence inflammatory reactions includes interleukin-1 (IL-1), interleukin-6 (IL-6), interleukin-15 (IL-15), interleukin-18 (IL-18), tumor necrosis factor (TNF, also known as cachectin), and IFN-γ (Table 4). IL-1 and TNF have membrane-associated and secreted forms, and seem to be directly or indirectly responsible (in conjunction with IL-6) for the acute phase reaction associated with acute inflammatory processes, as well as for the systemic metabolic abnormalities and circulatory collapse characteristic of shock associated with severe infections.

Interleukin-1

IL-1 exists in two molecular forms, IL-1α and IL-1β, encoded by two separate genes and displaying only 20% homology to one another. In spite of this structural difference, both forms

TABLE 4 Proinflammatory Cytokines

Cytokine	Predominant source	Main targets	Biological activity
IL-1	Macrophages, monocytes, and other cell types	T and B lymphocytes; many other cells	Stimulates T cells; activates several types of cells; proinflammatory mediator; pyrogen
IL-6	B and T lymphocytes, macrophages	B and T lymphocytes, others	B cell differentiation factor; polyclonal B cell activator; proinflammatory mediator; pyrogen
IL-15	Macrophages, APC	NK cells, T lymphocytes, macrophages, synovial cells	NK cell differentiation; increases and sustain TNF and interferon-γ synthesis by macrophages and NK cells; chemotactic for T cells
IL-18	Macrophages, APC	Macrophages, neutrophils, NK cells, endothelial cells	Stimulates interferon-γ synthesis; enhances Th1 and NK cell maturation
TNF (cachectin)	APCs, CD4$^+$ T cells	Multiple	Cytotoxic for some cells; cachexia; septic shock mediator; B lymphocyte activator; pyrogen
Interferon-γ	Activated T cells (esp. CD4$^+$ Th1 cells) and NK cells	T cells, phagocytic cells, endothelial cells	Downregulates Th2 and B cells; Activates macrophages; induces ICAM-1 in endothelial cells

Abbreviations: APC, antigen-presenting cells; ICAM, intercellular adhesion molecules; IL, interleukin; NK, natural killer; Th, helper T; TNF, tumor necrosis factor.

of IL-1 bind to the same receptor and share identical biological properties. IL-1α tends to remain associated to cell membranes, while IL-1β, synthesized as an inactive precursor, is released from the cell after being processed post-translationally by a cysteine–asparagin protease (Caspase-1 or interleukin converting enzyme). IL-1β is the predominant form in humans.

Tumor Necrosis Factor

TNF is produced by a variety of cells, including activated T lymphocytes and activated macrophages, and has multiple targets. Its original designation was derived from the fact from its cytotoxic effects on malignant cells.

Biological Properties of Interleukin-1 and Tumor Necrosis Factor

These ILs have effects at three different levels. At the metabolic level, IL-1 and TNF induce the synthesis of many proteins such as alpha-1 antitrypsin, fibrinogen, and C-reactive protein in the liver. These proteins are known generically as acute phase reactants because of their increase in situations associated with inflammatory reactions. In case of prolonged and severe infections, protracted TNF production may result in negative protein balance, loss of muscle mass, and progressive wasting (cachexia).

At the vascular level IL-1β and TNF cause the upregulation of cell adhesion molecules, particularly P-selectin and E-selectin in vascular endothelial cells. This upregulation promotes the adherence of inflammatory cells, which eventually egress to the extravascular space, where they form tissue inflammatory infiltrates. One of the possible consequences of the adherence of activated endothelial cells and inflammatory cells is endothelial cell damage. This is a major component of Gram-negative septic shock and of toxic shock syndrome; both are dramatic examples of the adverse effects of massive stimulation of cells capable of releasing excessive amounts of ILs (see Chapter 13).

At the central nervous system level IL-1 and TNF do not cross the blood brain barrier, but act on the periventricular organs, where the blood brain barrier is interrupted. They interact with a group of nuclei in the anterior hypothalamus, causing fever (secondarily to stimulation of prostaglandin synthesis) and sleep, and increase the production of adreno-corticotrophic hormone ACTH (Table 5).

Interleukin-6

IL-6, synthesized primarily by monocytes, macrophages, and other APCs, has proinflammatory and hematopoietic activities. Its role as a proinflammatory cytokine is similar to those of IL-1 and TNF, particularly in the induction of the synthesis of acute phase response proteins by the liver.

Interferon-γ

IFN-γ, in concert with IL-1β, induces an increase in the expression of intercellular adhesion molecules (ICAM)-1 on the membrane of endothelial cells, enhancing T lymphocyte adherence

TABLE 5 Cellular Sources and Biological Effects of Interleukin-1 and Tumor Necrosis Factor

	IL-1	TNF
Cellular source	Monocytes, macrophages, and related cells	Monocytes, macrophages, and related cells; CD4$^+$ T lymphocytes
Biologic property		
Pyrogen	+	+
Sleep inducer	+	+
Shock	+	+
Synthesis of reactive proteins	+	+
T cell activation	+	+
B cell activation	+	+
Stem cell proliferation and differentiation	+	−

to the vascular endothelium, an essential first step for T lymphocyte egress from the vascular bed. In addition, IFN-γ induces the release of several α-chemokines, such as CXCL9, CXCL10, and CXCL11 (see later in the chapter). These three chemokines can attract activated T helper (Th) 1 cells, natural killer (NK) cells, macrophages, and dendritic cells. Therefore, because of the combined effects of IFN and CXC chemokines, large numbers of T lymphocytes will exit the vascular bed in areas near the tissues where activated T cells are releasing ILs and will form perivenular infiltrates, characteristic of delayed hypersensitivity reactions. It must be noted that excessive and protracted production of IFN-γ may have adverse effects. Hyperstimulated monocytes may become exceedingly cytotoxic and may mediate tissue damage in inflammatory reactions and autoimmune diseases.

Interleukin-12

IL-12, in conjunction with nitric oxide, stimulates the cytotoxic activity of NK cells, enhancing their release of IFN-γ. IFN-γ and IL-12 also have an important role in promoting Th1 lymphocyte differentiation.

Interleukin-15

IL-15 has properties very similar to IL-2, including the ability to activate T cells through the IL-2 receptor. However, it has other unique properties, such as inducing the development and differentiation of NK cells. IL-15, in concert with IL-12, induces the release of IFN-γ, TNF, and macrophage inflammatory proteins (MIP) 1a and 1b by NK cells.

Interleukin-18

IL-18, a recently discovered IL produced primarily by macrophages and related cells, was initially named "IFN-γ inducing factor," reflecting its major biological role. In many respects, it is similar to IL-1 and IL-12. IL-18 is produced and released by APCs and its main targets are Th0/Th1 CD4$^+$ T cells and NK cells. However, in combination with other cytokines and cell–cell interactions, it can also induce Th2 lymphocyte activation.

Chemokines

This designation is given to a group of cytokines with chemotactic properties. They are divided into two major groups, α and β, depending on their tertiary structure. In the α chemokines, one amino acid separates the first two cysteine residues (Cys-X aminoacid-Cys) and for that reason are also known as CXC chemokines, the preferred term in modern literature. In β chemokines, the first two cysteine residues are adjacent to each other and for that reason are also known as CC chemokines.

CXC Chemokines

IL-8 (neutrophil activating factor) is the most important of the CXC chemokines. It is released by T lymphocytes and monocytes stimulated with TNF or IL-1. It functions as a chemotactic and activating factor for granulocytes, the cell population with the highest level of IL-8 receptor expression. IL-8 recruits granulocytes to areas of inflammation and increasing their phagocytic and proinflammatory abilities. It has also been demonstrated to be chemotactic for T lymphocytes. In addition to IL-8, the CXC chemokines include the above-mentioned IFN-γ-inducible chemokines (CXCL9, CXCL10, and CXCL11).

CC Chemokines

CC chemokines include four major cytokines, which act predominantly on mononuclear cells, the cells that predominantly express the receptors for this group of cytokines:

1. CCL5 [Regulated on Activation, Normal T cell Expressed and Secreted (RANTES)], released by T cells, attracts T cells with memory phenotype, NK cells, eosinophils, and mast cells.
2. MIP, released by monocytes and macrophages, attract eosinophils, lymphocytes, NK, and lymphokine activated killer (LAK) cells.

3. Macrophage chemotactic proteins (MCP) produced by monocytes, macrophages, and related cells attract monocytes, eosinophils, NK, and LAK cells.
4. Eotaxin, a chemokine induced by IL-4 that recruits eosinophils and Th2 CD4$^+$ T cells to the sites of allergic inflammation.

Other cytokines and peptides with chemotactic activity but that are structurally different from classical chemokines have also been characterized. Migration-inhibition factor (MIF), whose structure is not fully known, is released by T cells, monocytes, and macrophages, keeps macrophages in the area where the reaction is taking place and contributes to their activation, promoting the release of TNF. Recently, it has been found that endotoxin stimulates the release of MIF by the pituitary gland, and its release seems associated with increased mortality in the postacute phase of septic shock. β-Defensins, released primarily by granulocytes, have also been characterized as chemotactic for T lymphocytes.

Natural Killer Cells

NK cells represent a bridge between innate and acquired immunity, where the two systems become closely related. NK cells were recognized for their ability to kill certain tumor cell lines and viral infected cells. They are also one of the main cell populations involved in antibody-dependent cell-mediated cytotoxicity (ADCC).

The physiological significance of NK cells results from the fact that these cells seem to fulfill the need for a rapid response to a viral infection. The mobilization of a T lymphocyte-mediated cytotoxic response is a relatively slow process. In a resting immune system, the cytotoxic T cell precursors exist in relatively low numbers ($<1/10^5$). Proliferation and differentiation are required to generate a sufficient number of fully activated effector CD8$^+$ T cells, even the response of a primed individual takes a few days. Thus, an effective primary antiviral cytotoxic T cell response is seldom deployed in less than five to six days and may take as long as two weeks. During this time, the host depends on the innate defenses, which can be deployed much more rapidly, such as the production of type I IFNs (α and β), initiated as soon as the virus starts replicating, and the activity of NK cells.

Natural Killer Cell Activation

NK cells receive activation signals from NK cells, T lymphocytes, and monocytes/macrophages. Those signals are mediated by cytokines released from those cells, particularly type I IFNs (α and β), IL-2, and IL-12. The activating effect of IL-2 is mediated by the interaction of this cytokine with a functional IL-2 receptor, predominantly constituted by the β chain (p75 subunit) expressed by NK cells. Because the α chain is not expressed, NK cells are, for the most part, CD25$^-$. However, this variant of the IL-2 receptor enables NK cells to be effectively activated by IL-2, without the need for any additional costimulating factors or signals. IL-2-activated NK cells are also known as LAK cells.

Type I IFNs enhance the cytotoxic activity of NK cells. Thus, the release of these IFNs from infected cells mobilizes nonspecific defenses before the differentiation of major histocompatibility complex (MHC) restricted cytotoxic T lymphocytes is completed. IL-12, produced at the same time as IFNs α and β, is believed to play a crucial role in the early activation of NK cells.

The mechanism of recognition of target cells by NK cells is totally different from the antigen recognition mechanisms of B and T lymphocytes. A major difference is that NK cells can recognize virus-infected cells and many different types of malignant cells without clonal restriction. Normal cells deliver both activating and down-regulating signals that neutralize each other. Neoplastic transformation and viral infection often result in lack of delivery of the inhibitory signal (see Chapter 10), causing the activation of NK cells. Viral infection and malignant transformation activate NK cells because these conditions are associated with changes in the constitution of membrane glycoproteins and often interfere with the interaction of human leukocyte antigen (HLA) molecules with the inhibitory receptor. The impaired delivery of downregulating signals to NK cells may result from the replacement of a self-peptide on HLA-C by a nonself peptide, or from the reduced expression of MHC-I molecules on the cell membrane, a phenomenon frequently associated with viral infection. In either case, the end result will be that the activating receptor will deliver a strong signal that is not counteracted by an equivalent signal from the inhibitory receptor. In all these circumstances, the activated NK cell will be able to cause the death of the target cell by mechanisms similar to those described for T lymphocyte-mediated cytotoxicity.

Natural Killer Cells and Antibody-Dependent Cell-Mediated Cytotoxicity

NK cells express the FcγRIII, a low-affinity Fc receptor that binds IgG-coated cells. IgG binding results in the activation of the NK cell and lysis of the target, a process known as antibody-dependent cellular cytotoxicity. ADCC dependent activation and killing is not inhibited by the natural killer inhibitory receptor (NKIR); details are given in Chapter 10.

NATURAL ANTIBODIES

Pre-existing antibodies may play a very important anti-infectious protecting role. Natural antibodies may arise as a consequence of cross-reactions, as exemplified in the classical studies concerning the isoagglutinins of the ABO blood group system. Circulating ABO isoagglutinins exist in individuals of blood groups O, A, or B and agglutinate erythrocytes carrying alloantigens of the ABO system different than those of the individual himself.

The origin of natural antibodies, in most cases, appears to be unsuspected cross-reactions. Experimentally, this seems to be the explanation for the production of agglutinins recognizing the human AB alloantigens by chickens. Interestingly, the isoagglutinins are only produced by chicks fed conventional diets; chicks fed sterile diets do not develop them. Furthermore, anti-A and anti-B agglutinins develop as soon as chicks fed sterile diets after birth are placed on conventional diets later in life. These observations pointed to some dietary component as a source of immunization. It was eventually demonstrated that the cell wall polysaccharides of several strains of enterobacteriaceae and the AB oligosaccharides of human erythrocytes are structurally similar. Thus, cross-reactive antibodies to enterobacteriaceae are responsible for the "spontaneous" development of antibodies to human red cell antigens in chickens.

Newborn babies of blood groups A, B, or O do not have neither anti-A nor anti-B isoagglutinins in their cord blood, but develop them during the first months of life, as they become exposed to common bacteria with polysaccharide capsules. However, newborns are tolerant to their own blood group substance, so they will only make antibodies against the blood group substance that they do not express. Blood group AB individuals never produce AB isoagglutinins.

Other mechanisms, such as the mitogenic effects of T-independent antigens and the non-specific activation of B cells by lymphokines, released by antigen-stimulated T lymphocytes, could explain the rise of "nonspecific" immunoglobulins that is observed in the early stages of the humoral response to many different antigens. It is only a matter of random probability that some of these "nonspecific" immunoglobulins may play the role of "natural antibodies" relative to an unrelated antigen.

Irrespectively of their origin, "natural" antibodies may play an important protective role, as shown by the experiments summarized in Figure 2. Antibodies elicited to *E. coli* K100 cross-react with the polyribophosphate of *Haemophilus influenzae* and can protect experimental animals against infection with the latter organism. It is logical to assume that such cross-immunizations may be rather common and play an important protective role against a variety of infectious agents.

PROTECTIVE ROLE OF ANTIBODIES

If a pathogen is not eliminated by nonimmunological means and continues to replicate, it will eventually spread through the blood and lymph, and will usually be trapped by macrophages and dendritic cells in the lymph nodes and spleen. These cells are able to internalize antigens interacting with receptors such as the mannose receptor (see earlier), process the antigen in the endosomic compartment, and express MHC-II-associated antigen-derived peptides. This

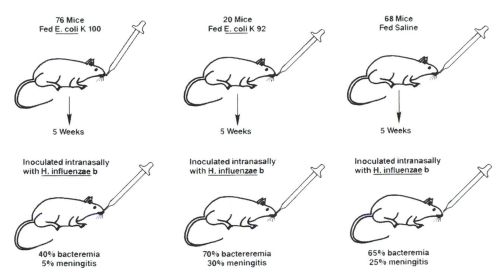

FIGURE 2 Diagrammatic representation of an experiment proving the anti-infectious protective role of cross-reactive "natural" antibodies. Three groups of mice were orally immunized with *Escherichia coli* K100, *E. coli* K92, and saline, as a control. Five weeks later, all animals were challenged with *Haemophilus influenzae* type b by the intranasal route. *E. coli* K100 has cross-reactivity with *H. influenzae* type b, but the same is not true for *E. coli* K92. The animals immunized with *E. coli* K100 showed significantly lower rates of bacteremia and meningeal infection than the animals immunized with *E. coli* K92 or controls fed with saline. *Source*: Based on Moxon ER, Anderson P. J Inf Diseases 1979; 140:471.

creates ideal conditions for the onset of a specific immune response: B lymphocytes can interact with membrane-bound antigen while helper T cells recognize MHC-II with antigen derived peptides presented by the same APC. The antigen-recognizing cells will interact and costimulate each other and after a time lag necessary for proliferation and differentiation of B cells into antibody-producing cells, circulating antibody will become detectable.

As described in Chapter 12, a primary immune response will take five to seven days (sometimes as long as two to three weeks) to be detected. The predominating isotype of the antibodies made early in a primary immune response is IgM and these antibodies are of relatively low affinity. In contrast, a secondary immune response has a shorter lag phase (as short as three to four days), and the predominant isotype of the antibodies is IgG, which have higher affinity. These different characteristics can be exploited for diagnostic purposes. The predominance of IgM or of low affinity antibodies indicates that a given immune response has been elicited recently and that the infection is recent or ongoing.

Antibody-Dependent Anti-infectious Effector Mechanisms

As soon as specific antibodies become available, they can protect the organism against infection by several different mechanisms.

Complement-Mediated Lysis
Complement-mediated lysis can result from the activation of the complete sequence of complement. However, as discussed later, both mammalian cells and most pathogenic microorganisms have developed mechanism that allows them to resist complement-mediated lysis.

Opsonization and Phagocytosis
Opsonization and phagocytosis are critically important. Several proteins can opsonize and promote phagocytosis, as discussed earlier, but IgG antibodies are the most efficient opsonins among the immunoglobulins. Opsonization becomes super-efficient when complement is activated as a consequence of the antigen–antibody reaction occurring on the surface of the

infectious agent and C3b and iC3b join IgG on the microbial cell membrane. This synergism is explained by the association of Fcγ and C3 receptors that are coexpressed on the membranes of all phagocytic cells. Killing through opsonization has been demonstrated for bacteria, fungi, and viruses, while phagocytosis of antibody/complement-coated unicellular parasites has not been clearly demonstrated.

The biological significance of phagocytic cells as ultimate mediators of the effects of opsonizing antibodies is obvious; the protective effects of antibodies are lost in patients with severe neutropenia or with severe functional defects of their phagocytic cells. Such patients have increased incidence of infections by a variety of opportunistic organisms.

Antibody-Dependent Cell-Mediated Cytotoxicity

Cells with Fc receptors may be able to participate in killing reactions that target antibody-coated cells. IgG1, IgG3, and IgE antibodies and cells with FcγR or FcεR are usually involved. Large granular lymphocytes or monocytes are the most common effector cells in ADCC, but in the case of parasitic infections, eosinophils play the principal role in cytotoxic reactions (Fig. 3). Different effector mechanisms are responsible for killing by different types of cells. Large granular lymphocytes kill through the release of granzymes and signaling for apoptosis; monocytes kill by releasing oxygen active radicals and nitric oxide; eosinophil killing is mostly mediated by the release of a "major basic protein," which is toxic for parasites.

Toxin Neutralization

Many bacteria release toxins, which are often the major virulence factors responsible for severe clinical symptoms. Antibodies to these toxins prevent their binding to cellular receptors and promote toxin elimination by phagocytosis.

Virus Neutralization

Most viruses spread from an initial focus of infection to a target tissue via the blood stream. Antibodies binding to the circulating virus can change its external configuration and prevent either its binding to cell receptors or its ability to release nucleic acid into the cell.

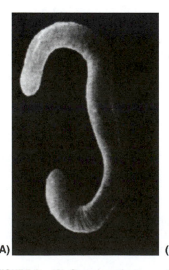 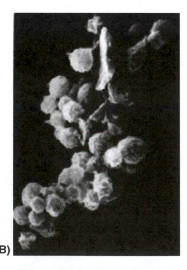

(A)   **(B)**

FIGURE 3   (**A**) Scanning electron microphotograph of a *Trichinella spiralis* larva incubated with eosinophils and complement-depleted normal (nonimmune) mouse serum for four hours; (**B**) Scanning electron microphotograph of a *T. spiralis* larva incubated with eosinophils and complement-depleted immune serum for four hours. Notice that the attachment of eosinophils happened only when eosinophils were added to *T. spiralis* larvae in the presence of immune sera containing antibodies directed against the parasite. *Source*: Reproduced from Kazura JW, Aikawa M. J Immunol 1980; 124:355.

Mucosal Protection

Secretory antibodies seem to confer their protective role by preventing the attachment and subsequent penetration of microbial agents through mucosal surfaces.

Factors Influencing the Effectiveness of an Anti-infectious Humoral Response

The effectiveness of the humoral immune response in preventing an infectious disease depends on the time differential between the incubation period of the disease and the time needed to mount the immune response. If antibodies can be synthesized before the organisms proliferate or before they secrete exotoxins, then the humoral response will prevent the infection's clinical manifestations.

If relevant antibodies are present in the circulation as a result of vaccination, previous infection, or cross-reaction between different microorganisms, then protection is most effective since the microorganism or its toxins will be almost immediately neutralized and the infection will remain subclinical.

If preformed antibodies are not present, protection will depend on whether antibody synthesis can take place before the "incubation period" (period of time during which the infectious agent is multiplying but has not yet reached sufficient mass to cause clinical disease) is over. Some infectious agents, such as the influenza virus, have very short incubation periods (about two to three days), and in such cases not even a secondary immune response is protective. In most infections, however, the duration of the incubation period is sufficiently long as to allow a secondary immune response to provide protective antibodies. Thus, for many infections, particularly the common viral diseases of childhood, previous exposure and acquisition of memory ensure that antibody will be produced in time to contain infection upon subsequent exposures. Thus, reinfection plays the role of natural "booster" doses, explaining the "immunity for life" associated with some of the most common childhood diseases. However, this effect appears to be lost when the spread of the infectious agent is limited as a consequence of vaccination, but not totally eliminated. Two examples of this situation are measles and whooping cough rarely seen in childhood but causing disease among young adults that have lost their immunity.

The goal of prophylactic immunization may vary from case to case. In diseases with very short incubation periods, it is essential to maintain the levels of neutralizing antibody in the circulation necessary to immediately abort infection. In most other diseases, it may be sufficient to induce immunological memory, since once memory has been induced, the immune system will be able to respond in time to prevent the development of clinical infection.

Finally, it must be noted that protection by humoral immunity is only possible if the infectious agent is easily available to the antibodies produced against it. Thus, intracellular pathogens are not easy to eliminate by antibodies. In addition, as discussed in detail later in this chapter, there are organisms able to change their antigenic make up during the course of an infection and that can persist in spite of a vigorous humoral response.

PROTECTIVE ROLE OF CELL-MEDIATED IMMUNITY

Many organisms have the ability to grow and replicate intracellularly. For some, it is an absolute requirement; for others, it is an option that allows them to survive after phagocytosis. Antibodies are largely ineffective against intracellular organisms, and T lymphocytes play a major role in their elimination. A cell-mediated immune response is indicated by the finding of lymphocytic infiltrates in tissues infected by intracellular infectious agents, such as viruses. The immune system has two basic options to eliminate intracellular organisms: to kill the infected cell, or to enhance the infected cell's ability to kill intracellular organisms. Either option requires the persistent activation of the Th1 subpopulation of helper cells.

Lymphocyte-Mediated Cytotoxicity

Lymphocyte-mediated cytotoxicity seems particularly significant for the elimination of viral-infected cells. It can be easily demonstrated that viral-infected cells are lysed as a consequence of their incubation with "immune" lymphocytes that are obtained from an animal previously exposed to the same virus. The sequence of events involves recognition of viral derived-peptides expressed in association with MHC-I molecules by $CD8^+$ lymphocytes, followed by differentiation into cytotoxic T cells specific for the same MHC-I/peptide complex that they recognized when initially activated. The differentiation usually requires Th1 help. The activation of Th1 cells usually requires recognition of MHC-II/peptide complexes. Considering that macrophages are common targets for most viral infections, they are likely to present viral peptides associated both with MHC-I and MHC-II molecules (see Chapter 4). This duality should allow the simultaneous activation of $CD4^+$ and $CD8^+$ T cells in close proximity, an ideal set-up for delivery of "help" to activate precursors of cytotoxic T cells.

Lymphocyte-Mediated Activation of Macrophages and Other Inflammatory Cells

Most intracellular bacteria and parasites infect tissue macrophages and fail to induce efficient cytotoxic reactivity. The persistence of the infection depends on a delicate balance between a state of relative inactivity by the macrophage and mechanisms that allow the infectious agent to escape proteolytic digestion once inside the cytoplasm (see subsequently). The immune system can react through a largely ineffective humoral response, or through a Th1-mediated inflammatory response, which may actually induce the elimination of the pathogen.

The effective response involves activation of $CD4^+$ Th1 lymphocytes as a consequence of their interaction with infected macrophages expressing MHC-II-associated peptides and releasing IL-12. The role of IL-12 appears to be critical, because IL-12 receptor deficiency is associated with the predisposition to develop tuberculosis, a classical example of intracellular infection. When properly activated by IL-12, Th1 lymphocytes release a variety of lympho-kines, particularly INF-γ that activates macrophages and enhances their ability to kill intracellular organisms (see Chapter 13), and granulocyte-monocyte colony stimulating factor (GM-CSF) that promotes differentiation and release of granulocytes and monocytes from the bone marrow. As a consequence of the delivery of activation signals, macrophages and lymphocytes enter in a complex cycle of self and mutual activation involving a variety of cytokines. In addition, several of these cytokines may activate other types of cells and have chemotactic properties (see Chapter 11). This group of cytokines, known as chemokines, includes IL-8, RANTES, MIP, MCP, MIF, and β-defensins. Collectively, the chemokines attract, activate, and retain leukocytes to the area where a cell-mediated immune reaction is taking place.

In concert with the release of chemotactic cytokines, the expression of cell adhesion molecules in neighboring microvasculature is upregulated, favoring adherence and migration of monocytes and granulocytes to the extravascular space. Inflammatory cells accumulate in the area of infection, and as a consequence of cross-activation circuits involving phagocytes and Th1 lymphocytes, the localized macrophages and granulocytes become activated. As a consequence, phagocytosis is enhanced, the enzymatic content of the granules increases, the respiratory burst is more vigorous, and the release of cytokines more pronounced.

The cytokines released by activated macrophages include IL-12, which continues to promote the differentiation of Th1 cells, as well as IL-1, IL-6, and TNF, which play the major role in inducing the metabolic effects characteristic of the inflammatory reaction.

IMMUNE DEFICIENCY SYNDROMES AS MODELS FOR THE STUDY OF THE IMPORTANCE OF IMMUNE DEFENSES AGAINST INFECTIONS IN HUMANS

Most of our information about the immune system in humans has been learned from the study of patients with immunodeficiency diseases (see Chapter 30). The most characteristic clinical features of immunocompromised patients are repeated or chronic infections, often caused by opportunistic agents. There are some characteristic associations between specific types of infections and generic types of immune deficiency that illustrate the physiological roles of the different components of the immune system.

1. Patients with antibody deficiencies and conserved cell-mediated immunity suffer from repeated and chronic infections with pyogenic bacteria.

2. Patients with primary deficiencies of cell-mediated immunity usually suffer from chronic or recurrent fungal, parasitic, and viral infections.
3. Neutrophil deficiencies are usually associated with bacterial infections caused by common organisms of low virulence that would normally be kept in check through nonimmune phagocytosis.
4. Isolated deficiencies of terminal complement components (C6–CC9) are also associated with bacterial infections, most frequently involving *Neisseria* sp, whose elimination appears to require formation of the cytolytic membrane attack complex.

ESCAPE FROM THE IMMUNE RESPONSE

Many infectious agents have developed the capacity to avoid the immune response. Several mechanisms are involved.

Complement Inhibitory Activity

Complement inhibitory activity has been characterized for bacterial capsules and membrane proteins of some bacteria, parasites, and enveloped viruses. Some pathogens can also acquire host complement inhibitory proteins from serum or cell membranes. Complement inhibitory activity on the pathogen surface results in a decreased level of opsonization by C3b and other complement fragments.

Resistance to Phagocytosis

Resistance to phagocytosis, either mediated by polysaccharide capsules that repel and inhibit the function of phagocytic cells, or by mechanisms that allow the pathogen to survive. Resistance to phagocytosis is characteristic of the group of bacteria known as facultative intracellular (*Mycobacteria, Brucella, Listeria,* and *Salmonella,* among others), as well as of some fungi and protozoa (*Toxoplasma, Trypanosoma cruzi,* and *Leishmania* sp.). Infectious agents have developed many different strategies to survive intracellularly. Some infectious agents secrete molecules that prevent the formation of phagolysosomes, allowing the infectious agent to survive inside phagosomes, relatively devoid of toxic compounds (e.g., *Mycobacterium tuberculosis, Legionella pneumophila,* and *Toxoplasma gondii*). Others have outer coats that protect the bacteria against proteolytic enzymes and free toxic radicals (such as the superoxide radical) or have developed mechanisms that allow them to exit the phagosome and survived unharmed in the cytoplasm (e.g., *T. cruzi*). Finally, others depress the response of the infected phagocytic cells to activating cytokines, such as IFN-γ.

Some organisms combine several of different mechanisms to survive intracellularly. For example, *Mycobacterium leprae* is coated with a phenolic glycolipid layer that scavenges free radicals and releases a compound that inhibits the effect of IFN-γ. In addition, the release of IL-4 and IL-10 by infected macrophages is enhanced, contributing to the downregulation of Th1 lymphocytes.

Ineffective Immune Responses

Some infectious agents appear to have acquired evolutionary advantage by not inducing effective immune responses. For example, polysaccharide capsules protect many bacteria and fungi against phagocytosis through physicochemical effects and also by the fact that their immonogenicity is not as strong as that of proteins. Polysaccharides are not presented to helper CD4 T cells and in the absence of adequate T cell help, the response to polysaccharides involves predominantly IgM and IgG2 antibodies, which are inefficient as opsonins (the FcγR of phagocytic cells recognize preferentially IgG1 and IgG3 antibodies). Another example is *Neisseria meningitides,* which often induces the synthesis of IgA antibodies. In vitro data suggests that IgA can act as a weak opsonin or induce ADCC (monocytes/macrophages and other leukocytes express Fcα receptors on their membranes), but the physiological protective role of IgA antibodies is questionable. Patient sera with high titers of IgA antibodies to *N. meningitides* fail to show bactericidal activity until IgA specific anti-*N. meningitides* antibodies are removed. This observation suggests that IgA antibodies may act as a "blocking factors," preventing opsonizing IgG antibodies from binding to the same epitopes.

Release of Soluble Antigens

Release of soluble antigens from infected cells that are able to bind and block antibodies before they can reach the cells have been demonstrated in the case of the hepatitis B virus. The circulating antigens act as a "deflector shield" that protects the infected tissues from "antibody aggression."

Loss and Masking of Antigens with Absorbed Host Proteins

Loss and masking of antigens with absorbed host proteins have been demonstrated with several worms, particularly schistosomula (the larval forms of schistosoma). The ability of parasitic worms to survive in the host is well-known and is certainly derived from the ability to evade the immune system.

Antigenic Variation

Antigenic variation has been characterized in bacteria (*Borrelia recurrentis*), protozoan parasites (trypanosomes, the agents of African sleeping sickness, *Giardia lamblia*), and viruses [human immunodeficiency virus (HIV)].

One of the best-studied examples is African trypanosomes. These protozoa have a surface coat constituted mainly of a single glycoprotein [variant-specific surface glycoprotein (VSG)], for which there are about 10^3 genes in the chromosome. At any given time, only one of those genes is expressed, the others remaining silent. For every 10^6 or 10^7 trypanosome divisions, a mutation occurs that replaces the active VSG gene on the expression site by a previously silent VSG gene. The previously expressed gene is destroyed, and a new VSG protein is coded, which is antigenically different. The emergence of a new antigenic coat allows the parasite to multiply unchecked. As antibodies emerge to the newly expressed VSG protein, parasitemia will decline, only to increase as soon as a new mutation occurs and a different VSG protein is synthesized. *G.lamblia* has a similar mechanism of variation, but the rate of surface antigen replacement is even faster (once every 10^3 divisions).

B. recurrentis, the agent of relapsing fever carries genes for at least 26 different variable major proteins (VMP) that are sequentially activated by duplicative transposition to an expression site. The successive waves of bacteremia and fever correspond to the emergence of new mutants, which, for a while, can proliferate unchecked until antibodies are formed.

HIV exhibits a high degree of antigenic variation that seems to be the result of errors introduced by the reverse transcriptase when synthesizing viral DNA from the RNA template. The mutation rate is relatively high (one in every 10^3 progeny particles), and the immune response selects the mutant strains that present new configurations in the outer envelope proteins, allowing the mutant to proliferate unchecked by pre-existing neutralizing antibodies.

Cell-to-Cell Spread

Cell-to-cell spread allows infectious agents to propagate without being exposed to specific antibodies or phagocytic cells. This strategy is commonplace for viruses, especially for Herpes viruses, retroviruses, and paramyxoviruses, and allows the fusion of infected cells with noninfected cells allowing viral particles to pass from cell-to-cell without exposure to the extracellular environment.

Some intracellular bacteria have also developed the ability to spread from cell-to-cell, with the best-known example being *Listeria monocytogenes*. After becoming intracellular, *L. monocytogenes* can travel along the cytoskeleton and promote the fusion of the membrane of an infected cell with the membrane of a neighboring noninfected cell, which is subsequently invaded.

Immunosuppressive Effects of Infection

Although immunosuppressive effects have been described in association with bacteria and parasitic infections, the best-documented examples of infection-associated immunosuppression are those described in viral infections. The effects of HIV on the immune system are described in detail in Chapter 30, but many other viruses have the ability to depress immune functions. For example, patients in the acute phase of measles are more susceptible to bacterial infections, such as pneumonia. Both delayed hypersensitivity responses and in vitro lymphocyte proliferation in response to mitogens and antigens are significantly depressed during the acute phase of measles and the immediate convalescence period, usually returning to normal after four weeks. It has also been shown that infection of monocytes/macrophages with the measles virus is associated with a downregulation of IL-12 synthesis, which can be a contributing factor to the depression of cell-mediated immunity associated with measles.

Mothers and infants infected with cytomegalovirus (CMV) show depressed responses to CMV, but normal responses to T cell mitogens, suggesting that in some cases the immunosuppression may be antigen-specific, while in measles it is obviously nonspecific.

Influenza virus has been found to depress CMI in mice, apparently due to an increase in the suppressor activity of T lymphocytes.

Epstein-Barr virus (EBV) releases a specific protein that has extensive sequence homology with IL-10. The biological properties of this viral protein are also analogous to those of IL-10; both are able to inhibit lymphokine synthesis by T cell clones.

ABNORMAL CONSEQUENCES OF THE IMMUNE RESPONSE

In the vast majority of situations, the immune response has a protective effect that allows the organism to recover from infection without major illness and without long-term sequelae. However, there are well-known examples of deleterious effects triggered by an exaggerated or misdirected immune response.

Activation of T Lymphocytes by Bacterial "Superantigens"

A variety of bacterial exotoxins, such as staphylococcal enterotoxins-A and -B (SE-A and SE-B), staphylococcal toxic shock syndrome Toxin-1 (TSST-1), exfoliating toxin, and streptococcal exotoxin A, as well as other unrelated bacterial proteins (such as streptococcal M proteins) have been characterized as "superantigens."

Superantigens are defined by their ability to stimulate T cells without being processed. The stimulation of T cells is polyclonal; thus the designation "superantigen" is a misnomer, but it has gained popularity and is widely used in the literature. The best-studied "superantigens" are the staphylococcal enterotoxins, which are potent polyclonal activators of murine and human T lymphocytes, inducing T cell proliferation and cytokine release. TSST-1 also appears to activate monocytes and is a potent B cell mitogen, inducing B cell proliferation and differentiation.

The stimulatory effects of "superantigens" are a consequence of the direct and simultaneous binding to the nonpolymorphic area of class II MHC on professional accessory cells (macrophages and related cells) and to the Vβ chain of the α/β T-cell receptors (TcR) (Fig. 4). For example, staphylococcal enterotoxins bind exclusively to specific subfamilies of Vβ chains that are expressed only by certain individuals. When expressed, these Vβ chain regions can be found on 2% to 20% of a positive individual's T cells, and the cross-linking of the TcR2 and of the APC by the enterotoxin, activates all T cells (both CD4 and CD8$^+$) expressing the specific Vβ region recognized by the enterotoxin. The massive T cell activation induced by superantigens results in the release of large amounts of IL-2, IFN-γ, lymphotoxin-α (LTα), and TNF. After the initial burst of cytokine release the stimulated T cells either undergo apoptosis or become anergic. This effect could severely disturb the ability of the immune system to adequately respond to bacteria releasing superantigens.

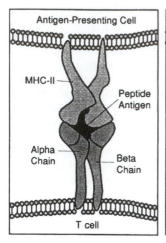 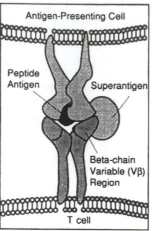

FIGURE 4 Diagrammatic comparison of the mechanisms of T cell stimulation by conventional antigens and staphylococcal enterotoxins. While conventional antigens are processed into oligopeptides, which bind to major histocompatibility complex-II (MHC-II) molecules and then bind specifically to a T-cell receptor (TcR) binding site (*left panel*), bacterial "superantigens" interact with nonpolymorphic areas of the Vβ chain of the TcR and of the MHC-II molecule on an antigen-presenting cells (APC) (*right panel*). Notice that "superantigen" binding overrides the need for TcR recognition of the MHC-II associated oligopeptide, and thus T cells of many different specificities can be activated. It is also important to note that both APC and T cells can be stimulated as a consequence of the extensive cross-linking of membrane proteins. *Source*: Modified from Johnson HM, Russell JK, Pontzer CH. Scientific American 1992; 266(4):92.

Patients infected by bacteria able to release large amounts of superantigens (e.g., *S. aureus* releasing enterotoxins or TSST-1 and Group A *Streptococcus* releasing exotoxin A) may develop septic shock as a consequence of the systemic effects of these cytokines. These systemic effects include fever, endothelial damage, profound hypotension, disseminated intravascular coagulation, multi-organ failure, and death.

Infection as a Consequence of the Uptake of Antigen–Antibody Complexes

The immune response, in some cases, facilitates the access of infectious agents to cells in which they will be able to proliferate. For example, macrophages are often infected by intracellular organisms that are ingested as a consequence of opsonization. *Leishmania* organisms are intracellular parasites that penetrate the host's cells after reacting with complement, particularly C3. EBV normally infects B cells through CR2, a complement receptor. However, if dimeric IgA reactive with the virus is produced and released into the mucosal secretions, the resulting IgA-EBV complex is able to infect mucosal cells through the poly-Ig receptor, which binds dimeric IgA (see Chapter 6). Mucosal infection in the nasopharynx can eventually acquire malignant characteristics.

Post-infectious Tissue Damage

Several examples of the pathogenic role of an anti-infectious immune response have been characterized. The following are some of the best-known examples:

Immune-Complex-Induced Inflammation

Antigen–antibody complexes, if formed in large amounts, can cause disease by becoming trapped in different capillary networks and leading to inflammation. The clinical expression of immune complex-related inflammation depends on the localization of the trapped complexes: vasculitis and purpura occurs when the skin is predominantly affected, glomerulonephritis if trapping takes place on the glomerular capillaries, and arthritis when the joints are affected (see Chapter 23). Viruses (particularly Hepatitis C virus) are often involved in the formation of circulating antigen–antibody complexes.

Immune Destruction of Infected Cells and Tissues

An immune response directed against an infectious agent may be the main cause of damage to the infected tissue. For example, in subacute sclerosing panencephalitis, a degenerative disease of the nervous system associated with persistent infection with the measles virus, the response against viral epitopes expressed in infected neurons is believed to be the primary mechanism of disease. Also, in some forms of chronic active hepatitis (see Chapter 17), the immune response directed against viral epitopes expressed by infected hepatocytes seems to cause more tissue damage than the infection itself.

Cross-Reactions with Tissue Antigens

Cross-reactions with tissue antigens have been proposed as the basis for the association of streptococcal infections with rheumatic carditis and glomerulonephritis. Antibodies to Type 1 streptococcal M protein cross-react with epitopes of myocardium and kidney mesangial cells and cause inflammatory changes in the heart and glomeruli, respectively.

Autoimmunity

The role of infectious agents as triggers of autoimmune reactions is discussed in detail in Chapters 3 and 16.

CONCLUSION

The outcome of an infectious process depends on a very complex set of interactions with the immune system. A successful pathogen is usually one that has developed mechanisms that avoid fast elimination by an immunocompetent host. These mechanisms allow the infectious agent to replicate, cause disease, and spread to other individuals before the immune response is induced. The immune response, on the other hand, is a powerful weapon that, once set in motion, may destroy friendly targets. Thus, a therapeutic strategy for infectious disease has to consider such questions as the particular survival strategy of the infectious agents, the effects of the infection on the immune system, and the possibility that the immune response may be more of a problem than the infection itself.

BIBLIOGRAPHY

Altare F, Durandy A, Lammas D, et al. Impairment of mycobacterial immunity in human interleukin 12 receptor deficiency. Science 1998; 280:1432.

Borst P, Graves DR. Programmed gene rearrangements altering gene expression. Science 1987; 235:658.

Cook DN, Beck M, Coffman TM, et al. Requirement of MIP-1a for an inflammatory response to viral infection. Science 1995; 269:1583.

De Smet K, Contreras R. Human Antimicrobial peptides: defensins, cathelicidins and histatins. Biotechnol Lett 2005; 27:1337–1347.

Fehniger TA, Caliguri MA. Interleukin 15: biology and relevance to human disease. Blood 2001; 97:14–32.

Ferri C, Giuggioli D, Cazzato M, Sebastiani M, Mascia MT, Zignego AL. HCV-related cryoglobulinemic vasculitis: an update on its etiopathogenesis and therapeutic strategies. Clin Exp Rheumatol 2003; 21(6 suppl 32):S78–S84.

Ganz T. Defensins and Host Defense. Science 1999; 286:420–421.

Gracie JA, Robertson SE, McInnes IB. Interleukin-18. J Leukoc Biol 2003; 73:213–224.

Hamerman JA, Ogasawara K, Lanier LL. NK cells in innate immunity. Curr Opin Immunol 2005; 17:29–35.

Karp CL, Wysocka M, Wahl LM, et al. Mechanism of suppression of cell-mediated immunity by measles virus. Science 1996; 273:228.

Kirk P, Bazan JF. Pathogen recognition: TLRs throw us a curve. Immunity 2005; 23:347–350.

Kraus W, Dale JB, Beachey EH. Identification of an epitope of type 1 streptococcal M protein that is shared with a 43-kDa protein of human myocardium and renal glomeruli. J Immunol 1990; 145:4089.

Lanier LL. NK cell recognition. Annu Rev Immunol 2005; 23:225–274.

Li H, Llera A, Malchiodi EL, Mariuzza RA. The structural basis of T cell activation by superantigens. Annu Rev Immunol 1999; 17:435.

Liu PT, Stenger S, Li H, et al. Toll-like receptor triggering of a vitamin D-mediated human antimicrobial response. Science 2006; 311:1770–1773.

Luster AD. Chemokines- Chemotactic cytokines that mediate inflammation. N Engl J Med 1998; 338:436.

Mauel J. Macrophage-parasite interactions in Leishmania infections. J Leukoc Biol 1990; 47:187.

Romagnani P, Lasagni L, Annunziato F, Serio M, Romagnani S. CXC chemokines: the regulatory link between inflammation and angiogenesis. Trends Immunol 2004; 25:201–209.

Tosi MF. Innate immune responses to infection. J Allergy Clin Immunol 2005; 116:241–249.

15 | Diagnostic Immunology

Virginia M. Litwin
MDS Pharma Services, Central Lab, North Brunswick, New Jersey, U.S.A.

Gabriel Virella
Department of Microbiology and Immunology, Medical University of South Carolina, Charleston, South Carolina, U.S.A.

INTRODUCTION

Scientists have exploited the exquisite sensitivity and specificity of antibody recognition for use in assays for both diagnostic and basic research applications. In the past few decades, technological advances in methods to generate antibodies and to detect antibody–antigen binding have transformed laboratory medicine and basic research in many fields. A variety of platforms make use of fluorescence or chemiluminescence to detect antigen–antibody interactions. These technologies are sensitive, specific, quantitative, and relatively rapid. Two of the most important technologies, immunoassays and flow cytometry, have replaced more laborious, less sensitive methods that relied on the detection of antigen–antibody aggregates in gel-based systems (immunodiffusion). The use of fluorescent and chemiluminescent detection systems in these newer technologies has all but replaced the use of radiation in the laboratory. Applications of these serologic and molecular methods are quite broad. They have been applied to the diagnosis of infectious diseases, the detection of previous infection, the monitoring of neoplasms and vaccine efficacy, the assay of hormones and drugs, and pregnancy diagnosis. In some cases, the antigen being measured is itself an antibody. Measurement of specific antibodies has found wide application in the diagnosis of infectious, allergic, autoimmune, and immunodeficiency diseases.

Serological Assays

Immunoserologic assays can be developed for antigen or antibody detection or quantitative assay. For antibody detection or measurement, a purified preparation of antigen must be available. For instance, when human serum is tested for antibody to diphtheria toxoid, a purified preparation of the toxoid must be available. Second, a method for detecting the specific antigen–antibody reaction must be developed. Conversely, to detect antigens in biological fluids, specific antibody must be available. In both types of assays, positive and negative controls are required for proper interpretation of the results.

Classical Assays
Radial Immunodiffusion
Radial immunodiffusion represents a hallmark in the evolution of immunoserology because it represents the first successful attempt to develop a precise quantitative assay suitable for routine use in the diagnostic laboratories. Radial immunodiffusion received its designation from the fact that a given antigen is forced to diffuse concentrically on a support medium to which antiserum has been incorporated (Fig. 1).

A polyclonal antiserum, known to precipitate the antigen, is added to molten agar and an agar plate containing the antibody is then prepared. Identical wells are cut in the antiserum-containing agar and those wells are filled with identical volumes of samples containing known amounts of the antigen (calibrators) and of unknown samples to which the antigen needs to be assayed. After 24 to 48 hours it is possible to measure the diameters of circular precipitates formed around the wells, where antigens were placed. Those diameters are directly proportional to antigen concentration. A plot of precipitation ring diameters versus

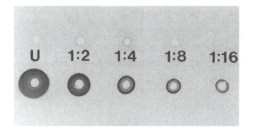

FIGURE 1   The principle of radial immunodiffusion. Five wells carved into antibody-containing agar were filled with serial dilutions of the corresponding antigen. The antigen diffused, reacted with antibody in the agar, and eventually precipitated in a circular pattern. The diameters or areas of these circular precipitates are directly proportional to the concentration of antigen in each well.

concentrations is made for the samples with known antigen concentrations. This plot, known as calibration curve, is used to extrapolate the concentrations of antigen in the unknown samples, based on the diameter of the corresponding precipitation rings.

Radial immunodiffusion can be applied to the assay of immunoglobulins, complement components, and, in general, of any antigenic protein that exists in concentrations greater than 5 to 10 mg/dL in any biological fluid.

Immunonephelometry

Immunonephelometry is nowadays preferred for the types of assays classically performed by radial immunofiffusion. The assay is also based on the formation of antigen–antibody aggregates, using constant concentrations of antibody and variable concentrations of antigen for calibration. The amount of complexes is measured by light dispersion (nephelometry). Immunonephelometry assays are more rapid and sensitive than radial immunodiffusion assays, and have the additional advantage of being automated.

Immunofixation (Immunoblotting)

An immunofixation study, illustrated in Figure 2, has several steps. In the first step, several aliquots of the patient's serum are simultaneously separated by electrophoresis. One of the separation lanes is stained as reference for the position of the different serum proteins (extreme right lane in the figure), while paper strips imbedded with different antibodies are laid over the remaining separation lanes. The antibodies diffuse into the agar and react with the corresponding immunoglobulins. After washing off unbound immunoglobulins and antibodies, the lanes where immunofixation take place are stained, revealing whether the antisera recognized the proteins they are directed against. In the figure, a monoclonal protein reacting with anti-IgG and anti-kappa antisera was revealed.

Western Blot

The Western blot (Fig. 3) is a variation of immunoblotting that was popularized by its use in the diagnosis of HIV infection. The first step in the preparation of an immunoblot is to separate the

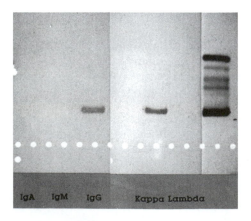

FIGURE 2   Use of the immunoblotting technique for typing a monoclonal protein. From right to left, the pictures show a reference lane in which the serum proteins were electrophoresed and stained, showing an homogeneous protein of gamma mobility, near the bottom of the separation. The next five lanes were blotted with the indicated antisera, washed, and then stained to reveal which antisera reacted with the homogeneous protein visualized in the reference lane. The results indicate that the homogeneous protein is a monoclonal protein of the IgG heavy chain isotype, with kappa light chains.

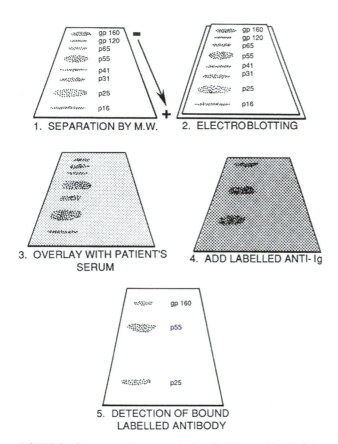

1. SEPARATION BY M.W.   2. ELECTROBLOTTING

3. OVERLAY WITH PATIENT'S SERUM   4. ADD LABELLED ANTI-Ig

5. DETECTION OF BOUND LABELLED ANTIBODY

FIGURE 3 Diagrammatic representation of a Western blot study to confirm the existence of anti-HIV antibodies. In the first step, a mixture of HIV antigens is separated by size (large antigens remain close to the origin where the sample is applied, smaller antigens move deep into the acrylamide gel used for the separation). In the second step, the separated antigens are electrophoresed into a permeable nitrocellulose membrane (electroblotting). Next, the patient's serum is spread over the cellulose membrane to which the antigens have been transferred. If antibodies to any of these antigens are present in the serum, a precipitate will be formed at the site where the antigen has been transferred. After washing excess of unreacted antigens and serum proteins, a labeled second antibody is overlaid on the membrane; if human antibodies precipitate by reacting with blotted antigens, the second antibody (labeled anti-human immunoglobulin) will react with the immunoglobulins contained in the precipitate. After washing off the excess of unreacted second antibody, labeled antibody bound to human antibody-viral protein complexes is revealed; its binding to an antigen–antibody precipitate can be detected either by adding a color-developing substrate or by measuring chemiluminescence, depending on the label.

different viral antigens (gp160 to p16) according to their molecular size (the numbers in front on "gp" or "p" refer to the protein mass in kilodaltons). This is achieved by performing polyacrylamide gel electrophoresis in the presence of a negatively charged detergent (such as sodium dodecyl sulfate) that becomes associated with the proteins and obliterates their charge differences, using as support for the separation a medium with sieving properties. The result is the separation of a protein mixture into components of different sizes. After the separation of the viral proteins is completed, it is necessary to transfer the separated proteins to another support, in order to proceed with the remaining steps. The proteins are then transferred or "blotted" onto polyvinyl membrane by a second electrophoresis step. The membrane is then incubated with the patient's serum. The patient's antibodies will bind to the viral antigen to which they are specific. Bound antibodies can then be detected and visualized by a variety of methods, most commonly using chemiluminescent or fluorescent secondary antibodies and digital imaging.

This technique has the advantage over other screening assays of not only detecting antibodies, but to identify the antigens against which the antibodies are directed. This results in increased specificity. The downside is the time consumed in running the assay, which requires very careful quality control, and needs to be carried out by specialized personnel in certified laboratories. To circumvent this problem, prepared western blot membranes can be purchased commercially. These specific blots (e.g., for HIV) only need to be probed with the patient serum and developed. Generally, positive and negative controls are included with the blots. Using these commercially available kits, the performance of sophisticated technology is accomplished with less time and training.

Agglutination Assays

Agglutination assays are used for a variety of purposes in bacteriology and diagnostic immunology.

Bacterial Agglutination

Bacterial agglutination is observed when a bacterial suspension is mixed with antibody directed to their surface determinants. Agglutination is rapid (takes a few minutes) and, being visible to the naked eye, does not require any special instrumentation other than a light box. Its disadvantages are the need for isolated organisms and poor sensitivity, requiring relatively large concentrations of antibody. In spite of its limitations, agglutination of whole microorganisms is commonly used for serotyping isolated organisms and for some rapid diagnostic tests.

Agglutination of Inert Particles Coated with Antigen or Antibody

Latex particles and other inert particles can be coated with purified antigen and will agglutinate in the presence of specific antibody. Conversely, specific antibodies can be easily adsorbed by latex particles and will agglutinate in the presence of the corresponding antigen. Semiquantitative analysis to determine the agglutinating antibody content of an antiserum involves dilution of the serum and determination of an end point, which is the last dilution at which agglutination can be observed. The reciprocal of this last agglutinating dilution is designated as antibody titer.

    This methodology is used both by clinical immunologists and clinical bacteriologists. For example, IgG-coated, latex particles are used for the detection of anti-immunoglobulin factors (such as the rheumatoid factor) in the rheumatoid arthritis (RA) test (Fig. 4). Also, rapid diagnosis tests for bacterial and fungal meningitis have been developed by adsorbing the relevant specific antibodies to latex particles. The antibody-coated particles will agglutinate if mixed with cerebrospinal fluid (CSF) containing the relevant antigen. This procedure allows a rapid etiologic diagnosis of meningitis that is essential for proper therapy to be initiated.

Red Cell Agglutination (Hemagglutination)

Red cell agglutination is the basis of a wide array of serological tests that can be subclassified as direct or indirect hemagglutination, depending on whether the assay involves a single step or two steps.

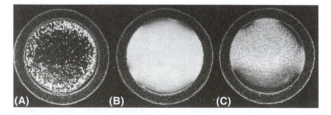

FIGURE 4 Detection of rheumatoid factor by the latex agglutination technique. A suspension of IgG-coated latex particles is mixed with a 1:20 dilution of three sera. (**A**) Obvious clumping is seen, corresponding to a strongly positive serum; (**B**) no clumping is seen, corresponding to a negative serum; (**C**) very fine clumping is seen, corresponding to a weakly positive serum.

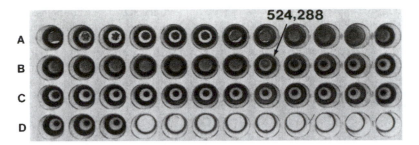

FIGURE 5 Detection of cold agglutinins by direct hemagglutination. The wells in the microtiter plate were first filled with serial dilutions of a patient's serum (rows A and B), serial dilutions of a control serum (row C), and saline (row D), and then with 0^+ red cells, incubated at $4°C$ and examined for agglutination. The normal control and saline control do not show agglutination. The patient's serum shows a prozone followed by agglutination up to a dilution of 1:524,288.

Direct Hemagglutination Tests

Direct hemagglutination tests are carried out with washed red cells that are agglutinated when mixed with IgM antibodies recognizing membrane epitopes. For example, direct agglutination tests are used for the determination of the ABO blood group and titration of isohemagglutinins (anti-A and anti-B antibodies), for the titration of cold hemagglutinins (IgM antibodies which agglutinate RBCs at temperatures below that of the body temperature, see Chapter 22), as illustrated in Figure 5, and for the Paul-Bunnell or monospot test, useful for the diagnosis of infectious mononucleosis. This last test detects circulating heterophile antibodies (cross-reactive antibodies that combine with antigens of an animal of a different species) that induce the agglutination of sheep or horse erythrocytes.

Indirect Hemagglutination

Indirect hemagglutination is used to detect antibodies that react with antigens present in the erythrocytes, but which by themselves cannot induce agglutination. Usually, these are IgG antibodies that are not as efficient agglutinators of red cells as polymeric IgM antibodies. A second antibody directed to human immunoglobulins is used to induce agglutination by reacting with the red-cell bound IgG molecules, and consequently, cross-linking the red cells. The best-known example of indirect agglutination is the antiglobulin or Coombs' test, which is used in the diagnosis of autoimmune hemolytic anemia (see Chapter 22).

Complement Fixation

When antigen and antibodies of the IgM or the IgG classes are mixed, complement is "fixed" to the antigen–antibody aggregate. If this occurs on the surface of a red blood cell, the complement cascade will be activated and hemolysis will occur. The method actually involves two antigen–antibody complement systems: a test system and an indicator system (Fig. 6).

1. The indicator system consists of red blood cells (RBC), which have been pre-incubated with a specific anti-red cell antibody in concentrations that do not cause agglutination, and in the absence of complement to avoid hemolysis; these are designated as "sensitized" red cells.
2. In the test system, patient's serum is first heated to $56°C$ to inactivate the native complement, and adsorbed with washed sheep RBC to eliminate broadly cross-reactive anti-red cell antibodies that could interfere with the assay. Then, the serum is mixed with purified antigen and with a dilution of fresh guinea pig serum, used as a controlled source of complement. The mixture is incubated for 30 minutes at $37°C$ to allow any antibody in the patient's serum to form complexes with the antigen and fix complement. "Sensitized" red cells are then added to the mixture. If the red cells are lysed, it indicates that there were no antigen specific antibodies in the serum of the patient, so complement was not consumed in the test system and was available to be used by the anti-RBC antibodies, resulting in hemolysis. This reaction is considered negative. If the red cells are not lysed, it indicates that antibodies specific to the antigen were present in the test

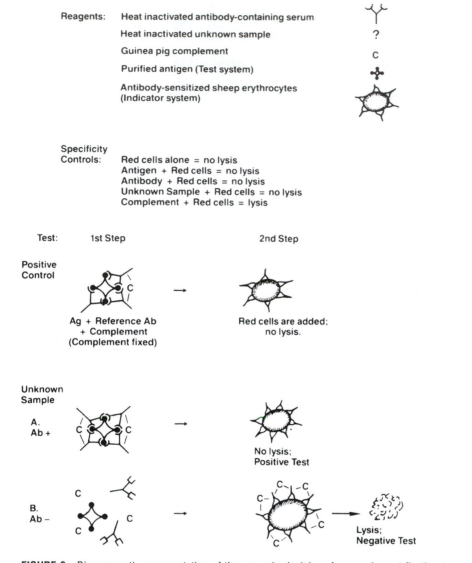

FIGURE 6 Diagrammatic representation of the general principles of a complement fixation test.

system, "fixed" complement, but none were available to be activated by the indicator system. This reaction is considered positive.

Complement fixation tests are widely applicable to the detection of antibodies to almost all antigens. Thus, complement fixation reactions have been widely used in a large number of tests designed to assist in the diagnosis of specific infections, such as the Wassermann test for syphilis and tests for antibodies to *Mycoplasma pneumoniae*, *Bordetella pertussis*, to many different viruses, and to fungi such as *Cryptococcus*, *Histoplasma*, and *Coccidioides immitis*. However, the methodology is difficult to execute, and complement fixation tests have been progressively replaced by other methods.

Tests Based on Immunofluorescence

The primary reaction between antibodies chemically combined with fluorescent dyes and cell or tissue-fixed antigens can be visualized in a suitable microscope. There are several variations

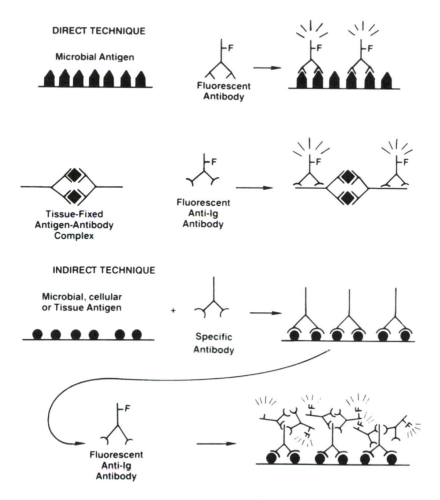

FIGURE 7 Diagrammatic representation of the general principles of direct and indirect immunofluorescence.

of immunofluorescence that can be used to detect the presence of antigens in cells or tissues and the presence of antibodies in patient's serum (Fig. 7).

Direct Immunofluorescence

Direct immunofluorescence visualizes antigen in a cell or tissue by direct labeling with fluorescent antibody. Similarly, tissue-deposited antigen–antibody complexes can be revealed by reaction with a fluorescent anti-immunoglobulin antibody.

Indirect Immunofluorescence

Indirect immunofluorescence (as all indirect tests) involves two steps. First, a substrate containing a fixed antigen (e.g., in a cell or tissue) is incubated with unlabeled antibody, which becomes associated with the antigen. After careful washing, a fluorescent antibody (e.g., fluorescent labeled anti-IgG) is added to the substrate. This second antibody will become associated to the first, and the complex antigen–antibody 1–antibody 2 can be visualized on a fluorescence microscope. The indirect method has the advantage of using a single labeled antibody to detect many different specific antigen–antibody reactions.

Immunofluorescence Tests in Microbiology

Immunofluorescence has been widely applied in diagnostic tests. In microbiology, it can be used to identify isolated organisms, to visualize infectious organisms in tissue biopsies or exudates, and also to diagnose an infection through the demonstration of the corresponding antibodies. A classical example is the use of the indirect fluorescence test for the diagnosis of syphilis. In the first step, the patient's serum is incubated with killed *Treponema pallidum*; in the second step, a fluorescent-labeled anti-human antibody is used to determine if antibodies from the patient's serum become bound to *Treponema*. Similar techniques have been used for the diagnosis of some viral diseases using virus-infected cells as substrate.

Using fluorescent antibodies specific for different immunoglobulin isotypes, it is possible to identify the class of a given antibody after it has been captured on an antigen-coated solid phase. While IgG antibodies can be present in circulation for extended periods of time, IgM antibodies are characteristic of the early stages of the primary immune response. Thus, tests specifically designed to detect IgM antibodies are particularly useful for the diagnosis of ongoing infections.

Immunofluorescence Tests for the Detection of Autoantibodies

Immunofluorescence is also the technique of choice for the detection of autoantibodies such as antinuclear antibodies. Classically, the suspect serum is incubated with an adequate tissue (rat kidney, HeLa cells), and indirect immunofluorescence is performed in a second step to detect antibodies fixed to the substrate. In a positive test, the nuclei of the cells used as substrate will be fluorescent. The pattern of nuclear fluorescence is variable and has diagnostic implications (see Chapter 18). Autoantibodies directed to a variety of tissue antigens can be detected by immunofluorescence and this is the basis for a variety of tests used in the evaluation of most organ-specific autoimmune diseases (see Chapter 17).

Anti-double stranded (ds) DNA antibodies can also be detected by immunofluorescence using a parasite (*Chritidia lucilliae*) that has a kinetoplast composed of pure dsDNA. Fixed parasites are incubated with patient's serum in the first step. Anti-dsDNA antibodies, if present, will bind to the kinetoplast and will be revealed with fluorescein-labeled anti-IgG antibody (Fig. 8). The assay has a specificity greater than 90%, but the sensitivity is relatively low, at around 60%.

Immunofluorescence Tests to Detect Tissue-Fixed Antigen–Antibody Complexes

Immunofluorescence assays have been extensively used by immunopathologists to detect immune complexes deposited in a variety of tissues. The technique usually involves performing a biopsy to obtain a tissue fragment that is then frozen and sectioned. The frozen sections are then incubated with fluorescent-labeled antibodies to immunoglobulins, C3, and fibrinogen (which is usually deposited in inflamed lesions).

Quantitative immunofluorescence assays have been developed as a result of the introduction of fluorometers. The principles are similar to those described for indirect fluorescence assays: antigen is bound to a solid phase, exposed to a serum sample containing specific antibody, unbound immunoglobulins are rinsed off, and a fluorescein-labeled antibody is added to

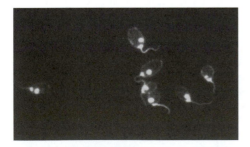

FIGURE 8   Positive immunofluorescence test for double-stranded (ds) DNA antibodies using *Crithidia lucilliae* as a substrate. This noninfectious flagellate has a kinetoplast packed with dsDNA. The test is done by incubating the flagellate with patient's serum in the first step, and, after washing, incubating with a fluorescent-labeled anti-human IgG antibody. After washing off the excess of fluorescent-labeled antibody, the test is read on the fluorescence microscope. Visualization of the kinetoplast reflects the binding of anti-dsDNA.

reveal the antibody which reacted specifically with the immobilized antigen. A fluorometer is used to assay the amount of fluorescence emitted by the second antibody. Since the amount of fluorescent antibody added to the system is fixed, the amount that remains bound is directly proportional to the concentration of antibody present in the sample. Thus, a quantitative correlation can be drawn between the intensity of fluorescence and the concentration of antibody added in the first step. These quantitative tests have been adapted to microbiological assays, because they can combine quantitative and analytical properties (e.g., distinguishing IgG from IgM antibodies).

Monoclonal Antibody-Based Assays

The previously discussed classical serological assays are based on the use of antibodies obtained from immunized animals, containing mixtures of clonal products reacting with different epitopes having different affinities (polyclonal antibodies). As a consequence, the specificity of the tests was not always ideal. The sensitivity of the early assays was also not ideal. Two factors led to the development of new, more specific assays: improved methodologies for detection of the antigen–antibody reaction, and the development of monoclonal antibodies— antibodies of a single specificity and high affinity.

Production of Monoclonal Antibodies

The methodology for production of monoclonal antibodies was first reported by Kohler and Milstein in the 1970s, and the Nobel prize was awarded to these investigators in recognition of the significance of their discovery.

The production of monoclonal antibodies involves two cell populations and three major steps: fusion, selection, and screening. Most commonly, spleen cells from a mouse immunized with the antigen-of-interest are fused with transformed murine plasma cells. This fusion results in the formation of hybrid cells (hybridomas) that proliferate like transformed cells. The B cell hybridomas produces the same antibody as the parental B cell (Fig. 9). The hybridomas are grown and selected in culture conditions, which support their growth but not that of the fusion partner or the nonfused splenocytes.

A lengthy screening process follows; the aim of which is to select from the large number of hybridomas produced by fusion, those that produce antibody against antigens of interest. Single cells are seeded (by manual limiting dilution or cell sorting by flow cytometry) into individual receptacles containing tissue culture medium and allowed to grow into clones producing antibody of a single specificity [monoclonal antibody (mAb)]. mAb generated in this process have a wide range of uses, including basic research, diagnostic purposes, and therapeutic protocols.

Cluster of Differentiation Nomenclature

Hundreds of monoclonal antibodies identifying different membrane markers on lymphocytes and other cell types have been generated. These cell surface antigens are complex molecules expressing many different epitopes. Accordingly, monoclonal antibodies raised in different laboratories often recognize slightly different parts of the same molecule. Historically, each laboratory would identify a molecule by a unique name, often the by the name of the mAb, recognizing the molecule or antigen. Soon the field became rather complicated; as each cell surface molecule was know in the literature by several different names. As a consequence, World Health Organization-sponsored workshops were developed in order to establish a standardized nomenclature for the molecules found on the surface of leukocytes. In these workshops, newly developed monoclonal antibodies are evaluated, the cellular antigen they recognize is verified, and a designation is given to the newly defined antigen. A given cellular antigen recognized by novel monoclonal antibodies is designated by the initials CD, for clusters of differentiation (a designation that recognizes the fact that each marker has multiple antigenic determinants), followed by a number. The numerical designations are assigned based partly on the order of discovery, and partly on the ontogenic order of appearance. For instance, the mAb recognizing what, at the time, was considered ontogenetically as the most primitive T lymphocyte membrane marker, was designated as CD1, and the T lymphocytes expressing

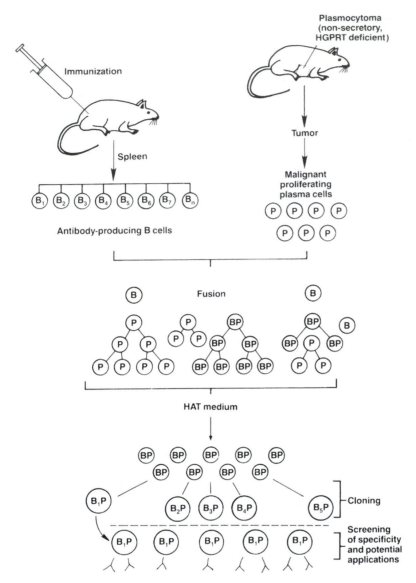

FIGURE 9 Schematic representation of the major steps involved in hybridoma production. First, antibody-producing lymphocytes are fused with nonsecretory malignant plasma cells, deficient in hypoxanthine guanine phosphoribosyl transferase (HGPRT). Nonfused lymphocytes do not proliferate, and nonfused plasma cells die in a hypoxanthine-rich medium. The HGPRT deficient plasma cells cannot detoxify hypoxanthine, while the hybrid cells have HGPRT provided by the antibody-producing B lymphocytes. The surviving hybrids are cloned by limiting dilution, and the resulting clones are tested for the specificity and potential value of the antibodies produced.

it are known as CD1$^+$. Some of the most common CD markers are described in Chapter 10. A complete up-to-date listing can be found at http://mpr.nci.nih.gov/prow.

Flow Cytometry

Flow cytometry has become one of the most important, if not the most important, and powerful technologies in immunology. A flow cytometer, as the name implies, is an instrument that measures cells (cytometry) in a fluid stream (flow) (Fig. 10). Within the flow cell, cells pass single-file in front of a laser light source, which allows for the measurement of multiple properties from individual cells. When the individual cells are intercepted by the laser light source, the light will be dispersed (or scattered); additionally, if the cells are labeled with fluorescent

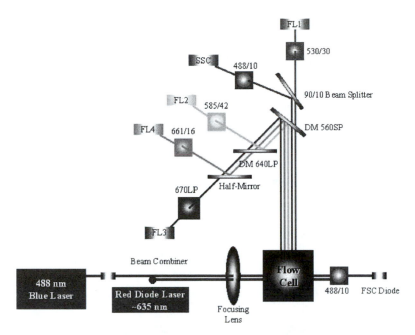

FIGURE 10   Diagrammatic representation of a typical flow cytometer. The key components of a flow cytometer are the fluidics system, the optical system, and the electronics system. The purpose of the fluidics is to focus the cells, single-file, in the center of a fluid stream, which is intercepted by the laser light source. This occurs within the flow cell. The optical components include the laser light source, a series of photomultiplier tubes (PMT), and a photodiode for collecting the light signals. In this figure, there is a photodiode for forward scatter light (FSC), a PMT for side scatter light (SSC), and four PMTs detect separate fluorescence signals (FL1, FL2, FL3, FL4). A series of mirrors and filters directs the fluorescence emission of the appropriate wavelength to the designated detector. The most commonly used fluorescent dyes are fluorescein isothiocyanate (FITC), phycoerythrin (PE), peridinin chlorophyll protein (PerCP), and allophycocyanin (APC), which are detected in FL1, FL2, FL3, and FL4, respectively. An electronic system converts optical signals into electronic impulses, which are in turn converted to digital values and sent to a computer.

dyes, the laser light will excite the fluorescent dyes and fluorescent energy will be emitted. The flow cytometer is equipped with multiple detectors to capture the light scatter and fluorescence emission signals, which allow for the simultaneous measurement of multiple characteristics of a single cell. Therein lies the true power of flow cytometry—multiparameter data acquisition/ analysis from individual cells. Data collected from the light scatter provides information about the size and complexity of the individual cells. Larger cells will disperse more light in the forward direction (forward scatter) and cells with greater internal complexity such as granulocytes will disperse more light in the 90° angle (side scatter). The most common instruments are equipped with two lasers and four detectors for fluorescence emission. This allows for the collection of six parameters (two light scatter measurements and four fluorescence measurements) of data from each individual cell.

Data acquisition is rapid, routinely 20,000 cells analyzed within a few seconds. The collection of such a large number of events eliminates the need for replicate analysis. Because multiple measurements are collected on each individual cell, mixed populations of cells can be assayed without prior physical separation. Later, during data analysis, cells with specific properties can be "electronically" separated or "gated" (Fig. 11).

Using a combination of membrane and intracellular probes, countless assays can be performed by flow cytometry. Flow cytometry allows us to gather information about the phenotype of a cell—the stage of development, the activation state of a cell, if a cell is dividing, or if a cell is undergoing cell death by apoptosis or necrosis. The newest instruments have up to four lasers and sixteen fluorescence detectors, which allows for more information to be gained on each cell type.

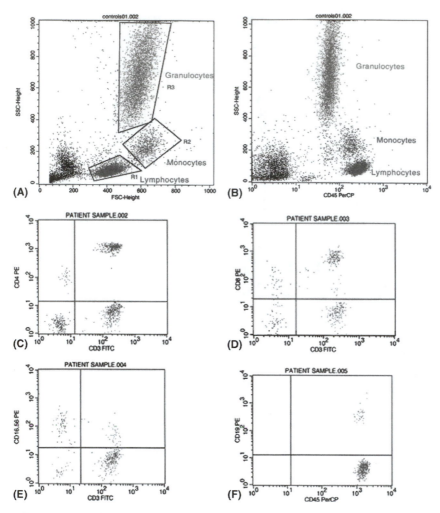

FIGURE 11 Lymphocyte Immunophenotyping. Whole blood is stained with two antibody cocktails each containing monoclonal antibodies directly conjugated to one of four fluorochromes: fluorescein isothiocyanate, phycoerythrin, peridinin chlorophyll protein, or allophycocyanin (Fig. 10). During data analysis lymphocytes are selected or gated from the other leucocytes based on their light scatter properties or a combination of light scatter and CD45 (common leukocyte antigen) expression (**A** and **B**). Next, lymphocyte subsets are characterized. T cells that express $CD3^+$ and $CD4^+$ are part of the T helper cell subset, while those that express $CD3^+$ and $CD8^+$ are part of the T cytotoxic cell subset (**C** and **D**). Natural killer cells are identified as $CD3^-$, and $CD16^+/CD56^+$ and B cells are identified as $CD3^-$, and $CD19^+$ (**E** and **F**).

Lymphocyte Immunophenotyping

One of the most common clinical applications of flow cytometry is to measure the absolute counts (cells/μL of whole blood) and the relative percentages of the major lymphocyte populations. This is a rather simple direct immunofluorescence procedure. Whole blood specimens are incubated directly with fluorescent-conjugated monoclonal antibodies specific for the major cell types (Table 1). Typically, about 50 μL of whole blood is added to each of the two tubes. One tube is incubated with antibodies to CD45, CD3, CD4, and CD8 and the other is incubated with antibodies to CD45, CD3, CD19, and CD56/16. Next, the RBCs are lysed and the white blood cells fixed in a hypotonic paraformaldehyde solution. The samples can be acquired on the flow cytometer without any wash steps or additional processing. For data analysis the data are first viewed in a two parameter plot (dot plot) of forward (FSC) and side scatter (SSC) (Fig. 11, panel A). The granulocytic neutrophils are the cells with the greatest SSC and the lymphocytes

TABLE 1 Typical Flow Cytometry Assays

Assay	Cell population/subset	Identifying markers
Lymphocyte immunophenotyping		
	T lymphocytes	SSC^{low}, $CD45^{bright}$, $CD3^+$
	Helper T lymphocytes (Th)	SSC^{low}, $CD45^{bright}$, $CD3^+$, $CD4^+$
	CTL	SSC^{low}, $CD45^{bright}$, $CD3^+$, $CD8^+$
	B lymphocytes	SSC^{low}, $CD45^{bright}$, $CD3^-$, CD19 or CD20 +
	NK cells	SSC^{low}, $CD45^{bright}$ $CD3^-$, $CD56^+/CD16^+$
Naive/memory cells		
	Th naive	$CD4^+$, $CD45RO^-$, $CCR7^+$
	Th central memory	$CD4^+$, $CD45RO^-$, $CCR7^+$
	Th effector memory	$CD4^+$, $CD45RO^+$, $CCR7^-$
	CTL naive	$CD8^+$, $CD45RO^-$, $CCR7^+$
	CTL central memory	$CD8^+$, $CD45RO^+$, $CCR7^+$
	CTL effector memory	$CD8^+$, $CD45RO^+$, $CCR7^-$
Cytotoxic cell panel		
	Lytic CTL	$CD3^+$, $CD8^+$, $CD107^+$
	Cytokine producing CTL	$CD3^+$, $CD8^+$, IFN-γ
	Lytic NK	$CD3^-$, $CD56^+/16^+/$, $D107^+$
	Cytokine producing NK	$CD3^-$, $CD56^+/16^+/$, IFN-γ
Th1/Th2 assessment		
	Th1 lymphocytes	$CD3^+$, $CD4^+$, IFN-γ
	Th2 lymphocytes	$CD3^+$, $CD4^+$, $_iIL-4/IL-10^+$

Abbreviations: SSC, side scatter light; CD, cluster of differentiation; Th, T helper; CTL, cytotoxic T lymphocytes; NK, natural killer; IFN, interferon; IL, interleukin.

the cells with the least FSC and SSC. Monocytes have intermediate FSC and SSC. The lymphocytes are then selected (or "gated") for subsequent analysis. A more accurate gating method is to view a dot plot of CD45 expression versus SSC (Fig. 11, panel B). In this case, the lymphocytes are the population of cells expressing the brightest CD45 and low SSC. The gated lymphocytes are then viewed in dot plots and the relative percentage of the major lymphocyte populations calculated (Fig. 11, panels C–F). An absolute cell count can be obtained directly from the flow cytometer if the blood is stained in the presence of quantitation beads or by using the absolute lymphocyte count obtained from a traditional hematology analyzer.

Most other assays for surface staining are carried out in a similar manner. In some cases it is necessary to add wash steps or to stain purified peripheral blood mononuclear cell (PBMC) as described later in the chapter.

Other Clinical Applications of Flow Cytometry

The applications of flow cytometry in the clinical and research laboratory are numerous. Monoclonal antibodies to cell surface antigens can be combined with mAb to intracellular proteins and nucleic acid-binding dyes. For intracellular protein and nucleic acid staining, cells are fixed and then permeabilized with detergent or alcohol solutions. Intracellular cytokine staining of CD4 lymphocytes can provide information about the disposition of an immune response; given that Th1 cells produce IFNγ and Th2 cells produce IL-4. Flow cytometry is routinely used to monitor CD4 counts in HIV disease progression and response to therapy. It is routinely used to in the diagnosis and subclassification of T and B cell neoplasia. Other common clinical applications include anti-platelet and anti-neutrophil antibody detection, HLA-B27 testing, and DNA content and cell cycle analysis. In the pharmaceutical industry and in oncology laboratories, cell-cycle analysis by flow cytometry provides information on precisely what part of the cell cycle a therapeutic agent is acting.

Cell Sorting

Some flow cytometers have the ability to collect populations of cells (sort) or individual cells (clone) expressing a given phenotype. This powerful combination of analysis and isolation has been invaluable to the field of immunology research. In particular, the study of hematopoiesis and lymphopoiesis has benefited from this technology. Researchers have been able to assess the differentiation potential of individual cloned progenitor cells in response to a variety of stimuli. Because the progenitor cells were sorted at the single-cell level (cloned), concerns regarding contaminating cell populations were lessened. This approach has limitations, including time consumption, cost, sharing of markers by different cell populations, and relatively low yields.

Another method for cell sorting uses immunomagnetic beads. This technique is more rapid and less expensive than sorting on a flow cytometer. The limitation is that single cell cloning is not possible. A mixed population of cells is incubated with monoclonal antibodies directed against the cell of interest. The antibodies can be directly conjugated to magnetic beads, or a secondary antibody directly conjugated to the magnetic bead can be used. Next, the cells bound to the immunomagnetic beads are isolated by placing the mixture in a magnetic field that attracts the labeled cells. Cells not recognized by the mAb remain in the flow-through and can be collected for further fractionation or can be discarded. When the magnetic field is removed, the positively selected cells can be used in functional assays. The use of magnetic column allows for the use of very small magnetic beads and eliminates the needs to remove the beads from the cells.

Immunohistochemistry

Immunohistochemistry (IHC) is the result of the application of monoclonal antibodies to the detection of antigens in tissues, and has replaced immunofluorescence in many applications due to the specificity of mAbs. What distinguishes this technique from flow cytometry is that the cells are evaluated within their physiological context. IHC is the only technique that preserves the tissue in its original microenvironment. Consequently, it is possible to observe the localization of the antigens of interest with regard to the neighboring cells and the cellular compartments (i.e., cytoplasm, nucleus, or membrane). IHC provides the pathologist with a new way of observing tissue specimens. In addition to the gross histology (changes in the cells), the pathologist can now also observe changes in specific proteins within the cells.

This approach has allowed oncologists to tailor specific medications for different cancer patients; there are now a growing number of IHC tests being used. This technique was the first proven method to deliver the promise of "personalized medicine." For example, Her2/neu$^+$ staining is an indication that breast cancer patients receive Herceptin, a monoclonal antibody therapy that specifically targets the Her2 receptor, weakly expressed in normal tissues and overexpressed in some breast cancer patients. It has been demonstrated that patients with high levels of this receptor benefit from the use of this drug. Several IHC tests have been developed that allow pathologists to measure Her2 receptors expression levels.

Highly Sensitive Immunoassays

Radioimmunoassay

The introduction of radiolabeled components into immunoassays was a very significant development, because it allowed developing assays combining high specificity and high sensitivity. The first radioimmunoassays (RIAs) were based on the principle of competitive binding: unlabeled antigen competes with radiolabeled antigen for binding to antibody with the appropriate specificity. Thus, when mixtures of constant amounts of radiolabeled and variable amounts of unlabeled antigen are incubated with fixed concentrations of the corresponding antibody, the amount of radiolabeled antigen that remains unbound is directly proportional to the quantity of unlabeled antigen in the mixture. One of the problems of the early assays was the separation of free antigen from antigen–antibody complexes. Usually, that was achieved by either cross-linking the antigen–antibody complexes with a second antibody or by means of the addition of reagents that promoted the precipitation of antigen–antibody complexes, such as ammonium sulfate or polyethylene glycol. Counting radioactivity in the precipitates allowed the determination of the amount of radiolabeled antigen coprecipitated with the antibody and a calibration curve was constructed by plotting the percentage of antibody-bound radiolabeled antigen against known concentrations of a standardized unlabeled antigen (Fig. 12). The concentrations of antigen in patient samples were extrapolated from that curve. A major technical development was the introduction of solid phase assays, in which antigens or antibodies (depending on the assay) were coupled to insoluble particles,

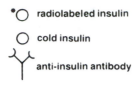

radiolabeled insulin

cold insulin

anti-insulin antibody

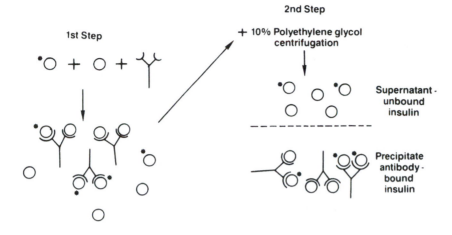

1st Step

2nd Step

+ 10% Polyethylene glycol centrifugation

Supernatant - unbound insulin

Precipitate antibody - bound insulin

Calibration: Displacement of radiolabeled insulin by known concentrations of "cold" insulin

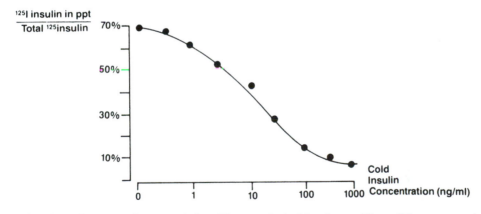

FIGURE 12 Diagrammatic representation of the general principles of competitive radioimmunoassay in fluid phase. In this type of assay (of which the assay of insulin levels is a good example), the free and antibody-bound antigens are separated either by physiochemical techniques, as shown in the diagram, or by using a second antibody (anti-immunoglobulin) to precipitate the insulin–antibody complexes formed in the first step of the assay.

paper disks, etc., thus allowing a much simpler and effective separation of bound and free-labeled compounds.

Noncompetitive solid phase RIA for the detection of specific antibodies was also developed, taking advantage of the solid phase technologies. The antigens were coupled to the solid phase, exposed to a sample-containing antibody, and a radiolabeled anti-human immunoglobulin was used to assay the antibody that becomes bound to the immobilized antigen.

The main drawbacks of RIA were the cost of equipment and reagents, short shelf-life of radiolabeled compounds, and the problems associated with the disposal of radiolabeled substances. In recent years, RIA has been virtually replaced by assays in which radiolabeled tags have been substituted by enzymes, fluorescence compounds, or chemiluminescent compounds. The basic principles of the assays, however, remained the same.

Enzymoimmunoassays

The second critical technology for the detection of antibody–antigen binding is the immunoassay originally referred to as the enzyme-linked immunosorbent assay (ELISA or EIA). The immunoassay is a very flexible platform for the detection of an unlimited number of antigens in a variety of matrices. This assay is most often performed in a 96-well plate format. In ELISA capture assays, (Fig. 13, panel A) an antibody (the capture antibody) is adsorbed to a polystyrene surface (i.e., the well of a 96-well plate). The sample, in liquid format (i.e., plasma, serum, tissue culture media, cell lysate) containing the analyte-of-interest is then added to the well and the antigen is allowed to bind the immobilized antibody. Given that the antigen–antibody complexes remain absorbed to the plate, the unbound proteins can be easily washed away. Bound antigen is then detected with a second antibody (the detection antibody) coupled to an enzyme, usually peroxidase or alkaline phosphatase. Usually, the second antibody recognizes a different epitope than the capture antibody, to avoid mutual interference between the capture antibody and the detection antibody. After unbound detection antibody is removed, a chromogenic, fluorogenic, or chemiluminescent, substrate is added to the well. The enzyme-coupled detection antibody hydrolyzes the substrate generating a colored, fluorescent, or chemiluminescent product, which can easily be detected in the appropriate plate reader. Immunoassays can be quantitative if an appropriate standard curve is incorporated into the assay. Immunoassays can be highly specific and sensitive in the nanomolar and picomolar range, when the correct configuration of high quality, highly specific, serological reagents (monoclonal or polyclonal) is incorporated into the assay. With the use of the 96-well plate format and automated pipetting devices, immunoassays can be high throughout. One of the most notable drawbacks with immunoassays can be a lack of specificity caused by cross-reactions and nonspecific reactions, leading to false positive results.

Various configurations of immunoassays have been used. In a competitive ELISA, a mixture of enzyme-labeled antigen and unlabeled antigen is added to a well coated with the

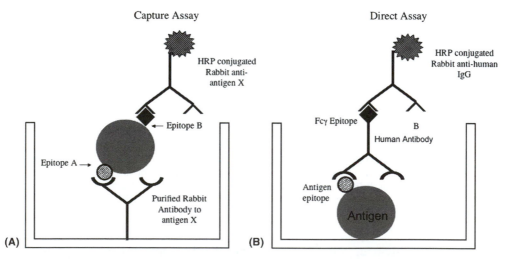

FIGURE 13 The principles of different types of enzymoimmunoassays. (**A**) in a capture assay a specific antibody is immobilized, reacts with the corresponding antigen, and a second enzyme-labeled antibody to a different epitope of the antigen is used to reveal its presence in the plate through a colorimetric reaction that takes place after adding a color-generating substrate to the enzyme coupled to the second antibody. The diagram illustrated the use of a horse-radish peroxidase (HRP)-conjugated second antibody. (**B**) In the direct assay, the antigen is adsorbed to the solid phase, antibodies to that antigen will become immobilized as a consequence of binding, and an enzyme-conjugated rabbit antibody to human IgG (or other immunoglbulin isotypes) is used to detect bound antibody. The intensity of color generated after adding a color-generating substrate will be proportional to the concentration of human antibody bound to the antigen and second labeled second antibody reacting with the human antibody.

capture antibody. The concentrations of labeled antigen and antibody are kept constant, and the concentration of unlabelled antigen is varied. After incubation and washing, the substrate is added. The substrate, upon reaction with the enzyme develops a color whose intensity can be measured by spectrophotometry. Color intensity is directly proportional to the amount of bound labeled antigen, which, in turn, is inversely proportional to the concentration of unlabelled antigen added to the mixture. In a non-competitive capture assay, also known as "sandwich assay" (Fig. 13, panel A), the second step consists of adding the antigen-containing samples to the plates coated with capture antibody. In a direct antibody assay, the second step is to add the antibody-containing samples to the antigen-coated wells (Fig. 13, panel B). In these two types of assays, the third step is basically the same: labeled antibody needs to be added. In the sandwich assay, the labeled antibody is of similar specificity to the antibody bound to the solid phase (antibodies reacting to different epitopes of the same antigen are preferred). In the direct antibody assay, the labeled antibody is an anti-immunoglobulin antibody. Finally, an enzyme-labeled component (antigen or antibody) is added, and after incubation and washing, a signal-generating substrate is added. Signal intensity is directly proportional to the concentration of the reactant that is being measured.

Clinical Applications of Enzyme-Linked Immunosorbent Assay

As a result of its relative simplicity and versatility, the immunoassays are very widely used. Commercially available ELISA kits have been developed for anti-microbial antibodies, antigen detection, hormone detection, and drug assay. In infectious diseases, immunoassays are used to distinguish disease specific IgG versus IgM responses. IgG antibodies can be present in circulation for extended periods of time; whereas, IgM antibodies are characteristic of the early stages of the primary immune response. Thus, assays specifically designed to detect IgM antibodies are particularly useful for the diagnosis of ongoing infections. Immunoassays for cytokines and soluble cytokine receptors are used to assess immune functions (see later).

Rapid Tests

One of the more innovative approaches to the immunoassay has been the development of the rapid diagnostic ELISA kits, which can be performed with minimal training and instrumentation at a physician's office and even at home by patients themselves. Rapid tests have been developed for pregnancy and a variety of infections including streptococcal sore throat, respiratory syncytial virus infections, viral influenza, and HIV.

The original rapid tests for pregnancy were sandwich assays that used two monoclonal antibodies recognizing two different, noncompeting epitopes in human chorionic gonadotrophin. One antibody was immobilized onto a solid phase, and its function was to capture the antigen (hCG). The second was labeled with an enzyme and would be retained on the solid surface, only if the antigen had been captured by the first antibody. The retention of labeled antibody was detected by a color reaction secondary to the breakdown of an adequate substrate. These tests usually involved two or more steps. One-step tests were later developed, but the manufacturers have not divulged their exact design.

Multiplex Assays

More recently, immunoassays have been adapted to formats that allow multiple simultaneous readings, known as multiplex assays. Two basic formats exist, a plate format and a microsphere format. The bead technology can be compared to an "ELISA-on-a-bead," the marriage of the ELISA and the flow cytometer. The capture antibody is conjugated to a fluorescent microsphere and all incubations are performed in solution. The bound antigen is detected with a fluorescent-conjugate detection antibody. The innovation of this method comes from the use of microspheres with varying levels of fluorescence and detection antibodies conjugated to different fluorochromes. This allows for multiplexing so that multiple antigens can be detected from the same sample in the same assay. While it is theoretically possible to measure 100 analytes from a single 50 µL plasma sample, in reality robust assays have been developed for about five to 10 analytes at a time. Challenges of this technology are to find the appropriate buffer conditions for multiple analytes. Furthermore, the assays are not as sensitive as some immunoassays for the detection of low levels of antigen. This technology has had great impact in the field of transplantation, where it is now routinely used to test for circulating anti-HLA antibodies in the recipients (see later).

In plate-based multiplex assays, antibodies of different sensitivities are chemically bound to 96-well assay plates (with round or square wells) and the bound analyte is revealed with an enzyme-labeled antibody. Although the maximum number of antibodies that can be spotted on each well has not been definitively set, 9 to 12 analytes/well formats are commonly used. The separate assay of the different analytes in each well requires that the antibodies are spotted precisely in the same positions in each well, and that the detection unit is able to measure the signal intensity of each spot without interference from nearby spots. These assays have been of special interest to clinical investigators interested in measuring cytokine profiles in their patients.

EVALUATION OF CELLULAR IMMUNE RESPONSES

Lymphocyte functional assays can be preformed directly in whole blood samples or in PBMC preparations, which include monocytes and lymphocytes. PBMC are prepared by density gradient centrifugation using a separation medium that has a specific gravity that lies between the density of erythrocytes/granulocytes and lymphocytes. Whole blood is layered over the separation medium and centrifuged. After centrifugation, the erythrocytes and granulocytes are below the separation medium, while the PBMC will rest on top of the separation medium, but below the platelet-rich plasma (Fig. 14). About 80% of the PBMC are lymphocytes and 20% are monocytes.

Laboratory Tests for Assessment of Lymphocyte Function Ex Vivo

The evaluation of cell-mediated immunity presents considerable more difficulties than the evaluation of the humoral immune responses. In vivo tests, such as skin tests with common antigens known to induce delayed hypersensitive reactions, are difficult to standardize. Ex vivo functional tests are difficult to execute, time consuming, and require specialized personnel and sophisticated equipment.

Ex Vivo Stimulation

Lymphocytes in whole blood samples or in purified PBMC can be stimulated ex vivo by specific antigens or by mitogenic substances. Ideally, specific antigens would be used to study lymphocyte function; however, given the fact that very few peripheral lymphocytes are specific for a given antigen this approach is difficult. Alternatively, mitogens, which stimulate lymphocytes by antigen-independent mechanisms, are commonly used for ex vivo stimulation. Typical endpoints used to assess ex vivo lymphocyte activation are proliferation, cytokine production, changes in membrane expression of activation markers, and immunoglobulin production by

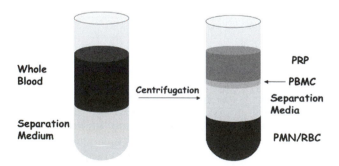

FIGURE 14 Diagrammatic representation of peripheral blood mononuclear cell (PBMC) isolation by density gradient centrifugation. Whole blood is carefully layered atop a dextran sucrose-based separation medium of approximately the same density as PBMC. After centrifugation, the cells with higher density [RBC and polymorphonuclear (PMN) cells] will sediment below the separation medium. PBMC will rest directly on top of the medium beneath the platelet rich plasma (PRP).

B cells. Technically, the assays to assess ex vivo are relatively simple to perform; however, the data can be difficult to interpret, given that reference values for the responses in healthy individuals have not been established and intrasubject variability in responses is high.

The common mitogens are lectins, such as phytohemagglutinin (PHA) and pokeweed mitogen (PWM). PWM stimulates both B cells and T cells, while PHA stimulates T cells only. A more physiologically relevant method is to stimulate the TCR directly with immobilized anti-CD3 monoclonal antibodies. The antigens most commonly used for ex vivo stimulation are purified protein derivative, *Candida albicans* antigens, keyhole limpet hemocyanin, and tetanus toxoid (which stimulates both T and B cells).

Proliferation Assays

Incorporation of tritiated thymidine into dividing cells was traditionally the most common endpoint used to measure lymphocyte proliferation. When tritiated thymidine [^{3}H-Tdr] is added after 72 hours of stimulation, it is incorporated into the newly synthesized DNA. The amount of ^{3}H-Tdr incorporated into the cells can be correlated for proliferation.

Using newer, innovative technologies the same information about immune function can be obtained in a simpler assay, without the use of radiation. Cylex^{TM} has developed a streamlined method to measure cell stimulation that requires only 18 hours incubation and does not require the use of radiation. This assay measures an early response to stimulation by detecting intracellular ATP synthesis, which increases within the cells responding to the stimulant and thus correlates to cellular activation. When this assay is preformed on isolated CD4 lymphocytes, which orchestrate global cell-mediated responses through immunoregulatory signaling, the results are thought to be an indicator of a patient's overall immune cell function. As the response to immunosuppressive therapy varies among individuals, assessment of a patient's immune cell function may provide useful information to the clinician in the course of individual patient management.

Cytokine Production Assays

Cytokine production from ex vivo stimulation assays can be measured by a variety of methods, such as ELISA, multiplex assays, intracellular cytokine staining by flow cytometry, or measurement of cytokine mRNA by quantitative real-time PCR. IL-2 production is probably the parameter choice for the evaluation of the initial stages of activation of the T helper cell population. Low or absent release of IL-2 has been observed in a variety of immunodeficiency states, particularly in patients with AIDS. Measurement of other cytokines such as IL-4, IL-5, IL-6, IL-10, IL-12, GM-CSF, TNF, LTα, and IFN-γ can provide a more complete picture of the functional response of T lymphocytes. For example, predominant release of IL-4, IL-5, or IL-10 is characteristic of Th2 responses, while predominant release of IFN-γ, IL-2, or GM-CSF is characteristic of Th1 responses (Table 1).

Expression of Activation Markers

Changes in membrane expression of activation markers by flow cytometry can also be used to evaluate ex vivo stimulation. Upregulation of CD25 and CD69, or a downregulation of CD62L is typical in activated lymphocytes.

Immunoglobulin Production

Immunoglobulin synthesis is the best indicator of B cell function. Changes in the levels of IgG and IgM after PWM stimulation can be easily measured in immunoassays.

Tetramer Assays

One of the developments with greater potential significance in the last few years has been the development of MHC/peptide tetramers. Both MHC-I and MHC-II tetramers able to bind specific peptides have been constructed, and those tetramers, once loaded with a peptide, interact specifically with CD8$^+$ or CD4$^+$ T cells with TCR being able to recognize the peptide–MHC combination in question. For example, MHC-I–peptide complexes loaded with peptides derived from melanoma-associated antigens have been shown to be able to bind specifically to CD8$^+$ lymphocytes from melanoma patients that can then be purified and shown to be able to lyse melanoma tumor cells in vitro. On the other hand, MHC-II tetramers loaded with an influenza hemagglutinin (HA) peptide have been shown to bind and activate HA-specific CD4$^+$ T cells. The potential for application of this technique to characterize normal and abnormal aspects of cell-mediated immune responses appears almost unlimited.

Assays for Cytotoxic Effector Cells

Traditionally, the functional evaluation of cytolytic activity in cytotoxic T lymphocytes (CTL) and natural killer cells (NK cells) was based on chromium (^{51}Cr) release cytotoxicity assays. Target cells pre-labeled with ^{51}Cr, were incubated with effector cells. Upon target cell lysis ^{51}Cr is release into the culture media. The amount of ^{51}Cr release correlates with the cytotoxic effector cell function. More recently a flow cytometric assay for cytolytic potential has been developed. This assay measures the level of CD107 on the plasma membrane (Table 1). In resting CTL or NK cell, CD107 is expressed intracellularly on the membrane of the cytotoxic granules. Upon activation-induced degranulation, CD107 can be detected on the cellular membrane, reflecting degranulation and loss of intracellular perforin. Thus, the CD107 positive CTL or NK cells represent the subset with lytic potential. This innovative assay is more rapid than a traditional cytotoxicity assay and does not require the use of radiolabelled materials.

The cellular targets for cytotoxic cells vary according to cytotoxic cell population to be evaluated. The evaluation of CTL requires mixing sensitized cytotoxic T cells with targets expressing the sensitizing antigen. NK cell activity is usually measured with tumor cell lines known to be susceptible to NK cell killing. Antibody dependent cell-mediated cytotoxicity (ADCC) is measured using antibody-coated target cells.

Laboratory Tests for Assessment of Lymphocyte Function In Vivo

While antigenic and mitogenic stimulation assays test lymphocyte reactions under more or less physiological conditions, the tested cells are those present in circulation, and it can be argued that the sampling does not adequately reflect the state of activation of their tissue counterparts. This is particularly problematic when the objective is to assess role of the T cell system in a patient with a hypersensitivity disease. Several groups have proposed that the assay of circulating cytokines or cytokine receptors (shed as a consequence of cell activation) are more reflective of the state of activation of T cells in vivo. It must be noted that these assays have not proven to be as useful as expected. A major limiting factor is their lack of disease specificity, which makes their correlation with specific clinical conditions rather difficult.

Plasma IL-2 levels have been measured as a way to evaluate the state of T lymphocyte activation in vivo. Increased levels of circulating IL-2 have been reported in multiple sclerosis, RA, and patients undergoing graft rejection, situations in which T cell hyperactivity would fit with the clinical picture. However, a significant problem with these assays is the existence of factors that interfere with the assay of IL-2 by ELISA, and the results may be inaccurate. Activated T cells shed many of their membrane receptors, including the IL-2 receptor (IL-2R). Elevated levels of circulating soluble receptors (shed by activated T lymphocytes) can be demonstrated in patients with hairy cell leukemia, AIDS, RA, graft rejection, etc. In general, the results of assays for IL-2R show parallelism with the results of assays for IL-2.

Urinary levels of IL-2 can also be measured in an immunoassay. Urine is a good matrix as it contains fewer interfering substances than plasma. Increased urinary levels of IL-2 have been reported in association with kidney allograft rejection and proposed as a parameter that may help differentiate acute rejection from cyclosporine A toxicity (see Chapters 26 and 27).

The measurement of serum IL-6 correlates with inflammatory reactions and B lymphocyte activity. High levels of IL-6 have been detected in patients with systemic lupus erythematosus and atherosclerosis—situations associated with tissue inflammation.

Laboratory Tests for Assessment of Phagocytic Cell Function

Phagocytic cell function tests can be performed with isolated peripheral blood neutrophils or directly in whole blood. Killing defects are the most frequent primary abnormalities of these cells, and can be tested in a variety of ways. Bacterial killing tests are not routinely available in diagnostic laboratories. Instead, tests based on the induction and measurement of the respiratory burst are used to investigate those defects. These tests are discussed in detail in Chapter 13.

BIBLIOGRAPHY

Betts MR, Brenchley JM, Price DA, et al. Sensitive and viable identification of antigen-specific CD8+ T cells by a flow cytometric assay for degranulation. J Immunol Methods 2004; 281:65–78.

Coligan JE, Kruisbeek AM, Margulies DH, Shevach EM, Strober W. Current Protocols in Immunology. New Jersey: Hoboken, 2005.

Robinson JP, Darzynkiewicz Z, Dean PN, et al. Current Protocols in Flow Cytometry. New Jersey: Hoboken, 2005.

Rose NR, Hamilton RG, Detrick B. Manual of Clinical Laboratory Immunology. Sixth Edition. Washington: ASM Press, 2002.

16 | Tolerance and Autoimmunity

George C. Tsokos
Beth Israel Deaconess Medical Center, Harvard Medical School, Boston, Massachusetts, U.S.A.

Gabriel Virella
Department of Microbiology and Immunology, Medical University of South Carolina, Charleston, South Carolina, U.S.A.

DEFINITION AND GENERAL CHARACTERISTICS OF TOLERANCE

Tolerance is best-defined as a state of antigen-specific immunological unresponsiveness. This definition has two important corollaries:

1. When tolerance is experimentally induced, it does not affect the immune response to antigens other than the one used to induce tolerance. This is a very important feature that differentiates tolerance from generalized immunosuppression, in which there is a depression of the immune response to a wide array of different antigens. Tolerance may be transient or permanent, whereas immunosuppression is usually transient.
2. Given the antigen-specificity that characterizes it, tolerance must be established at the clonal level. In other words, if tolerance is antigen-specific, it must involve the T and/or a B lymphocyte clone(s) specific for the antigen in question and not affect any other clones.

Mechanisms of Tolerance: Clonal Deletion

At the cellular level, tolerance can result from clonal deletion or from clonal anergy. Clonal deletion involves different processes for T and B lymphocytes. T lymphocytes are massively produced in the thymus and, once generated, will not rearrange their receptors. Memory T cells are long-lived, and there is no clear evidence that new ones are generated after the thymus ceases to function in early adulthood. Therefore, elimination of autoreactive T cells has been postulated to occur at the production site (thymus), at the time the cells are differentiating their T cell receptor (TcR) repertoire. Clonal deletion of T lymphocytes in the thymus is not a completely efficient process. The clones most likely to be eliminated are those that express T-cell receptors that interact with high affinity with self-peptides associated with major histocompatibility complex (MHC) molecules. This process assumes that auto-antigens are expressed in the thymus. Truly, mutation of the gene autoimmune regulator (AIRE) in both human and mice results in the so-called autoimmune polyendocrinopathy syndrome. AIRE protein is responsible for the expression in the thymus of proteins typically seen in peripheral organs. In the absence of thymic expression, T cells specific for these antigens escape negative selection (central tolerance), migrate to the periphery, and attack organs.

On the other hand, B lymphocytes are continuously produced by the bone marrow through life and initially express low-affinity IgM on their membranes. In most instances, interaction of these resting B cells with circulating self-molecules does neither activate them nor cause their elimination. Selection and deletion of autoreactive clones seem to take place in the peripheral lymphoid organs during the onset of the immune response. At that time, activated B cells can modify the structure of their membrane immunoglobulin as a consequence of somatic mutations in their germ-line immunoglobulin genes. B cells expressing self-reactive immunoglobulins of high affinity can emerge from this process, and their elimination takes place in the germinal centers.

Both T-cell and B-cell clonal deletion fail to eliminate all autoreactive cells. In the case of T cells, clonal deletion is very effective to eliminate autoreactive cells with high-affinity receptors for autoantigens, but autoreactive cells with moderate to low-affinity receptors will be spared. Other critical factors that determine the effectiveness of clonal deletion include the affinity and stability of the interaction of self-reactive peptides with MHC molecules and the level of expression of the MHC-peptide complexes. In other words, any condition that interferes with the effective presentation of a self-reactive peptide in association with an MHC molecule decreases the efficiency of clonal deletion. Clonal deletion will also not affect clones that recognize self antigens not expressed in the thymus. Furthermore, as the thymic function declines with age, alternative mechanisms have to be in place to ensure the inactivation of autoreactive clones emerging from the differentiation of lymphoid stem cells.

The causes of B cell escape from clonal deletion are not as well-defined, but they exist nonetheless. Thus, peripheral tolerance mechanisms must exist to ensure that autoreactive clones of T and B cells are neutralized after their migration to the peripheral lymphoid tissues.

Mechanisms of Tolerance: Clonal Anergy

One of the postulated peripheral tolerance mechanisms is known as clonal anergy, a process that incapacitates or disables autoreactive clones that escape selection by clonal deletion. Thus, anergy can be experimentally induced, after the ontogenic differentiation of immunocompetent cells has reached a stage in which clonal deletion is no longer possible.

By definition, anergic clones lack the ability to respond to stimulation with the corresponding antigen. Thus, the most obvious manifestation of clonal anergy is the inability to respond to proper stimulation. Anergic B cells carry IgM autoreactive antibody in their membrane, but are not activated as a result of an antigenic encounter. Anergic T cells express TcR for the tolerizing antigen, but fail to properly express the IL-2 and IL-2 receptor genes and to be proliferative in response to antigenic stimulation.

The mechanisms responsible for anergy have been the object of considerable interest. In a simplistic way, it can be stated that anergy results from either an internal block of the intracellular signaling pathways or from downregulating effects exerted by other cells. One major mechanism that is involved in anergy is the incomplete signaling of an immunocompetent cell. This may result in either a block of the intracellular activation pathways or in the developmental arrest of autoreactive clones, which fail to fully differentiate into mature clones of effector cells. As for immunoregulatory cells, emphasis has been placed on those that release IL-10 and/or TGF-β. Both mechanisms are discussed in detail later in this chapter.

As is often the case, when several mechanisms leading to a similar end result are defined, they end up not being mutually exclusive. Indeed, there is ample evidence suggesting that tolerance results from a combination of clonal deletion and clonal anergy. Both processes must coexist and complement each other under normal conditions, so that autoreactive clones, which escape deletion during embryonic development, may be downregulated and become anergic. The failure of either one of these mechanisms may result in the development of an autoimmune disease.

ACQUIRED TOLERANCE

Acquired tolerance can be induced in experimental animals, under the right conditions, known as tolerogenic conditions (Table 1). Several factors influence the development of tolerance. The clinical significance of understanding acquired tolerance is reflected in the need to reestablish tolerance in autoimmune diseases. Reestablishing tolerance limited only to antigens that lead

TABLE 1   Factors Influencing the Development of Tolerance

Host
Genetic predisposition
Soluble, small-sized antigen
Antigen structurally similar to self protein
Intravenous administration of antigen
High- or low-dose of antigen

to autoimmune pathology represents the only hope for specific treatment. Certain approaches that have claimed possible clinical effect are as follows:

1. Modulation of antigen receptors off the surface of B cells results in inability to bind auto-antigen and therefore to respond to it. Example: A tetramer of small DNA fragments binds to B cells expressing DNA antibody on their surface, forces the disappearance of surface antigen receptor, and subsequently the B cell does not recognize autoantigen.
2. Altering route of administration may suppress the response to the autoantigen. Oral administration of basic myelin or collagen, the suspected autoantigens in multiple sclerosis and arthritis, may lead to disease suppression.
3. Immunosuppressive drugs, if given at proper doses, may suppress the response of acti-vated cells, which, in an autoimmune disease, may represent the autoreactive immune cells. Excessive doses of immunosuppressive drugs may lead to immunosuppression rather than limited unresponsiveness to autoantigens.
4. On some occasions, the cells that respond to autoantigen may have additional distinguish-ing markers that can be targeted for depletion with proper antibodies. Or, the choice of B- or T-cell repertoire may be distinctive and therefore targetable.
5. Development of T- or B-cell receptor ligands that have altered (lower) avidity and through binding to the corresponding receptor induces anergy rather than a productive response.
6. Blockade of costimulation may result in T-cell anergy. For example, cytotoxic T cell late antigen (CTLA4) (in a soluble form fused to the Fc portion of IgG) blocks the delivery of costimulation through CD28 provided by CD80/86, blocking the immune response and causing the development of anergy.

EXPERIMENTAL APPROACHES TO THE DEFINITION OF THE MECHANISMS OF LYMPHOCYTE TOLERANCE

The understanding of the mechanisms involved in tolerance has received a significant boost through the use of transgenic mice. These mice are obtained by introducing a gene in the genome of a fertilized egg that is subsequently implanted in a pseudo-pregnant female in which it develops. The new gene introduced in the germ line is passed on, allowing the study of the acquisition of tolerance to a defined antigen under physiological conditions. Double transgenic mice, expressing a given antigen and antibody with predetermined speci-ficity, have been constructed by breeding transgenic mice. The tissue expression of the trans-gene can be manipulated by coupling a tissue-specific promoter to the gene in question.

B Lymphocyte Tolerance Models

The main characteristics of B-cell tolerance are summarized in Table 2. Experimental evidence supporting both anergy and clonal deletion as mechanisms leading to B-cell tolerance has been obtained in transgenic mouse models. One of the most informative models for the understand-ing of B-cell tolerance was obtained by breeding double transgenic mice from animals

TABLE 2 B-Cell Tolerance

B-cell anergy	Antigen is soluble
	Reactivation may occur
	Direct proof
	Double transgenic animals (soluble egg lysozyme and antiegg lysozyme Ab genes): B cells synthesize egg lysozyme but do not secrete antilysozyme Ab
	Transgenic animals (anti-DNA Ab gene on B cells): B cells do not secrete anti-DNA Ab
B-cell deletion	Antigen is surface bound
	Direct proof
	Double transgenic mice (genes coding for surface bound lysozyme and antilysozyme Ab): B cells do not produce lysozyme nor antilysozyme Ab
	Transgenic mice with B cells with genes coding for anti-H2-K^k antibody mated with H2-K^k mice produce offspring that lack H2-K^k antibody-positive B cells

Abbreviation: Ab, antibody.

transgenic for hen egg lysozyme, which develop tolerance to this protein during development, and animals of the same strain carrying the gene coding for IgM egg lysozyme antibody. The double transgenic F1 hybrids express the gene coding for egg lysozyme in nonlymphoid cells, and B lymphocytes of these mice also express IgM antiegg lysozyme antibody. These antibody-positive B lymphocytes are present in large numbers in the spleen. The predominance of B cells with membrane IgM specific for lysozyme is a consequence allelic exclusion: The insertion of a completely rearranged immunoglobulin transgene blocks rearrangement of the normal immunoglobulin genes.

The relevance of this model to the understanding of tolerance lies on the fact that the double transgenic F1 hybrids failed to produce antiegg lysozyme antibodies after repeated immunization with egg lysozyme. Thus, these animals have B lymphocytes carrying and expressing a gene that codes for a self-reactive antibody, but cannot respond to the antigen. Experiments on these cells suggests that one or several of the kinases activated during the response of a normal B cell to antigenic stimulation remain in an inactive state, interrupting the activation cascade.

Reversibility of B-Cell Anergy

By definition, a state of anergy should be reversible. Reversibility was experimentally proven by transferring lymphocytes from double transgenic F1 hybrids expressing the gene coding for antiegg lysozyme antibody to irradiated nontransgenic recipients of the same strain. In this new environment, from which egg lysozyme was absent, the transferred B lymphocytes produced antiegg lysozyme antibodies upon immunization. These experiments suggest that continuous exposure to the circulating self-antigen is necessary to maintain B-cell anergy.

Another approach to activate anergic cells is to separate peripheral blood B lymphocytes from an anergic animal and stimulate them in vitro with lipopolysaccharide, which is a polyclonal mitogen for murine B lymphocytes. As a consequence of this stimulation, the signaling block that characterizes anergy is overridden, and autoreactive B cells secreting antilysozyme antibody can be detected.

Models for B-Lymphocyte Clonal Deletion

Evidence supporting clonal deletion in B-cell tolerance has also been recently obtained in transgenic animal models. Experiments were carried out in F1 double transgenic mice, which were raised by mating animals that expressed egg lysozyme not as a soluble protein but as an integral membrane protein with transgenic mice of the same strain carrying the gene for IgM antiegg lysozyme antibody. In the resulting double transgenic F1 hybrids, B lymphocytes carrying IgM antiegg lysozyme antibody could not be detected.

Additional experiments have proven that stimulation of an immature IgM/IgD autoreactive B cell clone by a self-antigen abundantly expressed on a cell membrane leads to clonal deletion by apoptosis. The elimination of autoreactive clones seems to take place in the lymph node germinal centers.

Thus, the sum of experimental data suggests that B-cell tolerance can result both from clonal anergy and clonal deletion, and the choice of mechanism depends on whether the antigen is soluble or membrane-bound. Clonal deletion involves apoptosis of the self-reactive cells, but we do not know why only membrane-bound antigens appear to trigger apoptosis. B-cell anergy, on the other hand, is associated with a block in the transduction of the activating signal resulting from the binding of antigen to the membrane immunoglobulin, probably consequent to the lack of costimulatory signals usually delivered by activated Th2 cells (see Chapters 4 and 11). Experimental data suggests that the signal delivered to CD40[+] B cells by interacting with the CD40 ligand expressed by T cells is critically important for B-cell differentiation. In the absence of CD40 signaling, B cells are easy to tolerize.

T-Lymphocyte Tolerance Models

The main characteristics of T-cell tolerance are summarized in Table 3. As in the case of B-cell anergy, experimental evidence supporting both anergy and clonal deletion as mechanisms leading to T-cell tolerance has been obtained in transgenic mouse models.

TABLE 3 T-Cell Tolerance

Clonal deletion	Antigen presented in the thymus
	T cells die by apoptosis
	TcR repertoire bias
	Never absolute (residual autoreactive cells seem to persist)
Clonal anergy	Occurs in periphery
	Stimulation of T cells in the absence of proper costimulation leads to anergy

Abbreviation: TcR, T-cell receptors.

There is solid experimental evidence supporting clonal deletion as a mechanism involved in T-cell tolerance. Of seminal importance were the experiments in which transgenic mice were transfected with the gene coding for a TcR cloned from an MHC class I restricted CD8$^+$ cytotoxic T cell clone specific for the male HY antigen (Fig. 1). This TcR was able to mediate a cytotoxic reaction against any cell expressing the HY antigen. While female transgenic mice (HY$^-$) were found to have mature CD8$^+$ cells expressing the TcR specific for HY, none of the transgenic male animals (HY$^+$) had detectable mature CD8$^+$ cells expressing the anti-HY TcR. However, functionally harmless CD4$^+$ cells with the autoreactive TcR could be detected in male animals.

These observations were interpreted as meaning that those lymphocytes expressing the autoreactive TcR and the CD8$^+$ antigen interacted effectively with a cell presenting an immunogenic HY-derived peptide in association with an MHC-I molecule, and those cells were deleted. CD4$^+$ lymphocytes, even if carrying the same TcR, cannot interact effectively

**Transgenic mice with genes coding
for TCR specific for an
HY-derived peptide/MHC-D^b complex**

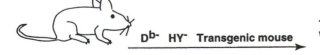

D^{b+} HY$^+$ Transgenic mouse

- Tolerant to HY;
No mature T cells reactive
with MHC-D^b/HY detected

T cell precursors interact with APC presenting MHC-Db/HY and are eliminated

D^{b+} HY$^-$ Transgenic mouse

- Reactive to HY;
Mature T cells reactive
with MHC-D^b/HY are detected

T cell precursors interact with the right MHC, but not with the HY peptide;
T cells with the transgenic TCR for D^b HY will differentiate

D^{b-} HY$^-$ Transgenic mouse

- No mature T cells reactive
with MHC-D^b/HY detected

T cell precursors with the transgenic TCR for Db/Hy fail to interact with MHC
and will not differentiate

FIGURE 1 Diagrammatic representation of an experiment in which transgenic animals expressing a T cell receptor specific for a HY-derived peptide–MHC-D^b complex were shown to become tolerant to the HY peptide, but only in D^{b+} animals. The tolerance in this model was apparently due to clonal deletion, since no mature T cells reactive with MHC-D^b/HY were detected in the tolerant animals. *Abbreviations*: MHC, major histocompatibility complex; TcR, T-cell receptor.

with MHC-I-associated HY-derived peptides and were spared (see Chapter 10). Similar experiments using mice transfected with genes coding for MHC class II restricted TcRs showed that the CD4$^+$ lymphocytes were selectively deleted, as expected from the fact that the reaction between a TcR and an MHC-II-associated peptide is stabilized by CD4 molecules. In other words, the role of CD4 and CD8, as stabilizers of the reaction between T lymphocytes and antigen-presenting cells (APCs), is not only important for antigenic stimulation but is also critical for clonal deletion.

Mechanisms of T-Cell Clonal Deletion

A common point to all types of clonal deletion is that cell death is due to apoptosis, involving interaction of the Fas molecule with its ligand. However, many details concerning the control of T-cell apoptosis remain unexplained, and, as discussed earlier, it is clear than clonal deletion is an imperfect mechanism that needs to be complemented by mechanisms ensuring that persisting autoreactive clones remain inactive.

T-Cell Anergy

Experimental models addressing the question of how do T cells become tolerant to tissue-specific determinants that are not expressed in the thymus have provided evidence for the role of clonal anergy. Transgenic mice were constructed in which the transgene was coupled to a tissue-specific promoter that directed their expression to an extrathymic tissue. For example, heterologous MHC class II (I–E) genes were coupled to the insulin promoter prior to their injection to fertilized eggs. Consequently, the MHC class II antigens coded by the transfected genes were expressed only in the pancreatic islet β cells. Class II (I–E) specific helper T cells were detectable in the transgenic animals, but they could not be stimulated by exposure to lymphoid cells expressing the transfected MHC-II genes. Thus, tolerance to a peripherally expressed MHC-II self-antigen can be due to clonal anergy.

Mechanisms of T-Cell Anergy

Proper stimulation of mature CD4$^+$ T lymphocytes requires at least two signals: one delivered by the interaction of the TcR with the MHC-II–antigen complex and the other delivered by the accessory cell. Both signals require cell–cell contact, involving a variety of surface molecules, and the release of soluble cytokines (see Chapters 4 and 11). When all these signals are properly transmitted to the T lymphocyte, a state of activation ensues. Several experiments suggest that the state of anergy develops when TcR-mediated signaling is not followed by costimulatory signals. For example, a state of anergy is induced when T lymphocytes are stimulated with chemically fixed accessory cells (which cannot release cytokines or upregulate membrane molecules involved in the delivery of costimulatory signals) or with purified MHC-II-antigen complexes (which also cannot provide costimulatory signals).

From the multitude of costimulatory pairs of molecules that have been described, the CD28/CTLA4-B7 family is the most significant in the physiology of T-cell anergy. CD28-mediated signals are necessary to induce the production of IL-2, which seems to be critical for the initial proliferation of Th0 cells and eventual differentiation of Th1 cells. CD28 engagement also results in a lower threshold for effective TcR activation and therefore may enhance the lower avidity interactions between TcR and autoantigens. If the interaction between CD28 and its ligand is prevented at the onset of the immune response, anergy and tolerance ensue. Also, if CD80/86 molecules interact with CTLA4 rather than CD28, a downregulating signal is delivered to the T lymphocyte (see Chapter 11). In contrast to the interactions involving CD28, those that involve CTLA4 may increase the threshold of T-cell activation and inhibit T-cell responses to low affinity autoantigens.

The molecular basis for T-cell anergy is emerging. On the one hand, there seems to be an inhibition of the mitogen-activated protein kinase pathway, resulting in decreased Jun and Fos induction or activation and, consequently, to a decreased expression of the genes regulated by NF-AT1, which include the IL-2 gene and many other cytokine genes. On the other hand, there is evidence suggesting that anergy is associated with the expression of cAMP-regulating elements that have a direct suppressive effect on the transcription of the IL-2 gene. A number of cell signaling molecules appear to be important in the maintenance of tolerance. The importance of these molecules emerges from studies in mice in which these molecules are genetically targeted.

Examples include the B-cell kinase lyn and Cbl (Casitas B-lineage lymphoma). Both of them have proven roles in negatively controlling the response and when absent, autoimmunity occurs.

In conclusion, clonal deletion seems extremely efficient during embryonic differentiation, but a large number of potentially autoreactive clones seems to escape deletion. Whether those autoreactive clones remain anergic or are activated may just depend on whether the autoantigens against which they are directed are ever presented in a context able to induce an active immune response; that is, by activated APC able to deliver costimulatory signals to the autoreactive T and/or B cells. Under normal physiologic conditions, the recognition of autoantigens is more likely to take place in the absence of costimulatory signals by helper T cells, conditions that are likely to contribute to the perpetuation of a state of T-cell anergy. The perpetuation of the anergic state by incomplete signaling of autoreactive clones is believed to be significant in the maintenance of tolerance in adult life.

Regulatory T Cells

Positive selection in the thymus implies that the circulating pool of T cells are to some extent autoreactive and therefore their control in the periphery is mandatory. T-cell anergy and deletion of autoreactive cells in the periphery (in addition to that occurring in the thymus) represent two control mechanisms of autoreactive cells.

T cells with regulatory function exist in the peripheral blood. They express constitutively high levels of CD25 on their surface, and when added to non-CD25 expressing cells in in vitro cultures, they limit their proliferation. Also, in a number of animal models of autoimmune diseases (diabetes and inflammatory bowel disease) when CD25 positive cells are administered intravenously, they suppress the expression of autoimmune disease. There are two caveats that should be considered:

1. CD25 is also expressed in high levels by activated T cells, and the definition of regulatory T cells (Tregs) exclusively based on the expression of CD25 may be problematic. On the other hand, most Tregs have been shown to express the transcription factor FoxP3 (of the Forkhead family of proteins), and this is certainly a valuable marker when it comes to enumerating Tregs. The significance of Foxp3 has been demonstrated in animal models and in humans. Mice deficient in FoxP3 do not have Tregs and develop autoimmunity. Humans with mutations in the FOXP3 gene develop a syndrome known as immune dysregulation, polyendocrinopathy, enteropathy, X-linked (IPEX).
2. It is not clear yet if they can be antigen-specific, although they can be generated following antigen stimulation.

How do Tregs exert their regulatory function? First, through direct cell contact, involving the CTLA4 molecule, and second, through the release of cytokines known to suppress immune cell function, such as IL-10, TGFβ and, to a lesser extent, IL-4.

MUCOSAL TOLERANCE

Ingested antigens seldom cause an immune response. If we consider the tons of potentially immunogenic proteins to which the digestive mucosae are exposed over a lifetime, the incidence of food allergies is miniscule, proof of the general lack of immunogenicity of ingested nonself-material. It is also well-documented that ingestion of proteins or nonreplicating organisms is not an efficient approach to immunization. On the other hand, reports of therapeutic benefit of oral administration of collagen to patients with rheumatoid arthritis raised considerable interest in the concept of oral tolerance.

The sum of experimental data collected so far suggests that the administration of large doses of oral antigen causes Th1 anergy-driven tolerance. However, this seems to be a rather exceptional mechanism, with little clinical application. In contrast, the administration of low doses of antigen is believed to stimulate Th2 responses and cause bystander suppression of autoreactive Th1 cells. A proposed framework for this type of suppression is as follows:

1. The ingested antigen (usually a protein) is transported to submucosal accessory cells in the Peyer's patches where it is processed and presented to Tregs (both of CD4$^+$ and CD8$^+$

phenotypes, including special subpopulations of $\gamma\delta$ CD4$^+$ and CD8$^+$ T cells), which after proliferation and differentiation become functionally suppressor. The suppressor effect is mediated by secretion of TGF-β, IL-10, and IL-4 after reexposure to the tolerizing antigen.

2. When antigen is introduced in small doses as a nasal aerosol, the main effect seems to be the stimulation of immunoregulatory $\gamma\delta$CD8$^+$ cells that cause a shift from a predominant and pathogenic Th1 response to a less harmful Th2 response.

3. The activated Tregs enter the circulation and are attracted to areas of ongoing reactivity. In the peripheral lymphoid tissues they may downregulate inmmune responses to the tolerizing antigen. In tissues where effector cells are causing inflammatory changes, the recruitment of activated Tregs releasing TGF-β and IL-10 may suppresses the activity of Th1 assisting the local immune response process, resulting in a downregulation of the inflammatory response.

The antigen used to induce oral tolerance does not need to be identical to that recognized by the autoreactive T cells in vivo, since the suppressor effects of IL-10 and TGF-β are nonspecific and can affect T cells reacting with other antigens (bystander suppression). However, the best results with oral tolerization protocols are obtained when antigens structurally related to the autoantigens are given orally. Thus, cross-reactivity between the two antigens may be important in localizing the activated suppressor CD8$^+$ cells to the right tissue.

TERMINATION OF TOLERANCE

A state of tolerance dependent on the downregulation of self-reactive clones can be terminated if those clones are adequately activated. Several possible scenarios can be envisaged and, in some cases, experimentally proven to explain the activation of anergic clones.

1. Exposure of anergic cells to an antigen that cross-reacts with a tolerogen may induce the activation of T helper lymphocytes specific for the cross-reacting antigen (molecular mimicry). As a consequence, the activated Th cells will provide autoreactive proinflammatory Th1 or B lymphocytes with the necessary costimulatory signals necessary to initiate a response against the tolerogen.

2. Proper stimulation of anergic T lymphocytes may re-establish the costimulatory pathways, terminate anergy, and initiate the autoreactive process. Experimental evidence supporting this concept was obtained in studies of transgenic mice expressing a lymphocytic choriomeningitis viral glycoprotein on the pancreatic cells. These transgenic mice have T lymphocytes that recognize the glycoprotein but remain anergic. However, the state of anergy in these transgenic mice can be terminated by an infection with the lymphocytic choriomeningitis virus. The infection stimulates the immune system, induces the overexpression of MHC-II-self peptide complexes and costimulatory signals, and previously unresponsive T cells are activated. Consequently, the previously tolerant animals develop inflammatory changes in the Langerhans islets (insulitis) caused by lymphocytes reacting with the viral antigen expressed on the pancreatic cells. Those changes precede the development of diabetes. This model supports the concept of tolerance resulting from the lack of costimulatory signals and also supports the role of infections, by generating a microenvironment favorable to the induction of an active immune response, as an initiating factor indirectly responsible for the activation of autoreactive clones.

3. Special type of infections that may be involved in termination of tolerance are those involving superantigen-producing organisms. Those superantigens react with most MHC-II molecules and with the TcR of specific variable region families. Those TcR families are expressed by as much as one-third of the total T-cell population. The cross-linking of TcRs on large numbers of T lymphocytes in close apposition with activated APCs delivers strong activating signals to T lymphocytes. The consequence is that previously anergic self-reactive T cells will be activated (as evidenced by the active expression of the IL-2 receptor gene) and a previously downregulated autoimmune response becomes active.

4. Perturbation in peripheral T-cell homeostasis can break tolerance and lead to autoimmunity. The survival of peripheral T cells—which by virtue of their positive selection in the

thymus are autoreactive—depends on their ability to "sense" thresholds for mere survival or activation. Therefore, changes in this balance can lead to response to autoantigen and autoimmunity. Clinical conditions that distinctly alter peripheral T-cell homeostasis such as lymphopenia may lead to autoimmunity.

AUTOIMMUNITY

Failure of the immune system to "tolerate" self antigens may result in the development of pathological processes known as autoimmune diseases. At the clinical level, autoimmunity is apparently involved in a variety of apparently unrelated diseases such as systemic lupus erythematosus (SLE), insulin-dependent diabetes mellitus (IDDM), myasthenia gravis, rheumatoid arthritis, multiple sclerosis, and hemolytic anemia. There are at least 40 diseases known or considered to be autoimmune in nature, affecting about 5% of the general population. Their distribution by sex and age is not uniform. As a rule, autoimmune diseases predominate in women and have a bimodal age distribution. A first peak of incidence is around puberty, whereas the second peak is in the 40s and 50s.

CLASSIFICATION OF THE AUTOIMMUNE DISEASES

There are several different ways to classify autoimmune diseases. Because several autoimmune diseases are strongly linked with MHC antigens, one of the proposed classifications, shown in Table 4, groups autoimmune diseases according to their association with class I or with class II MHC markers. It is interesting to notice that although autoimmune diseases may afflict both sexes, there is female preponderance for the class II-associated diseases and a definite increase in the prevalence of class I-associated diseases among males.

PATHOPHYSIOLOGY OF AUTOIMMUNE DISEASES

The autoimmune pathologic process may be initiated and/or perpetuated by autoantibodies, immune complexes containing autoantigens, and autoreactive T lymphocytes. Each of these immune processes plays a preponderant role in certain diseases or may be synergistically associated, particularly in multiorgan, systemic autoimmune diseases.

Pathogenic Role of Autoantibodies

B lymphocytes with autoreactive specificities remain nondeleted in the adult individuals of many species. In mice, polyclonal activation with lipopolysaccharide leads to production of autoantibodies. In humans, bacterial and viral infections (particularly chronic) may lead to the production of anti-immunoglobulin and antinuclear antibodies. In general, it is accepted that polyclonal B-cell activation may be associated with the activation of autoreactive B lymphocytes.

Autoantibody-associated diseases are characterized by the presence of autoantibodies in the individual's serum and by the deposition of autoantibodies in tissues. The pathogenic role of autoantibodies is not always obvious and depends on several factors, such as the availability and valence of the autoantigen and the affinity and charge of the antibody. Antibodies with high affinity for the antigen are considered to be more pathogenic, because they form stable immunity complexes (IC) that can activate complement more effectively. Other characteristics of the antibodies and corresponding agents may play a determinant pathogenic role. For example, anti-DNA antibodies, very prevalent in SLE, have a weak positive charge at physiological pH,

TABLE 4   Classification of Autoimmune Diseases

MHC class II-associated
Organ specific (autoantibody directed against a single organ or closely related organs)
Systemic (systemic lupus erythematosus-variety of autoantibodies to DNA, cytoplasmic antigens, etc.)
MHC class I-associated
HLA-B27-related spondyloarthropathies (ankylosing spondylitis, Reiter's syndrome, etc.)
Psoriasis vulgaris (which is associated with HLA-B13, B16, and B17)

Abbreviations: HLA, human leukocyte antigens; MHC, major histocompatibility complex.

TABLE 5 Pathogenic Mechanisms Triggered by Autoantibodies

Mechanism	Disease	Comments
C′-mediated cell lysis	Autoimmune cytopenias	C′-activating immunoglobulin binds to cell membrane antigen; C′ is activated; membrane attack complex is formed; cell is lysed.
Tissue destruction by inflammatory cells	SLE	Antinuclear antibodies bind to tissue-fixed antigens; C′ is activated; C3a and C5a are produced; PMNs are attracted; inflammation develops.
Blockage of receptor	Insulin-resistant diabetes mellitus (acanthosis nigricans)	Anti-insulin receptor antibodies bind to insulin receptor and compete with insulin.
Charge-facilitated	Lupus nephritis	Cationic anti-DNA tissue deposition; antibodies bind to glomerular basement membrane.
Activation of C′	Membrano-proliferative glomerulonephritis	Anti-C3bBb antibodies (nephritic factors) bind to and stabilize the C3 convertase (C3bBb), which cleaves C3.
Phagocytosis and intracellular lysis	Autoimmune cytopenias	Antibody binds to cell; may or may not activate C′; cell-antibody−(C3b,C3d) complexes are phagocytosed by Fc receptor and/or complement receptor-bearing cells.

Abbreviations: PMN, polymorphonuclear; SLE, systemic lupus erythematosus.

and bind to the negatively charged glomerular basement membrane, which also binds DNA. Such affinity of antigens and antibodies for the glomerular basement membrane creates the ideal conditions for in situ IC formation and deposition, which is usually followed by glomerular inflammation. Finally, autoantibodies may bind only to cells and tissues that have been exposed to a stressor, such as ischemia, activate complement and cause tissue injury. This may explain why titers of autoantibodies almost never correlate with autoimmune disease severity.

Autoantibodies may be directly involved in the pathogenesis of some diseases, while in others they may serve simply as disease markers without a known pathogenic role. For example, the anti-Sm antibodies that are found exclusively in patients with SLE are not known to play a pathogenic role. However, in many other situations, autoantibodies can trigger various pathogenic mechanisms leading to cell or tissue destruction (Table 5). This is particularly true of complement-fixing antibodies (IgG and IgM). If such antibodies react with red cell antigens, they may cause intravascular red cell lysis if the complement activation sequence proceeds all the way to the formation of the membrane attack complex, or may induce phagocytosis and extravascular lysis as a consequence of Fc-mediated phagocytosis and/or C3b-mediated phagocytosis if the sequence of complement activation is stopped at the C3 level. If the antigen-antibody reaction takes place in tissues, proinflammatory complement fragments (C3a, C5a) are generated and attract and activate granulocytes and mononuclear cells that can release proteolytic enzymes and toxic radicals in the area of IC deposition, causing tissue damage. Finally, other autoantibodies may have a pathogenic role dependent not on causing cell or tissue damage, but on the interference with cell functions resulting from their binding to physiologically important cell receptors.

Representative human autoimmune diseases in which autoantibodies are believed to play a major pathogenic role are listed in Table 6. It must be noted in some of these diseases, there is

TABLE 6 Antibody-Mediated Autoimmune Diseases

Disease	Antigen
Autoimmune cytopenias (anemia, thrombocytopenia, neutropenia)	Erythrocyte, platelet, or neutrophil cell surface determinant
Goodpasture's syndrome	Type IV collagen
Pemphigus vulgaris	Cadherin on epidermal keratinocytes
Myasthenia gravis	Acetylcholine receptor
Hyperthyroidism	Thyroid stimulating hormone receptor (Graves' disease)
Insulin resistant diabetes (acanthosis nigricans)	Insulin receptor
Pernicious anemia	Intrinsic factor, parietal cells

also a cell-mediated immunity component. For example, in myasthenia gravis, autoreactive T lymphocytes have been described, and both autoreactive cell lines and clones have been successfully established from patient's lymphocytes. These T lymphocytes may provide help to autoreactive B lymphocytes, producing antiacetylcholine receptor antibodies. In such cases, autoreactive T lymphocytes could be more central in the pathogenesis of the disease than autoantibody producing B lymphocytes. However, the pathogenic role of autoantibodies is evident from the fact that newborns to mothers with myasthenia gravis develop myasthenia-like symptoms for as long as they have maternal autoantibodies in circulation.

The Pathogenic Role of Immune Complexes in Autoimmune Diseases

In autoimmune diseases, there is ample opportunity for the formation of IC involving autoantibodies and self-antigens. Several factors determine the pathogenicity of IC, as discussed in greater detail in Chapter 23. They include the size of the IC (intermediate size IC are the most pathogenic), the ability of the host to clear IC (individuals with low complement levels or deficient Fc receptor and/or complement receptor function have delayed IC clearance rates and are prone to develop autoimmune diseases), and physicochemical properties of IC (which determine the ability to activate complement and/or the deposition in specific tissues). On many occasions, IC are formed in situ, activate the complement system, complement split products are formed, and neutrophils are attracted to the area of IC deposition where they will mediate the IC-mediated tissue destruction. SLE and polyarteritis nodosa are two classical examples of autoimmune diseases, in which IC play a major pathogenic role. In SLE, DNA and other nuclear antigens are predominantly involved in the formation of IC, whereas in polyarteritis nodosa, the most frequently identified antigens are hepatitis B-related.

The Role of Activated T Lymphocytes in the Pathogenesis of Autoimmune Diseases

Typical T cell-mediated autoimmune diseases are summarized in Table 7. T lymphocytes that are involved in the pathogenesis of such autoimmune diseases may be autoreactive and recognize self antigens, recognize foreign antigens associated with self determinants (modified self), or respond to foreign antigens but still induce self-tissue destruction by nonspecific mechanisms.

Cytotoxic CD8+ Lymphocytes

CD8+ lymphocytes play a pathogenic role in some autoimmune diseases, usually involving the recognition of nonself peptides expressed in the context of self MHC and destroying the cell expressing such "modified" self. For example, coxsackie B virus-defined antigens expressed on the surface of myocardial cells may induce CD8+-mediated tissue destruction, causing a viral-induced autoimmune myocarditis.

Activated CD4+ Helper Cells

CD4+ helper cells, particularly those of the Th1 phenotype, appear to be more frequently involved in cell-mediated autoimmune reactions than their CD8+ counterparts. Their pathogenic effects are mediated by the release of proinflammatory cytokines and chemokines. Th2 cells can also be involved, promoting the activation of autoreactive B lymphocytes.

TABLE 7 Examples of T Cell-Mediated Autoimmune Diseases

Disease	Specificity of T-cell clone/line	T cell involved[a]
Experimental allergic encephalomyelitis	Myelin basic protein	CD4+
Autoimmune thyroiditis	Thyroid follicular epithelial cells	?
Insulin-dependent diabetes mellitus	Pancreatic islet beta cells	CD8+ (CD4+)
Viral myocarditis	Coxsackie B virus	CD8+

[a]Derived from cells isolated from tissue lesions or peripheral blood of patients and animals affected by the experimental disease. Some of these T cell lines have been used for adoptive transfer of the disease. In experimental animals, treatment with anti-T cell antibodies may improve the clinical manifestations of the disease.

Pathogenic Factors Involved in the Onset of Autoimmune Diseases

Multiple factors have been proposed as participating in the pathogenesis of autoimmune diseases. These factors can be classified as immunologic, genetic, environmental, and hormonal. Each group of factors is believed to contribute in different ways to the pathogenesis of different diseases.

Abnormal Immunoregulation

Multiple lymphocyte abnormalities have been described in patients with autoimmune diseases. Prominent among them are B-lymphocyte overactivity, presence of spontaneously activated T and B lymphocytes, and decreased Treg function. These abnormalities are typified in SLE and will be discussed in Chapter 18.

Genetic Factors

Clinical observations have documented increased frequency of autoimmune diseases in families, and increased rates of clinical concordance in monozygotic twins. The basis for these associations seems to be complex, involving multiple sets of genes, only some of which have been identified. The same seems to be true in experimental animals. Study of congenic mice has shed some light into how different loci contribute, through positive and negative epistatic interactions, to loss of tolerance to autoantigens and the progressive establishment of a lupus-like disease. The number of genes involved in human lupus must be significantly higher. A similarly high number of loci have been proposed for diabetes and arthritis in humans and laboratory animals.

Single genetic traits though have been shown to lead to autoimmunity in mice and humans through distinct pathophysiologic processes:

1. Lack of AIRE (autoimmune regulator) leads to autoimmune polyendocrinopathy syndrome, because peripheral autoantigens are not expressed in the thymus to execute negative selection of T cells.
2. Lack of Fas and Fas ligand leads to autoimmune lymphoproliferative syndrome, because T and B cells are not eliminated through apoptosis.
3. Lack of C4 and C1q leads to lupus-like syndromes because of defective clearance of immune complexes.
4. Lack of FOXP3 causes IPEX because of failure to generate Tregs.
5. CTLA-4 mutations associate with Grave's disease type 1 diabetes and SLE because of failure in T-cell anergy and reduced activation threshold of self-reactive T cells.

Major Histocompatibility Complex Markers

Several studies have also documented associations between human leukocyte antigens (HLA) and various diseases (see Chapter 3). As stated earlier in this chapter, autoimmune diseases can be classified into two groups, one apparently associated with MHC-I genetic markers and the other associated with MHC-II genetic markers.

The classical example of linkage with MHC-I markers is the association between HLA-B27 and inflammatory spondyloarthropathies (ankylosing spondylitis, Reiter's syndrome, etc.). The pathogenic relevance of HLA-B27 is strongly supported by experiments with transgenic mice carrying the gene for HLA-B27. Those transgenic animals spontaneously develop inflammatory disease, involving the gastrointestinal tract, peripheral and vertebral joints, skin, nails, and heart. The disease induced in transgenic mice resembles strikingly the B27-associated disorders that afflict humans with that gene. It has been postulated that the autoimmune reaction is triggered by an infectious peptide presented by HLA-B27 and followed by cross-reactive lymphocyte activation by an endogenous collagen-derived peptide, equally associated with HLA-B27.

The linkage of autoimmunity with MHC-II markers is better understood. With the expanded definition of MHC-II alleles due to the development of antisera and DNA probes and because of the successful sequencing of the genes coding for the constitutive polypeptide chains of MHC-II molecules, the significance of MHC-II alelles has become clear. For example,

IDDM is strongly associated with serologically defined MHC-II markers (HLA-DR3 and HLA-DR4), but is even more strongly correlated with the presence of uncharged aminoacids at position 57 of the β chain of DQ (DQβ) (see Chapter 19). Those MHC-II molecules may be critically involved in the presentation of diabetogenic peptides to the immune system.

The exact mechanisms responsible for the association between HLA alleles and disease susceptibility are being actively investigated. Two have been hypothesized, based on the persistence and later activation of autoreactive clones.

Molecular Mimicry

Molecular mimicry is cross-reactivity between peptides derived from infectious agents and peptides derived from autologous proteins which are expressed by most normal resting cells in the organism. Anergic autoreactive T-cell clones would be activated by an immune response against an infectious agent due to this type of cross-reactivity.

Lack of Expression of MHC Alleles Able to Bind Critical Endogenous Peptides

This possibility has been documented in animal models of type I diabetes and multiple sclerosis. The MHC molecules associated with autoimmunity are either expressed in very low levels in differentiating cells and in resting cells of adult animals, or are associated with unstable peptides that are easily degraded and not efficiently presented. Under those circumstances, potentially autoreactive T-lymphocyte clones would not be eliminated and would remain available for later activation, due to an unrelated immune response or by the presentation of a cross-reactive peptide.

T-Cell Receptor Variable Region Types

The TcR repertoire of a given individual seems to be another important determinant of autoimmunity. Several autoimmune diseases show associations with specific TcR variable region types. This is not surprising, because the specific recognition of different oligopeptides by different T lymphocytes depends on the diversity of the TcR (see Chapters 10 and 11). Therefore, the development of an autoimmune response should require that the genome of an individual includes genes encoding a particular array of V region genes whose transcription resulted in the expression of TcR able to combine with a specific autologous peptide. In addition, the clones expressing such receptors must not be deleted during embryonic differentiation.

These postulates are supported by immunogenetic studies in different animals and humans with different manifestations of autoimmunity. Those studies suggest that linkages between specific TcR V region genes and specific autoimmune diseases may actually exist (e.g., IDDM, multiple sclerosis, and SLE). Experimental corollaries of the postulated positive association between specific TcR V region genes and disease are found in experimental allergic encephalomyelitis and murine collagen-induced arthritis. The lymphocytes obtained from arthritic joints of mice susceptible to collagen-induced arthritis have a very limited repertoire of Vβ genes. In mouse strains that do not develop collagen-induced arthritis, there are extensive deletions of Vβ genes, including those preferentially expressed by susceptible mice.

Even in identical twins, however, concordance for a particular autoimmune disease never exceeds 40%, suggesting that the presence of autoimmunity-associated TcR V region genes is not sufficient to cause disease by itself. Indeed, with certain exceptions, human autoimmune diseases are multigenic, and the number of the involved genes has not been determined.

Genes Related to the Inflammatory Process

The intensity of the inflammatory reaction triggered by the recognition of self epitopes is a key determinant of the development of pathological lesions and clinical symptoms. Autoimmunity is favored by overexpression of genes encoding proinflammatory cytokines (e.g., TNF) and under expression of genes encoding anti-inflammatory cytokines (e.g., IL-10) or membrane molecules associated with downregulation of activated T cells (e.g., CTLA-4).

Environmental Factors

The most important environmental factors are believed to be foreign antigens sharing structural similarity with self determinants. Exposure to these epitopes can trigger autoimmune reactions. The term molecular mimicry is used to describe identity or similarity of either amino acid sequences or structural epitopes between foreign and self antigens.

One of the best-known examples of autoimmunity resulting from the exposure to cross-reactive antigens is the cardiomyopathy that complicates many cases of acute rheumatic fever. Group A β-hemolytic streptococci have several epitopes cross-reactive with tissue antigens. One of them cross-reacts with an antigen found in cardiac myosin. The normal immune response to such a cross-reactive strain of *Streptococcus* will generate lymphocyte clones that will react with myosin and induce myocardial damage long after the infection has been eliminated.

Several other examples of molecular mimicry have been described, as summarized in Table 8, and additional ones await better definition. For example, molecular mimicry between the envelop glycolipids of gram-negative bacteria and the myelin of the peripheral nerves may explain the association of the Guillain-Barré syndrome with *Campylobacter jejuni* infections. Mimicry between LFA-1 and the *Borrelia burgdorferi* outer surface protein A is considered responsible for the rheumatic manifestations of Lyme's disease. Mimicry between glutamate decarboxylase, an enzyme concentrated in pancreatic beta cells, and coxsackie virus P2-C, an enzyme involved in the replication of coxsackie virus B, has been considered responsible for the development of insulin-dependent diabetes in humans and in murine models of this disease.

Infectious agents, particularly viruses, can precipitate autoimmunity by inducing the release of sequestered antigens. In autoimmune myocarditis associated with coxsackie B3 virus, the apparent role of the virus is to cause the release of normally sequestered intracellular antigens as a consequence of virus-induced myocardial cell necrosis. Autoantibodies and T lymphocytes reactive with sarcolemma and myofibril antigens or peptides derived from these antigens emerge, and the autoreactive T lymphocytes are believed to be responsible for the development of persistent myocarditis.

On the other hand, latent viral infections are believed to be responsible for the development of many autoimmune disorders. Latent infection is commonly associated with integration of the viral genome into the host chromosomes, and while integrated viruses very seldom enter a full replicative cycle and do not cause cytotoxicity, they can interfere, directly or indirectly, with several functions of the infected cells. For example, viral proteins may interfere with the function of proteins involved in the control of cell death and survival, such as p53 and bcl-2. In addition, viral proteins may mimic chemokine receptors or ligands and therefore mislead the function of immune cells. T-cell activation secondary to an inapparent viral infection has the potential to induce autoimmunity secondary to the release of interferon-γ and TNF, both known to be potent inducers of MHC-II antigen expression. The increased expression of class II MHC antigens would then create optimal conditions for the onset of an autoimmune response directed

TABLE 8 Human Proteins with Structural Homology to Human Pathogens

Disease	Human protein	Pathogen
Ankylosing spondylitis, Reiter's syndrome	HLA-B27	Klebsiella pneumoniae
Rheumatoid arthritis	HLA-DR4	Epstein–Barr virus
IDDM	Insulin receptor	Papilloma virus
	HLA-DR	Cytomegalovirus
	Glutamate decarboxylase	Coxsackie virus P2-C enzyme
Myasthenia gravis	Acetylcholine receptor	Poliovirus
Ro-associated clinical syndromes	Ro/SSA antigen	Vesicular stomatitis virus
Rheumatic heart disease	Cardiac myosin	Group A Streptococci
Celiac disease	A-gliadin or wheat gluten	Adenovirus type 12
Acute proliferative glomerulonephritis	Vimentin	*Streptococcus pyogenes* type 1
Lyme disease (rheumatic manifestations)	LFA-1	*Borrelia burgdoferi* outer surface protein-A

Abbreviations: HLA, human leukocyte antigens; IDDM, insulin-dependent diabetes mellitus; LFA, leukocyte function antigen; Ro/SSA, Ro/Sjogren's syndrome antigen A.

against MHC-II–self peptide complexes. Such a mechanism has been proposed to explain the onset of autoimmune thyroiditis. An unknown nonlytic virus would cause T-lymphocyte activation in the thyroid gland, followed by increased expression of MHC-II and thyroid derived peptides, and finally, an antithyroid immune reaction would develop.

Finally, physical trauma can also lead to immune responses to sequestered antigens. The classical example is sympathetic ophthalmia, an inflammatory process of apparent autoimmune etiology affecting the normal eye after a penetrating injury of the other. This process may not be limited to trauma; tissue injury induced by any cause may result in the generation of autoreactive T cells that recognize previously cryptic epitopes. Over time, this process will lead to expansion of the immune response by facilitating the onset of immune responses to additional epitopes. This process is known as "epitope spreading."

Unresolved Issues in Molecular Mimicry

There are still difficulties in proving that infections are the cause of autoimmune diseases. The infection may have resolved long before the appearance of disease or the infection may be inapparent, thus obscuring the temporal association between infection and autoimmunity. Alternatively, molecular mimicry may be the result rather than the cause of autoimmunity. The infectious process may result in the alteration of nonimmunogenic antigenic determinants as a consequence of tissue injury. The autoantibodies that appear when the disease is diagnosed may then be the result of tissue injury rather than the cause of it.

The increased frequency of autoimmune diseases in countries where infections have either been eradicated or are being effectively treated has advanced the argument that infections may also suppress autoimmunity. This is known as the "sterile" hypothesis of autoimmunity and there is experimental, besides epidemiologic, evidence to support it.

Animal Models of Autoimmunity

Our understanding of autoimmune disease has been facilitated by studies in animal models. Several animal models have been developed, each sharing some characteristics of a human disease of autoimmune etiology. These animal models often provide the only experimental approaches to the study of the pathogenesis of autoimmune diseases.

In some experimental models, injecting normal animals with antigens extracted from the human target tissues induces autoimmune diseases. A rapid onset and an acute course characterize the resulting diseases. These models have been particularly useful in the study of autoimmune thyroiditis and arthritis (collagen-induced arthritis). Most useful for the study of autoimmunity are animals that develop autoimmune disease spontaneously, whose course is protracted, and parallels closely the disease as seen in humans. Representative animal models of different autoimmune diseases are listed in Table 9.

TABLE 9 Representative Autoimmune Disease Models and their Human Analogs

	Animal model	Human disease analog
Antigen-induced		
Myelin basic protein	Experimental allergic ence phalomyelitis	Multiple sclerosis
Collagen type II	Collagen-induced arthritis	Rheumatoid arthritis
Induced by injecting mycobacterial extract	Adjuvant arthritis	Rheumatoid arthritis
Chemically-induced		
$HgCl_2$	Nephritis in rats	Nephritis
Spontaneous models		
NZB, (NZB × NZW)F_1	Murine lupus	Systemic lupus erythematosis
MRL lpr/lpr BXSB murine strains		
Nonobese diabetic mice and rats	Diabetes	Type 1 (autoimmune) diabetes
Inbred BB rats		
Transgenic animals		
HLA-B27 transgenic rats	Spondyloarthropathy	Inflammatory spondyloarthropathies

Abbreviations: HLA, human leukocyte antigens; MRL/lpr, MRL/lymphoproliferation; NZB, New Zealand black; NZW, New Zealand white.

Experimental Allergic Encephalomyelitis

Allergic encephalomyelitis in mice and rats is the best-characterized experimental model of multiple sclerosis. Immunizing animals with myelin basic protein and adjuvant induces the disease. One to two weeks later, the animals develop encephalomyelitis characterized by perivascular mononuclear cell infiltrates and demyelination. The mononuclear cell infiltrates show a predominance of $CD4^+$ T lymphocytes, which upon activation release cytokines that attract phagocytic cells to the area of immunological reaction; those cells are, in turn, activated and release enzymes that are responsible for the demyelination. $CD4^+$ T lymphocyte clones from animals with EAE disease can transfer the disease to normal animals of the same strain. Genetic manipulations leading to deletion of the genes coding for two specific variable regions of the TcR β chain (Vβ8 and Vβ13) prevent the expression of disease. These two Vβ regions must obviously be involved in the recognition of a dominant epitope of human myelin.

Diabetes

Diabetes develops spontaneously in inbred BB rats as well as in nonobese diabetic (NOD) mice. In both strains, the onset of the disease is characterized by T cell-mediated insulitis, which evolves into diabetes. This disease demonstrates H-2 linkage remarkably similar to that observed between human IDDM and HLA-DR3, DR4, and other MHC-II alleles. In NOD mice, a decreased expression of MHC-I genes, secondary to a TAP-1 gene deficiency, has also been characterized. Such deficiency would prevent these animals from deleting autoreactive cytotoxic T-cell clones during lymphocyte differentiation.

System Lupus Erythematosus

A number of murine strains spontaneously develop autoimmune disease that resembles human SLE.

1. [New Zealand block (NZB) × New Zealand white (NZW)]F$_1$ female mice develop glomerulonephritis, hemolytic anemia, and anti-DNA antibodies. Numerous alterations in T- and B-lymphocyte function, cytokine release, and macrophage functions have been described in these animals. It has also been demonstrated that this and other SLE and autoimmune-prone mouse strains, such as MRL/lymphoproliferation (MRL/lpr), BXSB, and NOD, express reduced levels of the inhibitory FcγRIIB receptor on activated B cells. The low expression of this receptor removes an important downregulating control for autoantibody producing cells.
2. MRL-lpr/lpr mice that lack Fas antigen and g/d mice that lack Fas ligand produce autoantibodies and develop arthritis and kidney disease, but they also develop massive lymphadenopathy which is not seen in human disease.
3. BXSB mice develop anti-DNA antibodies, nephritis, and vasculitis. In this strain, in contrast to the others, disease susceptibility is linked to the Y chromosome.

IMMUNOMODULATION IN THE TREATMENT OF AUTOIMMUNE DISEASES

Standard therapeutic approaches to autoimmune disease usually involve symptomatic palliation with anti-inflammatory drugs and attempts to downregulate the immune response. Glucocorticoids, which have both anti-inflammatory and immunosuppressive effects, have been widely used, as well as immunosuppressive and cytotoxic drugs. However, the use of these drugs is often associated with severe side effects and is not always efficient. Other therapeutic approaches that have been tried have had as their objective to downregulate the autoimmune response and, if possible, to induce tolerance.

Induction of Tolerance

Induction of tolerance to the responsible antigen is the most logical approach to the treatment of autoimmune disorders. This approach is hampered by the fact that the identity of the antigen is not known with certainty in many diseases and because of the individual variations to tolerization that will be encountered in humans, due to their high degree of genetic diversity. The need for well-defined tolerogens may not be an insurmountable obstacle, due to the phenomenon recently described as "bystander tolerance." For example, when a cross-reactive antigen is used to induce oral tolerance, immunoregulatory cells secreting IL-10 and TGF-β differentiate in the submucosa and migrate to lymphoid organs and inflamed site, where they suppress the activity of proinflammatory Th1 cells. The effects of regulatory cells are not antigen-specific, so they may extend to autoreactive T cells interacting with a peptide different from those generated by the orally-administered tolerogen. Examples of the beneficial effects of oral tolerization have been described, both in animal models and humans. In experimental animals, oral administration of basic myelin protein has been shown to decrease the severity of experimental allergic encephalitis. In patients with rheumatoid arthritis, oral administration of collagen type II was followed by clinical improvement.

B-cell tolerization has been tried in patients with SLE. A reportedly successful protocol involved administration of a construct of 4 short DNA fragments conjugated to a dextran backbone that caused cessation of DNA antibody synthesis. Apparently, the construct bound to B-cell surface immunoglobulins in DNA specific B cells and caused its internalization. The reason why this causes the interruption of antibody synthesis has not been clarified.

Elimination or downregulation of T cells by injection of monoclonal anti-T cell antibodies has been shown to be therapeutic in a number of animal models, as well as in human transplantation. Murine monoclonal antibodies are immunogenic and unsuitable for long-term use in humans. However, recombinant humanized monoclonal antibodies are better tolerated and increasingly preferred for therapeutic use. Humanized monoclonal antibodies are produced by cells engineered with recombinant genomes in which all immunoglobulin-coding genes minus those coding for the antibody binding site are of human origin, whereas the genes coding for the specific antibody binding site are obtained from a murine B-cell clone of known specificity. Because the immunogenic epitopes are predominantly located in the constant regions, which in these monoclonals are homologous, humanized monoclonals can be repeatedly administered to humans with low risk of inducing serum sickness. The clinical value of these antibodies in human autoimmune diseases is being evaluated.

The knowledge that costimulatory signals are essential for T-cell activation has led to attempts to induce anergy or tolerance by disrupting costimulatory interactions, with promising results in animal models (Table 10). For example, the interruption of the CD40/CD40 ligand interaction, essential both for the activation of CD4 T lymphocytes and for the full differentiation of B lymphocytes, in (NZB × NZW) F_1 female mice has been shown to delay the onset of nephritis as well as to induce the reversion of established nephritis. The delivery of downregulating signals with CTLA-4 Ig (hybrid molecules obtained by fusion of CTLA-4 and the Fc segment of human IgG) has also been met with success in tolerance-inducing protocols in mice, in the treatment of murine lupus, and in therapeutic trials carried out in patients with rheumatoid arthritis and psoriasis.

Disruption of the action of cytokines using monoclonal antibodies or soluble recombinant receptors has been shown to be very effective in patients with rheumatoid arthritis. Humanized monoclonal antibodies to TNF (infliximab and adalimumab, see Chapter 24) as well as a recombinant, soluble TNF receptor produced by a hybrid genome in which the TNF receptor gene was fused to a human IgG Fc gene (etarnecept) have been approved by the FDA for use as an anti-inflammatory agents in the treatment of rheumatoid arthritis. The addition of the

TABLE 10 Summary of Interventions Aimed at Disrupting Costimulation of T cells in Animal Models of Autoimmune Diseases

Model	Anti-CD80 Ab	Anti-CD86	CTLA4-Ig
SLE-like disease in (NZB × NZW)F1 mice			Benefit
Insulin-dependent diabetes in NOD mice	Worsening	Prevention	
Experimental allergic encephalomyelitis	Benefit ($\uparrow$ Th2)	Worsening	

Abbreviations: Ab, antibody; SLE, systemic lupus erythematosus.

IgG constant region genes in recombinant proteins, such as CTLA4–Ig and etarnecept, has the effect of prolonging the half-life of the recombinant protein in circulation.

Injection of Normal Pooled Immunoglobulins

Injection of normal pooled immunoglobulins (IVIg) has been tried in a number of human autoimmune diseases and proved to be of definite help in a form of pediatric vasculitis (Kawasaki's syndrome), as well as in many cases of idiopathic thrombocytopenic purpura. The mechanism of action is believed to involve B-cell downregulation, as a consequence of the simultaneous cross-linking of membrane immunoglobulins by anti-idiotypic antibodies contained in the IVIg preparations and of FcγRIIb receptors. The consequence of this downregulation is a decreased synthesis of autoantibodies.

Reestablishment of a Perturbed Th1/Th2 Lymphokine Balance

Reestablishment of a Perturbed Th1/Th2 lymphokine balance has been successful in a number of animal models. Th2 diseases (such as lupus) would benefit from blockade of the action of Th2 cytokines such as IL4, whereas Th1 diseases (such as EAE) would benefit from the administration of IL-4. However, the effects of cytokines are pleiotropic, and the expected outcome of these interventions in humans may not be accomplished without undesirable side effects.

Plasmapheresis

It consists of pumping the patient's blood through a special centrifuge to separate plasma from white and red cells. The red cells and plasma substitutes are pumped back into the patient while the plasma is discarded. The rationale for plasmapheresis in the treatment of autoimmune diseases is to remove pathogenic autoantibodies and immune complexes from the circulation.

BIBLIOGRAPHY

Agarwal P, Oldenburg MC, Czarneski JE, et al. Comparison study for identifying promoter ellelic polymorphism in interleukin 10 and tumor necrosis factor alpha genes. Diagn Mol Path 2000; 9:158.

Albert LJ, Inman RD. Molecular mimicry and autoimmunity. N Engl J Med 2000; 341:2068.

Blackman M, Kapler J, Marrack P. The role of the T lymphocyte receptor in positive and negative selection of developing T lymphocytes. Science 1990; 248:1335.

Christen U, von Herrath MG. Infections and autoimmunity–good or bad? J Immunol 2005; 174:7481–7486.

Faria AMC, Weiner HL. Oral tolerance: mechanisms and therapeutic applications. Adv Immunol 1999; 73:153.

Goodnow GC. Transgenic mice and analysis of B-cell tolerance. Annu Rev immunol 1992; 10:489.

Goodnow CC, Sprent J, de St Groth BF, Vinuesa CG. Cellular and genetic mechanisms of self tolerance and autoimmunity. Nature 2005; 435:590.

Jiang H, Chess L. An integrated view of suppressor T cell subsets in immunoregulation. J Clin Invest 2004; 114:1198.

Mayer L. Oral tolerance: new approaches, new problems. Clin Immunol 2000; 94:1.

McGaha TL, Sorrentino B, Ravetch JV. Restoration of tolerance in lupus by targeted inhibitory receptor expression. Science 2005; 307:590.

Ohashi PS. T-cell signalling and autoimmunity: molecular mechanisms of disease. Nat Rev Immunol 2002; 2:427.

Plotz PH. The autoantibody repertoire: searching for order. Nat Rev Immunol 2003; 3:73.

Powell JD, Lerner CG, Ewoldt GR, Schwartz RH. The -180 site of the IL-2 promoter is the target of CREB/CREM binding in T cell anergy. J Immunol 1999; 163:6631.

Seamons A, Sutton J, Bai D, et al. Competition between two MHC binding registers in a single peptide processed from myelin basic protein influences tolerance and susceptibility to autoimmunity. J Exp Med 2003; 197:1391.

Shevach EM. Regulatory/suppressor T cells in health and disease. Arthritis Rheum 2004; 50:2721.

Theofilopoulos AN, Dummer W, Kono DH. T cell homeostasis and systemic autoimmunity. J Clin Invest 2001; 108:335.

Theofilopoulos AN, Kono DH. The genes of systemic autoimmunity. Proc Assoc Am Phys 1999; 111:228.

Thomson CB. Distinct roles for the costimulatory ligands B7-1 and B7-2 in helper cell differentiation. Cell 1995; 81:979.

Tsokos GC, Fleming SD. Autoimmunity, complement activation, tissue injury and back. Curr Dir Autoimmun 2004; 7:149.

Ueda H, Howson JM, Esposito L, et al. Association of the T-cell regulatory gene CTLA4 with susceptibility to autoimmune disease. Nature 2003; 423:506.

Von Herrath MG, Harrison LC. Antigen-induced regulatory T cells in autoimmunity. Nat Rev Immunol 2003; 3:223.

Wucherpfenning KW. Mechanisms for the induction of autoimmunity by infectious agents. J Clin Invest 2001; 108:1097.

17 | Organ-Specific Autoimmune Diseases

Gabriel Virella
*Department of Microbiology and Immunology, Medical University of South Carolina,
Charleston, South Carolina, U.S.A.*

George C. Tsokos
Beth Israel Deaconess Medical Center, Harvard Medical School, Boston, Massachusetts, U.S.A.

INTRODUCTION

Autoimmune diseases can be roughly divided into organ-specific and systemic, based both on the extent of their involvement and the type of "autoantibodies" present in the patients. The systemic forms of autoimmune diseases, best-exemplified by systemic lupus erythematosus (SLE) and rheumatoid arthritis (RA), are discussed in Chapters 18 and 19. Less generalized autoimmune processes may affect virtually every organ system (Table 1); in many instances, only certain cell types within an organ system will be affected in a particular disease, that is, gastric parietal cells in pernicious anemia. In this chapter, we restrict our discussion to the major autoimmune diseases that affect specific organs and the associated autoantibodies, with the understanding that in many cases these antibodies are not the cause of the disease, but just a secondary manifestation. Our understanding of the pathogenesis of most organ-specific autoimmune disorders is schematically illustrated in Figure 1. The key cells are autoreactive T cells, which under the right circumstances become activated. The activated T cells can be controlled by T regulatory cells (Tregs), but if they manage to overcome the downregulating effects of those cells, then, both directly and through activated macrophages, they are able to cause the death of cells expressing the autoantigens that triggered the reaction.

AUTOIMMUNE DISEASES OF THE THYROID GLAND

Autoimmune factors have been implicated in two major thyroid diseases, Graves' disease and Hashimoto's disease.

Graves' Disease

Graves' disease, also known as thyrotoxicosis, diffuse toxic goiter, and exophthalmic goiter, is the result of the production of antibodies against the thyrotrophic hormone (TSH) receptor (thyroid receptor antibodies). The TSH receptor antibodies detected in patients with Graves' disease stimulate the activity of the thyroid gland. For that reason, they have been known by a variety of descriptive terms, including long-acting thyroid stimulator, thyroid-stimulating immunoglobulin (TSI), or thyroid stimulating antibodies.

Thyroid stimulating antibodies are detected in 80% to 90% of the patients with Graves' disease, are usually of the IgG isotype, and have the capacity to stimulate the production of thyroid hormones by activating the adenylate cyclase system after binding to the TSH receptor. Biopsy of the thyroid gland shows diffuse lympho-plasmocytic interstitial infiltration.

Pathogenesis
Role of Lymphocytes and Macrophages Cells Infiltrating the Thyroid
Activated B lymphocytes seem to play a key role in the pathogenesis of Graves' disease. The thyroid gland is heavily infiltrated with lymphocytes, most of which can be identified as Th1 (helper T cells) lymphocytes, but Th2 and B lymphocytes displaying activation markers, plasma cells, as well as CD8$^+$ T cells and activated macrophages, are also present in the

TABLE 1   Representative Examples of Organ-Specific and Systemic Autoimmune Diseases

Disease	Target tissue	Antibodies mainly against
Organ-specific diseases:		
Graves' disease	Thyroid	TSH receptor
Hashimoto's thyroiditis	Thyroid	Thyroglobulin
Myasthenia gravis	Muscle	Acetylcholine receptors
Pernicious anemia	Gastric parietal cells	Gastric parietal cells IF B12-IF complex
Addison's disease	Adrenals	Adrenal cells microsomal antigen
Insulin-dependent diabetes mellitus	Pancreas	Pancreatic islet cells; insulin
Primary biliary cirrhosis	Liver	Mitochondrial antigens
Autoimmune chronic active hepatitis	Liver	Nuclear antigens, smooth muscle, liver-kidney microsomal antigen, soluble liver antigen, and so on
Autoimmune hemolytic anemia	RBC	RBCs
Idiopathic Thrombocytopenic Purpura	Platelets	Platelets
Systemic diseases:		
Systemic lupus erythematosus	Kidney, skin, lung, brain	Nuclear antigens, microsomes, IgG, and so on
Rheumatoid arthritis	Joints	IgG, nuclear antigens
Sjögren's syndrome	Salivary and lachrymal glands	Nucleolar mitochondria
Goodpasture's syndrome	Lungs, kidneys	Basement membranes

Abbreviations: IF, human leukocyte antigen; IgG, immunoglobulin G; RBC, red blood cell; TSH, thyrotrophic hormone.

thyroid infiltrates. The activated macrophages, together with thyroid endothelial cells, produce IL-6 that seems to promote intra-thyroidal B cell differentiation. Thus, B cells receive sufficient costimulatory signals to differentiate and produce TSI and other autoantibodies and it is believed that the majority of the autoantibody in patients with Graves' is produced in the thyroid. Animal models of thyrotoxicosis have shown dependency on both interferon-γ (IFNγ) and IL-4 production, in what is one of the many examples of diseases that do not show a clear-cut Th1–Th2 dichotomy. The IFN-producing CD4$^+$ and CD8$^+$ T cells in the thyroid tissue express the chemokine receptor CXCR6 indicating that they have been recruited selectively from the periphery. Their critical role is based on the activation of macrophages by IFNγ. Activated macrophages are the most likely cells responsible for the progressive destruction of the thyroid tissue.

Graves' Ophthalmopathy

One of the clinical hallmarks of Graves' disease is exophthalmos (protrusion of the eyeball). Exophthalmos can be unilateral or bilateral and may be associated with proptosis, conjunctivitis and/or periorbital edema. Exophthalmos is secondary to retro-orbital accumulation of fibroblasts, adipocytes, and muscle cells, all of which exhibit TSH receptor antigen to which TSI binds and alters their function.

Clinical Presentation

Graves' disease has its peak incidence in the third to fourth decade and has a female to male ratio of 4–8 : 1. Patients usually present with diffuse goiter and 60% to 70% of patients have ocular disturbances. Symptoms of hyperthyroidism include increased metabolic rate with weight loss, nervousness, weakness, sweating, heat intolerance, and loose stools. Abnormalities on physical examination include diffuse and nontender enlargement of the thyroid, tachycardia, warm and moist skin, tremor, exophthalmos, and pretibial edema.

Diagnosis

The diagnosis is usually investigated on patients with hyperthyroidism, found to have increased levels of thyroid hormones (triiodothyronine, T_3 and thyroxine, T_4) and increased uptake of T_3. The diagnosis is confirmed by demonstration of anti-thyroid receptor antibodies that can be done with two types of assays. Some assays are based on the inhibition of TSH binding by TSI antibodies (TSH-binding inhibition assay), while others are based on the

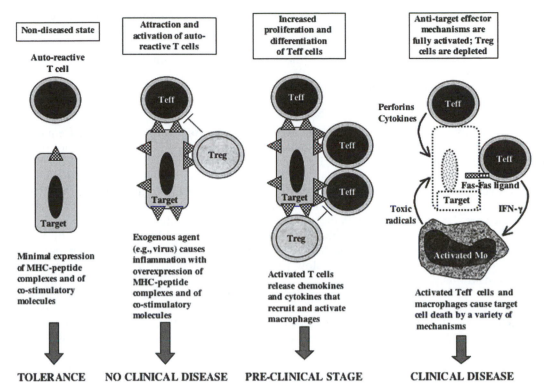

FIGURE 1 Pathogenesis of organ-specific autoimmunity. In normal, tolerant conditions, autoreactive clones remain inactive because the cells expressing the corresponding autoantigens express them in low density and do not provide costimulatory signals. A combination of genetic and environmental factors, such as a viral infection leading to inflammatory changes and activation of accessory cells, might lead to the breaking of self-tolerance and activation of autoreactive T cells. Further inflammation might attract more such cells, for example, if a virus persists or autoantigens are being presented in a chronic manner. The ultimate outcome is determined by the magnitude of the autoreactive response. Many aggressive T cells, such as cytotoxic T lymphocytes (CTL) and Th1 lymphocytes will enhance progression, whereas the presence of (autoreactive) Tregs will dampen inflammation. Penetrance of clinical disease is directly correlated with the amount of target cell (organ) destruction and is determined by this balance of Tregs to pro-inflammatory (Th1) and cytotoxic T cells. The cytotoxic effects on target cells can be directly mediated by activated T effector cells or by activated macrophages. *Abbreviations*: MHC, major histocompatibility complex; Th1, helper T cell; Treg, T regulatory cells. *Source*: Modified from a figure contributed by Dr. Matthias von Herrath, La Jolla CA.

functional consequences of thyroid receptor antibody binding to TSH such as increased adenylate-cyclase activity and increased levels of CyclicAMP (cAMP).

Therapy
Therapy is directed at reducing the thyroid's ability to respond to stimulation by antibodies. This can be achieved surgically, by subtotal thyroidectomy, or pharmacologically, either by administration of radioactive iodine (^{131}I) (which is difficult to dose), or by the use of antithyroid drugs such as propylthiouracil and methimazole, which are useful but slow in their effects.

Hashimoto's Thyroiditis (Autoimmune Thyroiditis)
Hashimoto's thyroiditis is believed to be a consequence of a cell-mediated autoimmune reaction triggered by unknown factors. Several lines of evidence support this conclusion:

1. The inflammatory infiltrate of the thyroid gland shows predominance of activated, lymphokine-secreting T lymphocytes. Numerous plasma cells can also be seen. IL-1 predominates among the cytokines released by activated mononuclear cells, and it has been shown that this cytokine can induce the expression of Fas in thyroid cells, which also

express Fas ligand (FasL). It has been postulated that this dual expression of Fas and FasL sets the stage for exaggerated apoptosis and may explain the slowly progressive decline of thyroid function in these patients.

2. Infusing lymphocytes from sick to healthy laboratory animals can easily transfer thyroiditis.
3. Infants of mothers with active disease carrying IgG antibodies (which cross the placenta) are unaffected.

Whether or not autoantibodies against thyroglobulin and microsomal antigens, frequently detected in those patients, play any pathogenic role is unclear. The main argument supporting their involvement is a good correlation between their titers and disease activity. However, this relationship is also expected if those antibodies arise as a consequence of the activation of helper T cells and presentation of high levels of major histocompatibility complex (MHC)-II/ endogenous peptide complexes to previously tolerant B lymphocytes. Furthermore, these auto-antibodies are detected in low titers in up to 15% of the normal adult female population.

Hashimoto's thyroiditis is the most common form of thyroiditis, and it usually has a chronic evolution. Its incidence peaks during the third to fifth decades, with a female/male ratio of 10:1. It is characterized by a slow progression to hypothyroidism, and symptoms develop insidiously.

The diagnosis is usually confirmed by the detection of anti-thyroglobulin antibodies. Sixty to seventy-five percent of the patients show a positive reaction by passive hemagglutina-tion using thyroglobulin-coated erythrocytes (titers higher than 25, while normal individuals usually have titers up to five). Although, these antibodies are also found in other autoimmune disorders such as pernicious anemia, Sjogrën's syndrome, and in 3% to 18% of normal individuals, the titer of autoantibodies is lower in all other groups with the exception of patients with Sjogrën's syndrome.

In the early stages glucocorticoids may be used as mild immunosuppressants, with the aim of reducing the autoimmune response and extending the asymptomatic phase. When patients develop hypothyroidism, thyroid hormone replacement is indicated.

ADDISON'S DISEASE (CHRONIC PRIMARY HYPOADRENALISM)

Addison's disease can either be caused by exogenous agents (e.g., infection of the adrenals by *Mycobacterium tuberculosis*) or by idiopathic form. The idiopathic form is believed to have an immune basis, since 50% of patients have been found to have antibodies to the microsomes of adrenal cells (as compared to 5% in the general population) by immunofluorescence. The autoantibodies directed against the adrenal react mainly in the zona glomerulosa, zona fasci-culata, and zona reticularis 'and are believed to play the main pathogenic role in this disease, causing its atrophy and loss of function of the adrenal cortex. Biopsy of the adrenal glands shows marked cortical atrophy with an unaltered medulla. Abundant inflammatory mono-nuclear cells are seen between the residual islands of epithelial cells.

The diagnosis is confirmed by demonstration of anti-adrenal antibodies by indirect immunofluorescence in the presence of clinical and laboratory hypoadrenalism.

AUTOIMMUNE POLYGLANDULAR SYNDROMES

Autoimmune polyglandular syndrome (APS)-I is a rare childhood disease with Mendelian recessive inheritance mode. The three major components are chronic mucocutaneous candidia-sis, hypoparathyroidism, and autoimmune Addison's disease. Other endocrine glands may be involved. The entity is also known as autoimmune polyendocrinopathy-candidiasis, ectoder-mal dystrophy. The molecular basis for this entity has been established. These patients lack autoimmune regulator (AIRE), a transcriptional regulator that is believed to control the expression of tissue-specific genes in the thymus. Therefore, autoreactive T cells do not see self-antigens in the thymus and they are not deleted during the negative selection process. The second variant of APS, APS-II, is more common than APS-I and afflicts young adults.

Main features include diabetes and Addison's disease. Some patients may have vitiligo, pernicious anemia celiac disease, and other autoimmune diseases. It is proper, therefore, that patients presenting with diabetes or Addison's disease be screened for other autoimmune diseases.

AUTOIMMUNE DIABETES MELLITUS (TYPE 1A)

Autoimmune diabetes mellitus (DM) is a multi-organ disease with multiple etiologies, and certainly with more than one basic abnormality. The critical defect of type 1A DM (insulin-dependent DM, IDDM) is a decreased to absent production of insulin secondary to β cell destruction. In type 1B diabetes, considerably less frequent than type 1A diabetes, the patients (usually of African, Hispanic, or Asian origin) have permanent insulin deficiency, suffer from episodic ketoacidosis, but lack immunological evidence for β cell autoimmunity. Genetic factors play the key role in this form of diabetes that is strongly inherited, but is not human leukocyte antigen (HLA)-associated. In type 2 diabetes, there is a decrease of the effect of insulin at the target cell level, but pancreatic function is essentially normal. In this chapter, we will limit our discussion to type 1A diabetes, in which autoimmune mechanisms play a key pathogenic role.

Pathogenesis

The original body of evidence on which the concept that the majority of cases of type 1 diabetes are the consequence of an autoimmune disease was based is the detection of many different types of autoantibodies in patients with this disease. These antibodies, however, do not seem to play a major pathogenic role, at least as initial pathogenic insults, but they seem to reflect the intensity of the underlying autoimmune reaction against the islet cell β cells. The autoantibodies can be detected before diabetes becomes clinically evident, and the number of different autoantibodies that are detected seems to be inversely correlated with the length of the disease-free interval in positive individuals.

Autoantibodies
The following are the major types of autoantibodies detected in patients with type 1 diabetes:

1. Anti-islet cell antibodies (ICA) are classically detected by indirect immunofluorescence and react against membrane and cytoplasmic antigens of the islet cells. These antibodies are detected in as many as 90% of type 1 diabetic patients at the time of diagnosis, but they diminish in frequency to 5% to 10% in patients with long-standing DM. Other interesting characteristics of ICA are their isotype distribution, with predominance of subclasses IgG2 and/or IgG4 (which have limited complement activating properties), and their detection months or years before the appearance of clinical symptoms.
2. Antibodies to β cell antigens. The best-characterized islet cell antigens against which antibodies have been demonstrated in type 1 diabetics and individuals predisposed to develop the disease are IA-2α and IA-2β (phogrin), two closely related β cell-associated tyrosine phosphatases. About two-thirds of the patients have antibodies to IA-2α and about 60% of the patients have antibodies to IA-2β. Epitope mapping studies suggest that the immunogenic epitopes are located in the intracytoplasmic segment of these enzymes. Antibodies to glutamic acid decarboxylase are also present in a large proportion of newly diagnosed diabetics (84%).
3. Anti-insulin autoantibodies are responsible for a rare form of diabetes known as insulin autoimmune syndrome, or Hirata's disease, characterized by the combination of fasting hypoglycemia, high concentration of total serum immunoreactive insulin, and presence of autoantibodies to native human insulin in serum. The combination of anti-insulin antibodies with insulin alters the pharmacokinetics and bioavailability of insulin, causing a dissociation between the activity of insulin and blood glucose levels. This disease has been reported in Japan and has no relation with the common form of type 1 diabetes, characterized by permanent insulin deficiency.

Anti-insulin antibodies are detected in as many as 92% of noninsulin-treated patients with type 1 diabetes at the time of diagnosis, but their pathogenic significance is not clear.

Induced anti-insulin antibodies can be found in all diabetic patients treated with insulin. The incidence of these antibodies was greater when bovine or porcine insulin was used. However, anti-human insulin antibodies can also be detected (less frequently) in patients treated with recombinant human insulin, whose tertiary configuration differs from that of the insulin released by the human pancreas. The antibodies directed against therapeutically administered insulin appear to be predominantly of the IgG2 and IgG4 isotypes and may cause insulin resistance, similar to what is observed in Hirata's disease, but in a much milder form.

Cell-Mediated Immunity

Cell-mediated immunity is believed to be the main pathogenic factor causing islet cell damage. One major argument in favor of the involvement of cell-mediated mechanisms is the fact that the pathological hallmark of recent onset diabetes is the mononuclear cell infiltration of the islet cells, known as insulitis. Similar observations can be made in animals with experimentally induced forms of diabetes. The predominant cells in the islet cell infiltrates are T lymphocytes, including both activated $CD4^+$ and $CD8^+$ T lymphocytes. Activated macrophages are also present in the infiltrates. The major pathogenic role seems to be played by $CD4^+$ T cells, with a Th0-Th1 cytokine secreting pattern. Those cells secrete large amounts of IL-2 and IFNγ.

The significance of increased IL-2 secretion may lie in the fact that it causes the upregulation of MHC-II in islet β cells, thus creating favorable conditions for the induction of autoreactive cells. In experimental animal models, this change precedes the development of insulitis. IFN-γ on the other hand, activates macrophages causing the release of cytokines, such as IL-1, IL-12, and toxic radicals. IL-1 has been shown to lead to β cell damage by indirect mechanisms. IL-12 may promote the differentiation and activation of additional Th1 cells as well as the activation of cytotoxic T cells and natural killer cells. Toxic radicals, such as superoxide and nitric oxide, are known to damage islet cells in vitro. Recently, it has been shown that IFN-γ can also activate the synthesis of oxygen active radicals and nitric oxide in β cells. These compounds can react with each other forming peroxinitrate, which is highly toxic. Activated $CD8^+$ cells may also be involved in monocyte activation through the secretion of IFNγ. The main question that remains unanswered is the nature of the epitopes that are recognized by these cells and trigger their activation.

Of crucial importance to our understanding of the pathogenesis of DM is the definition of the insult(s) that may activate autoreactive T lymphocytes and trigger the disease. It is generally accepted that an environmental insult, most likely a viral infection (rubella virus and coxsackie virus B4 have been repeatedly suggested as culprits), plays the initiating role, causing β cell cytotoxicity. Experimental data suggest several possible pathways for the pathogenic effects of viral infections. Infected cells in the pancreas can present viral-derived peptides to the $CD8^+$ cytotoxic T lymphocytes and in this way initiate the immune response. However, experimental studies suggest that this is a rather ineffective pathway, and evidence suggesting the need for activation of accessory cells has been accumulating. One mechanism proposed for such activation would involve the interaction of viral particles with toll-like receptors (TLR), particularly TLR-3. Mononuclear cells activated in this way release IFN-α that can facilitate β-cell destruction either directly or indirectly, upregulating the expression of MHC-I in β cells, thus rendering them more susceptible to T cell-mediated cytotoxicity. Another possible mechanism of activation of accessory cells is the engulfment of dead cells, killed as a consequence of viral replication.

There is suggestive evidence supporting the pathogenic role of viral infections in some patient populations. For example, 12% to 15% of patients with congenital rubella develop type I diabetes, particularly when they are DR3 or DR4 positive. But for the majority of diabetic patients, a link with any given viral infection remains elusive.

Whatever the initial insult to the β cell may be, it can be postulated that damaged β cells are ingested by macrophages, which will express islet-cell derived peptides in association with MHC-II, thus creating conditions for the initiation of an autoimmune T cell response. In addition, macrophages activated as a consequence of phagocytosis, will release cytokines, such as IL-1 and IL-12, which activate T cells. Activated T cells, in turn, will release IFN-γ

which activates macrophages and induces MHC-II expression. The mutual activation of macrophages and T cells results in the development of insulitis, causing persistent β cell destruction through the release of cytokines and toxic compounds and the differentiation of cytotoxic T cells. β-cell death seems to result both from necrosis and apoptosis.

Nature of the Epitopes Recognized by Autoreactive T Cells

The nature of the epitopes recognized by autoreactive T cells is still being investigated but published data suggest that proinsulin, insulin, glutamic acid decarboxylase (GAD), and IA-2α and β are the source of peptides recognized by autoreactive T cells. The overall evidence suggests that the T cell autoimmune response is polyclonal.

Using tetramer technology, autoreactive Th1 lymphocytes recognizing proinsulin and GAD-derived peptides have been found in circulation of at-risk patients, which are also positive for ICA and insulin antibodies. Whether the identification of self-reactive T cells in this patient population has greater prognostic significance is not known.

Genetic Factors

Type 1 DM is a polygenic disease. Eighteen to twenty different chromosomal regions possibly influencing the development of this form of diabetes have been identified. Of those, two have been better characterized.

1. The IDDM1 region, which includes the major histocompatibility complex (MHC) genes determining resistance/susceptibly to diabetes, is considered to be the major genetic determinant of predisposition for the development of diabetes. Several DP and DQ alleles are associated with predisposition or resistance to diabetes (Table 2).
   a. Ninety-five percent of diabetics express DR3 (HLA-DRB1*03) and/or DR4 (HLA-DRB1/04), compared to 42% to 54% of nondiabetics. This corresponds to a relative disease risk of two to five. It has been proposed that this association is due, at least in part, to linkage disequilibrium between DR and DQ.
   b. Several haplotypes that include different DQ and DRB1 alleles are associated with susceptibility or resistance to diabetes. The nomenclature of these haplotypes is complex. Because both alpha and beta chains are polymorphic, alleles have a dual nomenclature indicating to which A and B chains they correspond. For example, the haplotypes HLADRB1*0401-DQA1*0301-DQB1*0302 and HLADRB1*0301-DQA1*0501-DQB1*0201 are associated with a high risk for the development of diabetes. A heterozygous individual expressing both of these haplotypes has a risk of 25% to 40% to develop type 1 diabetes. Other haplotypes seem to be associated with resistance to type 1 diabetes. In Caucasians, resistance is associated with a DQ 3.1 heterodimer (DQA1*0102-DQB1*0602), characterized by the presence of aspartate (a negatively charged amino acid) in position 57 of the β chain (DQB1*0602 allele). The presence

TABLE 2   Insulin-Dependent Diabetes-Related Major Histocompatibility Complex Markers

Markers associated with protection	Markers associated with predisposition
DR2	DR3 (DRB1*0301)[a]
DR5	DR4 (DRB1*0401, 0405)[a]
DQA1*0102-DQB1*0602[b,d]	DQA1*0301-DQB1*302[c,e]
	DQA1*0501-DQB1*0201[e]
	DQA1*0401-DQB1*0402[e]
	DQA1*0101-DQB1*0501[e]

[a]Association secondary to linkage disequilibrium between DR and DQ; Maximal risk in DR3/DR4 heterozygous individuals.
[b]DQ3.1 heterodimer.
[c]DQ8 heterodimer.
[d]Contains an Aspartic acid residue on DQB57; Maximal protection is associated with expression of two aspartate (Asp) 57[+] DQB alleles.
[e]Maximal predisposition is associated either with the expression of two Asp[−]57 alleles of DR3 or DR4 or with the expression of an Asp 57[−], Arg52[+] DQ3.1 heterodimer.

of a neutral amino acid in that same position, as well as the presence of arginine in position 52 of DQα are characteristic of susceptibility alleles Individuals with two susceptibility-determining Asp⁻DQ3.1 alleles have the highest degree of predisposition to develop DM. it is also worth noting that the protection or susceptibility to develop diabetes associated with DQ8 haplotypes (DQB1*0302) is influenced by the DR4 alleles linked to them. In fact, the same DQ8 haplotype can either be protective or not depending on its association with different DR4 alleles (Fig. 2).

2. MHC-I genes associated with predisposition to develop diabetes have also been identified. These MHC-I molecules are believed to be involved in the presentation of "diabetogenic" peptides to $CD8^+$ cells, as supported by the finding of activated $CD8^+$ T cells in the infiltrates surrounding the islets. Two additional sets of genes may play significant roles in determining whether $CD8^+$ T cells are activated or not:

   a. Loci coding for proteasome components, which influence the type of peptides generated from autologous proteins. The generation of endogenous "diabetogenic" peptides, therefore, may depend on the nature of proteasomes.

   b. Loci coding for the synthesis of transport-associated proteins (TAP proteins) responsible for the transport of endogenous peptides to the endoplasmic reticulum, where those peptides become associated with MHC-I peptides.

      i. The Tap genes are located in chromosome 6, near the MHC-region, and may be transmitted in linkage disequilibrium with MHC-II genes.

      ii. One Tap-2 gene allele (Tap-2*0101) is associated with susceptibility to diabetes (relative risk of 3.4) while another has been defined as protective in relation to diabetes.

3. The IDDM2 region has been mapped to a variable number of tandem repeats (VNTR) that flank the insulin gene and the insulin-growth factor II genes on chromosome 11. The VNTR are highly polymorphic and their structure seems to influence the expression of the

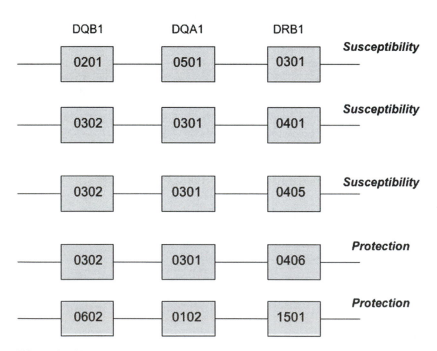

FIGURE 2 Diagrammatic representation of some major histocompatibility complex-II haplotypes associated with susceptibity or protection relative to type 1 diabetes mellitus. DR3 (DRB1*0301) and DR4 (DRB1*04) alleles are commonly associated with suceptibility while the DQ3.1 haplotype containing the DQB1*602 allele is associated with resistance. Note that the effect of the DQ8 haplotype DQA1*0301-DQB1*0302 is closely related to the DRB1 allele linked to it. While the association with DRB1*0405 determines susceptibility to type 1 diabetes, the association with DRB1*0406 determines resistance. *Source*: Modified from Undlien et al. Trends in Genetics 2001; 17:93.

adjacent genes, particularly the insulin gene in the thymus. Those VNTR alleles that are associated with low expression of the insulin gene in the thymus would impair the ability to develop central tolerance to insulin-derived peptides. As a consequence, these alleles would predispose to the development of type I diabetes.

4. Several other regions are linked to diabetes predisposition with variable consistency. These include regions where loci coding for insulin-growth factor-binding proteins (chromosome 2), which appear to be linked with predisposition to develop diabetes, particularly in females and the Cytotoxic T cell late antigen-4 (CTLA4) gene (also in chromosome 2), which is believed to play a significant role in the induction of peripheral tolerance. Recent data suggest that high level of CTLA4 expression is associated with protection from diabetes, the reverse also being true.

How Genetic Factors Influence the Development of Diabetes

Several hypotheses have been advanced to explain how MHC molecules, proteasomes, and TAP proteins influence the development of diabetes, all of them hinging on their ability to generate and present in association with MHC-molecules β cell-derived peptides involved in the elicitation of the autoimmune response resulting in diabetes (diabetogenic peptides). One of the many interpretations that has been put forward as the basis for the MHC-II role in protection or predisposition for type 1 DM is related to the differential ability to bind diabetogenic peptides generated from the ingestion of β cells undergoing spontaneous apoptosis or viral-induced cell death and present them to the immune system. Protective MHC-II molecules would present diabetogenic petides to the immune system, inducing central and/or peripheral tolerance (it is possible that the insulin gene is expressed in thymic cells during differentiation) while predisposing MHC-II molecules would not.

The emergence of IDDM seems to be related to an abnormally low expression of the MHC-II molecules associated to IDDM predisposition by all types of APCs and thymic epithelial cells. Consequently, neither central nor peripheral tolerance will develop and the predisposed individual will retain the ability to react with diabetogenic peptides.

Later on, a viral infection that causes β cell damage and ingestion of damaged cells by APCs, will result in APC activation and upregulated expression of MHC-II molecules whose binding sides may be occupied by diabetogenic peptides generated in the phagolysosomes where the β cell debris are digested. The MHC-II-peptide complexes generated in this way should be expressed with sufficient density as to activate a vigorous CD4$^+$ T cell response from individuals no longer tolerant. Activated CD8$^+$ T cells are also present in the infiltrates surrounding the islets of diabetic patients and diabetic experimental animals. Those cells must be activated by recognizing MHC-I expressed diabetogenic peptides, generated in patients with the proper conjunction of MHC-I molecules, proteasomes, and TAP proteins.

Finally, whether or not an individual carrying predisposing genes develops diabetes or not may depend on whether all the cells necessary to start an active autoimmune response receive the correct activation signals, and on the lack of activation of counter-regulatory cells that otherwise would keep the autoreactive clones in check.

Sequence of Pathogenic Events Leading to the Development of IDDM

Based on our current knowledge of the control of immunological responses and tolerance and on data accumulated from studies of IDDM patients and experimental animal models, the following hypothetical sequence of events leading to the development of IDDM can be proposed. First, one has to admit that autoreactive T cell clones potentially able to be engaged in autoimmunity against pancreatic β cells persist in adult life. In normal conditions, even if the MHC-II molecules associated with predisposition and respective diabetogenic peptides were recognized by self-reactive TcR, their expression in resting APCs unable to deliver co-stimulatory signals would result in tolerogenic or apoptotic signaling of the autoreactive T cells.

A viral infection affecting the β cells or neighboring tissues has the potential to cause the activation of accessory cells and of Th cells involved in the anti-viral response. Those cells will deliver co-stimulatory signals to the autoreactive Th cells, pushing them into a state of activation rather than anergy. Other cytokines will act on β cells, increasing their susceptibility to immune destruction. Thus, IFN-α released by activated accessory cells enhances the expression of MHC-I molecules, while IL-2 and other cytokines released by activated T cells induce the expression of MHC-II and cell adhesion molecules (CAMs).

The activated auto-reactive T cells accumulate in the pancreatic islets and release chemotactic cytokines and IFN-γ, which will attract and activate monocytes/macrophages to the area, where interactions with islet cells overexpressing CAMs will contribute to their fixation in the islets. The activated monocytes/macrophages release cytokines such as IL-1, IL-12, TNF, and toxic compounds such as oxygen active radicals and nitric oxide. The cytokines contribute to the damage by increasing the level of activation of Th1 cells (IL-12), monocytes, and macrophages (IL-1, TNF) In addition, IL-1 and IFN-γ (released by activated Th1 cells) induce the expression of Fas on islet cells. Islet cell death is a consequence of several mechanisms, including Fas–FasL apoptosis signaling and the release of toxic radicals that lead to oxidative changes of cell and organelle membrane lipids.

Immunotherapy

Two main approaches to immunotherapy have been evaluated, one involving the use of immunosuppressants, and the other involving tolerization.

Among immunosuppressants, cyclosporin A received considerable attention in trials with the goal of preventing the full development of type 1A DM. To be effective, immunosuppressive therapy needs to be instituted to recently diagnosed patients with residual β cell function, but the treatment is only effective while cyclosporin A is administered. In the vast majority of cases progression to diabetes is seen soon after immunosuppressive therapy is discontinued.

Induction of tolerance by administration of insulin either by aerosol or by the oral route was investigated. Aerosol administration seems to result in the induction of γ/δ CD8$^+$ T cells that secrete IL-10 and IL-4 and, in experimental animal models, are able to prevent the development of diabetes. Oral administration seems to generate a similar set of γ/δ CD4$^+$ regulatory cells that secrete large amounts of transforming growth factor (TGF)-β in addition to IL-4 and IL-10. However, clinical trials have not shown any evidence of clinical effectiveness of these protocols on children identified at risk of developing type 1A DM.

ACANTHOSIS NIGRICANS

Acanthosis nigricans is a rare syndrome that received its name because of thickening and hyperpigmentation of the skin in the flexural and intertriginous areas, in which patients develop a particularly labile form of diabetes associated with antibodies directed against the insulin receptor. These antibodies block the binding of insulin to the receptor. If the antibodies themselves are devoid of activating properties they induce insulin-resistant diabetes. On the other side, the antibodies may stimulate the insulin receptor and cause hypoglycemia.

The clinical symptoms can be rather variable, depending on the biological properties of the predominant antibody population. Blocking antibodies to the insulin receptor cause hyperglycemia that does not respond to the administration of insulin (insulin-resistant diabetes). In contrast, insulin receptor antibodies with stimulating properties may induce the cellular metabolic effects usually triggered by insulin, albeit in an abnormal and unregulated fashion. The clinical picture is one of hyperinsulinism. The same patient may undergo cycles of predominance of hypo and hyperinsulinism-like symptoms, mimicking an extremely brittle and difficult to control form of diabetes.

AUTOIMMUNE DISEASES OF THE GASTROINTESTINAL TRACT AND LIVER
Pernicious Anemia

Pernicious or megaloblastic anemia is a severe form of anemia secondary to a special type of chronic atrophic gastritis associated with lack of absorption of vitamin B12. Pathologically, the disease is associated with chronic atrophic gastritis and with defective production and/or function of intrinsic factor (IF), which is required for the absorption of vitamin B12. Three types of autoantibodies have been described in patients with this disease:

1. Type I (blocking) antibodies, present in 75% of patients, bind to IF and prevent its binding to vitamin B12.
2. Type II (binding) antibodies react with the IF-vitamin B12 complex and inhibit IF action. The type II antibody is found in 50% of patients, and it does not occur in the absence of antibody I.
3. Type III (parietal canalicular) antibodies, present in the microvilli of the canalicular system of the gastric mucosa, are detected in 85% to 90% of patients and react with the parietal cell, inhibiting the secretion of IF.

Animal Models of Pernicious Anemia

Animal models of pernicious anemia strongly implicate Th1 $CD4^+$ T cells in the pathogenesis of the disease. Autoreactive $CD4^+$ T cell that have escaped thymic selection and recognize gastric epithelial cell antigens (in mice H/K ATPase) home the gastric mucosa, where they secrete cytokines such as IFNγ and IL-10. Macrophages also are present in the early mucosal infiltrates. The action of the effector $CD4^+$ T cells is, under normal conditions, under the control of $CD4^+CD25^+$ Treg cells. Experimental depletion of these cells allows the expression of the disease, whereas their presence blocks the expression of the disease.

In 10% to 15% of patients with pernicious anemia no antibody can be detected with currently available techniques. Other autoimmune diseases such as thyroiditis and Addison's disease are diagnosed with abnormally high frequency in patients with pernicious anemia.

Severe neuropathy and megaloblastic anemia dominate the clinical picture in patients with vitamin B12 deficiency. The development of neuropathy is a consequence of the fact that vitamin B12 is an essential coenzyme for the metabolism of homocysteine, the metabolic precursor of methionine and choline. Choline is required for the synthesis of choline-containing phospholipids, and methionine is also needed for the methylation of basic myelin.

Treatment

Treatment involves intramuscular injection of vitamin B12 that will correct both hematological and neurological manifestations.

Chronic Active Hepatitis

Chronic active hepatitis (CAH) is a disease characterized by persistent hepatic inflammation, necrosis, and fibrosis, which often lead to hepatic insufficiency and cirrhosis. It can be subclassified by its etiology as viral-induced, drug- or chemically-induced, autoimmune, and cryptogenic (cases that do not fit into any of the other groups).

Viral Chronic Active Hepatitis

Viral CAH can be caused by a variety of hepatotropic viruses, namely hepatitis B, C, and D viruses. The liver disease is often accompanied by extrahepatic manifestations suggestive of immune complex disease, such as athralgias, arthritis, skin rash, vasculitis, and glomerulonephritis. These manifestations are believed to result from chronic viral antigen release, eliciting an antibody response and consequent immune complex formation and deposition in different tissues and organs.

Autoimmune Chronic Active Hepatitis

Autoimmune CAH is characterized by the presence of autoantibodies and by lack of evidence of viral infection. Based on the pattern of autoantibodies detected in different patients, CAH can be subclassified into four types. The best-characterized in the classic autoimmune chronic hepatitis (also known as "lupoid hepatitis") is defined by the detection of antinuclear antibodies. The term "lupoid" is used to stress the common feature (i.e., antinuclear antibodies) between this type of CAH and SLE. The antinuclear antibodies in autoimmune CAH are heterogeneous and are not directed against any specific nuclear antigen. In addition, autoantibodies to liver membrane antigens and to smooth muscle are also detected in patients with this type of CAH. The other types of autoimmune chronic active hepatitis are characterized by different patterns of detection of autoantibodies to smooth muscle, liver–kidney microsomal antigens, and soluble liver antigens.

The autoimmune form of CAH affects predominantly young or postmenopausal women. A genetic predisposition is suggested by the strong association with certain MHC-II antigens, particularly HLA-DRB1 alleles of DR3 and DR4. In addition, relatives may suffer from a variety of "autoimmune" diseases, such as thyroiditis, DM, autoimmune hemolytic anemia, and Sjögrën's syndrome. Evidence suggesting a dysregulation of the immune system in these patients includes marked hypergammaglobulinemia and detection of multiple autoantibodies.

Pathogenesis

Liver damage in all forms of CAH is believed to be the result of a cell-mediated immune response against altered hepatocyte membrane antigens. Both circulating and liver-derived lymphocytes from these patients have been shown to be cytotoxic for liver cells in vitro. Antibody-dependent cell-mediated cytotoxicity has also been suggested as playing a pathogenic role.

In the case of viral infections, the expression of viral proteins in the cell membrane of infected cells could be the initiating stimulus for the response. The trigger of most autoimmune forms of CAH remains unknown. In some cases, drugs, particularly α-methyldopa, may play the initiating role. α-methyldopa is believed to modify membrane proteins of a variety of cells and induce immune responses, which cross-react with native membrane proteins and perpetuate the damage, even after the drug has been removed.

The pathogenesis of cryptogenic CAH, in which there is no evidence of viral infection, exposure to drugs known to be associated with CAH, or autoimmune responses, remains unknown. It is possible that most of these cases may have been caused by an undetected viral infection or by exposure to an unsuspected drug or chemical agent.

Diagnosis

Diagnosis of CAH is usually established by liver biopsy. Typically, the biopsy will reveal a picture of "piecemeal necrosis," characterized by marked mononuclear cell infiltration of the periportal spaces and/or paraseptal mesenchymal–parenchymal junctions, often expanding into the lobules. Plasma cells are often prominent in the infiltrate. There is also evidence of hepatocyte necrosis at the periphery of the lobules, with evidence of regeneration and fibrosis. It is believed that this picture reflects an immune attack of the infiltrating lymphocytes directed against the periportal and paraseptal lymphocytes. In one-quarter to one-half of the patients (depending on the study), evidence of postnecrotic cirrhosis is detected; and in some patients, the evolution toward cirrhosis is progressive.

Treatment

Treatment involves administration of glucocorticoids in the autoimmune forms and anti-viral agents in cases associated with viral infection. α-IFN administration seems beneficial for patients with viral CAH, which can complete several months of therapy without severe side effects. In some cases IFN administration is associated with the emergence of anti-nuclear antibodies, which usually disappear after therapy is discontinued, but rarely may evolve toward a complete picture of autoimmune CAH requiring glucocorticoid therapy.

AUTOIMMUNE DISEASES OF THE NEUROMUSCULAR SYSTEMS
Myasthenia Gravis

Myasthenia gravis is a chronic autoimmune disease caused by a disorder of neuromuscular transmission. Two main pathological findings are characteristic of myasthenia gravis: the production of anti-nicotinic-acetylcholine receptor antibodies, detected in 85% to 90% of the patients, and a 70% to 90% reduction in the number of acetylcholine receptors in the neuromuscular junctions.

The reduction in the number of acetylcholine receptors is believed to be due to their destruction by the immune system. This could be a consequence of direct cytotoxicity by complement, opsonization, ADCC, activation of phagocytic cells, or T cell-mediated cytotoxicity. Cell-mediated immunity has been suggested as playing the major pathogenic role due to the lymphocytic infiltration, which is often seen at the neuromuscular junction level, and because blast transformation can be achieved in vitro by stimulating T lymphocytes, isolated from myasthenia gravis patients with acetylcholine receptor protein. However, the lymphocytic infiltrates are not detected in a significant number of patients clinically indistinguishable from those with infiltrates.

Thymic abnormalities are frequent in myasthenia gravis. Seventy percent of the patients have increased numbers of B-cell germinal centers within the thymus, which some authors have suggested to be the source of autoantibodies. About 10% of the patients develop malignant tumors of the thymus (thymomas).

Symptoms

Symptoms of myasthenia gravis include increased muscular fatigue and weakness especially becoming evident with exercise. The diagnosis is confirmed by the finding of anti-acetylcholine receptor antibodies.

Treatment

Treatment is based on the administration of acetylcholinesterase inhibitors, such as neostigmine and pyridostigmine (Mestinon), in combination with atropine. Virtually, complete or partial relief of symptoms can be achieved with medical treatment in a significant number of patients.

Thymectomy

Thymectomy is undertaken with improvement in 75% of patients and with remission in the other 25%, although it may be several months after surgery when clinical improvement starts to be obvious.

Those patients who do not respond to either forms of therapy may be treated with glucocorticoids, which can induce clinical improvement in 60% to 100% of the patients, depending on the series.

Plasmapheresis and Thoracic Duct Drainage

Plasmapheresis and thoracic duct drainage can also be effective by removing circulating antibodies. However, the benefits of this type of therapy are very short-lived, unless the synthesis of autoantibodies is curtailed with glucocorticoids or immunosuppressive drugs.

Multiple Sclerosis

Multiple sclerosis (MS) is an autoimmune disease that results from the destruction of the myelin sheath in the central nervous system (CNS). MS lesions observed at autopsy are characterized by areas of myelin loss surrounding small veins in the deep white matter. A perivenous cuff of inflammatory cells is associated to acute lesions but is absent from old lesions, where gliosis replaces myelin and the oligodendrocytes that produce and support it.

The inflammatory cells found in MS lesions are a mixture of T and B lymphocytes and macrophages (which are known as microglial cells in the CNS). The T lymphocytes are mostly $CD4^+$, express IL-2R and secrete IL-2 and IFN-γ. A smaller proportion of $CD4^+$ lymphocytes produce IL-4 and IL-10, suggesting that Th1 activity predominates over Th2 activity. A few $CD8^+$ lymphocytes are also present in the lesions. Two main lines of evidence support the importance of T lymphocytes in the pathogenesis of MS. First, experimental allergic encephalomyelitis, the best animal model for MS, is transferred by $CD4^+$ T lymphocytes but not by serum. Injection of T cell clones specific for the immunodominant epitope of myelin basic protein (MBP) derived from sick animals is the most efficient protocol to transmit the disease to healthy animals.

Second, MBP-specific CD4 clones can be established from lymphocytes isolated from the spinal fluid of MS patients. These clones generally recognize an epitope located at amino acids 87 to 99 but clones specific for other groups of 12 aminoacids in the MBP molecule and to other myelin components, such as proteolipid protein and myelin associated glycoprotein, are also expanded. Therefore, many different T cell clones with different TcRs appear to be involved in the autoimmune response.

The T cells present in MS lesions are clonally restricted, suggesting a role for autoantigen in the process. Autoreactive cells specific for MBP can be found in the peripheral blood of MS patients. The cell type that is involved is that of Th1 type (IFN γ, TNFα and lymphotoxin), which appears to migrate from the periphery to CNS. The MBP-reactive T cells express a number of chemokines and chemokine receptors, including MCP-1, RANTES, CCR5 and CXCR3, which apparently enable their migration to the CNS. They also express a series of adhesion molecules such as intercellular adhesion molecules-1 and leukocyte function antigen-1 that allow adhesion and inappropriate homing around microglial cells, which, in MS patients, have been found to express adhesion molecules.

MS occurs mostly in young adults between the ages of 16 and 40 with a three to one female predominance. As in many other autoimmune diseases, the role of genetic factors was suggested by the finding that some HLA alleles are overrepresented among MS patients, particularly HLA-DR2 and HLA- DQ1, which are found in up to 70% of the patients. These class-II MHC molecules are likely to be involved in peptide presentation to CD4$^+$ lymphocytes. It has been demonstrated that normal individuals have myelin specific T cells in their blood, suggesting that MBP-specific T lymphocytes are not deleted during differentiation, probably because myelin antigens are not expressed in the thymus. However, many of the normal individuals having myelin specific T cells in their blood do not develop MS, even when they express HLA-DR2. Thus, in normal individuals these clones remain in a state of anergy or tolerance.

Very little is known about what activates previously tolerant MBP-specific clones and other autoreactive clones involved in MS. Viral infections have been proposed as the trigger for MS, perhaps as a consequence of molecular mimicry. In fact, many viral antigens from Corona viruses, Epstein-Barr virus, Hepatitis B virus, Herpes Simplex virus, and others, have sequences identical to MBP epitopes. Consequently, the immune response to the virus would activate a set of T cells whose TcR would cross-react with MBP peptides. Another possibility is that a viral superantigen could accidentally activate an MBP specific T lymphocyte, and cause its expansion.

In any case, autoreactive T lymphocytes, by themselves, are incapable of damaging the myelin sheath. However, autoreactive T lymphocytes secrete IFN-γ that activates the macrophages found in the lesions. Some of these activated macrophages are seen attached to the myelin sheath that they actively strip and phagocytose, becoming lipid laden. In addition, once they have engulfed myelin, they present myelin-derived antigens to T cells, contributing to the perpetuation of the immune reaction.

Clinical Manifestations

Frequent symptoms at diagnosis include visual abnormalities, abnormal reflexes, sensory, and motor abnormalities. This variety of manifestations reflects the fact that lesions can occur any-where in the white matter of the brain, cerebellum, pons, or spinal cord, at any time. The multiplicity and progression (both in number and extent) of MS lesions is the major clinical diagnostic criterion for this disease.

The course of MS is characterized by relapses and remissions in about 60% of the patients, but each new attack may bring additional deficits when the myelin sheaths are incompletely or imperfectly replaced. Frequently, after 5 to 15 years of evolution, these patients enter a phase of relentless chronic progression and become wheelchair bound, bedridden, and totally dependent for all activities of daily living. In the remaining 40% of the cases MS is chronic, progressive from onset.

The diagnosis of MS may be assisted by magnetic resonance imaging (MRI), which demonstrates breakdown of the blood–brain barrier that is always present at the beginning of a new attack and spinal fluid electrophoresis, which may detect oligoclonal bands (multiple electrophoretically homogeneous bands) of IgG in the spinal fluid.

Treatment

The treatment of MS is not satisfactory. Glucocorticoids have been used extensively during the past 20 years. Usually, high doses are required (to seal the blood-brain barrier), not suitable for long-term administration. In addition, glucocorticoid administration does not affect significantly disease progression.

Recombinant IFN β b and the closely related IFN β1a are recommended for the treatment of relapsing–remitting MS. These IFNs act by downregulating IFN-γ production and class-II expression on APC. IFN β administration has been shown to slow down the progression of MS.

Copolymer-1 (Cop-1, Copaxone), a synthetic basic copolymer of four amino acids designed to resemble MBP epitopes, without the ability to induce T cell proliferation, has been used with some success. Administration of this product reduces the frequency of relapses of MS, lessens disease activity as measured by MRI, and can induce neurological improvement. Two mechanisms of action have been proposed for Copaxone based on studies carried out in experimental animals:

1. Cop-1 is a TCR antagonist of the immunodominant 82 to 100 epitope of MBP, thus turning off the immune response to MBP.
2. Oral Copaxone administration may lead to a tolerant state by down regulating T cell immune responses to MBP. This effect is supposed to be mediated by IL-10–secreting Treg lymphocytes.

In humans, administration of Copaxone is associated with an elevation of serum IL-10 levels and profound changes in T lymphocyte activity, including suppression of TNF mRNA and elevation of TGF-β and IL-4 mRNA. These results suggest that Copaxone may induce a shift from Th1 to a Treg cytokine profile, possibly associated with bystander suppression of the autoreactive immune response.

AUTOIMMUNE DISEASES OF THE BLOOD CELLS

Virtually, all types of blood cells can be affected by autoantibodies. Autoimmune hemolytic anemia is discussed in detail in Chapter 22.

Autoimmune Neutropenia

The reduction of the total number of neutrophils is the most frequent cause of infection due to defective phagocytosis. Although there are congenital forms of neutropenia of variable severity, most frequently neutropenia is secondary to a variety of causes, particularly iatrogenic (administration of cytotoxic dugs is the most frequent cause). Autoimmune neutropenia can be seen in patients with RA, usually in association with splenomegaly (Felty's Syndrome).

Idiopathic Thrombocytopenic Purpura

Idiopathic thrombocytopenic purpura (ITP) is an autoimmune disease related to low platelet counts (thrombocytopenia). The low platelet counts result from a shortened platelet half-life caused by anti-platelet antibodies, which cannot be compensated by increased release of platelets from the bone marrow.

Anti-platelet autoantibodies have been detected in 60% to 70% of patients with the "immunoinjury" technique that relies on the release of platelet factors, such as serotonin, following exposure to sera containing such antibodies. Competitive binding assays and antiglobulin assays can also be used to demonstrate anti-platelet antibodies.

Clinical Presentation

ITP can present itself as an acute or a chronic form. Acute ITP is due to the formation of immune complexes containing viral antigens that become adsorbed to the platelets or to the production of anti-viral antibodies that cross-react with platelets. Platelet destruction can be due to irreversible aggregation caused by immune complexes, or when anti-platelet antibodies are involved, to complement-induced lysis or phagocytosis.

Chronic ITP is caused by autoantibodies that react with platelets and lead to their destruction by phagocytosis. Clinically, ITP is characterized by easy and exaggerated bleeding mucosal and subcutaneous bleeding secondary to thrombocytopenia.

The acute forms of ITP are seen mainly in children, often in the phase of recovery after a viral exanthem or an upper respiratory infection, and are usually self-limited. In contrast, chronic ITP is an adult disease, often associated with other autoimmune diseases. The bone marrow is usually normal, but in some cases an increase in megakaryocytes may be seen, representing an attempt to compensate for the excessive destruction in the peripheral blood. The spleen may be enlarged due to platelet sequestration by phagocytic cells.

Treatment

The treatment of ITP can be surgical or medical. Splenectomy is usually reserved for patients in whom the spleen is the major site for platelet sequestration and destruction. The removal of the spleen is often associated with prolonged platelet survival. Glucocorticoids have been used in cases in which splenectomy is not indicated or has not been beneficial. However, the efficiency of glucocorticoids in severe cases of ITP is questionable.

Intravenous Gammaglobulin

Intravenous gammaglobulin (IVIg) has become the therapy of choice. Its administration is associated with a prolongation of platelet survival and improvement in platelet counts. Several mechanisms have been proposed to explain this effect of IVIg in ITP:

1. Competition with immune complexes for the binding to platelets (immune complexes would cause irreversible aggregation or complement-mediated cytolysis, while IVIg would not)
2. Blocking of Fc receptors in phagocytic cells, which would inhibit the ingestion and destruction of antibody-coated platelets (for which there is experimental documentation). This mechanism is most likely to explain the rapid increase in platelet counts, seen after therapy with IVIg is initiated.
3. The long-term, beneficial effects of IVIg administration are apparently a consequence of the downregulation of autoreactive B cells caused coligation of membrane immunoglobulins (by anti-idiotypic antibodies reactive with the mIg of autoreactive B cells) and FcIIγR (by the Fc region of partially denatured IgG contained in IVIg). This coligation is believed to even be able to induce B cell apoptosis. The end result is a decrease of the titers of antiplatelet antibodies.
4. Scavenging of complement fragments produced during complement activation, including C4b, C3b, and the anaphylotoxins C3a and C5a, has also been proposed as a mechanism of action of IVIg.

BIBLIOGRAPHY

Arnason BG. Immunologic therapy of multiple sclerosis. Ann Rev Med 1999; 50:291.
Amrani A, Verdaguer J, Thiessen S, et al. IL-1α, IL-1β and IFN-γ mark β cells for Fas-dependent destruction by diabetogenic CD4+ T lymphocytes. J clin Invest 2000; 105:459.
Bach JF. A toll-like trigger for autoimmune diseases. Nat Med 2005; 11:120.
Basta M, Van Goor F, Luccioli S, et al. F(ab)'2-mediated neutralization of C3a and C5a anaphylatoxins: a novel effector function of immunoglobulins. Nat Med 2003; 9:431–438.
Eisenbarth GS, ed. Immunology of Diabetes, 2nd ed. Adv Exp Med Biol 2004; 552:1–335.
Eisenbarth GS. Type 1 diabetes: molecular, cellular and clinical immunology. Adv Exp Med Biol 2004; 552:306–310.
Green EA, Flavell RA. The initiation of autoimmune diabetes. Curr Opin Immunol 1999; 11:663.
Kelly MA, Rayner ML, Mijovic CH, Barnett AH. Molecular aspects of type 1 diabetes. Mol Pathol 2003; 56:1–10.
Koelman BPC, Lie BA, Undlien DE, et al. Genotype effects and epistasis in type 1 diabetes and HLA-DQ trans dimer associations with disease. Genes Immun 2004; 5:381–388.
Lemark A. Selecting culprits in β-cell killing. J clin Invest 1999; 104:1487.
Lindstrom J, Shelton D, Fujii Y. Myasthenia gravis. Adv Immunol 1988; 42:233.
McDougall IR. Graves' disease. Current concepts. Med Clin North Am 1991; 75:79.

Nakayama M, Abiru N, Moriyama H, et al. Prime role for an insulin epitope in the development of type 1 diabetes in NOD mice. Nature 2005; 435(7039):220–223.

Rapoport B. Pathophysiology of Hashimoto's thyroiditis and hypothyroidism. Ann Rev Med 1991; 42:91.

Redondo MJ, Fain PR, Eisenbarth GS. Genetics of type 1A diabetes. Recent Prog Horm Res 2001; 56:69–89.

Undlien DJ, Lie BA, Thorsby E. HLA complex genes in type 1 diabetes and other autoimmune diseases. Which genes are involved? Trends Genet 2001; 17:93–100.

von Herrath M, Tsokos GC. Animal models of autoimmune disease. In: Rose NR, Mackay IR, eds. The Autoimmune Diseases. 4th ed. Mosby, 2005.

Wong FS, Karttunen J, Dumont C, et al. Identification of an MHC class-I restricted autoantigen in type 1 diabetes by screening an organ-specific cDNA library. Nat Med 1999; 5:1026.

18 | Systemic Lupus Erythematosus

George C. Tsokos
Beth Israel Deaconess Medical Center, Harvard Medical School, Boston, Massachusetts, U.S.A.

INTRODUCTION

Systemic lupus erythematosus (SLE) is a generalized autoimmune disorder associated with multiple cellular and humoral immune abnormalities and protean clinical manifestations. It is most common in females of childbearing age.

CLINICAL MANIFESTATIONS

The clinical expression of SLE varies among different patients. The kind of organ (vital vs. non-vital) that becomes involved determines the seriousness and the overall prognosis of the disease. The average frequency of some main clinical manifestations of SLE that may be observed during the entire course of SLE is shown in Table 1.

Diagnosis

The diagnosis is based on the verification that any four of the clinical and/or laboratory manifestations that listed in Table 2 are present simultaneously or serially during a period of observation.

Course

Exacerbations and remissions, heralded by the appearance of new manifestations and worsening of pre-existing symptoms, give the disease its fluctuating natural history. Although high levels of autoantibodies and low levels of serum complement (C3, C4) may accompany clinical disease activity, there is no laboratory marker as of yet that can reliably predict an upcoming flare.

Overlap Syndromes

Occasionally, physicians observe clinical situations in which the differentiation between SLE and another connective tissue disease is difficult. In some patients, the distinction may be impossible, and are classified as having an overlap syndrome. This syndrome represents the association of SLE with another disorder such as scleroderma or rheumatoid arthritis. On the other hand, some patients have symptoms and laboratory findings that are reminiscent of lupus; yet, a formal diagnosis (defined by the criteria listed in Table 2) cannot be made. Patients who take certain drugs (hydralazine, procainamide, etc.) may present with incomplete picture of lupus known as drug-induced lupus. Other patients may present with an incomplete picture of lupus that may remain stable over a period of years or evolve with the appearance of additional manifestations.

IMMUNOLOGICAL ABNORMALITIES IN SYSTEMIC LUPUS ERYTHEMATOSUS
Autoantibodies

The lupus erythematosus (LE) cell is a peculiar-looking polymorphonuclear leukocyte, which has ingested nuclear material. It is possible to reproduce this phenomenon in vitro by incubating normal neutrophils with damaged leukocytes, preincubated with sera obtained from SLE patients. Investigations concerning the nature of this phenomenon led to the discovery of

TABLE 1   Main Clinical Manifestations of Sytemic Lupus Erythematosus

Manifestation	% of patients
Musculoarticular	95
Renal disease	60
Pulmonary disease (pleurisy, pneumonitis)	60
Cutaneous disease (photosensitivity, alopecia, etc.)	80
Cardiac disease (pericarditis, endocarditis)	20
Fever of unknown origin	80
Gastrointestinal disease (hepatomegaly, ascites, etc.)	45
Hematologic/Reticuloendothelial (anemia, leukopenia, splenomegaly)	85
Neuropsychiatric (organic brain syndrome seizures, peripheral neuropathy, etc.)	20

antibodies directed against nuclear antigens can promote the formation of LE cells, and subsequently to the definition of a heterogeneous group of antinuclear antibodies (ANAs).

Antinuclear Antibodies

ANAs are detected by indirect immunofluorescence using a variety of tissues and cell lines as substrates. A positive result is indicated by the observation of nuclear fluorescence after incubating the cells with the patient's serum and, after thorough washing to remove unbound immunoglobulins (Igs), with an anti-human Ig serum labeled with fluorochrome. Four patterns of fluorescence can be seen, indicating different types of ANAs (Table 3). The test for ANAs is not very specific, but is very sensitive. A negative result virtually excludes the diagnosis of SLE (95% of patients with SLE are ANA positive), while high titers are strongly suggestive of SLE but not confirmatory. ANAs can be detected in other conditions including other systemic autoimmune/collagen diseases and chronic infections as well as in normal individuals, albeit in low titers.

DNA Antibodies

DNA Antibodies are the most important in SLE. They can react with single stranded DNA (ssDNA) or with double stranded DNA (dsDNA). Two-thirds of patients with SLE have circulating anti-DNA antibodies. Although anti-ssDNA may be found in many diseases besides SLE, anti-dsDNA antibodies are found almost exclusively in SLE (40–60% of the patients). Most commonly they are detected by immunofluorescence, using as a substrate a noninfectious flagellate, *Crithidia lucilliae*, which has a kinetoplast packed with double-stranded DNA (see Chapter 15). This test is very specific, and the antibodies can be semiquantitated by titration of the serum (to determine the highest serum dilution associated with visible fluorescence of the kinetoplast after addition of a fluorescent-labeled anti-IgG antibody). Most laboratories nowadays use enzyme-linked immunosorbent assay (ELISAs) to detect DNA antibodies.

TABLE 2   Diagnostic Features of Systemic Lupus Erythematosus[a]

Facial erythema (butterfly rash)
Discoid lupus
Photosensitivity
Oral or nasopharyngeal ulcers
Arthritis without deformity
Pleuritis, or pericarditis
Psychosis, or seizures
Hemolytic anemia, leukopenia, lymphopenia, or thrombocytopenia
Heavy proteinuria, or cellular casts in the urinary sediment
Positive lupus erythematosus cell preparation, positive anti-dsDNA, anti-Sm antibodies, false positive syphilis serology, and positive anti-cardiolipin antibodies
Antinuclear antibody

[a]Established by the American College of Rheumatologists.

TABLE 3 Immunofluorescence Patterns of Antinuclear Antibodies

Pattern	Antigen	Disease association(s)
Peripheral	Double-stranded DNA	SLE
Homogeneous	DNA-histone complexes	SLE and other connective tissue diseases
Speckled	Non-DNA nuclear antigens	
	Sm	SLE
	Ribonucleoprotein	Mixed connective tissue disease, SLE, scleroderma, etc.
	SS-A, SS-B	Sjögren's disease
Nucleolar	Nucleolus-specific RNA	Scleroderma

Abbreviations: SLE, systemic lupus erythematosus; SS, Sjögren's syndrome.

Antibodies to the DNA–Histone Complex

Antibodies to the DNA–histone complex are present in over 65% of patients with SLE. The use of ELISA has permitted the identification of antibodies to all histone proteins including H1, H2A, H2B, H3, and H4. Anti-histone antibodies are also present in patients with drug-induced SLE, most frequently associated with hydralazine and procainamide treatment.

Antibodies to Non-Histone Proteins

Antibodies to non-histone proteins that have been characterized best include:

1. Anti-Sm: Antibodies to the Sm (Smith) antigen are present in one-third of patients with SLE but not in other conditions. The antigenic determinant is on a protein that is conjugated to one of six different small nuclear RNAs(snRNA).
2. Anti-U1-RNP: The antigenic epitope is on a protein conjugated to U1-RNA. Antibodies to this antigen are present in the majority of patients with SLE and mixed connective tissue disease, which represents an overlap syndrome.
3. Anti-Sjogren's syndrome-A/Ro (Anti-SS-A/Ro): These antibodies are present in one-third of patients with SLE and two-thirds of patients with Sjogren's syndrome (SS). Antibodies to the Ro antigen is frequently found in patients with SLE who are ANA-negative. Babies born to mothers with Ro antibodies may have heart block, leukopenia, and/or skin rash.
4. Anti-Sjogren's syndrome-B/La (Anti-SS-B/La): The antigenic epitope recognized by this antibody is on a 43°kDa protein conjugated to RNA. Antibodies to La antigen are present in about one-third of patients with SLE and in approximately one-half of the patients with SS.

Cardiolipin and Phospholipid Antibodies

Patients with SLE frequently have anti-phospholipid antibodies and anti-cardiolipin antibodies. The anti-cardiolipin antibodies recognize a cryptic epitope on β2-glycoprotein I, that is exposed after it binds to anionic phospholipids. A related group of antibodies are the phospholipid antibodies that react with phospholipids and are apparently implicated as one of the causes of clotting disorders in SLE.

Lupus Anticoagulant

Lupus anticoagulant is detected by prolongation of in vitro clotting assays. It represents a major form of anti-phospholipid antibodies with some overlap with the ELISA-detected anti-phospholipid antibodies.

Pathogenic Role of Autoantibodies in Systemic Lupus Erythematosus

There are three groups of autoantibodies. Those that have not been assigned a role in pathogenesis and are not helpful in diagnosis; those that are helpful in diagnosis or are associated with a particular clinical manifestation but they have not been shown to cause certain pathology (Sm antibody); and those that cause, or at least initiate, a pathologic process (anti-erythrocytic antibody causes red cell destruction). Increasingly though, antibodies are assigned new roles such as entering live cells and altering cell biochemistry, binding cell surface membranes and altering cell function, binding to cells that have already been stressed or injured, and activating complement.

Anti-T Cell Antibodies

Anti-T cell Antibodies are believed to bind and eliminate certain subsets of T cells (suppressor-inducer). As a consequence, the normal negative feedback circuits controlling B-cell activity may not be operational, explaining the uncontrolled production of autoantibodies by the B cells. Also, T cell antibodies may alter the function of T cells; for example, they cause decreased production of IL-2.

Anitbodies Against Complement Receptor 1 and C3 Convertase

Antibodies against complement receptor 1 (CR1) and against the C3 convertase are occasionally detected. CR1 antibodies may block the receptor and interfere with the clearance of immune complexes (CI). Antibodies to the C3 convertase, by stimulating its function, may contribute to increased C3 consumption.

Anti-red cell antibodies and anti-platelet antibodies are the cause, respectively, of hemolytic anemia and thrombocytopenia.

Autoantibodies directed against central nervous system antigens may be detected in the serum and the cerebrospinal fluid of patients with SLE who have CNS involvement and have also been considered, but not proven, pathogenic.

Anti-DNA Antibodies

DNA antibodies form immune complexes (IC) by reacting with DNA and are implicated in the pathogenesis of glomerulonephritis (see below).

Cardiolipin Antibodies, Phospholipid Antibodies, and Lupus Anticoagulant

Cardiolipin antibodies, phospholipid antibodies, and lupus anticoagulant are detected frequently in SLE patients. The cardiolipin antibodies cause false positivity in serological tests for syphilis. Cardiolipin and phospholipid antibodies are also associated with miscarriages, thrombophlebitis and thrombocytopenia, and various CNS manifestations, secondary to vascular thrombosis. The constellation of these symptoms is known as anti-phospholipid antibody syndrome and although it was first recognized in lupus patients, the majority of the cases do not fulfill the diagnostic criteria for SLE.

Anti-Ro Antibodies

Ro antibodies, when present in mothers with SLE, seem associated with the development of heart block in their babies. Ro antibodies may interfere with the electrophysiology of the cells involved with the conductance within the heart.

Diagnostic Value of Autoantibodies

Some autoantibodies may not be linked with any specific clinical manifestations but are very useful as disease markers. For example, dsDNA and Sm antibodies are diagnostic of SLE. Most other autoantibodies are present in more than one clinical disease or syndrome.

PATHOGENESIS OF SYSTEMIC LUPUS ERYTHEMATOSUS

Multiple environmental, hormonal, genetic, and immunoregulatory factors are involved in the expression of the disease. In any given patient, different factors contribute variably to the expression of the disease.

Genetic Factors

The understanding of the pathogenic mechanisms underlying the progression of SLE has been facilitated by the discovery of spontaneously occurring disease in mice that resembles SLE in many respects. During the inbreeding of mice, it was observed that the F1 (first generation) hybrids obtained by mating white and black mice from New Zealand [(NZBxNZW) F1] spontaneously developed a systemic autoimmune disease, involving a variety of organs and systems. Throughout the course of their disease, the mice develop hypergammaglobulinemia, reflecting a state of hyperactivation of the humoral immune system. The animals have a variety of autoantibodies and manifestations of autoimmune disease and IC disease similar to those seen in humans with SLE. As the disease progresses, they develop nephritis and lymphoproliferative disorders and die.

The importance of genetic factors in the development of disease in NZB mice is underlined by the observation that the parental NZB mice have a mild form of the disease manifested by autoimmune hemolytic anemia, but that the introduction of the NZW genetic background causes the disease to appear earlier and in severe form. Genetic linkage studies and microsatelite gene marker analysis indicate that many of the immunologic abnormalities are under multigenic control, one gene(s) controlling the animal's ability to produce anti-DNA antibodies, another the presence of anti-erythrocyte antibodies, and still other genes controlling high levels of IgM production and lymphocytic proliferation.

Two other mouse strains that develop a SLE-like disease spontaneously have been identified: MRL *lpr/lpr* and MRL *gld*. The first strain has a defect in the Fas gene, whereas the second has a defect in the Fas ligand gene. The products of these two genes are responsible for programmed cell death, also known as apoptosis, which is critical for the control of undesirable immune responses. Only rare patients with lupus have structural defects of the Fas/Fas ligand proteins.

Several pieces of evidence indicate that genetic factors also play a role in the pathogenesis of human SLE. Serum DNA and T cell antibodies as well as cellular abnormalities are present in healthy relatives of lupus patients. There is moderate degree of clinical disease concordance among monozygotic twins. The fact that the clinical concordance between twins is only moderate strongly indicates that genetic factors alone may not lead to the expression of the disease and that other factors are needed. The genes, which could play a role, probably in synergy with environmental factors, have not been identified. Current evidence indicates that in humans, as in mice, these genes are probably linked to the major histocompatibility complex (MHC). For example, the human leukocyte antigen-DR2 (HLA-DR2) haplotype is over-represented in patients with SLE. Also, as mentioned before, an SLE-like disease develops frequently in individuals with C4 and C2 deficiencies (C4 and C2 genes are located in chromosome 6, in close proximity to the MHC genes). Also, individuals lacking C1q are also prone in developing lupus. Recently, genome-wide searches for "lupus" genes have been undertaken. These studies have reported various genome areas to be associated with lupus. Interestingly, many of these areas are found in 6p and 1q.

Immune Response Abnormalities

SLE is a disease associated with profound immunoregulatory abnormalities, affecting both humoral and cellular responses.

B-Cell Abnormalities

Increased numbers of B cells and plasma cells are detected in the bone marrow and peripheral lymphoid tissues secreting Igs spontaneously. The hyperactive status of B cells and plasma cells in SLE seems to result from several factors (Fig. 1).

Signals derived from the occupation of B-cell receptors (BCR, sIgM or sIgD) lead to significantly enhanced production of tyrosine-phosphorylated cellular proteins and to increased formation of inositol triphosphate, when compared to B-cell responses from either normal or disease-control individuals. These events are followed by a significantly increased free Ca^{2+} flux in the cytoplasm, which is contributed primarily by the intracellular calcium stores (Fig. 2). Thus, the responses are more vigorous than normal. In addition, the modulation of B-cell responses by costimulatory molecules is also abnormal. The coactivation signals derived from the occupation of complement receptor type 2 (CR2, a complex of CD21, CD19, and CD81) and the lowering of the threshold of B-cell activation secondary to the cross-linking

Health   **Disease**

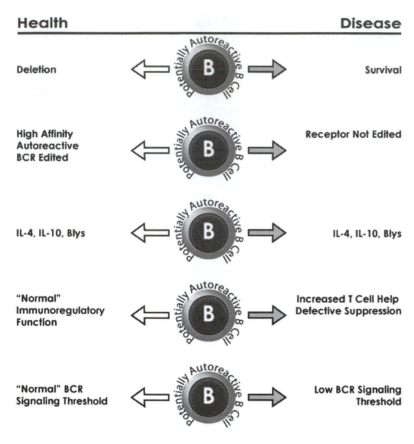

FIGURE 1   Diagrammatic summary of B cell abnormalities associated with systemic lupus erythematosus.

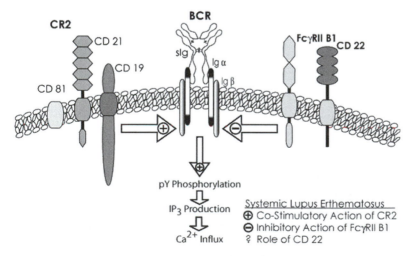

FIGURE 2   An outline of the antigen receptor-mediated signal transduction aberrations encountered in lupus B-cells, and possible contributions from B-cell surface coreceptors. Signals derived from B-cell receptor occupancy are significantly enhanced, due to enhanced activity of complement receptor-2 and defective activity of the negative regulatory coreceptor FcγRIIB1. This results in enhanced phosphorylation of signaling proteins and increased free Ca2+ flux in the cytoplasm. The end result is B-cell hyper-reactivity to antigen stimulation. *Source*: Modified from Liossis SNC, Tsokos GC. B cell abnormalities in systemic lupus erythematosus. 7th ed. In: Wallace DJ, Hahn BH, eds. Dubois' Lupus Erythematosus. Baltimore, Maryland: Lippincott Williams and Wilkins, 2006.

of CR2 and BCR (which co-cross linking are enhanced in SLE, as a consequence of the abundance of circulating CR2 ligands (C3d, C3dg, and iC3d). On the other hand, feedback mechanisms believed to assist in the down regulation of B-cell responses appear to be deficient in SLE. Normally, the B-cell FcγRIIB1 coreceptor causes an early termination of B-cell receptor-initiated signals when co-cross linked with sIg (i.e., when antigen is presented to B cells in the form of IC). In SLE, the function of Fc receptors is defective, and this down-regulating effect is depressed.

The number of activated B-cells and plasma cells correlates with disease activity. Only a limited number of light and heavy chain genes are used by autoantibodies, demonstrating that the autoantibody response involves only a few of all B-cell clones available. Furthermore, the changes appearing in their sequence over time strongly suggest that they undergo affinity maturation, a process that requires T cell help. It also suggests that a few antigens drive the response.

Immunosuppressive drug treatment of both murine and human lupus causes clinical improvement associated with decreased B-cell activity. Any infection that induces B-cell activation is likely to cause a clinical relapse in patients with inactive SLE.

T Cell Abnormalities

From our knowledge of the biology of the immune response, it can be assumed that the production of high titers of IgG anti-dsDNA antibodies in patients with SLE must depend upon excessive T cell help and/or insufficient control by regulatory T cells. Support to this theory is provided by the following observations:

1. In both human and murine lupus, a new subset of CD3$^+$ cells that express neither CD4 nor CD8 has been found to provide help to autologous B-cells synthesizing DNA antibodies.
2. The finding of anti-T cell antibodies in the serum of (NZBxNZW) F1 mice and in the sera of humans with SLE raised the possibility that the deletion of a specific subset of regulatory cells could contribute to the inordinate B-cell activity associated with the development of autoimmunity.
3. In humans, the anti-T cell antibodies are also responsible for the lymphopenia that is frequently seen in patients with SLE. This lymphopenia is often associated with findings suggestive of a generalized depression of cell-mediated immunity, such as decreased lymphokine production (IL-1 and IL-2) and lack of reactivity (anergy) both in vivo and in vitro to common recall antigens, particularly during active phases of human SLE. The impairment of cell-mediated immunity may explain the increased risk of viral and opportunistic infections in patients with SLE.
4. Extensive deletions in the T cell repertoire have been found in NZW mice, in which the Cβ2 and Dβ2 genes of the T cell antigen receptor are missing. These deletions could be associated with a faulty establishment of tolerance to self-MHC during intrathymic ontogeny.
5. In humans, restriction fragment length polymorphism studies of the constant region of the T cell receptor (TcR) demonstrated an association between TcRα chain polymorphism and SLE and TcRβ chain polymorphism, and production of anti-Ro antibodies. More recently, sequence information of the TcR chains of pathogenic human T cell clones demonstrated bias in the T cell repertoire selection process.

Dendritic Cell Abnormalities

Plasmacytoid dendritic cells may present autoantigen to T and B-cells at increased rates in patients with SLE. Interferon$-\alpha$ and circulating IC (acting through Fc receptors and Toll-like receptor 9) stimulate dendritic cell function in SLE.

Immune Complexes in Systemic Lupus Erythematosus

The pathogenic role of IC in SLE has been well established. As summarized in Figure 3, this pathogenic role is a result of a variety of abnormal circumstances. First, marked elevations in the levels of circulating IC can be detected in patients with SLE sera during acute episodes of the disease by a variety of techniques (see Chapter 25). Since patients with active SLE have

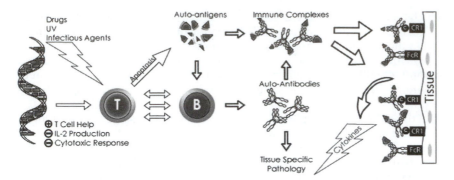

FIGURE 3 Diagrammatic overview of the pathogenesis of systemic lupus erythematosus: multiple genetic, environmental, and hormonal factors influence the function of T and B-lymphocytes. T cells display a wide spectrum of abnormalities including decreased cytotoxic responses and increased ability to help B-cells to produce antibodies. Lupus B-cells with the help of T cells produce autoantibodies that bind to autoantigens found on cells and tissues and others released in the circulation by apoptotic cells. The resulting immune complexes are not cleared effectively because, besides the fact that they are produced at increased rates, the receptors that are responsible for their clearance, that is, Fc and complement receptors are deficient either in numbers or in function. Once deposited in tissues, IC initiate a cascade that eventually results in tissue injury (see Chapter 23).

high levels of free circulating DNA and most have also DNA antibodies, DNA-anti-DNA IC are likely to be formed either in circulation or in collagen-rich tissues and structures such as the glomerular basement membrane, which have avidity for DNA. Besides the fact that IC are formed at increased rates in patients with SLE, the clearance rate of circulating IC is decreased, as a consequence of several factors.

1. IC are cleared by the Fc receptor bearing cells of the reticuloendothelial system. Many patients with lupus nephritis have alleles of Fc receptors that bind IgG with less avidity. This results in slower immune complex clearance.
2. IC often have adsorbed complement components and split products, including C3b, which reacts with CR1. Consequently, IC are transported to the reticuloendothelial system by red blood cells, which bind them through their CR1. Patients with SLE have decreased numbers of CR1, a fact that may compromise the clearance of IC and contribute to the development of IC-induced inflammatory reactions.
3. IC are partially solubilized as a consequence of complement activation, a process that contributes to their inactivation and clearance. Individuals with C4 deficiency develop a disease with clinical features resembling those of SLE. This observation can be explained by the fact that IC are cleared at slower rates in C4-deficient individuals, perhaps due to the role of C4 fragments in the solubilization and clearance of circulating IC.

The proinflammatory properties of IC in SLE are suggested by a variety of observations. First, rising levels of DNA antibodies in conjunction with falling serum C3 levels (reflecting consumption by antigen–antibody complexes) are associated with disease flares. Second, patients with IgG1 and IgG3 (complement fixing) DNA antibodies develop lupus nephritis more frequently than those patients in whom DNA antibodies are of other isotypes do. Glomerulonephritis, cutaneous vasculitis, arthritis, and some of the neurologic manifestations of SLE are fully explainable by the development of local inflammatory lesions secondary to the formation or deposition of IC. What remains unclear is whether tissue-fixed IC are circulating IC that eventually become deposited in tissues or if they result from the formation of antigen–antibody complexes in situ.

In SLE patients, immune complex deposits have also been noted on the dermo-epidermal junction of both inflamed skin and normal skin, appearing as a fluorescent "band" when a skin biopsy is studied by immunofluorescence with anti-sera to Igs and complement components (band test).

Glomerulonephritis

Immunofluorescence studies indicate that the capillary tufts of renal glomeruli in patients with lupus nephritis contain deposits of Igs and complement. Several lines of evidence support the conclusion that those deposits represent IC and that these IC are likely to play a primary pathogenic role. DNA and DNA antibodies can be eluted from the kidneys of lupus patients, confirming that they correspond to antigen–antibody complexes. The deposition of IC in the glomerular basement membrane can be explained in four different ways:

1. Deposition of soluble, circulating IC (as discussed in Chapter 23)
2. Formation of IC in situ. DNA has affinity to glomerular basement membranes and, once immobilized, may react with circulating DNA antibodies to form antigen–antibody complexes.
3. Cross-reaction of DNA antibodies with collagen and cytoskeleton proteins.
4. Anti-C1q antibodies, highly associated with nephritis, cause renal damage if IC have already been deposited. This experimental fact suggests a cascade of events that involves the deposition of IC, autoantiboby, and complement leading to renal injury.

The pathogenic role of IC deposited in the kidney is supported by ample evidence for complement activation via the classic and the alternative pathway in patients with active nephritis. Circulating levels of C3 and C4 are usually decreased, whereas plasma levels of complement breakdown products such as C3a, C3d, and Bb are increased. C1q, C3b, and complement split products such as C3d, C3bi, and C3c can be detected attached to circulating IC.

Nonimmune Factors Influencing the Course of Systemic Lupus Erythematosus

In addition and in close interplay with genetic and immunological factors, a variety of other factors have an apparent effect on the evolution of the disease.

Hormonal Effects

The expression of the genetic and immunologic abnormalities characteristic of murine lupus-like disease is influenced by female sex hormones. For example, in (NZBxNZW) F1 mice, the disease is more severe in females. Administration of estrogens aggravates the evolution of the disease, which is only seen in castrated male mice and not in complete males.

The extent of the hormonal involvement in human SLE cannot be proven directly, but the large female predominance (9:1 female:male ratio) as well as the influence of puberty and pregnancies at the onset of the disease, or the severity of the disease's manifestations, indicates that sex hormones play a role in the modulation of the disease. Estrogens and prolactin administered to animals promote anti-DNA antibody synthesis.

Environmental Factors

Several environmental insults have been related to the onset or relapse of SLE. Sunlight exposure was the first environmental factor influencing the clinical evolution of human SLE to be identified. Exposure to sunlight may precede the clinical expression of the disease or disease relapse. This could be related to the fact that the Langerhans cells of the skin and keratinocytes release significant amounts of interleukin-1 upon exposure to UV light, and could thus represent the initial stimulus tipping off a precarious balance of the immune system. Infections also seem to play a role. The normal immune response to bacterial and viral infections may spin-off into a state of B-cell hyperactivity, triggering a relapse. Infection, through the so-called molecular mimicry, can initiate an autoimmune response. Also, various infections may suppress the autoimmune response and in their absence autoimmune manifestations may occur at increased rates.

Drugs, particularly those with DNA binding ability, such as hydantoin, isoniazide, and hydralazine, can cause a drug-induced lupus-like syndrome. These drugs are known to cause DNA hypomethylation. Because hypomethylated genes are transcribed at higher rates, it is theoretically possible that they cause SLE by increasing the transcription rate of genes that are involved in the expression of the disease. ANA antibodies appear in 15% to 70% of patients treated with any of these drugs for several weeks. These ANA antibodies belong, in most cases, to the IgM class and react with histones. Only when the antibodies switch from IgM to IgG does the patient become symptomatic. ANA usually disappear after termination of the treatment. Patients with drug-induced SLE usually have a milder disease, without significant vital organ involvement.

TREATMENT

Improvement of our understanding of the pathogenesis of SLE has led to reasonable therapeutic strategies that have improved dramatically the well-being and life expectancy of patients with SLE whose 10 year survival rate is now 80%. The therapeutic approach to each patient is determined by the extent of the disease and, most importantly, by the nature and extent of organ involvement. Careful avoidance of factors implicated in the induction of relapses, such as high-risk medications, exposure to sunlight, infections, and so on, is always indicated but in most cases, administration of anti-inflammatory and immunosuppressive drugs is essential.

Glucocorticoids

Glucocorticoids combine anti-inflammatory effects with a weak immunosuppressive capacity. The anti-inflammatory effect is probably beneficial in disease manifestations secondary to immune complex deposition, while the immunosuppressive effect may help to curtail the activity of the B-cell system.

Nonsteroidal Anti-Inflammatory Drugs

These are frequently used in order to control arthritis and serositis.

Immunosuppressive Drugs

Immunosuppressive drugs are often used in the treatment of patients with vital organ involvement (i.e., glomerulonephritis, and CNS involvement). Cyclophosphamide, given intravenously, has been successfully used to prolong adequate renal function with only few side-effects. Maximal benefit is achieved when long-term treatment is started early, with relatively good renal function. In some patients, clinical effects require the administration of high (nonablative) doses of cyclophosphamide. Infections, sterility, and malignancies are frequent side effects.

Experimental Therapeutic Approaches

Experimental therapeutic approaches are under study in patients with SLE. These new approaches capitalize on information that has been generated from the study of the pathogenesis of the disease.

As discussed earlier much of the produced autoantibody is the result of cognate interaction between helper T cells and B-lymphocytes. Therefore, the interruption of this interaction by either humanized antibodies (see Chapter 24) or fusion proteins (recombinant molecules constituted by the binding site of a receptor or ligand and the Fc portion of IgG to prolong serum half life) is expected to have therapeutic value. Such reagents include anti-CD40 ligand antibody and the CTLA4-Ig.

Complement activation mediates significant pathology in human lupus. An anti-C5 antibody that disrupts complement activation is currently in clinical trials to determine its role in the treatment of lupus.

Anti-CD20 antibody, able to deplete B-cells, and antibodies blocking the effect of B-cells stimulating cytokines/factors appear to have significant therapeutic value. Additional trials will determine the possibility of curing, or setting back the lupus clock, by ablating (by means of administration of large doses of cytotoxic drugs or total body irradiation) the patient's own immune system and reinfusing autologous hematopoietic stem cells.

BIBLIOGRAPHY

Boumpas DT, Fessler BJ, Austin HA III, Balow JE, Klippel JH, Lockshin MD. Systemic lupus erythematosus: emerging concepts. Part 1: Renal, neuropsychiatric, cardiovascular, pulmonary, and hematologic disease. Ann Intern Med 1995; 121:940.

Boumpas DT, Fessler BJ, Austin HA III, Balow JE, Klippel JH, Lockshin MD. Systemic lupus erythematosus: emerging concepts. Part 2: Dermatologic and joint disease, the antiphospholipid antibody syndrome, pregnancy and hormonal therapy, morbidity and mortality, and pathogenesis. Ann Intern Med 1995; 123:42.

Davidson A, Diamond B. Autoimmune diseases. N Engl J Med 2001; 345:340–350.

Kammer GM, Perl A, Richardson BC, Tsokos GC. Abnormal T cell signal transduction in systemic lupus erythematosus. Arthritis Rheum 2002; 46:1139–1154.

Kono DH, Theofilopoulos AN. Genetic susceptibility to spontaneous lupus in mice. Curr Dir Autoimmun 1999; 1:72–98.

Kyttaris V, Tsokos G. Uncovering the genetics of systemic lupus erythematosus: implications for therapy. Am J Pharmacogenomics 2003; 3:193–202.

Liossis SNC, Tsokos, GC. B-cell abnormalities in systemic lupus erythematosus. In: Wallace DJ, Hann BH, eds. Dubois lupus erythematosus, 7th ed. Lippincott Williams and Wilkins, Baltimore, MD 2006.

McClain MT, Heinlen LD, Dennis GJ, Roebuck J, Harley JB, James JA. Early events in lupus humoral autoimmunity suggest initiation through molecular mimicry. Nat Med 2005; 11:85–89.

Theofilopoulos AN, Baccala R, Beutler B, Kono DH. Type I interferons (alpha/beta) in immunity and autoimmunity. Annu Rev Immunol 2005; 23:307–335.

Wakeland EK, Liu K, Graham RR, Behrens TW. Delineating the genetic basis of systemic lupus erythematosus. Immunity 2001; 15:397–408.

19 | Rheumatoid Arthritis

George C. Tsokos
Beth Israel Deaconess Medical Center, Harvard Medical School, Boston, Massachusetts, U.S.A.

Gabriel Virella
Department of Microbiology and Immunology, Medical University of South Carolina, Charleston, South Carolina, U.S.A.

INTRODUCTION

Rheumatoid arthritis (RA) is a chronic autoimmune disease characterized by inflammatory and degenerative lesions of the distal joints, frequently associated with multi-organ involvement. This disease affects just under 1% of the population and its etiology is complex; immunologic, genetic, and hormonal factors are thought to determine its development. RA waxes and wanes for many years, but the attacks progressively run into one another, setting the stage for the chronic form of the disease, which is associated with deformity and functional impairment.

CLINICAL AND PATHOLOGICAL ASPECTS OF RHEUMATOID ARTHRITIS
Localized Disease: Clinical Presentation

A chronic inflammatory process of the joints that progresses through different stages of increasing severity (Table 1) characterizes RA. The damage is reversible until cartilages and bones become involved (stages 4 and 5). At that time the changes become irreversible and result in severe functional impairment.

The most common clinical presentation of RA is the association of pain, swelling, and stiffness of the metacarpo-phalangeal and wrist joints, often associated with pain in the sole of the foot, indicating metatarso-phalangeal involvement. The disease is initially limited to small distal joints. With time, it progresses from the distal to the proximal joints so that in the late stages, joints such as the ankles, knees, and elbows may become affected.

Pathological Manifestations of Localized Disease

In the early stages, the inflammatory lesion is limited to the lining of the normal diarthrodial joint. A thin membrane composed of two types of synoviocytes, the type A synoviocyte, which is a phagocytic cell of the monocyte-macrophage series with a rapid turnover, and the type B synoviocyte, which is believed to be a specialized fibroblast, constitutes the normal synovial lining. This cellular lining sits on top of a loose acellular stroma that contains many capillaries.

The earliest pathologic changes, seen at the time of the initial symptoms, affect the endothelium of the microvasculature, whose permeability is increased, as judged by the development of edema and of a sparse inflammatory infiltrate of the edematous subsynovial space, in which polymorphonuclear leukocytes predominate. Several weeks later, hyperplasia of the synovial lining cells and perivascular lymphocytic infiltrates can be detected.

In the chronic stage, the size and number of the synovial lining cells increases and the synovial membrane takes a villous appearance. There is also subintimal hypertrophy with massive infiltration by lymphocytes, plasmablasts, and granulation tissue (forming what is known as pannus). This thick pannus behaves like a tumor and in the ensuing months and years continues to grow, protruding into the joint. The synovial space becomes filled by exudative fluid, and this progressive inflammation causes pain and limits motion. With time, the

TABLE 1   The Stages of Rheumatoid Arthritis

Stage	Pathologic process	Symptoms	Physical signs
1	Antigen presentation to T lymphocytes	None	None
2	Proliferation of T and B lymphocytes	Malaise, mild joint stiffness	Swelling of small joints
3	Neutrophils in synovial fluid; synovial cell proliferation	Joint pain and morning stiffness, malaise	Swelling of small joints
4	Invasive pannus; degradation of cartilage	Joint pain and morning stiffness, malaise	Swelling of small joints
5	Invasive pannus; degradation of cartilage; bone erosion	Joint pain and morning stiffness, malaise	Swelling of small joints; deformities

cartilage is eroded and there is progressive destruction of bones and tendons, leading to severe limitation of movement, flexion contractures, and severe mechanical deformities.

Systemic Involvement: Clinical Presentation

It is frequent to observe some signs and symptoms more indicative of a systemic disease, particularly those that are indicative of vasculitis. The most frequent sign is the formation of the rheumatoid nodules over pressure areas, such as the elbows. These nodules are an important clinical feature because with rare exceptions, they are pathognomonic of RA in patients with chronic synovitis, and generally indicate a poor prognosis.

Systemic Involvement: Pathological Manifestations

In contrast with the necrotizing vasculitis associated with systemic lupus erythematosus (SLE), due almost exclusively to immune complex (IC) deposition, the vasculitis seen in RA is associated with granuloma formation. This indicates that cell-mediated immune processes are also likely to be involved. Regardless of the exact pathogenesis of the vasculitic process, rheumatoid patients with vasculitis usually have persistently elevated levels of circulating IC, and generally, a worse prognosis.

Histopathological studies of rheumatoid nodules show fibrinoid necrosis at the center of the nodule surrounded by histiocytes arranged in a radial palisade. The central necrotic areas are believed to be the seat of IC formation or deposition. When the disease has been present for some time, small brown spots may be noticed around the nail bed or associated with nodules. These indicate small areas of endarteritis.

Overlap Syndrome

The overlap syndrome describes a clinical condition in which patients show variable degrees of association of RA and SLE. The existence of this syndrome suggests that the demarcation between SLE and RA is not absolute, resulting in a clinical continuum between both disorders.

Clinically, these patients present features of both diseases. Histopathological studies also show lesions characteristic of the two basic pathologic components of RA and SLE (necrotizing vasculitis and granulomatous reactions). Serological studies in patients with the overlap syndrome demonstrate both antibodies characteristically found in SLE (e.g., anti-double-stranded DNA) and antibodies typical of RA [rheumatoid factor (RF), see later].

Other Related Diseases
Sjögren's Syndrome
Sjögren's syndrome can present as an isolated entity or in association with RA, SLE, and other collagen diseases. It is characterized by dryness of the oral and ocular membranes (Sicca syndrome); and the detection of RF is considered almost essential for the diagnosis, even for those cases without clinical manifestations suggestive of RA.

Felty's Syndrome

Felty's syndrome is an association of RA with neutropenia caused by anti-neutrophil antibodies. The spleen is often enlarged, possibly reflecting its involvement in the elimination of antibody-coated neutrophils.

AUTOANTIBODIES IN RHEUMATOID ARTHRITIS
Rheumatoid Factor and Anti-immunoglobulin Antibodies

The classical serological hallmark of RA is the detection of RF and other anti-immunoglobulin (Ig) antibodies. By definition, classical RF is an IgM antibody to autologous IgG. The more encompassing designation of anti-Ig antibodies is applicable to anti-IgG antibodies of IgG or IgA isotypes. As a rule, the affinity of IgM RF for the IgG molecule is relatively low and does not reach the mean affinity of other IgM antibodies generated during an induced primary immune response.

RFs from different individuals show different antibody specificity, reacting with different determinants of the IgG molecule. In most cases, the antigenic determinants recognized by the antigen-binding sites of these IgM antibodies are located in the Cγ2 and Cγ3 domains of IgG; some of these determinants are allotype-related. Circulating RF reacts mostly with IgG1, IgG2, and IgG4; in contrast, RF detected in synovial fluid reacts more frequently with IgG3 than with any other IgG subclasses. The significance of these differences is unknown, but suggest that different B cell clones may produce circulating RF and synovial RF. Other RF react with determinants that are shared between species, a fact that explains the reactivity of the human RF with rabbit IgG as well as with IgG from other mammalians.

The frequent finding of RF reactive with several IgG subclasses in a single patient suggests that the autoimmune response leading to the production of the RF is polyclonal. This is supported by the fact the idiotypes of RF are heterogeneous, being obviously the product of several different variable (V) region genes.

Methods Used for the Detection of Rheumatoid Factor

RF and anti-Ig antibodies can be detected in the serum of affected patients by a variety of techniques.

1. The Rose-Waaler test is a passive hemagglutination test, which uses sheep or human erythrocytes coated with anti-erythrocyte antibodies as indicators. The agglutination of the IgG-coated red cells to titers greater than 16 or 20 is considered as indicative of the presence of RF. These tests detect mostly the classic IgM RF specific for IgG.
2. The latex agglutination test, in which IgG-coated polystyrene particles are mixed with serum suspected of containing RF or anti-Ig antibodies (see Chapter 15). The agglutination of latex particles by serum dilutions greater than 1:20 is considered as a positive result. This test detects anti-Ig antibodies of all isotypes.

Diagnostic Specificity of Anti-immunoglobulin Antibodies

As with many other autoantibodies, the titers of RF are a continuous variable within the population studied. Thus, any level intending to separate the seropositive from the seronegative is arbitrarily chosen to include as many patients with clinically-defined RA in the seropositive group, while excluding from it as many nonrheumatoid subjects as possible.

Even with these caveats, RF is neither specific nor diagnostic of RA. First, it is found in only 70% to 85% of RA cases, while it can be detected in many other conditions, particularly in patients suffering from Sjögren' syndrome. Also, RF screening tests can be positive in as many as 5% of apparently normal individuals, sharing the same V-region idiotypes (and by implication, the same V-region genes) as the antibodies detected in RA patients.

Physiological Role of Anti-immunoglobulin Antibodies

The finding of RF in normal individuals raise the concept that RF may have a normal, physiological role-such as to ensure the rapid removal of infectious antigen–antibody complexes from circulation. The synthesis of anti-Ig antibodies in normal individuals follows some interesting rules:

1. Anti-Ig antibodies are detected transiently during anamnestic responses to common vaccines, and in these cases, are usually reactive with the dominant Ig isotype of the antibodies produced in response to antigenic stimulation.
2. Anti-Ig antibodies are also found in relatively high titers in diseases associated with persistent formation of antigen–antibody complexes such as subacute bacterial endocarditis, tuberculosis, leprosy, and many parasitic diseases.
3. The titers of vaccination-associated RF follow very closely the variations in titer of the specific antibodies induced by the vaccine; similarly, the levels of RF detected in patients with infections associated with persistently elevated levels of circulating IC decline once the infection has been successfully treated. In contrast, the anti-Ig antibodies detected in patients with RA persist indefinitely, reflecting their origin as part of an autoimmune response.
4. Infection-associated RF binds to IgG molecules whose configuration has been altered as a consequence of binding to exogenous antigens. The resulting RF–IgG–Ag complexes are large and quickly cleared from circulation. The adsorption of IgG to latex particles seems to induce a similar conformational alteration of the IgG molecule as antigen-binding, and, as a result, IgG-coated latex particles can also be used to detect this type of RF.

The transient nature of anti-Ig antibodies in normal individuals suggests that the autoreactive clones responsible for the production of autoantibodies to human Igs are not deleted during embryonic differentiation. The persistence in adult life of such autoreactive clones is supported by the observation that the bone marrow contains precursors of RF-producing B cells. Their frequency is surprisingly high in mice, where it is relatively easy to induce the production of RF in high titers after polyclonal B cell stimulation. Human bone marrow B lymphocytes can also be stimulated to differentiate into RF-producing plasmablasts by mitogenic stimulation with pokeweed mitogen or by infection with Epstein-Barr virus. In addition, tolerance to self-IgG must be ensured by a strong negative feedback mechanism(s), since tolerance is broken only temporarily.

Phenotype of B Cell Precursors of Rheumatoid Factor-Producing Plasmablasts
Both in mice and humans, the B lymphocytes capable to differentiate into RF-producing plasmablasts express CD5 in addition to the classical B cell markers, such as membrane IgM and IgD, CR2, CD19, and CD20. CD5 is expressed by less than 2% of the B lymphocytes of a normal individual and was first detected in patients suffering from very active RA. It is considered as a marker characteristic of autoimmune situations.

Pathogenic Role of Rheumatoid Factor and Anti-immunoglobulin Antibodies
RF titers are highly variable, even in patients with full-blown RA, and do not seem to correlate very closely with the activity of the disease. However, high titers of RF tend to be associated with a more rapid progression of the articular component and with systemic manifestations, such as subcutaneous nodules, vasculitis, intractable skin ulcers, neuropathy, and Felty's syndrome. Thus, the detection of RF in high titers in a patient with symptomatic RA is associated with a poor prognosis.

The pathogenic properties of RF are likely to be derived from the biological characteristics of the antibodies involved. Classical IgM RF activates complement via the classical pathway and the ability of RF to fix complement is of pathogenic significance, because it may be responsible, at least in part, for the development of rheumatoid synovitis.

The source of the anti-Ig antibodies that are likely to play an important role in causing the arthritic lesions is predominantly the synovium of the affected joints. The joints are the principal sites of RF production in RA patients, and it should also be noted that in some individuals, the locally produced anti-Ig antibodies are of the IgG isotype. When this is the case, the joint disease is usually more severe, because anti-IgG antibodies of the IgG isotype have a higher affinity for IgG than their IgM counterparts; consequently, they form stable IC, which activate complement very efficiently.

Seronegative Rheumatoid Arthritis

Some patients with RA may have negative results on the screening tests for RA. True seronegative RA cases exist, particularly among agammaglobulinemic patients. In spite of their inability to synthesize antibodies, these patients develop a disease clinically indistinguishable from RF-positive RA. This is a highly significant observation since it argues strongly against the role of the RF or other serologic abnormalities as a major pathogenic insult in RA and suggests that the inflammatory response in the rheumatoid joint could be largely cell-mediated. However, in many instances negative serologies in patients with RA are falsely negative. Four different mechanisms may account for false negative results in the RA test:

1. The presence of anti-Ig antibodies of isotypes other than IgM, less efficient than IgM RF in causing agglutination (particularly in tests using red cells) and, therefore, more likely to be overlooked.
2. The reaction between IgM RF and endogenous IgG results in the formation of soluble IC that, if the affinity of the reaction is relatively high, will remain associated when the RF test is performed. Under these conditions, the RF binding sites are blocked, unable to react with the IgG coating indicator red cells or latex particles.
3. RF may be present in synovial fluid but not in peripheral blood.

In clinical practice, it is very seldom necessary to investigate these possibilities, since a positive test is not necessary for the diagnosis.

Anticollagen Antibodies

Antibodies reacting with different types of collagen have been detected with considerable frequency in connective tissue diseases such as scleroderma. In RA, considerable interest has been aroused by the finding that antibodies elicited by injection of type II collagen with complete Freund's adjuvant into rats are associated with the development of a rheumatoid-type disease. However, the frequency of these antibodies in RA patients has been recently estimated to be in the 15% to 20% range, which is not compatible with a primary pathogenic role. It is probable that the anticollagen antibodies in RA arise as a response to the degradation of articular collagen that could yield immunogenic peptides.

Anticitrullinated Protein Antibodies

The recently described autoantibodies to citrullinated proteins such as filaggrin and its circular form [cyclic citrullinated peptide (CCP)] are highly sensitive and specific for RA. Citrullinated proteins, mostly fibrins, are localized in the synovial tissue of patients with RA and the corresponding antibodies are locally produced in the joints. CCP antibodies have been proposed as a serologic marker for early diagnosis of RA. Also, CCP antibody levels seem to have prognostic prediction of joint destruction.

Antinuclear Antibodies

Antibodies against native, dsDNA are conspicuously lacking in patients with classical RA, but the antibodies against single-stranded DNA (ssDNA) can be detected in about one-third of the patients. The epitopes recognized by anti-ssDNA antibodies correspond to DNA-associated proteins. The detection of anti-ssDNA antibodies does not have diagnostic or prognostic significance because these antibodies are neither disease-specific nor involved in IC formation.

The reasons for the common occurrence of anti-ssDNA in RA and in many other connective tissue diseases are unknown. However, these antibodies may represent an indicator of immune abnormalities due to the persistence of abnormal B lymphocyte clones, which have escaped the repression exerted by normal tolerogenic mechanisms and which are able to produce autoantibodies of various types.

GENETIC FACTORS IN RHEUMATOID ARTHRITIS
Human Leukocyte Antigen-Associations

The incidence of familial RA is low, and only 15% of the identical twins are concordant for the disease. However, 70% to 90% of Caucasians with RA express the human leukocyte antigens (HLA) DR4 antigen that is found in about 15% to 25% of the normal population. Individuals expressing this antigen are 6 to 12 times more at risk of having RA but HLA-DR1 was also found to increase susceptibility to RA and wide fluctuations in the frequency of these markers are seen between different patient populations.

Human Leukocyte Antigen-DR4 Subtypes

DNA sequencing of the β chain of the DR4 and DR1 molecules defined 5 HLA-DR4 subtypes: Dw4, Dw10, Dw13, Dw14, and Dw15. While Dw4, Dw10, Dw13, and Dw15 differ from each other in amino acid sequence at positions 67, 70, and 74 of the third hypervariable region of the β1 domain of the β chain, Dw4 and Dw14 have identical amino acid sequences at these positions and are associated with RA. The same amino acids are present in the Dw1 subtype of HLA-DR1. The prevalence of Dw4, Dw14, or Dw1 in the general population is 42%. Of these individuals, 2.2% develop RA. In contrast, the frequency of RA in individuals negative for these markers is only 0.17%, a 12.9 fold difference. Since most humans are heterozygous, a given individual may inherit more than one susceptibility allele. Individuals having both Dw4 and Dw14 have a much higher risk (seven to one) of developing severe RA. In contrast, individuals with the Dw10 and Dw13 markers, whose sequence differs in the critical residues (Table 2), seem protected against RA.

The interpretation of these findings hinges on the fact that amino acids 67 to 74 are located on the third hypervariable region of the DR4 and DR1 β chains. This region is part of a helical region of the peptide-binding pouch of the DRβ chain (see Chapter 3) that interacts both with the side chains of antigenic peptides and with the T cell receptor (TcR). Its configuration, rather than the configuration of any other of the hypervariable regions of the DR4 and DR1 β chains, seems to determine susceptibility or resistance to RA, depending on the charge of amino acids located on critical positions. In the case of Dw1 and DW14 the sequence of the 70–74 motif is identical (QRRAA), while the homologous sequence in Dw4 (QKRAA) shows one single substitution (a basic arginine by an equally basic lysine). In contrast, the sequence of the same stretch of aminoacids in protective alleles shows a higher degree of divergence. In Dw10 aspartic acid and glutamic acid replace the first two aminoacids (glutamine and arginine or lysine) resulting in a total change in the charge and affinity of the peptide-binding pouch. In the case of Dw13, glutamic acid replaces alanine at position 74, again resulting in a marked charge difference relatively to Dw1, 4, and 14.

It has been postulated that the structure of those DR4 and DR1 molecules that are associated with increased risk for the development of RA is such that they bind very strongly an "arthritogenic epitope" derived from an as yet unidentified agent. Bacterial antigens, including heat-shock proteins, microbial proteins from *Proteus mirabilis*, Epstein-Barr (EB) virus, or retroviruses, as well as autologous proteins such as type II collagen or cartilage glycoprotein gp39 have been proposed as candidate sources for these peptides. The consequence of the binding of immunogenic peptides would be a strong and prolonged immune response that would be the basis for the inflammatory response in the joints. Obviously, the predominant localization of the inflammatory reaction to the peri-articular tissues implies that the level of expression of

TABLE 2 Human Leukocyte Antigen-DR Subtypes and Rheumatoid Arthritis

Subtype	Critical residues on the third diversity region of β1				Predisposition to rheumatoid arthritis
	67	70	71	74	
DRB1*0101 (Dw1)	L	Q	R	A	+
DRB1*0401 (Dw4)	L	Q	K	A	+
DRB1*0404 (Dw14)	L	Q	R	A	+
DRB1*0403 (Dw13)	L	Q	R	E	−
DRB1*0402 (Dw10)	I	D	E	A	−

Abbreviations: A, Ala; D, Asp; E, Glu; I, IsoLeu; K, Lys; L, Leu; Q, Gln; R, Arg.

the peptides in question must be higher in those tissues. The reverse would be the case for those DR4 molecules associated with protection against the development of RA.

Supporting this interpretation are several observations concerning the severity of the disease in patients bearing those HLA antigens and subtypes. For example, DR4 positivity reaches 96% in patients suffering from Felty's syndrome, the most severe form of the disease. More recent studies showed that RA patients who are DR4–Dw14 positive have a faster progression to the stages of pannus formation and bone erosion.

The most significant discrepancy in this apparent consensus sequence between DR sequence and RA susceptibility was found in African-Americans with RA; in this group, only 20% are DR4$^+$. In this ethnic group predisposition and severity appear independent of the presence and dose of the "arthritogenic" DR alleles identified in Caucasians.

IMMUNOLOGICAL FACTORS IN THE PATHOGENESIS OF RHEUMATOID ARTHRITIS
Cell-Mediated Immunity Abnormalities in Rheumatoid Arthritis

It is accepted that cell-mediated immune mechanisms play the main pathogenic role in RA. This conclusion is based on studies performed in the synovial fluid and on the hypertrophic synovium of the rheumatoid joints, both easily accessible to study by needle biopsy or aspiration. All the essential cellular elements of the immune response are present in the joint, and the main challenge is to reconstitute the sequence of events that leads to the progressive destruction of joint tissues.

Critical Role of T Lymphocytes
Immunohistologic studies of the inflammatory infiltrates of the synovial membrane show marked lymphocytic predominance (lymphocytes may represent up to 60% of the total tissue net weight). Among the lymphocytes infiltrating the synovium, CD4$^+$ helper T (Th) lymphocytes outnumber CD8$^+$ lymphocytes in a ratio of 5:1. The critical pathogenic role for Th lymphocytes is suggested by two important observations:

1. RA is associated with specific DR alleles (see above), and it is well accepted that major histocompatibility complex (MHC)-II molecules present immunogenic peptides to Th lymphocytes.
2. Increased concentrations of many lymphocyte-released cytokines are measurable in the synovial fluid, probably reflecting the activated state of infiltrating lymphocytes.

Most of the infiltrating CD4$^+$ lymphocytes have the phenotype of a terminally differentiated memory Th cell (CD4$^+$, CD45RO$^+$), which represent 20% to 30% of the mononuclear cells in the synovium. They also express class-II MHC, consistent with chronic T cell activation, but only 10% express CD25, suggesting that they do not proliferate actively in the synovial tissues. In situ hybridization studies performed in biopsies of synovial tissue obtained at late stages of the disease, disclosed that these chronically activated T cells express mRNAs for interleukin (IL)-2, IFN-γ, IL-7, IL-13, IL-15, and granulocyte macrophage-colony stimulating factor (GM-CSF). One conspicuously missing IL is IL-4, suggesting that the CD4$^+$, CD45RO$^+$ T lymphocytes in the synovial tissues are predominantly of the Th1 type, which produces predominantly IL-2 and IFN-γ. A variety of chemokines (RANTES, MIP1-α, MIP1-β, and IL-8), most of them produced by lymphocytes, can also be detected in the synovial fluid. These chemokines are probably responsible for the attraction of additional T lymphocytes, monocytes, and neutrophils to the rheumatoid joint. T cells in the RA synovium also express CD40L, and are, therefore, able to deliver costimulating signals to B cells and dendritic cells (DC) (see later).

A most significant question that remains unanswered is; what is the nature of the stimulus responsible for the activation of the T lymphocytes found in the synovial infiltrates? Studies of the TcR Vβ genes expressed by the infiltrating T lymphocytes has shown that the repertoire is limited, that is, only some T cell clones appear to be activated and the same clones are found in several joints of the same patient. An even more restricted profile was observed when the analysis was confined to the Ag-binding area of the Vβ chain (the so-called CDR3 region).

These findings suggest that antigenic stimulation through the TcR plays a critical role. However, a defined correlation between the Vβ chains expressed by the infiltrating T lymphocytes and the patient's MHC-II alleles has not yet been found. Such correlation is expected because of the role played by the MHC molecules in selecting the T cell repertoire of any given individual (see Chapter 11). Thus, HLA-linked RA susceptibility alleles could introduce a first bias in TCR selection, but there is no evidence supporting this hypothesis.

The long-term goal of these approaches, to identify the actual targets of the immune attack, remains elusive at this time. A major obstacle is our limited knowledge about the immunogenic peptides recognized by different TcR Vβ region families. Until some breakthrough happens in that area, our understanding will remain fragmentary and highly speculative.

Antigen Presentation and the Dendritic Cells

The autoimmune response that underlies the pathogenesis of RA is mostly localized to the synovial tissue and fluid in the synovial space. Fully differentiated DC can be found in the synovial tissue, surrounding small vessels and in close association with T cells and B cell follicles. These DC appear to be derived from circulating precursors, attracted to the synovium by chemokines such as MIP-1α, monocyte chemotactic protein and RANTES (see Chapter 11), a process made possible by the expression of cell adhesion molecules induced by tumor necrosis factor (TNF) and IL-1. On reaching the synovium, DC undergo differentiation and activation under the influence of T cells expressing the CD40L and of some of the cytokines present in high concentrations in the synovial fluid, such as GM-CSF, TNF, and IL-1. Their differentiation in the synovium seems associated with an increased ability to present self-antigen, and, therefore, to stimulate autoimmune responses. Activated and differentiated DC are also known to secrete IL-18, which, as discussed later in the chapter, has pro-inflammatory activity, synergizes with IL-12 in the expansion of Th1 cells, and induces the synthesis and release of interferon-γ by activated Th1 cells.

B Cells as Local Amplificators of the Autoimmune Response

B cells expressing RF on their membrane can be found in the synovium of chronically inflamed joints. These RF$^+$ B cells can bind IC by the Fc portion of the antibodies, a process that results in B-cell activation and peptide presentation to T cells. In this role as antigen-presenting cells (APCs), RF$^+$ B cells can activate multiple T-cell clones recognizing a wide variety of endogenous and exogenous peptides internalized as IC. Thus, RF$^+$ B cells amplify intra-synovium immune responses and contribute to the exacerbation of the local inflammatory process.

Multiple Roles of Synovium Macrophages

The synovial infiltrates are rich in activated monocytes, macrophages, and macrophage-derived synoviocytes that are believed to play several critical pathogenic roles. One of the significant roles played by these cells is antigen presentation to CD4$^+$ lymphocytes. It is not unusual to see macrophage–lymphocyte clusters in the inflamed synovial tissue and in those clusters in which CD4$^+$ lymphocytes are in very close contact with large macrophages expressing high levels of class II MHC antigens. In addition IL-12 and IL-18 mRNA and secreted IL-12 and IL-18 are found at biologically active concentrations, and could play an important role in Th2 expansion and differentiation.

The other critical role of synovial monocytes and macrophages is to induce and perpetuate local inflammatory changes. Several lines of evidence support this role. First, the synovial fluid of patients with RA contains relatively large concentrations of phospholipase A2 (PLA2), an enzyme that has a strong chemotactic effect on lymphocytes and monocytes. Moreover, this enzyme is actively involved in the metabolism of cell membrane phospholipids, particularly in the early stages of the cyclooxygenase pathway, which leads to the synthesis of eicosanoids such as PGE2, one of a series of pro-inflammatory mediators generated from the breakdown of arachidonic acid. Thus, it is possible that these high levels of PLA2 reflect a hyperactive state of infiltrating macrophages, engaged in the synthesis of prostaglandin E2 and other eicosanoids. Other factors locally released by activated macrophages include transforming growth factor-β (TGF-β), GM-CSF, and IL-18.

Transforming Growth Factor-β

TGF-β has the potential to favor the predominance of Th2 activity over TH1 activity at the inflammatory sites.

Granulocyte Macrophage-Colony Stimulating Factor

GM-CSF induces the proliferation of several cell types in the monocyte–macrophage family, including DC. It has been suggested that this overproduction of GM-CSF by all CD4 cells (macrophages and T lymphocytes) is responsible for the relatively large number of DC found in the inflammatory lesion. This is a significant finding, because activated DC release a variety of pro-inflammatory lymphokines, such as IL-1. Another prominent role of GM-CSF is to be a very strong inducer of the expression of MHC-II molecules (stronger than IFN-γ). Increased MHC-II expression is believed to be an important factor leading to the development of autoimmune responses, and could help perpetuate a vicious circle of anti-self immune response by facilitating the persistent activation of Th2 cells and, consequently, the stimulation of synovial cells, monocytes, and DC.

Interleukin-18

IL-18, in addition to promoting differentiation of Th2 cells in synergism with IL-12, promotes the synthesis of IFN-γ, thus contributing indirectly to macrophage activation. In addition, mononuclear cells activated by IL-18 release GM-CSF, TNF, and PGE2, and show increased expression of inducible nitric oxide synthase. Therefore, IL-18 can be classified as a pro-inflammatory cytokine.

Finally, activated macrophages secrete a variety of metalloproteinases (including collagenase, elastase, stromelysin, matrylisin, and gelatinase B), particularly when stimulated with IL-1 and TNF-α. Studies of biopsies of the rheumatoid synovium discussed earlier found these 2 cytokines at levels high enough to deliver such stimulatory signals to monocytes and fibroblasts. The subsequent release of metalloproteinases is believed to have a primary role in causing tissue damage in the inflamed joints.

A SUMMARY OVERVIEW OF THE PATHOGENESIS OF RHEUMATOID ARTHRITIS
Predisposing Factors

Two important types of factors seem to have a strong impact in the development of RA.

Genetic Factors

The link to HLA-DR4, and particularly with subtypes Dw4 and 14, as well as with the structurally related Dw1 subtype of HLA-DR1, has been previously discussed in this chapter. It is currently accepted that such DR subtypes may be structurally fitted to present a peptide to auto-reactive or cross-reactive Th lymphocytes, thus precipitating the onset of the disease.

Hormonal Factors

The role of hormonal factors is suggested by two observations:

1. RA is three times more frequent in females than in males, predominantly affecting women from 30 to 60 years of age.
2. Pregnancy produces a remission during the third trimester, sometimes followed by exacerbation after childbirth.

These observations suggest that hormonal factors may have a significant effect on the development of RA. However, to this day the responsible factors have not been defined. On the other hand, a possible mechanism by which pregnancy would cause an improvement in the clinical picture has been recently suggested by the observation that estrogens potentiate

B lymphocyte responses in vitro. This increased B cell activity is likely to reflect a shift of predominant Th activity from Th1 to Th2, which is considerably less pro-inflammatory.

Precipitating Factors

Three main mechanisms responsible for the escape from tolerance that must be associated with the onset of RA have been proposed.

1. Decreased activity of downregulating T cells
2. Nonspecific B cell stimulation by microbial products (e.g., bacterial lipopolysaccharide) or infectious agents (e.g., viruses).
3. Stimulation of self-reactive T lymphocytes as a consequence of the presentation of a cross-reactive peptide (possibly of infectious origin) by an activated antigen-presenting cell (e.g., DC or RF^+ B cell).

The genetic linkages discussed earlier in this chapter support the last theory. Also, the key role of T lymphocytes is supported by histological data (discussed earlier) and by the observations that HIV infection and immunosuppression for bone marrow transplantation, two conditions that depress Th lymphocyte function very profoundly, are associated with remissions of RA.

Self-Perpetuating Mechanisms

Once Th cells are activated, a predominantly Th1 response develops (Fig. 1). Activated Th1 cells release IFN-γ and GM-CSF that activate macrophages and related cells, inducing the expression of MHC-II molecules, creating conditions for continuing and stronger stimulation of Th lymphocytes. As this cross-stimulation of Th1 lymphocytes and macrophages continues, chemotactic factors are released and additional lymphocytes, monocytes, DC, and granulocytes are recruited into the area. As inflammatory cells become activated, they release proteases and pro-inflammatory mediators, such as PGE2. The release of proteases will cause the damage on the synovial and peri-sinovial tissues, while the activation of osteoblasts and osteoclasts by mediators released by activated lymphocytes and macrophages (particularly IL-1 and IL-6) is the cause of bone damage and abnormal repair.

What Are the Initiating Factors of Rheumatoid Arthritis?

While our understanding of the basic immune abnormalities and of the self-perpetuating circuits involved in RA has become more complete, there is considerable uncertainty about the factor(s) that may be responsible for the initiation of the disease. There is also very little knowledge about the factors that localize the disease to the joints on the initial stages. For example, there is experimental evidence supporting a critical role of DC, probably by promoting autoreactive T cell activation, but there is no logical way to explain how the DC would be initially activated and localized to the synovial tissue. There are observations in animal models suggesting that arthritis can develop in the absence of autoreactivity to joint antigens, a model that could explain the association with infections such as those caused by *P. mirabilis* and EB virus. What this model fails to provide is an explanation for the localization of the ensuing autoimmune reaction to the joints. In addition, the MHC molecules linked to RA appear to be able to recognize peptides derived from joint tissue proteins. If this is proven to be unquestionably the case, what remains to be explained is what triggers the initial activation of APCs in the joints to an extent that the recognition of self-peptides takes place in an environment conducive to the development of an immune response rather than maintaining the normal state of anergy.

THERAPY

It is not surprising that our very incomplete knowledge of the pathogenesis of RA is reflected at the therapeutic level. Most of our current therapeutic approaches are palliative, aiming to reduce joint inflammation and tissue damage. Under these conditions, RA therapy is often a frustrating experience for patients and physicians.

Nonsteroidal Anti-inflammatory Drugs

This heterogeneous group of anti-inflammatory drugs includes, among others, aspirin, ibuprofen, naproxen, indomethacin, and the recently introduced COX-2 inhibitors. These compounds have as common mechanism of action the inhibition of the cyclooxygenase pathway of arachidonic acid metabolism, which results in a reduction of the local release of prostaglandins. Their administration is beneficial in many patients with RA.

Glucocorticoids

In more severe cases, in which the nonsteroidal anti-inflammatory drugs are not effective, glucocorticoids are indicated. However, the use of glucocorticoids in RA raises considerable problems, because in most instances, their administration masks the inflammatory component only as long as it is given. Thus, glucocorticoid therapy needs to be maintained for long periods of time at doses exceeding 20 mg/day, exposing the patient to very serious side effects, include muscle and bone loss and may become more devastating than the original arthritis.

Disease-Modifying Drugs

A variety of potent drugs have been used in attempts to reduce the intensity of the autoimmune reaction and/or the consequent inflammatory reaction and attenuate the clinical manifestations of the disease. This group includes a series of drugs that seems mainly to have anti-inflammatory effects, such as auranofin and gold salts, hydroxychloroquine, minocycline, sulfasalazine, D-penicillamine, and a group of cytotoxic/immunosuppressive drugs that include methrotrexate, azathioprine, chlorambucil, cyclophosphamide, leflunomide, and cyclosporine A. All these agents have side effects, some more severe than others. Usually less toxic compounds are used first and more toxic agents are introduced if the patient continues to deteriorate. Some authors have claimed that methrotrexate, administered in low weekly doses, is not associated with long-term side effects while controlling the inflammatory component of the disease and delaying the appearance of the chronic phase. The use of agents specifically directed at reducing T cell activation levels, such as cyclosporine A and leflunomide has also met with some successes, by themselves or in association (e.g., leflunomide plus methrotrexate).

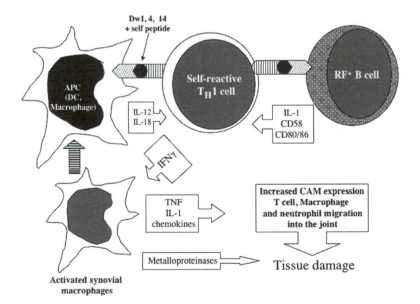

FIGURE 1 Diagrammatic representation of the pathogenesis of rheumatoid arthritis. In this diagram it is postulated that helper Th1 lymphocytes play the central role in the sequence of events that leads to the activation of synovial macrophages, which is the main effector system mobilized by this Th subpopulation. Not shown in the diagram is the role of rheumatoid factor as the mediator for complement and neutrophil-mediated articular and extrarticular inflammation.

Biological Response Modifiers

Considerable interest has been devoted in recent years to the use of biological response modifier (BRM) agents (discussed in detail in Chapter 24). Two basic types of BRMs have been used: those that try to suppress activated T cell populations and those that have the neutralization of pro-inflammatory cytokines as their major mechanism of action. To this date, there has been very limited success with BRMs targeting activated T cells, while the opposite has been true with BRMs that downregulate the effects of pro-inflammatory cytokines. Among the latter, recombinant humanized anti-TNF (infliximab) and a recombinant form of a soluble TNF receptors (etarnecept) have been most successful in clinical trials and have received FDA approval. Other BRMs, such as monoclonal antibodies directed to IL-6 and IL-6 receptors, CD4, and ICAM-1 are still being evaluated.

B cell depletion using an anti-CD20 antibody proved to be efficacious in the treatment of patients with RA who fail anti-TNF antibody treatment. It should be noted that clinical responses do not necessarily correlate with serum antibody levels although the numbers of circulating B cells decrease. The clinical results have demonstrated that B cells are important in the pathogenesis of RA by virtue of presenting autoantigen to T cells

CTLA4-Ig, a fusion construct between the inhibitory co-receptor, CTLA4 and the Fc portion of Ig, proved of clinical value in the treatment of RA. This important clinical observation demonstrates the value of costimulation in the pathogenesis of RA.

It seems possible that maximal clinical benefit for RA patients may be obtained from the combination of more than one type of therapeutic agent. For example, the combination of infliximab and methrotexate seems particularly effective.

Reinduction of Tolerance

Attempts to reinduce tolerance to cartilage antigens postulated to be involved in the autoimmune response by feeding animal cartilage extracts to RA patients have yielded promising results. However, the clinical benefits reported so far have been observed in short-term studies, and research is necessary to determine if the benefits persist in the long run. Also, additional studies are needed to better define the mechanism(s) involved in oral tolerization.

BIBLIOGRAPHY

Auger I, Toussirot E, Roudier J. Molecular mechanisms involved in the association of HLA-DR4 and rheumatoid arthritis. Immunol Res 1997; 16:121.

de Vries-Bouwstra JK, Dijkmans BA, Breedveld FC. Biologics in early rheumatoid arthritis. Rheum Dis Clin North Am 2005; 31:745–762.

Feldman M, Maini RN. The role of cytokines in the pathogenesis of Rheumatoid Arthritis. Rheumatology 1999; 38(suppl 3):3.

Firestein GS. Immunologic mechanisms in the pathogenesis of rheumatoid arthritis. J Clin Rheumatol 2005; 11(suppl):S39–S44.

Mimori T. Clinical significance of anti-CCP antibodies in rheumatoid arthritis. Int Med 2005; 44:1122–1126.

Savage C, St Clair EW. New therapeutics in rheumatoid arthritis. Rheum Dis Clin North Am 2006; 32:57–74.

Schur PH. Serologic tests in the evaluation of rheumatic diseases. Immunol Allergy Pract 1991; 13:138.

Sokka T, Hannonen P, Mottonen T. Conventional disease-modifying antirheumatic drugs in early arthritis. Rheum Dis Clin North Am 2005; 31:729–744.

Struik L, Hawes JE, Chatila MK, et al. T cell receptors in rheumatoid arthritis. Arthritis Rheum 1995; 38:577.

Thomas R, MacDonald KPA, Pettit AR, et al. Dendritic cells and the pathogenesis of rheumatoid arthritis. J Leukoc Biol 1999; 66:286.

Tsokos GC. B cells, Bc gone. B-cell depletion in the treatment of rheumatoid arthritis. N Eng J Med 2004; 350: 2546–2548.

Turesson C, Matteson EL. Genetics of rheumatoid arthritis. Mayo Clin Proc 2006; 81:94–101.

Walsh NC, Crotti TN, Goldring SR, Gravallese EM. Rheumatic diseases: the effects of inflammation on bone. Immunol Rev 2005; 208:228–251.

Winchester R. The molecular basis of susceptibility to rheumatoid arthritis. Adv Immunol 1994; 56:389.

Yocum DE. T cells: pathogenic cells and treatment targets in rheumatoid arthritis. Semin Arthritis Rheum 1999; 29:27.

Ziff M. The rheumatoid nodule. Arthritis Rheum 1990; 33:768.

20 | Hypersensitivity Reactions

Gabriel Virella
*Department of Microbiology and Immunology, Medical University of South Carolina,
Charleston, South Carolina, U.S.A.*

INTRODUCTION

The immune response of vertebrates has evolved as a mechanism to eradicate infectious agents that succeed in penetrating natural anti-infectious barriers. However, in some instances the immune response can be the cause of disease, both as an undesirable effect of an immune response directed against an exogenous antigen, or as a consequence of an autoimmune reaction. These undesirable immune responses define what is known as hypersensitivity, that is, as an abnormal state of immune reactivity that has deleterious effects on the host. A patient with hypersensitivity to a given compound suffers pathologic reactions as a consequence of exposure to the antigen to which one is hypersensitive. The term "allergy" is often used to designate a pathological condition resulting from hypersensitivity, particularly when the symptoms occur shortly after exposure.

Hypersensitivity reactions can be classified as immediate or as delayed, depending on the time elapsed between the exposure to the antigen and the appearance of clinical symptoms. They can also be classified as humoral or cell-mediated, depending on the arm of the immune system predominantly involved. A classification combining these two elements was proposed in the 1960s by Gell and Coombs; and, although, many hypersensitivity disorders may not fit well into their classification, it remains popular because of its simplicity and obvious relevance to the most common hypersensitivity reactions.

The Gell's and Coombs' classification of hypersensitivity reactions considers four types of reactions. Type I, II, and III reactions are basically mediated by antibodies with or without participation of the complement system; type IV reactions are cell-mediated (Table 1). While in many pathological processes mechanisms classified in more than one of these types of hypersensitivity reactions may be operative, the subdivision of hypersensitivity states into four broad types aids considerably in the understanding of their pathogenesis.

TYPE I HYPERSENSITIVITY REACTIONS (IMMUNOGLOBULINE-MEDIATED HYPERSENSITIVITY, IMMEDIATE HYPERSENSITIVITY)
Historical Overview

Much of our early knowledge about immediate hypersensitivity reactions was derived from studies in guinea pigs. Guinea pigs immunized with egg albumin frequently suffer from an acute allergic reaction upon challenge with this same antigen. This reaction is very rapid (observed within a few minutes after the challenge) and is known as an anaphylactic reaction. It often results in the death of the animal in anaphylactic shock. If serum from a guinea pig sensitized seven to ten days earlier with a single injection of egg albumin and adjuvant is transferred to a nonimmunized animal that is challenged 48 hours later with egg albumin, this animal develops an anaphylactic reaction and may die in anaphylactic shock. Because hypersensitivity was transferred with serum, this observation suggested that antibodies play a critical pathogenic role in this type of hypersensitivity.

The passive transfer of hypersensitivity can take less dramatic aspects if the reaction is limited to the skin. To study what is known as passive cutaneous anaphylaxis, nonsensitized animals are injected intradermally with the serum from a sensitized donor. The serum from the sensitized donor contains homocytotropic antibodies that become bound to the mast cells in and around the area where serum was injected. After 24 to 72 hours the antigen in question is injected intravenously, mixed with Evans blue dye. When the antigen reaches the area of

TABLE 1 General Characteristics of the Four Types of Hypersensitivity Reactions as Defined by Gell and Coombs

Type	Clinical manifestations	Lag between exposure and symptoms	Mechanism
I (immediate)	Anaphylaxis, asthma, urticaria, hay fever	Minutes	Homocytotropic Ab (IgE)
II (cytotoxic)	Hemolytic anemia, cytopenias, Goodpasture's syndrome	Variable	Complement-fixing/opsonizing Ab (IgG, IgM)
III	Serum sickness, Arthus reaction, vasculitis	6 hr[a]	Immune complexes containing complement-fixing Ab (mostly IgG)
IV (delayed)	Cutaneous hypersensitivity, graft rejection	12–48 hr	Sensitized lymphocytes

[a]For the Arthus reaction.
Abbreviations: Ab, antibody; IC, immune complex; Ig, immunoglobulin.

the skin where antibodies were injected and became bound to mast cells, a localized type I reaction takes place, characterized by a small area of vascular hyperpermeability that results in edema and redness. When Evans blue is injected with the antigen, the area of vascular hyperpermeability will have a blue discoloration due to the transudation of the dye.

The Prausnitz-Kustner reaction is a reaction with a similar principle that was practiced in humans and contributed to our understanding of the immediate hypersensitivity reaction. Serum from an allergic patient was injected intradermally into a nonallergic recipient. Twenty-four to forty-eight hours later, the area of skin where the serum was injected was challenged with the antigen that was suspected to cause the symptoms in the patient. A positive reaction consisted of a wheal and flare appearing a few minutes after injection of the antigen. The reaction can also be performed in primates, which are injected intravenously with serum of an allergic individual and challenged later with intradermal injections of a battery of antigens that could be implicated as the cause of the allergic reaction. Both of these reactions are no longer used for any clinical purpose.

Clinical Manifestations of Immediate Hypersensitivity

A wide variety of hypersensitivity states can be classified as immediate hypersensitivity reactions. Some have a predominantly cutaneous expression (hives or urticaria), others affects the airways (hay fever, asthma), while still others are of a systemic nature. The latter are often designated as anaphylactic reactions, of which anaphylactic shock is the most severe form.

The expression of anaphylaxis is species-specific. The guinea pig usually has bronchoconstriction and bronchial edema as predominant expression, leading to death in acute asphyxiation. In the rabbit, on the contrary, the most affected organ is the heart, and the animals die of right heart failure. In man, allergic bronchial asthma in its most severe forms closely resembles the reaction in the guinea pig.

Most frequently, human type I hypersensitivity has a localized expression, such as the bronchoconstriction and bronchial edema that characterize bronchial asthma, the mucosal edema in hay fever, and the skin rash and subcutaneous edema that defines urticaria (hives). The factor(s) involved in determining the target organs that will be affected in different types of immediate hypersensitivity reactions are not well defined, but the route of exposure to the challenging antigen seems an important factor. For example, allergic (extrinsic) asthma and hay fever are usually associated with inhaled antigens while urticaria is seen as a frequent manifestation of food allergy. However, the manifestations of food allergy are very diverse, and, in addition to hives, can include a variety of symptoms affecting different organs and systems (Table 2).

Systemic Anaphylaxis

Systemic anaphylaxis is usually associated with antigens that are directly introduced into the systemic circulation, such as in the case of hypersensitivity to insect venom or to

TABLE 2 Common Manifestations of Food Allergy

Nausea
Diarrhea
Abdominal cramps
Pruritic rashes
Angioedema
Asthma/rhinitis
Vomiting
Hives
Laryngeal edema
Anaphylaxix

systemically-administered drugs, such as penicillin. However, seafood and peanuts can also elicit anaphylactic reactions. Systemic anaphylactic reactions in humans can present in diverse forms, affecting different organs and systems (Table 3). Cardiovascular involvement is associated with the highest mortality rates.

Atopy

Some individuals have an obvious tendency to develop hypersensitivity reactions. The term atopy is used to designate this tendency of some individuals to become sensitized to a variety of allergens (antigens involved in allergic reactions) including pollens, spores, animal danders, house dust, and foods. These individuals, when skin tested, are positive to several allergens and successful therapy must take this multiple reactivity into account. A genetic background for atopy is suggested by the fact that this condition shows familial prevalence.

Pathogenesis

Immediate hypersensitivity reactions are a consequence of the predominant synthesis of specific IgE antibodies by the allergic individual; these IgE antibodies bind with high affinity to the membranes of basophils and mast cells. When exposed to the sensitizing antigen, the reaction with cell-bound IgE triggers the release of histamine through degranulation, and the synthesis of leukotrienes C4, D4, and E4 [this mixture constitutes what was formerly known as slow-reacting substance of anaphylaxis-A]. These substances are potent constrictors of smooth muscle and vasodilators and are responsible for the clinical symptoms associated with immediate hypersensitivity (see Chapter 23). In recent years, it has been shown, mainly through animal studies, that IL-13, released by Th2 cells, can induce clinical manifestations of asthma, independently of IgE and eosinophils. Thus, cell-mediated, IgE-independent mechanisms may also play a pathogenic role in type I hypersensitivity reactions (Chapter 21).

TABLE 3 Common Clinical Manifestations of Anaphylaxis

Cardiovascular
    Tachycardia then hypotension
    Shock: $\leq$50% intravascular volume loss
    Myocardial ischemia
Lower respiratory
    Bronchoconstriction
    Wheezing
    Cough
    Shortness of breath
Upper respiratory
    Laryngeal/pharyngeal edema
    Rhinorrhea

Source: Adapted from Fisher MM. Anaesth Intens Care 1986; 14:17–21.

CYTOTOXIC REACTIONS (TYPE II HYPERSENSITIVITY)

This second type of hypersensitivity involves, in its most common forms, complement-fixing antibodies (IgM or IgG) directed against cellular or tissue antigens. The clinical expression of type II hypersensitivity reaction depends largely on the distribution of the antigens recognized by the responsible antibodies.

Autoimmune Hemolytic Anemia and Other Autoimmune Cytopenias

Autoimmune hemolytic anemia, autoimmune thrombocytopenia, and autoimmune neutropenia (discussed in greater detail in Chapters 19, 20, and 24) are clear examples of type II (cytotoxic) hypersensitivity reactions in which the antigens are unique to cellular elements of the blood. Autoimmune hemolytic anemia is the best understood of these conditions.

Patients with autoimmune hemolytic anemia synthesize antibodies that are directed to their own red cells. Those antibodies may cause hemolysis by two main mechanisms:

1. If the antibodies are of the IgM isotype, complement is activated up to C9, and the red cells can be directly hemolysed (intravascular hemolysis).
2. If, for a variety of reasons, the antibodies (usually IgG) fail to activate the full complement cascade, the red cells will be opsonized with antibody (and possibly C3b) and are taken up and destroyed by phagocytic cells expressing FcγR and C3b receptors (extravascular hemolysis).

Intravascular hemolysis is associated with release of free hemoglobin into the circulation (hemoglobinemia), which may be excreted in the urine (hemoglobinuria). Massive hemoglobinuria can induce acute tubular damage and kidney failure, usually reversible. In contrast, extravascular hemolysis is usually associated with increased levels of bilirrubin, derived from cellular catabolism of hemoglobin. All hemolytic reactions usually lead to the mobilization of erythrocyte precursors from the bone marrow, to compensate for the acute loss. This is reflected by reticulocytosis, and in severe cases, by erythroblastosis (see Chapter 22).

Goodpasture's Syndrome

The classical example of a type II hypersensitivity reaction in which the antibodies are directed against tissue antigens is Goodpasture's syndrome. The pathogenesis of Goodpasture's syndrome involves the spontaneous emergence of basement membrane autoantibodies that bind to antigens of the glomerular and alveolar basement membranes. Those antibodies are predominantly of the IgG isotype. Using fluorescein-conjugated antisera, the deposition of IgG and complement in patients with Goodpasture's syndrome usually follows a linear, very regular pattern, corresponding to the outline of the glomerular or alveolar basement membranes.

Two types of observations support the pathogenic role of antibasement membrane antibodies:

1. Elution studies yield Ig-rich preparations that, when injected into primates, can induce a disease similar to human Goodpasture's syndrome.
2. Goodpasture's syndrome recurs in patients who receive a kidney transplant and the transplanted kidney shows identical patterns of IgG and complement deposition along the glomerular basement membrane.

Once antigen–antibody complexes are formed in the kidney glomeruli or in the lungs, complement will be activated and, as a result, C5a and C3a will be generated. These complement components are chemotactic for polymorphonuclear (PMN) leukocytes; C5a also increases vascular permeability directly or indirectly (by inducing the degranulation of basophils and mast cells) (see Chapter 9). Furthermore, C5a can upregulate the expression of cell adhesion molecules (CAMs) of the CD11b/CD18 family (see Chapter 13) in PMN leukocytes and monocytes, promoting their interaction with ICAM-1 expressed by endothelial cells, thus facilitating the migration of inflammatory cells into the extravascular space. In the extravascular space

PMN leukocytes will recognize the Fc regions of basement membrane-bound antibodies, as well as C3b bound to the corresponding immune complexes (IC), and will release their enzymatic contents that include a variety of metalloproteinases, including collagenases and plasminogen activator. Plasminogen activator converts plasminogen into plasmin, which in turn can split complement components and generate bioactive fragments, enhancing the inflammatory reaction. Collagenases and other metalloproteinases cause tissue damage (i.e., destruction of the basement membrane) that eventually may compromise the function of the affected organ.

The pathological sequence of events after the reaction of antibasement membrane antibodies with their corresponding antigens is indistinguishable from the reactions triggered by the deposition of soluble IC or by the reaction of circulating antibodies with antigens passively fixed to a tissue, considered as type III hypersensitivity reactions.

Nephrotoxic (Masugi) Nephritis

This experimental model of immunologically mediated nephritis, named after the scientist who developed it, is induced by injection of heterologous antibasement membrane antibodies into healthy animals. Those antibodies combine with basement membrane antigens, particularly at the glomerular level, and trigger the development of glomerulonephritis.

This experimental model has been extremely useful to demonstrate the pathogenic importance of complement activation and of neutrophil accumulation. For example, if instead of complete antibodies, one injects Fab or F(ab')2 fragments generated from antibasement membrane antibodies that do not activate complement, the accumulation of neutrophils in the glomeruli fails to take place, and tissue damage will be from minimal to nonexistent. Similar protection against the development of glomerulonephritis is observed when animals are rendered C3 deficient by injection of cobra venom factor prior to the administration of antibasement membrane antibodies, or when those antibodies are administered to animals rendered neutropenic by administration of cytotoxic drugs or of antineutrophil antibodies.

IMMUNE COMPLEX-INDUCED HYPERSENSITIVITY REACTIONS (TYPE III HYPERSENSITIVITY)

In the course of acute or chronic infections, or as a consequence of the production of autoantibodies, antigen–antibody complexes (IC) are likely to be formed in circulation or in tissues to which the pertinent self antigens or microbial antigens are expressed or have been adsorbed. Both scenarios can lead to inflammatory changes, which are characteristic of the so-called IC diseases (see Chapter 23).

Circulating IC are usually adsorbed to red cells and cleared by the phagocytic system (see Chapters 13 and 23). In most cases, this will be an inconsequential sequence of events, but in cases where there is massive formation of circulating IC (e.g., serum sickness), the clearance capacity of the phagocytic system is exceeded, and inflammatory reactions can be triggered by the deposition of those IC in tissues. A simplified sequence of events leading to immune complex-induced inflammation is shown in Figure 1.

The in situ formation of IC is a more likely scenario as far as triggering tissue inflammation in conditions other than serum sickness. The adsorption of circulating antigens of microbial origin or released by dying cells to a variety of tissues seems to be a relatively common event. If the same antigens trigger a humoral immune response, immune complex formation may take place in the tissues where the antigens are adsorbed, in which case clearance by the phagocytic system may become impossible. In fact, tissue–bound IC are very strong activators of the complement system and of phagocytic cells, which triggers a sequence of events leading to tissue inflammation virtually identical to that observed in cases of in situ immune reactions, involving the reaction of tissue antigens with the corresponding antibodies.

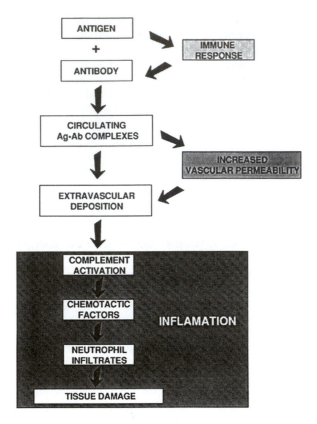

FIGURE 1 Diagrammatic representation of the sequence of events triggered by the deposition of soluble immune complexes that eventually results in inflammation and tissue damage.

Special Manifestations of Type III Hypersensitivity
The Arthus Reaction

Arthus, who observed that the intradermal injection of antigen into an animal previously sensitized results in a local inflammatory reaction, first described this reaction at the turn of the century. A human equivalent of this reaction can be observed in some reactions to immunization boosters in individuals who have already reached high levels of immunity.

The Arthus reaction is triggered by the combination of complement-fixing IgG antibodies (characteristically predominating in hyperimmune states in most species) and tissue-fixed antigens. The lag time between antigen challenge and the reaction is usually six hours, which is considerably longer than the time lag of an immediate hypersensitivity reaction, but considerably shorter than that of a delayed hypersensitivity reaction.

Arthus reactions are typically elicited in the skin. They are usually edematous in the early stages, but later can become hemorrhagic, and, eventually, necrotic. Deep tissues can also be affected, because the same pathogenic mechanisms can lead to deep tissue inflammation whenever the antigen, although intrinsically soluble, is unable to diffuse freely and remains retained in or around its penetration point (e.g., the perialveolar spaces for inhaled antigens).

Because it is easily induced in a variety of laboratory animals, the Arthus reaction is one of the best-studied models of immune complex disease. Immunohistological studies have shown that soon after antigen is injected in the skin, IgG antibody and C3 will appear in perivascular deposits at the site of injection. This is followed by massive influx of granulocytes, believed to result from activation of the complement system by the in situ-formed IC. The importance of granulocytes was confirmed in experiments in which investigators tried to induce the Arthus in laboratory animals rendered neutropenic by administration of nitrogen mustard or of anti-neutrophil serum. Under these experimental conditions the inflammatory reaction is prevented and the reactions does not develop.

In spite of their pathogenic role, granulocytes will actively engulf and catabolize the tissue-deposited IC, eliminating the trigger for the inflammatory reaction. As the IC are eliminated, the cellular infiltrate changes from a predominance of neutrophils and other granulocytes to a predominance of mononuclear cells, which is usually associated with the healing stage. The degree of healing depends on whether the exposure to the triggering antigen is a discrete event or repeated over time. Single or widely spaced exposure is usually followed by complete healing, while chronic or frequently repeated exposure(s) tend to lead to irreversible damage.

Serum Sickness

In the pre-antibiotic era, the treatment of rabies, bacterial pneumonia, diphtheria and other infections involved the administration of heterologous antisera as a way to transfer immunity to the offending agents. In many instances, serotherapy appeared to be successful, and the patient improved, but a week to ten days after the injection of heterologous antiserum, the patient developed what was termed as "serum sickness": a combination of cutaneous rash (often purpuric), fever, arthralgias, mild acute glomerulonephritis, and carditis. Currently, serum sickness as a complication of passive immunotherapy with heterologous antisera is seen after injection of heterologous antisera to snake venom, after the administration of mouse monoclonal antibodies in cancer immunotherapy, and after the administration of heterologous (monoclonal or polyclonal) antilymphocyte sera in transplanted patients. However, it can also be a side effect of some forms of drug therapy, particularly with penicillin and related drugs.

Serum sickness is extremely easy to reproduce in experimental animals through the injection of heterologous proteins. Basically, two types of experimental serum sickness can be induced:

1. Acute, after a single immunization with a large dose of protein
2. Chronic, after repeated daily injections of small doses of protein

While acute serum sickness is reversible, the chronic form, which closely resembles human glomerulonephritis, is usually associated with irreversible damage.

In all types of serum sickness, the initial event is the triggering of a humoral immune response, which explains the lag period of 7 to 10 days between the injection of heterologous protein (or drug) and the beginning of clinical symptoms. The lag period is shorter and the reaction more severe if there has been presensitization to the antigen in question.

As soon as the antibodies are produced in sufficient amounts, they combine with the antigens (which at that time are still present in relatively large concentrations in the serum of the injected individual or experimental animal). Initially, the antigen–antibody reaction will take place in conditions of great antigen excess, and the resulting complexes are too small to activate complement or to be taken up by phagocytic cells, and will remain in circulation without major consequences. As the immune response progresses and increasing amounts of antibody are produced, the antigen–antibody ratio will be such that intermediate-size IC will be formed. The intermediate-size IC are potentially pathogenic; they are large enough to activate complement and small enough to cross the endothelial barrier (particularly if vascular permeability is increased as a consequence of complement activation and release of C3a and C5a). Once they reach the extravascular space, inflammatory cells are recruited and activated and initiate the chain of events leading to tissue inflammation. As in the case of the Arthus reaction, the inflammatory changes associated with serum sickness do not take place or are very mild if complement or neutrophils are depleted.

The deposition of IC can take place in different organs, such as the myocardium (causing myocardial inflammation), skin (causing erythematous rashes), joints (causing arthritis), and kidney (causing acute glomerulonephritis). Soluble IC can also be absorbed by formed elements of the blood, particularly erythrocytes, neutrophils, and platelets. Although red cell absorption is usually a protective mechanism (see Chapter 9), if the amounts and characteristics of RBC-absorbed IC are such that the regulatory function of CR1 is overridden, hemolysis may take place. Thrombocytopenia and neutropenia can also result from the activation of the complement system by cell-associated IC. Purpuric rashes due to thrombocytopenia are frequently seen in serum sickness.

DELAYED (TYPE IV) HYPERSENSITIVITY REACTIONS

In contrast to the other types of hypersensitivity reactions discussed earlier, type IV or delayed hypersensitivity is a manifestation of cell-mediated immunity. In other words, this type of hypersensitivity reaction is due to the activation of specifically sensitized T lymphocytes rather than to an antigen–antibody reaction.

Tuberculin Test as a Paradigmatic Type IV Reaction

Intradermal injection of tuberculin or PPD into an individual that has been previously sensitized (by exposure to *Mycobacterium tuberculosis* or by Bacillus Calmette Guérin vaccination) is followed, 48–72 hours after the injection, by a skin reaction at the site of injection characterized by redness and induration. Histologically, the reaction is characterized by perivenular mononuclear cell infiltration, often described as "perivascular cuffing." Macrophages can be seen infiltrating the dermis. If the reaction is intense, a central necrotic area may develop. The cellular nature of the perivascular infiltrate, which contrasts with the predominantly edematous reaction in a cutaneous type I hypersensitivity reaction, is responsible for the induration.

Experimental Studies

Experiments carried out with guinea pigs investigating the elements involved in transfer of delayed hypersensitivity were critical in defining the involvement of lymphocytes in delayed hypersensitivity. When guinea pigs are immunized with egg albumin and adjuvant, not only do they become allergic, as discussed earlier, but they also develop cell-mediated hypersensitivity to the antigen. This duality can be demonstrated by passively transferring serum and lymphocytes from sensitized animals to nonsensitized recipients of the same strain and challenging the passively immunized animals with egg albumin. The animals that received serum will develop an anaphylactic response immediately after challenge, while those that received lymphocytes will only show signals of a considerably less severe reaction after at least 24 hours have elapsed from the time of challenge.

Most of our knowledge about the pathogenesis of delayed hypersensitivity reactions derives from experimental studies involving contact hypersensitivity. Experimental sensitization through the skin is relatively easy to induce by percutaneous application of low molecular weight substances such as picric acid or dinitrochlorobenzene. The initial application leads to sensitization, a second application will elicit a delayed hypersensitivity reaction in the area where the antigen is applied. In some cases, perhaps as a consequence of retention of the sensitizing substance in the dermis, a delayed reaction can be seen about one week after the contact. These instances may represent responses after primary sensitization.

Induction of Contact Hypersensitivity

The compounds used to induce contact hypersensitivity are not immunogenic by themselves. It is believed that these compounds couple spontaneously to an endogenous carrier protein, and as a result of this coupling, the small molecule will act as a hapten, while the endogenous protein will play the role of a carrier. A common denominator of the sensitizing compounds is the expression of reactive groups, such as Cl, F, Br, and SO_3H, which enable them to bind covalently to the carrier protein.

Spontaneous sensitization to drugs, chemicals, or metals, is believed to involve diffusion of the haptenic substance into the dermis mostly through the sweat glands (hydrophobic substances appear to penetrate the skin more easily than hydrophilic substances) and once in the dermis, the haptenic groups will react spontaneously with "carrier" proteins to which they become covalently bound. By a pathway that has not been defined, antigen-presenting cells in the dermis (Langerhans cells, dendritic cells) take up the hapten–carrier conjugates, transport them to a draining lymph node, where a sensitizing peptide is presented in association with major histocompatibility complex-II molecules to the $CD4^+$ T lymphocytes in the environment. The predominant involvement of T lymphocytes in the anti-hapten responses of cutaneous expression is paradoxical if we consider that in most experimentally induced hapten–carrier responses, the hapten is recognized by B lymphocytes. Since the carrier protein is autologous and the T cell receptors are not known to react with haptenic compounds, it seems likely that the reaction is triggered by a sensitizing peptide derived from an autologous protein carrier, containing the covalently associated sensitizing compound, which somehow must modify the configuration of the autologous peptide, rendering it immunogenic.

Effector Mechanisms

The initial sensitization results in the acquisition of immunological memory. Later, when the sensitized individual is challenged with the same chemical, sensitized T cells will be stimulated into functionally active cells, releasing a variety of cytokines, which include IL-8, RANTES, and macrophage chemotactic proteins that attract and activate monocytes/macrophages, lymphocytes, basophils, eosinophils, and neutrophils. Other cytokines released by activated lymphocytes, particularly tumor necrosis factor (TNF) and IL-1, upregulate the expression of CAMs in endothelial cells, facilitating the adhesion of leukocytes to the endothelium, a key step in the extravascular migration of inflammatory cells. As a result of the release of chemokines and of the upregulation of CAMs a cellular infiltrate predominantly constituted by mononuclear cells (but also including granulocytes) forms in the area where the sensitizing compound has been re-introduced, 24 to 48 hours after exposure. The tissue damage that takes place in this type of reaction is likely to be due to the effects of active oxygen radicals and enzymes (particularly proteases, collagenase, and cathepsins) released by infiltrating monocytes and tissue macrophages, activated by the chemokines and other cytokines.

In severe cases, a contact hypersensitivity reaction may take an exudative, edematous, highly inflammatory character. The release of proteases from monocytes and macrophages may trigger the complement-dependent inflammatory pathways by directly splitting C3 and C5; C5a will add its chemotactic effects to those of chemokines released by activated mononuclear cells, and will also cause increased vascular permeability—a constant feature of complement-dependent inflammatory processes. It is not surprising, therefore, that a reaction which at the onset is cell-mediated and associated to a mononuclear cell infiltrate, may, in time, evolve into a more classical inflammatory process with predominance of neutrophils and a more edematous character, less characteristic of a cell-mediated reaction.

Contact Hypersensitivity in Humans

Contact hypersensitivity reactions are observed with some frequency in humans due to spontaneous sensitization to a variety of substances:

1. Plant catechols are apparently responsible for the hypersensitivity reactions to poison ivy and poison oak.
2. A variety of chemicals can be implicated in hypersensitivity reactions to cosmetics and leather.
3. Topically used drugs, particularly sulfonamides, often cause contact hypersensitivity.
4. Metals such as nickel can be involved in reactions triggered by the use of bracelets, earrings, or thimbles.

The diagnosis of contact hypersensitivity is usually based on a careful history of exposure to potential sensitizing agents and on the observation of the distribution of lesions that can be very informative about the source of sensitization. Patch tests using small pieces of filter paper impregnated with suspected sensitizing agents, which are taped to the back of the patient can be used to identify the sensitizing substance.

Jones-Mote Reaction

Following challenge with an intradermal injection of a small dose of a protein to which an individual has been previously sensitized, a delayed reaction (with a lag of 24 hours), somewhat different than a classical delayed hypersensitivity reaction, may be seen. The skin appears more erythematous and less indurated, and the infiltrating cells are mostly lymphocytes and basophils, the latter sometimes predominating. The reaction has also been described, for this reason, as cutaneous basophilic hypersensitivity. Experimentally, it has been demonstrated that this reaction is triggered as a consequence of the antigenic stimulation of sensitized T lymphocytes.

Homograft Rejection

A most striking clinical manifestation of a delayed hypersensitivity reaction is the rejection of a graft. In classical chronic rejection, the graft recipient's immune system is first sensitized to peptides derived from alloantigens of the donor. After clonal expansion, activated T lymphocytes will reach the target organ, recognize the alloantigen-derived peptides against which they became sensitized, and initiate a sequence of events that leads to inflammation and eventual necrosis of the organ. This topic will be discussed in detail in Chapter 25.

Systemic Consequences of Cell-Mediated Hypersensitivity Reactions

While type IV hypersensitivity reactions with cutaneous expression usually have no systemic repercussions, cell-mediated hypersensitivity reactions localized to internal organs, such as the formation of granulomatous lesions caused by chronic infections with *Mycobacterium* sp., may be associated with systemic reactions. Cytokines released by activated lymphocytes and inflammatory cells play a major pathogenic role in such reactions. Pro-inflammatory cytokines, particularly IL-1, induce the release of prostaglandins in the hypothalamic temperature-regulating center and cause fever, thus acting as a pyrogenic factor. TNF is also pyrogenic, both directly and by inducing the release of IL-1 by endothelial cells and monocytes. In addition, these two cytokines activate the synthesis of acute phase proteins (e.g., C-reactive protein) by the liver.

Prolonged release of TNF, on the other hand, may have deleterious effects since this factor contributes to the development of cachexia. Cachexia develops because TNF inhibits lipoprotein lipase, and as a consequence, there is an accumulation of triglyceride-rich particles in the serum and a lack of the breakdown of triglycerides into glycerol and free fatty acids. This results in decreased incorporation of triglycerides into the adipose tissue, and, consequently, in a negative metabolic balance. The cells continue to breakdown stored triglycerides by other pathways to generate energy, and the used triglycerides are not replaced. Cachexia is often a preterminal development in patients with severe chronic infections

BIBLIOGRAPHY

Cavani A. Breaking tolerance to nickel. Toxicology 2005; 209:119–121.
Collins T. Adhesion molecules in leukocyte emigration. Sci Am Med 1995; 2(6):28.
Fisher MM. Clinical observations on the pathophysiology and treatment of anaphylactic cardiovascular collapse. Anaesth Intensive Care 1986; 14:17–21.
Graft DF. Insect sting allergy. Med Clin North Am 2006; 90:211–232.
Kaplan AP, Kuna P, Reddigari SR. Chemokines and the allergic response. Exp Dermatol 1995; 4:260.
Kavanaugh A. Adhesion molecules as therapeutic targets in the treatment of allergic and immunologially mediated disorders. Clin Immunol Immunopathol 1996; 80(Pt 2):S40.
Meyers CM, Geanacopoulos M, Holzman LB, Salant DJ. Glomerular disease workshop. J Am Soc Nephrol 2005; 16:3472–3476.
Nagata M. Inflammatory cells and oxygen radicals. Curr Drug Targets Inflamm Allergy 2005; 4:503–504.
Nangaku M, Couser WG. Mechanisms of immune-deposit formation and the mediation of immune renal injury. Clin Exp Nephrol 2005; 9:183–191.
Nankivell BJ, Chapman JR. Chronic allograft nephropathy: current concepts and future directions. Transplantation 2006; 81:643–654.
Schroeder JT, Kagey-Sobotka A, Lichtenstein LM. The role of the basophil in allergic inflammation. Allergy 1995; 50:463.
Schwiebert LA, Beck LA, Stellato C, et al. Glucocorticosteroid inhibition of cytokine production: relevance to antiallergic actions. J Allergy Clin Immunol 1996; 97:143.
Semple JW, Freedman J. Autoimmune pathogenesis and autoimmune hemolytic anemia. Semin Hematol 2005; 42:122–130.
Vliagoftis H, Befus AD. Mast cells at mucosal frontiers. Curr Mol Med 2005; 5:573–589.
Wills-Karp M, Luyimbazi J, Xu X, et al. Interleukin-13: cental mediator of allergic asthma. Science 1998; 282:2258.

21 | Immunoglobulin E-Mediated (Immediate) Hypersensitivity

Albert F. Finn, Jr.
National Allergy, Asthma, and Urticaria Centers of Charleston, Medical University of South Carolina, Charleston, South Carolina, U.S.A.

Gabriel Virella
Department of Microbiology and Immunology, Medical University of South Carolina, Charleston, South Carolina, U.S.A.

INTRODUCTION

Immunoglobulin (Ig) E-mediated hypersensitivity reactions are also known as immediate hypersensitivity reactions because of the short time lag (seconds to minutes) between antigen exposure and the onset of clinical symptoms. This is because the initial symptoms of immediate hypersensitivity depend on the release of preformed mediators stored in cytoplasmic granules of basophils and mast cells; the release is triggered by the cross-linking of membrane-bound IgE with the corresponding antigen (also known as allergen, by being involved in allergic reactions).

MAJOR CLINICAL EXPRESSIONS

Immediate hypersensitivity or allergic reactions can have a variety of clinical expressions, including anaphylaxis, asthma, urticaria (hives), and rhinitis (hay fever). Table 1 summarizes the morbidity and mortality data for the two most severe types of allergic reactions, anaphylaxis, and asthma.

Anaphylaxis

Anaphylaxis is an acute life-threatening IgE-mediated reaction usually affecting multiple organs. The time lag between exposure to the allergen and the onset of symptoms depends on the level of hypersensitivity, nature of the antigen, intensity of exposure, and site of exposure to the antigen. In a typical case, manifestations begin within 5 to 10 minutes after antigenic challenge. Reactions that appear more slowly tend to be less severe. Latency longer than two hours after antigen exposure leaves the diagnosis of anaphylaxis open to question.

Multiple organ systems are usually affected in anaphylactic reactions, including the skin (pruritus, flushing, urticaria, and angioedema), respiratory tract (bronchospasm and laryngeal edema), and cardiovascular system (hypotension, cardiac arrhythmias, and myocardial infarction).

As a rule, most of the acute manifestations subside within one or two hours. However, similar symptoms of variable intensity may occur 6 to 12 hours later. This late-phase reaction results from cytokine release from activated basophils and mast cells, secondary immune cell activation, and further synthesis and release of mediators of inflammation.

When death occurs, it is usually due to laryngeal edema, intractable bronchospasm, hypotensive shock or cardiac arrhythmias developing within the first two hours.

Atopy

Atopy is defined as a genetically determined state of IgE-related disease. Its most common clinical manifestations include asthma, rhinitis, urticaria, and atopic dermatitis.

TABLE 1   Morbidity and Mortality from Systemic Anaphylaxis and Bronchial Asthma in the United States

	Morbidity	**Mortality**
Systemic anaphylaxis		
Caused by antibiotics	10–40: 100,000 injections	1: 100,000 injections
Caused by insect bites	10: 100,000 persons/yr	10–80/yr
Asthma	More than 15 million persons (5–8.9% of U.S. population)	All ages: 1.7/100,000/yr >60 yr of age: 7.0/100,000/yr

Allergic Asthma

Allergic asthma, by its potential severity and frequency, is the most important manifestation of atopy. However, not all cases of asthma are of proven allergic etiology. The differential characteristics of allergic (extrinsic) and nonallergic (intrinsic) asthma are summarized in Table 2. The major difference between both is the strong association of allergic asthma with demonstrable clinical allergy to relevant respirable allergens. These airborne allergens are inspired and reach the lower airways, where they cause chronic allergic inflammation.

Food Allergies

Food allergies are common, can be caused by a variety of food stuffs (Table 3), and have multiple clinical presentations (Table 4). Shellfish and peanuts are often involved in the most severe reactions to food antigens, including anaphylactic reactions.

PATHOGENESIS

The pathogenesis of immediate hypersensitivity reactions involves a well-defined sequence of events:

1. Induction of the immune response and synthesis of specific IgE antibodies.
2. Binding of IgE antibodies to high affinity $Fc_\varepsilon I$ receptors on basophils and mast cells. Once bound, IgE remains associated to the cell membrane and acts as an antigen receptor.
3. Cross-linking of receptor-bound IgE by multivalent antigens. This initiates the release of preformed vasoactive compounds and their synthesis, and later release, of cytokines [e.g., Interleukin (IL)-4, IL-5, and IL-13] and other mediators of inflammation.
4. The preformed substances released by basophils and mast cells have significant effects on target tissues, such as smooth muscle, vascular endothelium, and mucous glands. They also act as chemoattractants and may elicit central nervous system-mediated reflexes (e.g., sneezing).
5. Furthermore, activated basophils and mast cells can synthesize and release IL-4 and IL-13, and express the CD40 ligand. IL-4 synthesis and the expression of CD40L are both essential

TABLE 2   Characteristics of Allergic (Extrinsic) and Nonallergic (Intrinsic) Asthma

Symptoms: Dyspnea with prolonged expiratory phase; may be associated with cough and sputum
Chest X-rays: Hyperlucency with increased AP distance (reflecting impaired expiratory capacity with air trapping), bronchial thickening

	Allergic	*Nonallergic*
Blood	Eosinophilia	Normal eosinophil count
Sputum	Eosinophilia	No eosinophils
Total IgE	Raised	Normal
Antigen-specific IgE	Raised	None
Pathology	Obstruction of airways due to smooth muscle hypertrophy with constriction and mucosal edema; hypertrophy of mucous glands; eosinophil infiltration	
Frequency	Children: 80%[a] Adults: 60%[a]	20% 40%

[a]% of total number of bronchial asthma cases seen in each age range.
Abbreviation: AP, antero-posterior.

TABLE 3   Common Allergenic Foods

Legumes (peanuts and soybeans)
Mollusks (snails, mussels, oysters, scallops, clams, and squid)
Milk
Eggs
Fish (cod, salmon, haddock, etc.)
Crustacea (shrimp, crawfish, lobster, etc.)
Wheat
Tree nuts (almonds, walnuts, Brazil nuts, etc.)
Selected food additives

factors to stimulate IgE synthesis (see Chapter 11). The synthesis and release of IL-13 can facilitate processes that cause many of the symptoms associated with persistent reactions, particularly chronic allergic asthma.

Immunoglobulin-E Antibodies

Prausnitz and Kustner in 1921 published the first demonstration that serum contains a factor capable of mediating specific allergic reactions. The injection of serum from a fish-allergic person (Kustner) into Dr. Prausnitz's skin, and subsequent exposure of Dr. Prausnitz to fish antigen injected in the same site resulted in an allergic wheal and flare response.

In 1967, Ishizaka et al. isolated a new immunoglobulin class, IgE, from the serum of ragweed-allergic individuals. Several patients with IgE-producing plasmocytomas were subsequently discovered and provided a source of very large amounts of monoclonal IgE that greatly facilitated further studies of IgE structure and the production of anti-IgE antibodies.

Immunoglobulin-E Antibody Response

IgE is predominantly synthesized in perimucosal lymphoid tissues of the respiratory and gastrointestinal tract. In developing countries, the main antigenic stimuli for IgE synthesis are parasites (particularly nematodes). Levels of circulating IgE considered as normal in a developing country with endemic parasitism are two to three orders of magnitude higher than in the western world. The vast majority of allergens, which are either ingested or inhaled, stimulate the same perimucosal cells. In the perimucosal tissues only B lymphocytes with membrane IgE will differentiate into IgE-producing plasma cells. Those IgE-carrying B cells are only a small fraction of the total B cell population in the submucosa, but are over-represented in the perimucosal lymphoid tissues compared to other lymphoid territories.

During the primary immune response to an allergen or a parasite, most of the IgE synthesized appears to be of low affinity. The changes, occurring after a second exposure, select out the synthesis of IgE of progressively higher affinity, probably as a consequence of somatic hypermutations (see Chapters 7 and 12) and apoptosis. The expansion of affinity-optimized clones may be the reason why allergic reactions very seldom develop after the first exposure to an allergen. When an immediate hypersensitivity reaction appears to develop after what seems to be a first exposure to any given allergen, one must consider the possibility of

TABLE 4   Clinical Manifestations of Food Allergy

Nausea
Diarrhea
Abdominal cramps
Pruritic rashes
Angioedema
Asthma/rhinitis
Vomiting
Hives
Laryngeal edema
Anaphylactic shock

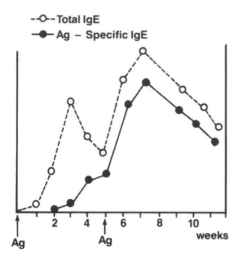

FIGURE 1 Longitudinal evolution of total immunoglobulin E (IgE) and antigen-specific IgE levels during an immune-response to an allergen.

cross-reaction between a substance to which the individual was previously sensitized and the substance which elicits the allergic reaction. Such cross-reactions are usually due to molecular mimicry (see Chapter 18) and can be quite unpredictable.

Repeated exposures to parasites or allergens will stimulate the differentiation of memory cells, and the proportion of circulating high affinity antigen-specific IgE will also increase (Fig. 1). In patients suffering from severe seasonal allergies due to pollen, antigen-specific IgE may constitute up to 50% of the total IgE.

Genetic Control of Immunoglobulin-E Synthesis

The study of total IgE levels in normal nonallergic individuals shows a distribution in three groups: high, intermediate, and low producers (Fig. 2). Family studies further suggested that the ability to produce high levels of IgE is a recessive trait, controlled by unknown genes independent of the human leukocyte antigen (HLA) system. A candidate gene has been localized to chromosome 5(5q31–q33)—in close vicinity to the genes for IL-4, IL-5, and IL-13. The gene in question seems to influence not only the synthesis of IgE but also determines bronchial hyper-responsiveness to histamine and other stimuli.

On the other hand, the tendency to develop allergic disorders in response to specific allergens is HLA-linked. For instance, the ability to produce antigen-specific-IgE after exposure to the Ra5 antigen of ragweed is observed more often in HLA B7, DR2 individuals than in the general population. Recent studies suggest that various major histocompatibility complex (MHC) class II antigens are associated with high responses to many different allergens. The biological basis for the association between MHC-II molecules and the IgE-mediated allergic immune reaction is believed to be one of the many expressions of the control exerted by

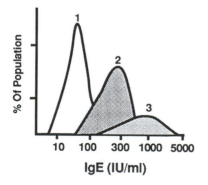

FIGURE 2 Distribution of IgE levels in a population of nonallergic individuals. Three subpopulations appear to exist: one constituted by low-responder individuals, one by high responder individuals (3), and a third population of individuals with intermediate levels of IgE (2). *Abbreviation*: IgE, Immunoglobulin E.

MHC-II–expressing antigen-presenting cells on the immune response. This theory is based on the assumption that the MHC-II repertoire determines what antigen-derived peptides are most efficiently presented to helper T cells.

The genes controlling high IgE levels and high IgE antibody synthesis after exposure to allergens appear to have synergistic effects. For example, an HLA B7, DR2 individual who is also genetically predisposed to produce high levels of IgE is likely to have a more severe allergic disorder than an individual without this genetic combination.

T–B Cell Cooperation in Immunoglobulin-E Antibody Responses

The role of activated Th2 cells in type I hypersensitivity reaction is critically important. Production of high levels of IgE has been shown to be dependent on the activation of IL-4–producing Th2 cells, as well as on the delivery of coactivating signals involving CD28/CD80 and CD40/CD40L. IL-4 has been demonstrated to promote IgE synthesis by activated B lymphocytes. IL-5, which is produced at the same time by the same activated CD4 lymphocytes, is believed to play a role in the late phase of allergic reactions, which is discussed later in this chapter.

Both in humans and animal models the production of allergen-specific IgE persists long after the second exposure. This may result from the capture of IgE-containing immune complexes by dendritic cells, which express the Fc$_\varepsilon$RII (CD23). Membrane-bound immune complexes are known to persist for longer periods of time, constantly stimulating B cells and promoting the persistence of secondary immune responses and the differentiation of antibodies with increased affinity (see Chapter 12). At the same time, the internalization and processing of immune complexes containing the same antigen(s) and IgG antibody is likely to be the source of allergen-derived peptides that will continue to activate the Th2 subpopulation.

Interaction of Immunoglobulin-E with Cell Surface Receptors

Two types of Fc receptors reacting with IgE molecules have been characterized. A unique high affinity receptor designated as Fc$_\varepsilon$ RI is expressed on the surface of basophils and mast cells. Most IgE antibodies interact with this receptor and become cell-associated soon after secretion from plasma cells. This sequestration is partially responsible for the short, circulating half-life of IgE as a free molecule.

The structure of the Fc$_\varepsilon$RI is unique among the well-characterized immune cell receptors. It is composed of three subunits: a heterodimer formed by the interaction of two chains (α and β), and a homodimer of a third type of chain (γ chain). The whole molecule is therefore designated as $\alpha\beta\gamma_2$ (Fig. 3). The external domain of the α chain binds the Fc portion of IgE. The β and

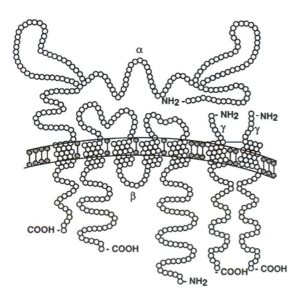

FIGURE 3 Diagrammatic representation of the primary structure of the Fc$_\varepsilon$RI. *Source*: Modified from Metzger H. Clin Exp Allergy 1991; 21:1.

γ chains function as signal transduction units. Both of them contain immunoreceptor tyrosine-based activation motifs (ITAM) (see Chapter 4). Cross-linking of the Fc_ε RI results in activation of the protein kinase Lyn, which phosphorylates ITAM tyrosines, leading them to the activation of other protein kinases, such as Syk, as well as of the integral membrane linker molecule LAT (see Chapter 11). The phosphorylation of Syk and LAT is followed by activation of signaling cascades, which eventually lead to the release of preformed granules and to the expression of a variety of genes coding for cytokines, enzymes, and so on.

The interaction between the $Fc_\varepsilon RI$ and IgE is characterized by a very high affinity (association constants range from 10^8 to $10^{10}\,M^{-1}$). Because of this high affinity, IgE binds rapidly and very strongly to cells expressing $Fc_\varepsilon RI$ and is released from these cells very slowly. Passively transferred IgE remains cell-bound for several weeks in the skin of normal humans. Because the mast cells and basophils do not produce IgE molecules, there is no clonal restriction at the mast cell/basophil level. Therefore, if the patient produces IgE antibodies to more than one allergen, each basophil or mast cell may bind IgE antibodies of different specificities.

The interaction between IgE and $Fc_\varepsilon RI$ does not result in cell activation, as there is no cross-linking of receptors. IgE serves as an antigen-receptor for mast cells and basophils. Receptor-bound IgE discriminates among antigens, binding exclusively those allergens to which the patient has become sensitized.

Receptor-bound IgE must be cross-linked for basophils and mast cells to release their intracellular mediators (Fig. 4). The physiological cross-linking agent is the allergen, which needs to be multivalent. Cross-linking of receptor bound IgE can also be induced with anti-IgE antibodies or with their divalent F(ab')2 fragments. Unoccupied receptors may be cross-linked with aggregated Fc fragments of IgE. In contrast, mast cells and basophils with IgE-antihapten antibodies on their membranes cannot be stimulated by soluble, univalent, haptens, because they are unable to cross-link membrane IgE molecules. Stimulation is only possible when carrier-bound haptens are used, because those can cross-link many IgE molecules. All the types of cross-linking listed earlier are equally efficient in activating IgE-carrying mast cells and basophils. Activation results in the release of granule contents into the extracellular compartment and activation of the synthesis of additional mediators.

Other receptors can be involved in basophil/mast cell activation, leading to the liberation of mediators. Basophils and mast cells also respond to C3a, C5a, basic lysosomal proteins, kinins, opioids, ionophores, and autoantibodies of the IgG isotype directed against the α subunit of the $Fc_\varepsilon RI$ (these autoantibodies are detected in 40% of the patients with chronic idiopathic urticaria). It is apparent that there are multiple pathways for mast-cell activation and that the participation of cell-bound IgE is not always needed.

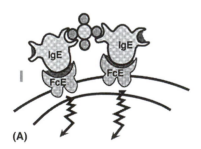

(A)

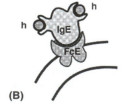

(B)

FIGURE 4 Diagrammatic depiction of the conditions required for stimulation of mediator release by mast cells and basophils. (**A**) the reaction of membrane-bound immunoglobulin E (IgE) with a polyvalent antigen, leading to cross-linking of IgE molecules, is represented. This type of reaction leads to mediator release. (**B**) the reaction of membrane-bound IgE with a monovalent hapten is illustrated. This reaction does not lead to mediator release.

A second receptor for IgE, Fc$_\varepsilon$RII (CD23), is expressed on the membrane of lymphocytes, platelets, eosinophils, and dendritic cells and binds IgE to receptors with lower affinity than Fc$_\varepsilon$RI. The role of Fc$_\varepsilon$RII on dendritic cells has been previously discussed and it is supposed to be involved in targeting eosinophils to parasites in one of the different variations of antibody dependent cell-mediated cytotoxicity (ADCC); its role on platelets and lymphocytes is unclear.

Early and Late Phases in Type I Hypersensitivity
Early Phase
After cross-linking of Fc-receptor associated IgE, mast cells and basophils undergo a series of biochemical and structural changes. The first change to be detected is the polymerization of microtubules, which is energy-dependent (inhibited by 2-deoxyglucose), enhanced by the addition of 3–5 guanosine monophosphate (GMP), and inhibited by the addition of 3–5 adenosine monophosphate (AMP) and colchicine. The polymerization of microtubules allows the transport of the cytoplasmic granules to the cell membrane to which they fuse. This is followed by the opening of the granules that contain a variety of preformed mediators (Table 5). In vitro, the sequence of events leading to the release of histamine, platelet activating factor (PAF), and eosinophil–chemotactic factors for anaphylaxis (ECFA) into the surrounding medium takes 30 to 60 seconds.

Histamine is the mediator responsible for most of the symptoms observed during the early phase of allergic reactions. Since the constricting effect of histamine on the smooth muscle lasts only one or two hours, this phase stops shortly after most of the granules have been emptied.

A second mediator involved in the early phase of the reaction is PAF, which is a phospholipid whose effects include platelet aggregation, chemotaxis of eosinophils, release of vasoactive amines, and increased vascular permeability (due to a direct effect and to the release of vasoactive amines). PAF is released by basophils, mast cells, neutrophils, and other cells.

TABLE 5 Mediators of Immediate Hypersensitivity Produced by Mast Cells and Basophils

Mediators	Structure	Actions
Stored		
Histamine	5-β-imidazolylethylamine (MW 111)	Smooth muscle contraction; increased vascular permeability; many others
ECF-A	Acidic tetrapeptides (MW 360–390); Others (MW 500–3000)	Chemotactic for eosinophils
Proteolytic enzymes	Tryptase, chymase, and other enzymes in human mast cells	Actions in vivo unknown, possibly include C′ activation
Heparin	Acidic proteoglycan (MW $\approx$ 750,000)	Anticoagulant; C′ inhibitor
Neutrophil chemotactic factor	Poorly characterized activity with MW >750,000	Chemotactic for neutrophils
Other granuloproteins	Numerous poorly characterized peptides	In vivo significance not yet known
Newly synthesized (upon stimulation of mast cells or basophils)		
SRS	Leukotrienes C4, D4, E4 (derived from arachidonic acid, MW 439–625)[a]	Smooth muscle contraction; increased vascular permeability; glandular hypersecretion
Prostaglandin D2	Cyclooxygenase product of arachidonic acid[b]	Smooth muscle contraction
PAF	Phospholipid (MW 300–500)[c]	Platelet aggregation and release reaction; increased vascular permeability; eosinophil chemotaxis
Leukotriene B4	Eicosotetraenoate product of arachidonic acid (MW 336)	Chemotactic for eosinophils and neutrophils; neutrophil aggregation

[a]Also released by activated eosinophils.
[b]Produced exclusively by mast cells.
[c]Also stored as a preformed mediator.
Abbreviations: ECFA, eosinophil-chemotactic factors of anaphylaxis; MW, molecular weight; PAF, platelet activating factor; SRSA, slow-reacting substance of anaphylaxis.

It may exist in preformed stores, but de novo synthesis is very rapid, so release takes place in a matter of seconds to a few minutes after cell stimulation.

Late Phase
The cells remain viable after degranulation and proceed to synthesize other substances, which will be released at a later time, causing the late phase of a type I hypersensitivity reaction. The mediators responsible for the late phase of the response are not detected until several hours after release of histamine and other preformed mediators. The long latency period between cell stimulation and detection of these mediators suggest that they are synthesized by mast cells after stimulation and/or by cells attracted by the previously mentioned chemotactic factors.

The main mediators involved in the late phase are the leukotrienes (LT) C4, D4, and E4 (LTC4, LTD4, LTE4). This mixture of LT previously known as slow-reacting substance of anaphylaxis (SRS-A) reaches effective concentrations only five to six hours after challenge and have effects on target cells lasting for several hours. LTC4 and LTD4 are several times more potent than histamine in causing smooth muscle contraction, bronchovascular leak, and mucous hypersecretion in human bronchi.

Role of Eosinophils in the Late Phase
Eosinophils are attracted to the site where an immediate hypersensitivity reaction is taking place by chemotactic factors released by basophils, mast cells, and Th2 lymphocytes including:

1. ECFA and PAF, preformed chemotactic factors released during basophil or mast-cell degranulation.
2. LTB4, synthesized and released by stimulated basophils/mast cells.
3. IL-5, released by activated Th2 lymphocytes, mast cells, and eosinophils.

In many cases, the appearance of eosinophils signals the onset of internal negative feedback and control mechanisms that terminate the immediate hypersensitivity reaction. This effect is associated with the production and release of enzymes, particularly histaminase (which degrades histamine) and phospholipase D (which degrades PAF). Active oxygen radicals released by stimulated granulocytes, including eosinophils and perhaps neutrophils (which are also attracted by ECF-A and LTB4) cause the breakdown of LT. Histamine itself can contribute to the downregulation of the allergic reaction by binding to a type II histamine receptor expressed on basophils—the occupancy of this receptor leads to an intracellular increase in the level of cyclic AMP (cAMP) which inhibits further release of histamine (negative feedback).

In contrast, persistent eosinophil infiltrates are associated with intense inflammation that causes prolongation of symptoms. For example, asthmatic patients may develop a prolonged crisis during which the symptoms remain severe, and breathing becomes progressively more difficult, leading to a situation of increasing respiratory distress, which does not respond to the usual treatment.

In these patients, it is frequent to find very heavy peribronchial cellular infiltrates of the epithelium and lamina propria, with a prominent eosinophilic component, but containing also T lymphocytes, neutrophils, and plasma cells. The infiltrating lymphocytes are mostly activated CD4, CD25[+] T lymphocytes, whose cytokine mRNA pattern is typical of the Th2 subpopulation.

Three major cytokines released primarily by Th2 cells are believed to play significant roles in immediate hypersensitivity reactions, particularly in bronchial asthma:

1. IL-4, which is a critical factor in promoting Th2 cell differentiation, B cell activation, and switch to IgE synthesis.
2. IL-13, a cytokine related to IL-4, has been shown in experimental animal models to induce the pathophysiological features of asthma in an IgE and basophil-independent manner. It has also been shown that basophils also release this cytokine. These observations raise the interesting possibility that asthma symptoms may be triggered independently of the histamine pathway, and that activated Th2 cells may play a significant role in its pathogenesis (Fig. 5).

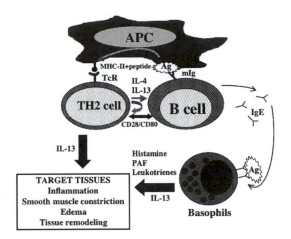

FIGURE 5 Diagrammatic representation of the pathways involved in immediate hypersensitivity. The classical pathway involves recognition of the allergens by B cells, synthesis of IgE antibodies favored by the predominant release of IL-4 and IL-13 by activated Th2 cells. The IgE antibodies bind to high-affinity receptors on basophils and mast cells, and when cross-linked by the sensitizing antigen as a consequence of an ulterior exposure, degranulate and release histamine and other mediators, including IL-13. The IL-13 released by activated Th2 cells can also stimulate inflammatory cells in target tissues, inducing the same general symptoms of hypersensitivity without participation of histamine. *Abbreviations*: APC, antigen-presenting cells; IgE, Immunoglobulin E; IL, interleukin; MHC, major histocompatability; PAF, platelet activating factor; TcR, T cell receptor.

3. IL-5 released from the infiltrating activated Th2 lymphocytes seems to attract, retain, and activate eosinophils.

Activated eosinophils release LT and several toxic proteins: eosinophilic cationic protein (ECP), eosinophil-derived neurotoxin (EDN), eosinophil peroxidase (EPO), and major basic protein (MBP). ECP and MBP can cause ciliary dysfunction, bronchial epithelium injury, nonspecific bronchial hyper-responsiveness, and cellular denudation. This is believed to be a critical step in the pathogenesis of chronic airways inflammation that after decades may lead to chronic obstructive pulmonary disease with irreversible remodeling of the airways.

The severity of the clinical symptoms in an immediate hypersensitivity reaction is directly related to the amount of mediators released and produced, which in turn is determined by the number of "sensitized" cells stimulated by the antigen. The expression of early and late phases can be discriminated clinically. In the case of a positive immediate reaction elicited by a skin test, the early phase resolves in 30 to 60 minutes, the late phase generally peaks at six to eight hours and resolves at 24 hours. In the case of an asthma crisis, the early phase is characterized by shortness of breath and nonproductive cough and lasts four to five hours. If the exposure to the responsible airborne allergen is very intense, life-threatening bronchospasm may develop. With less intense or chronic exposure, the initial symptoms of wheezing and dry cough will linger for a few hours.

Around the sixth hour, the cough starts to produce sputum, signaling the onset of the late phase during which the dyspnea may become more severe. In very severe cases, death may occur at this late stage because of persistent bronchoconstriction, marked peribronchial inflammation associated with diffused cellular infiltration of the airway mucosa, and increased mucous secretion, all of which contribute to severe airflow obstruction.

DIAGNOSTIC TESTS FOR IMMEDIATE HYPERSENSITIVITY
Immunoglobulin-E levels and Immediate Hypersensitivity

The total IgE concentration, even in allergic individuals, is extremely low and generally not detectable by most routine assays used for the assay of IgG, IgA, and IgM. The concentration of specific IgE antibody to any given allergen is a very small fraction of the total IgE. The assay

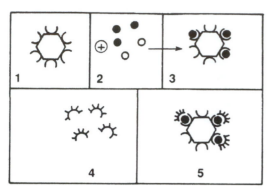

1. **Anti-IgE coupled to paper disc**
2. **Serum IgE**
3. **Binding of Serum IgE to paper disc**
4. **Radiolabeled anti-IgE**
5. **Binding of the Radiolabel to disc-bound IgE**

FIGURE 6 Diagrammatic representation of the general principles of the radioimmunosorbent test for immunoglobulin E (IgE) quantitation.

of such low concentrations became possible with the development of highly sensitive immunoassays.

The paper disc radioimmunosorbent test was one of the first solid-phase radioimmunoassays (see Chapter 15) introduced in diagnostic medicine. This assay, diagrammatically summarized in Figure 6, measures total serum IgE. In brief, a serum sample is added to a small piece of adsorbent paper to which anti-IgE antibodies are covalently bound. The immobilized antibody captures IgE and ^{125}Iodine-labeled anti-IgE antibodies are subsequently added and will react with the paper-bound-IgE. The radioactivity counted in the solid phase is directly related to the IgE level in the serum tested. Later, sensitive enzyme immunoassays and quantitative fluorescence assays were developed that are equally able to measure total IgE levels without the need for use of radiolabelled compounds.

The results of IgE assays are expressed in ng/mL (1 ng = 10^{-6} mg), or in International Units (1 IU = 2.5 ng/mL); 180 IU/mL is considered as the upper limit for normal adults. Allergic individuals often have elevated levels of IgE. However, some asymptomatic individuals may also have elevated IgE levels. Therefore, a diagnosis of immediate hypersensitivity cannot be based solely on the determination of abnormally elevated IgE levels.

Assays for Specific Immunoglobulin-E Antibodies
Radioallergosorbent Test
The radioallergosorbent test (RAST), diagrammatically summarized in Figure 6, was the first solid phase radioimmunoassay that determined antigen-specific IgE, which, from the diagnostic point of view, is considerably more relevant than the measurement of total serum IgE levels. In brief, a given allergen (ragweed antigen, penicillin, β-lactoglobulin, and so on) is covalently bound to polydextran beads. Patient's serum is added to beads coated with a single antigen—the antigen-specific IgE, if present, will bind to the immobilized antigen. After washing off unbound Igs, radiolabeled anti-IgE is added. The amount of bead-bound radioactivity counted after washing off unbound labeled antibody is directly related to the concentration of antigen-specific IgE present in the serum. This test has also been replaced by nonisotopic antigen-specific IgE assays, which follow the same principle but use enzyme-labeled anti-IgE antibodies.

Skin Tests
Although the antigen-specific IgE assays are helpful in screening tests, they are expensive, and lack clinical specificity and sensitivity. Further, the range of antigens for which there are tests available is limited. As such, some authors have questioned the biological and clinical relevance of the antigen-specific IgE assay results. The alternative method for diagnosis of specific

allergies is provocation skin tests, which allow testing to a wider array of antigens. Although positive skin tests depend on the existence of allergen-specific IgE antibodies, they do not allow a direct quantitative assay of such antibodies; rather, they provide clinical information about their ability to mediate the hypersensitivity reaction in an individual patient. This explains the opinion of many specialists that the results of skin tests correlate better with clinical data than the results of the antigen-specific IgE laboratory assays.

The skin tests for immediate hypersensitivity are performed by introducing small amounts of purified allergens percutaneously or intradermally, in known patterns. The patients are then observed for about 30 minutes to one hour. Classical IgE-mediated hypersensitivity reactions present as a wheal and flare at the site of the allergen exposure, which develops in a matter of minutes. In highly sensitized individuals, there is always a risk of anaphylaxis, even after minimal challenge. Because of this risk, trained professionals should always perform these tests in a properly equipped clinical facility.

PREVENTION AND THERAPY
Prevention
Environmental Control
Environmental control, trying to prevent exposure to the allergen, is possible for individuals sensitized to a limited number of allergens; however, it cannot be easily achieved by individuals sensitized with multiple or ubiquitous allergens.

Hyposensitization
Hyposensitization (systemic allergen immunotherapy) is the standard of care in individuals with insect venom IgE-mediated hypersensitivity, and has beneficial results in patients suffering from pollen and perennial allergies (i.e., dust mites and cat dander). Hyposensitization is achieved by subcutaneous injection of very small quantities of the sensitizing antigen, starting at the nanogram level, and increasing the dosage on a weekly basis. This induces the production of IgG blocking antibodies, and an increase in the number of regulatory cells able to turn off the production of IgE antibodies, as reflected by a decline of serum IgE levels. Because both effects tend to be simultaneous, they appear to correlate with a decrease of the allergic symptoms (Fig. 7). Conceptually, blocking antibodies of the IgG class in the systemic vascular and interstitial compartments should have a protective effect by combining with the antigen before it reaches the cell-bound IgE. In fact, a significant clinical improvement correlates better with an increase in blocking IgG than with a decrease antigen-specific IgE. Recent observations do suggest the shifting of the T helper response from a Th2 pattern (predominant release of IL-4 and IL-13) to a Th1 profile (predominant release of IFN-γ) following hyposensitization.

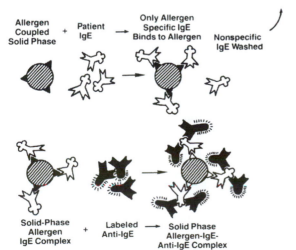

FIGURE 7 Diagrammatic representation of the general principles of the radioallergosorbent test for quantitation of specific immunoglobulin E (IgE) antibodies.

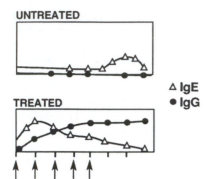

UNTREATED

TREATED

△ IgE
● IgG

FIGURE 8 Evolution of allergen-specific immunoglobulin (Ig) E and IgG levels in patients submitted to hyposensitization (treated) and control patients (untreated).

Anti-immunoglobulin-E Monoclonal Antibodies

Omalizumab (Xolair) is a humanized monoclonal antibody that has been used successfully in the treatment of chronic asthma not responsive to conventional therapy. Patients treated with this antibody show a marked decrease on the number of FcεRI receptors on basophils and mast cells as well as a marked decrease of serum IgE levels. Functional tests based on the measurement of ragweed-induced nasal volume response also show improvements 35 to 42 days after initiation of therapy.

Drug Therapy

Various drugs are used to treat or prevent immediate hypersensitivity reactions. Some inhibit or decrease mediator's release by mast cells or basophils; others block or reverse the effect of mediators. The complex interactions of different drugs able to influence mediator release are summarized in Figure 9.

Treatment of Localized Allergic Reactions

Localized allergic reactions [seasonal rhinitis (hay fever), perennial rhinitis, and urticaria] respond to antihistaminic compounds, which compete with histamine in the binding to their type I receptors at the target cell level, as well as LT antagonists that block the effects of LT (see later). Systemic reactions often require very aggressive and urgent measures, particularly the administration of epinephrine (see later).

Treatment of Allergic Asthma

Bronchial asthma presents very complex therapeutic problems. Current therapy is based upon the understanding that an initial acute bronchoconstrictive attack is followed by progressive inflammation in the airways and, later, by increased bronchial responsiveness. Each phase requires a different treatment. In the early phase, relief of bronchial obstruction is the initial therapeutic goal. β-adrenergic agonists, methylxanthines, and anticholinergic compounds are the main drugs used.

β-Adrenergic Receptor Agonists

β-adrenergic receptor agonists (epinephrine, isoproterenol, and albuterol) increase cAMP levels by stimulating membrane adenylcyclase directly, inhibiting further degranulation of mast cells and basophils. As stated earlier, epinephrine is the drug of choice for treatment of severe allergic reactions such as anaphylaxis. Patients at risk of developing anaphylactic reactions are advised to carry a portable pressurized injecting device able to deliver a therapeutic dose of epinephrine by intramuscular injection on the thigh across clothes, if necessary. Epinephrine causes vasoconstriction with an increased heart rate, as well as bronchodilation. This results in an improvement in cardiovascular and respiratory function. However, the use of epinephrine and other β-adrenergic receptor agonists in allergic asthma is limited by the fact that these compounds do not affect eosinophils, so that when patients have significant peribronchial eosinophilic inflammation, administration of β-agonists will have diminishing benefits. The patient will have a tendency to increase their use to try to achieve symptomatic

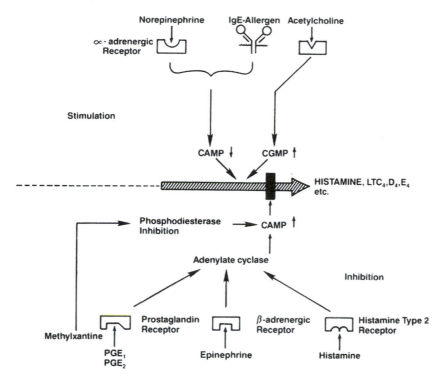

FIGURE 9 Diagrammatic representation of the major pathways leading to stimulation and inhibition of mediator-release by basophils and mast cells. *Abbreviations*: CAMP, cyclic adenosine monophosphate; CGMP, cyclic guanosine monophosphate; PG, prostaglandin E1, E2. *Source*: David J, Rocklin RE. Immediate hypersensitivity. In: Rubinstein E, Federman DD, eds. Section 6, ch. IX. Sci Am Med. New York: Sci Am Inc., 1983.

relief. But since eosinophils and other immune cells are unaffected, the inflammation progresses and can reach a stage at which the patient is at risk of death or near death. A patient's increasing need for β-agonists should be considered an ominous sign of worsening lower airway inflammation.

Methylxanthines
Methylxanthines (e.g., theophylline) block phosphodiesterases, leading to a persistently high intracellular level of cAMP, which, in turn, inhibits histamine release. However, recent studies have led to question this interpretation because the levels of serum methylxanthine reached during the treatments are much lower than those needed to inhibit phosphodiesterases.

Anticholinergic Drugs
Most cholinergic agents, raising intracellular levels of cyclic GMP, have an enhancing effect on mediator release: Their use must be avoided in asthmatic patients since they aggravate the symptoms. On the other hand, anticholinergic drugs that block vagal cholinergic tone may be useful, but are not as efficient as β-agonists for bronchodilation.

In persistent asthma, treatment needs to focus on the chronic inflammatory reaction that no longer responds to the agents useful for treatment in the early phase. Therefore, the treatment's goals are quite different and will include locally administered corticosteroids, cromolyn, and LT-modifying drugs.

Glucocorticoids
Glucocorticoids have no direct action on IgE synthesis or mast-cell degranulation in the lung but strongly inhibit eosinophil degranulation and the elaboration of proinflammatory cytokines. Thus, they have an excellent anti-inflammatory effect that inhibits the progression of the late phase, preventing or reducing bronchial hyper-responsiveness. These effects can be

achieved safely through the administration of glucocorticoids by aerosol, delivering small intrabronchial concentrations that result in local anti-inflammatory effects with low daily doses. This lessens the risk of systemic side effects previously incurred with chronic systemic (oral or parenteral) administration. Glucocorticoids administered by inhalation are now recommended for the treatment of chronic persistent asthma, irrespectively of its severity. Systemic administration of glucocorticoids is reserved for the treatment of severe acute episodes, trying to prevent the development of the severe late phase reactions, or for the treatment of severe recalcitrant asthma.

Disodium Cromoglycate

Disodium cromoglycate (cromolyn) and nedocromil sodium, not shown in Figure 8, are examples of prophylactic drugs. Their mechanism of action is still being investigated; however, it is believed that these drugs attenuate mast-cell degranulation. Objectively, they decrease bronchoconstriction and have proven valuable in helping to reduce the needs for glucocorticoids.

Leukotriene-Modifying Drugs

LT-modifying drugs are being employed in the treatment of asthma. These agents include lipoxygenase enzyme inhibitors that downregulate the production of LT (zileuton) and LT receptor antagonists that block the effects of LT (montelukast, zafirlukast). Presently they are used in mild forms of asthma, exercise-induced bronchospasm or as adjuncts to inhaled-glucocorticoids.

BIBLIOGRAPHY

Abramovits W. Atopic dermatitis. J Am Acad Dermatol 2005; 53(suppl 1):S86–S93.
Borish L. Allergic rhinitis: systemic inflammation and implications for management. J Allergy Clin Immunol 2003; 112:1021–1031.
Chiu AM, Kelly KI. Anaphylaxis: drug allergy, insect stings, and latex. Immunol Allergy Clin North Am 2005; 25:389–405.
Gruchalla RS, Pirmohamed M. Antibiotic allergy. N Engl J Med 2006; 354:601–608.
Haitchi HM, Holgate ST. New strategies in the treatment and prevention of allergic diseases. Expert Opin Investig Drugs 2004; 13:107.
Kon OM, Kay AB. T cells and chronic asthma. Int Arch Allergy Immunol 1999; 118:133.
Li XM. Beyond allergen avoidance: update on developing therapies for peanut allergy. Curr Opin Allergy Clin Immunol 2005; 5:287–292.
Mannino DM, Homa DM, Akinbami LJ, Moorman JE, Gwynn C, Redd SC. Surveillance for asthma—United States, 1980-1999. CDC Surveillance Summaries, March 29, 2002. MMWR Morb Mortal Wkly Rep 2002; 51:1–13.
National asthma education and prevention program expert panel report: guideline for the diagnosis and management of asthma, update of selected topics-2002. J Allergy Clin Immunol 2002; 110(5 suppl): S141–S219.
Plaut M, Valentine MD. Allergic rhinitis. N Engl J Med 2005; 353:1934–1944.
Poole JA, Matangkasombut P, Rosenwasser LJ. Targeting the IgE molecule in allergic and asthmatic diseases: review of the IgE molecule and clinical efficacy. J Allergy Clin Immunol 2005; 115:S376–S385.
Postma D, Bleekeer ER, Amelung PJ, et al. Genetic susceptibility to asthma-bronchial hyperresponsiveness coinherited with a major gene for atopy. N Eng J Med 1995; 333:894.
Salvi SS, Krishna MT, Sampson AP, Holgate ST. The anti-inflammatory effects of leukotriene-modifying drugs and their use in asthma. Chest 2001; 119:1533–1546.
Weller PF. The immunobiology of eosinophils. N Eng J Med 1991; 324:1110.
Wills-Kapp M, Luyimbazi J, Xu X, et al. Interleukin-13: central mediator of allergic asthma. Science 1998; 282:2258.
Yssel H, Abbal C, Pene J, Bousquet J. The role of IgE in asthma. Clin Exp Allergy 1998; 28(suppl 5):104.
Yssel H, Groux H. Characterization of T cell subpopulations involved in the pathogenesis of asthma and allergic diseases. Int Arch Allergy Immunol 2000; 121:10.

22 | Immunohematology

Gabriel Virella and Armand Glassman
Department of Microbiology and Immunology, Medical University of South Carolina, Charleston, South Carolina, U.S.A.

INTRODUCTION: BLOOD GROUPS
ABO System

The first human red cell antigen system to be characterized was the ABO blood group system. Specificity is determined by the terminal sugar in an oligosaccharide backbone structure. The terminal sugars of the oligosaccharides defining groups A and B are immunogenic. In group O, the precursor H oligosaccharide is unaltered. The red cells express either A, B, both A and B, or neither. Antibodies to antigens not expressed in the red cells of a given individual are detected in circulation, as shown in Table 1.

The ABO group of specific individuals is determined by testing both cells and serum. The subjects' red cells are mixed with serum containing a known antibody, and their serum is tested against cells possessing a known antigen. For example, the cells of group A individuals are agglutinated by anti-A serum but not by anti-B serum, and their serum agglutinates type B cells but not type A cells. The typing of cells as group O is done by exclusion (a cell not reacting with anti-A or anti-B is considered to be of blood group O).

The anti-A or anti-B antibodies (known as isoagglutinins) are synthesized as a consequence of cross-immunization with enterobacteriaceae that have outer membrane oligosaccharides strikingly similar to those that define the A and B antigens (see Chapter 14). For example, a newborn with group A blood will not have anti-B in his serum, since it has had no opportunity to undergo cross-immunization. When the newborn's intestine is eventually colonized by the normal microbial flora, the infant will start to develop anti-B, but will not produce anti-A because of its tolerance to its own blood group antigens (Table 1).

The inheritance of the ABO groups follows simple Mendelian rules, with three common allelic genes: A, B, and O (A can be subdivided into A_1 and A_2), of which any individual will carry two, one inherited from the mother and one from the father. The ABO system is the most important blood system for consideration in transfusion medicine, as incompatible transfusions can result in immediate and fatal transfusion reactions.

Rh System

In the late 1930s, it was discovered that the sera of most women who gave birth to infants with hemolytic disease of the newborn contained an antibody that reacted with the red cells of their infants and with the red cells of 85% of Caucasians. A year later, it was discovered that a reagent produced by injecting blood from the monkey *Macacus rhesus* into rabbits and guinea pigs agglutinated rhesus red cells and appeared to have the same specificity as the neonatal antibody. Individuals whose cells reacted with the reagent were termed Rh-positive (for the rhesus monkey); those whose cells were not agglutinated were termed Rh-negative. The Rh system is the second most important blood system in transfusion medicine.

Antigens of the Rh System

The Rh system is now known to have many antigens in addition to the one originally described, and several nomenclature systems were developed. For practical purposes, the Fisher–Race nomenclature is now used almost exclusively. Fisher and Race originally postulated that the *Rh* gene complex is formed by combinations of three pairs of allelic genes: *Cc*, *Dd*, and *Ee*. This was later modified to a model that proposed a single genetic locus with three subloci. The possible combinations are: *Dce, DCe, DcE, DCE, dce, dCe, dcE,* and *dCE*. Thus, a *DCe/DcE*

TABLE 1 ABO System

Red cell antigen	Serum isoagglutinins	Blood group
A	anti-B	A
B	anti-A	B
A and B	None	AB
None	anti-A and B	O

individual can only pass *DCe* or *DcE* to his offspring and no other combination. The original antigen discovered is called D, and people who possess it are called Rh-positive. The allele "d" has never been discovered, so the symbol "d" is used to denote the absence of D. All individuals lacking the D antigen are termed Rh-negative. The most frequent genotype of D-negative individuals is *dce/dce*.

Recent studies analyzing DNA from donors of different Rh phenotypes have found that there are neither three loci nor one locus governing Rh, but that there are two structural loci governing Rh in Rh (D) positive individuals and only one present in Rh-negative persons. Therefore, one gene appears to encode the D protein and the other governs the presence of the C, c, E, and e antigens. Since most Rh-negative persons completely lack a *D* gene and have nothing in its place, and the few others appear to have a partial or inactive *D* gene, it is easier to understand why a "d" antigen does not exist.

Other Blood Groups

Several other blood group systems with clinical relevance have been characterized. Most transfusion reactions other than those caused by clerical error are due to alloimmunization to antigens of the Kell, Duffy, and Kidd systems, of which the Kell system is the most polymorphic. Occasionally, antibodies to these antigens may cause hemolytic disease of the newborn. On the other hand, most cases of autoimmune hemolytic anemia involve autoantibodies directed to public antigens (antigens common to most, if not all, humans), such as the I antigen or core Rh antigens.

There are over 200 blood group antigens in addition to those of the ABO and Rh systems. Some of the most important blood groups are seen in Table 2. Blood group antigenic determinants are either carbohydrate or protein in nature. Upon exposure to foreign carbohydrate antigens, IgM antibodies are predominantly produced while IgG antibodies predominate after immunization to protein borne blood group antigens. Many IgM antibodies have a low-thermal amplitude (i.e., react better at temperatures below normal body temperature) and may lack clinical significance.

Many of the proteins recognized as blood group antigens are important to the integrity of the red blood cell. This does not appear to be true of the carbohydrate antigens. Some blood

TABLE 2 Characteristics of Some Common Blood Group Antigens and Antibodies

Blood group	Antigen structure	Usual antibodies	Clinical significance	
			HTR	HDN
ABO	Carbohydrate	anti-A, B	Yes	Yes (mild)
Rh	Protein	anti-D, E, c	Yes	Yes
Kell	Protein	anti-K	Yes	Yes
Kidd	Protein	anti-Jk^a, Jk^b	Yes	Few
Duffy	Glycoprotein	anti-Fy^a, Fy^b	Yes	Yes
MNS	Glycoprotein	anti-M	Few	Few
P	Carbohydrate	anti-P$_1$	Rare	No
Lewis	Carbohydrate	anti-Le^a, Le^b	Few	No
I	Carbohydrate	autoanti-I	No*	No*

*The clinical significance of anti-I antibodies relates to a special form of autoimmune hemolytic anemia, known as cold agglutinin disease.
Abbreviations: HDN, hemolytic disease of the newborn; HTR, hemolytic transfusion reaction.

groups have known associated biological functions such as the Duffy glycoprotein that is the receptor for *Plasmodium vivax*, which causes malaria. The Duffy glycoprotein also has recently been shown to be a chemokine receptor able to bind both C—X—C and C—C chemokines (see Chapter 11) and, for this reason, has been renamed as Duffy antigen receptor for chemokines (DARC). Its function on the mature red cell membrane is not known. Another known function of some blood groups is transport. The Kidd protein is the urea transporter. Many carbohydrate antigens bind bacteria, such as the P antigen that binds *Escherichia coli* and the Lewis system Le^b antigen on gastric epithelial cells, which binds *Helicobacter pylori*, the organism implicated in gastritis, gastric ulcers, and gastric carcinoma.

SEROLOGICAL PRINCIPLES OF BLOOD TRANSFUSION
Laboratory Determination of Blood Types
Reagents
Most reagents used for blood group typing consist of monoclonal antibodies, usually of mouse origin, used individually or blended, directed against the different blood group antigens. A major advantage of the use of monoclonal antibodies is their specificity, minimizing the possibility of false positive reactions due to additional contaminating antibodies found in human serum reagents. An important disadvantage derives from the fact that monoclonal antibodies react with a single epitope and the blood group antigens have multiple epitopes. Thus, individuals missing the epitope recognized by the antibody may be typed as negative. Using a blend of monoclonal antibodies, each one of them recognizing a different epitope of a given antigen, significantly reduces this problem.

Tests
Direct Hemagglutination
Direct hemagglutination is the simplest, preferred test. It is easy to perform with typing reagents containing IgM antibodies that directly agglutinate cells expressing the corresponding antigen. Reagents containing IgG antibodies can also be used in a direct hemagglutination test. Protein is added in relatively high concentration to the reagent with the purpose of dissipating the repulsive forces that keep the red cells apart. As a consequence, IgG antibodies can directly agglutinate the red cells.

In general, reagents containing IgG antibodies are used in an indirect antiglobulin test (see next), as a way to induce the agglutination of red cells coated with the corresponding antibodies. The advent of monoclonal reagents has made it possible to type many red cell antigens by direct agglutination, which previously required the indirect antiglobulin test in the past when only IgG human source reagents were available.

Direct and Indirect Antiglobulin (Coombs') Tests
In 1945, Coombs, Mourant, and Race described the use of antihuman globulin serum to detect red cell bound nonagglutinating antibodies. There are two basic types of antiglobulin or Coombs' tests.

The direct antiglobulin test is performed to detect in vivo sensitization of red cells or, in other words, sensitization that has occurred in the patient (Fig. 1). The test is performed by adding antihuman IgG (and/or antihuman complement, to react with complement components bound to the red cells as a consequence of the antigen-antibody reaction) to the patient's washed red cells. If IgG antibody (and/or complement) is/are bound to the red cells, agglutination (positive result) is observed after addition of the antiglobulin reagent and centrifugation. The direct antiglobulin test is an aid in diagnosis and investigation of hemolytic disease of the newborn, autoimmune hemolytic anemia, drug-induced hemolytic anemia, and hemolytic transfusion reactions.

The indirect antiglobulin test detects in vitro sensitization, that is, sensitization that has been allowed to occur in the test tube under optimal conditions (Fig. 2). Therefore, the test is used to investigate the presence of nonagglutinating red cell antibodies in a patient's serum. The test is performed in two steps (hence the designation of indirect). In the first step, a serum suspected of containing red cell antibodies is incubated with normal type O red

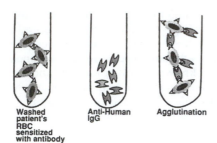

FIGURE 1 Diagrammatic representation of a direct Coombs' test using anti-IgG antibodies.

blood cells. In the second step, after washing unbound antibodies, antihuman IgG (and/or anticomplement) antibodies are added to the red cells as in the direct test. The indirect antiglobulin test is useful in detecting and characterizing red cell antibodies using test cells of known antigenic composition (antibody screening), cross-matching, and phenotyping blood cells for antigens not demonstrable by other techniques.

Compatibility Testing

Before a blood transfusion, a series of procedures need to be done to establish the proper selection of blood for the patient. Basically, those procedures try to establish the ABO and Rh systems compatibility between donor and recipient, and to rule out the existence of antibodies in the recipient's serum that could react with transfused red cells. To establish this compatibility between donor and recipient, both the recipient and the blood to be transfused are typed. To rule out the existence of antibodies (other than anti-A or anti-B), a general antibody screening test is performed with group O red cells of known composition. The O$^+$ cells are first incubated with the patient's serum to check for agglutination; if this test is negative, an indirect antiglobulin (Coombs') test is performed.

Cross-Match

The most direct way to detect antibodies in the recipient's serum that could cause hemolysis of the transfused red cells is to test the patient's serum with the donor's cells (major cross-match). The complete cross-match also involves the same tests as the antibody screening test described earlier.

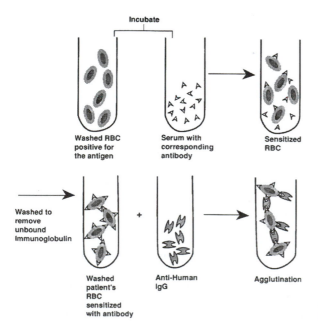

FIGURE 2 Diagrammatic representation of an indirect Coombs' test.

An abbreviated version of the cross-match is often performed in patients with a negative antibody screening test. This consists of immediately centrifuging a mixture of patient's serum and donor cells to detect agglutination; this primarily checks for ABO incompatibility.

The minor cross-match, which consists of testing a patient's cells with donor serum, is of little significance and rarely performed, since any donor antibodies would be greatly diluted in the recipient's plasma and rarely cause clinical problems.

Alternatives to Tube Testing

Newer methods that represent alternatives to the traditional tube test are being increasingly utilized in larger blood banks. These methods require little training, offer greater standardization, and use a micro sample. The reactions are stable and may be rechecked by another technologist.

Gel Test

The gel test uses six microtubes in a card, replacing six test tubes. In each microtube, a column of dextran acrylamide gel particles functions as a filter that traps agglutinates upon centrifugation. This technique may be used for antiglobulin tests, where gels containing antiglobulin serum are used to trap sensitized but unagglutinated red cells. The red cells in a negative test will all centrifuge to the bottom of the microtube. The gel test is adaptable to typing, antibody screening, antibody identification, and cross-matching.

Solid-Phase Red Cell Adherence Tests

Solid-phase red cell adherence tests use immobilized antibody for the direct test. Adding the red cells to be typed to antibody-coated wells in a polystyrene tray does the test. The red cells will adhere in a monolayer across the well in a positive test and will settle to the bottom in a negative test. The indirect test uses red cells of known composition, which are immobilized in a monolayer. In order to demonstrate that a patient's serum has an antibody directed against a red cell sample, indicator red cells coated with anti-IgG are added, and the cells will efface across the well. Antibody screening and identification may be done by the indirect test. Automated solid phase techniques are being used by some blood centers.

Implications of Positive Antibody Screening for Transfusion

Donor blood found to contain clinically significant red cell antibodies is generally not transfused. If a patient (recipient) has a positive antibody screening test due to a clinically significant antibody, the antibody is identified using a panel of cells of known antigenic composition, and antigen negative blood is selected for transfusion.

BLOOD TRANSFUSION REACTIONS

Transfusion reactions may occur due to a wide variety of causes (Table 3). Among them, the most severe are those associated with hemolysis, which may be life threatening. A list of the causes of fatal transfusion reactions reported to the FDA from 1985 to 1987 is reproduced in Table 4.

The most frequent cause is an ABO mismatch due to clerical error, resulting in the transfusion of the wrong blood. Transfusion of blood incompatible for other blood groups to a patient previously sensitized during pregnancy or as a consequence of earlier transfusions can also cause a hemolytic reaction.

TABLE 3   Immunological Classification of Transfusion Reactions

Nonimmune
Immune
Red cell incompatibility
Incompatibilities associated with platelets and leukocytes
Incompatibilities due to antiallotypic antibodies (anti-Gm or -Am antibodies)

TABLE 4 Summary of Fatal Transfusion Reactions

Causes	No.
Hemolytic reactions	
ABO incompatible transfusions	29
Collection errors	7
Blood bank clerical errors	8
Blood bank technical errors	1
Nursing unit errors	11
Undetermined	2
Non-ABO incompatible transfusions[a]	6
No detectable antibody	3
Glycerol	1
Nonhemolytic reactions	26
Bacterial contamination	11[b]
Acute respiratory distress	9
Anaphylaxis	6

Note: Reported to the Food and Drug Administration from 1985–1987.
[a]Including anti-Jk[b], -c, Fy[a], and -K.
[b]In nine cases, the source of contamination was a platelet preparation.
Source: Adapted form Beig K, Calhoun A, Petz LD. ISTB & AABB Joint Congress. Los Angeles, CA, 1990, Abstract S282.

Intravascular Hemolytic Reactions ("Immediate" Transfusion Reactions)

The binding of preformed IgM antibodies to the red cells triggers intravascular hemolytic transfusion reactions. IgM antibodies are very effective in causing the activation of the complement system. Massive complement activation by red cell antibodies causes intravascular red cell lysis, with release of hemoglobin into the circulation. Most intravascular reactions are due to ABO incompatibility. The direct antiglobulin test may be negative if all donor cells are quickly lysed.

Due to the massive release of soluble complement fragments (e.g., C3a and C5a) with anaphylotoxic properties, the patient may suffer generalized vasodilatation, hypotension, and shock. Because of the interrelationships between the complement and clotting systems, disseminated intravascular coagulation may occur during a severe transfusion reaction. As a consequence of the nephrotoxicity of free hemoglobin or the action of released cytokines, the patient may develop acute renal failure, usually due to acute tubular necrosis.

Extravascular Hemolytic Reactions ("Delayed" Transfusion Reactions)

Extravascular hemolytic reactions are caused by the opsonization of red cells with IgG antibodies. IgG red cell antibodies can activate complement but do not cause spontaneous red cell lysis. Red cells opsonized with IgG (often with associated C3b) are efficiently taken up and destroyed by phagocytic cells, particularly splenic and hepatic macrophages.

These reactions are usually less severe than intravascular transfusion reactions. In addition, transfusion reactions may be delayed when an anamnestic response in a patient with undetectable antibody is the precipitating factor. Typically, a positive direct antiglobulin (Coombs') test will be noted after transfusion in association with a rapidly diminishing red cell concentration.

Clinical Presentation of Transfusion Reactions

The most common initial symptom in a hemolytic transfusion reaction is fever, frequently associated with chills. Red or wine-colored urine (due to hemoglobinuria) may be noted. With progression of the reaction, the patient may experience chest pains, dyspnea, hypotension, and shock. Renal damage is indicated by back pain, oliguria and, in most severe cases, anuria.

During surgery, the only symptom may be bleeding and/or hypotension. Generalized bleeding is the most serious manifestation of disseminated intravascular coagulation. Treatment includes immediate cessation of the transfusion, support of vital signs, and active prevention of possible renal failure.

Laboratory Investigation

Immediately after a hemolytic transfusion reaction is suspected, the following procedures must be done:

1. A clerical check to detect any errors that may have resulted in the administration of a unit of blood to the wrong patient.
2. Confirmation of intravascular hemolysis by visual or photometric comparison of pre- and postreaction plasma specimens for free hemoglobin (the prereaction specimen should be light yellow, and the postreaction sample should have a pink/red discoloration).
3. Direct antiglobulin (Coombs') test on pre- and postreaction blood samples.

If any of these procedures gives a positive result supporting a diagnosis of intravascular hemolysis, additional serological investigations are indicated, including the following:

1. Repeat ABO and Rh typing on patient and donor samples
2. Repeat antibody screening and cross-matching
3. If a red cell antibody is detected, determine its specificity using a red cell panel, in which group O red cells of varied antigenic composition are incubated with the patient's serum to determine which RBC antigen(s) are recognized by the patient's antibody(ies).

Additionally, one or several of the following confirmatory tests may be performed.

1. Measurement of unconjugated bilirubin on blood drawn five to seven hours after transfusion (the concentration should rise as the released hemoglobin is processed).
2. Determination of free hemoglobin and/or hemosiderin in the urine (neither is normally detected in the urine).
3. Measurement of serum haptoglobin (if hemolysis is not apparent upon visual inspection of the serum).
4. Culture of the unit(s) for bacterial contamination.

Nonhemolytic Immune Transfusion Reactions
Antileukocyte Antibodies

When a patient has antibodies directed to leukocyte antigens, a transfusion of any blood product containing cells expressing those antigens can elicit a febrile transfusion reaction. Leukocyte-depleted blood products should be used for transfusions in patients with recurrent febrile reactions.

Special problems are presented by patients requiring platelet concentrates that have developed antihuman leukocyte antigen (HLA) antibodies or antibodies directed to platelet-specific antigens (human platelet antigens, HPA). In such cases, it will be necessary to give HLA- or HPA-matched platelets, since platelets will be rapidly destroyed if given to a sensitized individual with circulating antibodies to the antigens expressed by the donor's platelets.

Transfusion of blood products containing antibodies to leukocyte antigens expressed by the patient receiving the transfusion can induce intravascular leukocyte aggregation. These aggregates are usually trapped in the pulmonary microcirculation, causing acute respiratory distress and, in some cases, noncardiogenic pulmonary edema. This condition is recognized clinically as transfusion related acute lung injury. A similar situation may emerge when granulocyte concentrates are given to a patient with antileukocyte antibodies reactive with the transfused granulocytes.

Anti-IgA Antibodies

The transfusion of any IgA-containing blood product into a patient with preformed anti-IgA antibodies can cause an anaphylactic transfusion reaction. Transfusion reactions are not usually observed when the antibody titers (determined by passive hemagglutination) are low. Anti-IgA antibodies are mostly detected in immunodeficient individuals, particularly those with IgA deficiency.

It is very important to test for anti-IgA antibodies in any patient with known IgA deficiency that is going to require a transfusion, even if the patient has never been previously transfused. If an anti-IgA antibody is detected, it is important to administer packed red cells with all traces of plasma removed by extensive washing. If plasma products are needed, they should be obtained from IgA deficient donors.

HEMOLYTIC DISEASE OF THE NEWBORN (ERYTHROBLASTOSIS FETALIS)
Pathogenesis

Immunological destruction of fetal and/or newborn erythrocytes is likely to occur when IgG antibodies are present in the maternal circulation directed against the corresponding antigen(s) present on the fetal red blood cells (only IgG antibodies can cross the placenta and reach the fetal circulation).

The two types of incompatibility most usually involved in hemolytic disease of the newborn are anti-D and anti-A or B antibodies. Anti-A or B antibodies are usually IgM, but in some circumstances, IgG antibodies may develop (usually in group O mothers). This can be secondary to immune stimulation (some vaccines contain blood group substances or cross-reactive polysaccharides), or may occur without apparent cause for unknown reasons.

Mechanisms of Sensitization

Although the exchange of red cells between mother and fetus is prevented by the placental barrier during pregnancy, about two-thirds of all women have fetal red cells in their circulation after delivery (or miscarriage).

If the mother is Rh-negative and the infant Rh-positive, the mother may produce antibodies to the D antigen. The immune response is usually initiated at term, when large amounts of fetal red cells reach maternal circulation. In subsequent pregnancies, even the small number of red cells crossing the placenta during pregnancy is sufficient to elicit a strong secondary response, with production of IgG antibodies. As IgG antibodies are produced in larger amounts, they will cross the placenta, bind to the Rh-positive cells, and cause their destruction in the spleen through Fc-mediated phagocytosis. Usually, the first child is not affected, since the red cells that cross the placenta after the 28th week of gestation do so in small numbers and are unlikely to elicit a primary immune response.

IgG anti-D antibodies do not appear to activate the complement system, perhaps because the D antigenic sites on the red cell surface are too separated to allow the formation of IgG doublets with sufficient density of IgG molecules to induce complement activation. Complement, however, is not required for phagocytosis that can be mediated by the Fc receptors in monocytes and macrophages.

Epidemiology

Prior to the introduction of immunoprophylaxis, the frequency of clinically evident hemolytic disease of the newborn was estimated to be about 0.5% of total births, mostly due to anti-D, with a mortality rate close to 6% among affected newborns. Recent figures are considerably lower: 0.15% to 0.3% incidence of clinically evident disease, and the perinatal mortality rate appears to be declining to about 4% of affected newborns. Due to the introduction of immunoprophylaxis, the proportion of cases due to anti-D antibodies decreased, whereas the proportion of cases due to other Rh antibodies, and to antibodies to antigens of other systems, increased proportionately.

Clinical Presentation

The usual clinical features of this disease are anemia and jaundice present at birth or, more frequently, in the first 24 hours of life. In severe cases, the infant may die in utero. Unless treated appropriately, other severely affected children who survive until the third day develop signs of central nervous system damage, attributed to the high concentrations of unconjugated bilirubin (kernicterus). The peripheral blood shows reticulocytes and circulating erythroblasts (hence the term "erythroblastosis fetalis").

Immunological Diagnosis

A strongly positive direct Coombs' (antiglobulin) test on cord RBC is invariably found in cases of Rh incompatibility, although 40% of the cases with a positive reaction do not require treatment. In ABO incompatibility, the direct antiglobulin test is usually weakly positive and may be confirmed by eluting antibodies from the infant's red cells and testing the eluate with A and B cells.

Prevention

Rh hemolytic disease of the newborn is rarely seen when mother and infant are incompatible in the ABO systems. In such cases, the ABO isoagglutinins in the maternal circulation appear to eliminate any fetal red cells, before maternal sensitization occurs. This observation led to a very effective form of prevention of Rh hemolytic disease of the newborn, achieved by the administration of anti-D IgG antibodies (Rh Immune Globulin) to Rh-negative mothers.

The therapeutic anti-D preparation is manufactured from the plasma of previously immunized mothers with persistently high titers or from male donors immunized against Rh-positive RBC. Its mechanism of action is not entirely clear, but a recently proposed mechanism to explain the immunotherapeutic effect of intravenous gamma globulin in idiopathic thrombocytopenia has some interesting parallels. According to this postulate, it is possible that Rh immune globulin may downregulate anti-D-producing B cells as a consequence of coligation of surface immunoglobulin (by anti-idiotypic specificities present in the Rh immune globulin) and FcIIγR (by the Fc region of red-cell bound anti-D).

The schedule of administration involves two separate doses. Antepartum administration of a full dose of Rh immune globulin at the 28th week of pregnancy is recommended, in addition to postpartum administration. The rationale for this approach is to avoid sensitization due to prenatal spontaneous or post-traumatic bleeding. Prenatal anti-D prophylaxis is also indicated at the time that an Rh-negative pregnant woman is submitted to amniocentesis and must be continued at 12-week intervals until delivery to maintain sufficient protection. The postpartum dose is administered in the first 72 hours after delivery of each Rh incompatible infant (before sensitization has had time to occur). The risk of immunization with a postpartum dose alone is 1% to 2%. Antepartum administration decreases the risk to 0.1%.

The recommended full dose is 300 μg IM that can be increased if there is laboratory evidence of severe feto-maternal hemorrhage (by tests able to determine the number of fetal red cells in maternal peripheral blood, from which one can calculate the volume of feto-maternal hemorrhage). Smaller doses (50 μg) should be given after therapeutic or spontaneous abortion in the first trimester.

Treatment

To prevent serious hemolytic disease of the newborn in their infants, pregnant women who have a clinically significant antibody in the maternal circulation directed against a fetal antigen are carefully monitored. Amniocentesis is usually performed if the titer of antibody is greater than 16 or if the woman has a history of a previously affected child. The amniotic fluid is examined for bile pigments at appropriate intervals, and the severity of the disease is assessed according to those levels. An alternate approach is to monitor the fetus by percutaneous umbilical blood sampling, which allows for direct hematologic and biochemical measurements by removing blood from the umbilical vessel using ultrasound guidance.

If fetal maturity has been established, labor may be induced, and, if necessary, the baby can be exchange-transfused after delivery. If fetal lung maturity is inadequate (judged by the lecithin/sphyngomyelin ratio in amniotic fluid), intrauterine transfusion may be performed by transfusing O, Rh-negative red cells to the fetus.

IMMUNE HEMOLYTIC ANEMIAS

The designation of hemolytic anemias includes a heterogeneous group of diseases whose common denominator is the exaggerated destruction of red cells (hemolysis). In this chapter, we will discuss only the hemolytic anemias, in which an abnormal immune response plays the major pathogenic role.

Autoimmune Hemolytic Anemia (Warm Antibody Type)

This is the most common form of autoimmune hemolytic anemia. It can be idiopathic (often following overt or subclinical viral infection) or secondary, as shown in Table 5.

Pathogenesis
Warm autoimmune hemolytic anemia is due to the spontaneous emergence of IgG antibodies that may have a simple Rh specificity such as anti-e, or uncharacterized specificities common to almost all normal red cells ("public" antigens, thought to be the core of the Rh substance). In many patients, one can find antibodies of multiple specificities. The end result is that the serum from patients with autoimmune hemolytic anemia of the warm type is likely to react with most, if not all, of the red cells tested. These antibodies usually cause shortening of red cell life due to the uptake and destruction by phagocytic cells in the spleen and liver.

Diagnosis
Diagnosis relies on the demonstration of antibodies coating the red cells or circulating in the serum. RBC-fixed antibodies are detected by the direct antiglobulin Coombs' test. The test can be done using anti-IgG antiglobulin, anticomplement, or polyspecific antiglobulin serum that has both anti-IgG and anticomplement. The polyspecific or broad-spectrum antiglobulin sera produce positive results in higher numbers of patients, as shown in Table 6.

The search for antibodies in serum is carried out by the indirect antiglobulin test. Circulating antibodies are only present when the red cells have been maximally coated, and the test is positive in only 40% of the cases tested with untreated red cells. A higher positivity rate (up to 80%) can be achieved by using red cells treated with enzymes such as trypsin, papain, ficin,

---

TABLE 5   Immune Hemolytic Anemias

AIHA
  Warm antibody AIHA
    Idiopathic (unassociated with another disease)
    Secondary (associated with chronic lymphocytic leukemia,
      lymphomas, systemic lupus erythematosus, etc.)
  Cold antibody AIHA
    Idiopathic cold hemagglutinin disease
    Secondary cold hemagglutinin syndrome
    Associated with *Mycoplasma pneumoniae* infection
    Associated with chronic lymphocytic leukemia, lymphomas, etc.
Immune drug-induced hemolytic anemia
Alloantibody-induced immune hemolytic anemia
  Hemolytic transfusion reactions
  Hemolytic disease of the newborn

Abbreviation: AIHA, autoimmune hemolytic anemia.
Source: Modified from Petz LD, Garraty G. Laboratory Correlations in immune hemolytic anemias. In Laboratory Diagnosis of Immunologic Disorders. Vyas GN, Stites DP, Brechter G, Eds. New York: Grune & Stratton, 1974.

TABLE 6　Typical Results of Serological Investigations in Patients with Autoimmune Hemolytic Anemia

	Cells			Serum	
	Direct Coombs' test				
	Antibody to	**Positivity rate (%)**	**Antibody isotype**	**Serologic characteristics**	**Ab specificity**
Warm AIHA	IgG	30	IgG	Positive indirect Coombs' test (40%)	Rh system antigens ("public")
	IgG + C′	50		Agglutination of enzyme-treated RBC (80%)	
Cold agglutinin disease	C′	20			
	C′		IgM	Monoclonal IgMk agglutinates RBC to titers >1024 at 4°C	I antigen

Abbreviation: AIHA, autoimmune hemolytic anemia.
Source: Modified from Petz LD, Garraty G. Laboratory correlations in immune hemolytic anemias. In Laboratory Diagnosis of Immunologic Disorders. Vyas GN, Stites DP, Brechter G, Eds. New York: Grune & Stratton, 1974.

and bromelin in the agglutination assays. The treatment of red cells with these enzymes increases their agglutinability by either increasing the exposure of antigenic determinants or by reducing the surface charge of the red cells. In the investigation of warm-type autoimmune hemolytic anemias (AIHA), all tests are carried out at 37°C.

Cold Agglutinin Disease and Cold Agglutinin Syndromes
Pathogenesis
The cold agglutinins are classically IgM antibodies (very rarely IgA or IgG) and react with red cells at temperatures below normal body temperature.

Chronic, Idiopathic, and Cold Agglutinin Diseases
In chronic, idiopathic, cold agglutinin disease, the antibodies are in the vast majority of cases of the IgMk isotype and react with the I antigen. This is a public antigen in adults. The fetus expresses the "I" antigen, common to primates and other mammalians, which is the precursor of the "i" specificity. The newborn expresses "I" predominantly over "i"; in the adult, the situation is reversed.

Postinfectious Cold Agglutinin Syndrome
In postinfectious cold agglutinin syndrome, the antibodies are also predominantly IgM, but contain both κ and λ light chains, suggesting their polyclonal origin. The cold agglutinins that appear in patients with *Mycoplasma pneumoniae* infections are usually reactive with the "I" antigen, whereas those that appear in association with infectious mononucleosis usually react with the "i" antigen.

Hemolysis in patients with postinfectious cold agglutinin disease is usually mild. In those cases, the cold agglutinins are present in relatively low titers and have low thermal amplitude; that is, do not react at temperatures close to normal body temperature, and hemolysis is due to opsonization of red cells through C3b receptors. In severe cases of idiopathic cold agglutinin disease, cold agglutinins are present in high titers and react at temperatures close to normal body temperature (i.e., 35°C). Under those circumstances, the cold agglutinins cause intravascular hemolysis and ischemia of cold-exposed areas. Intavascular hemolysis can cause the release of large concentrations of hemoglobin and lead to acute renal failure. Cold-induced ischemia is caused by massive intracapillary agglutination areas where the temperature drops below the critical level for agglutination.

Clinical Presentation
Hemolysis is usually mild, but, in some cases, may be severe leading to acute tubular necrosis. In most cases, the clinical picture is dominated by symptoms of cold sensitivity (Raynaud's phenomenon, vascular purpura, and tissue necrosis in exposed extremities).

Laboratory Diagnosis

Testing for cold agglutinins is usually done by incubating a series of dilutions of the patient's serum (obtained by clotting and centrifuging the blood at 37°C immediately after drawing) with normal group O RBC at 4°C. Titers up to the thousands or even millions can be observed in patients with cold agglutinin disease. Intermediate titers (below 1000) can be found in patients with *M. pneumoniae* infections (postinfectious cold agglutinins). Low titers (less than 64) can be found in normal asymptomatic individuals.

Drug-Induced Hemolytic Anemia

Three different types of immune mechanisms may play a role in drug-induced hemolytic anemias, as summarized in Table 7. It is important to differentiate between drug-induced hemolytic anemia and warm autoimmune hemolytic anemia, since cessation of the drug alone will usually halt the drug-induced hemolytic process.

Immune Complex Mechanism (Drug-Dependent Antibody Mechanism)

Traditionally this mechanism has been thought to be due to the formation of soluble immune complexes between the drug and the corresponding antibodies that is followed by nonspecific adsorption to red cells and complement activation. Alternatively, the neoantigen concept proposes that the drug binds transiently with the red cell, forming a "nonself" epitope that stimulates antibody formation. The distinction between this mechanism and the drug adsorption mechanism, where a stable bond is formed between the drug and the cell membrane, may be more apparent than real. When IgM antibodies are predominantly involved, intravascular hemolysis is frequent, and the direct Coombs' test is usually positive if anticomplement antibodies are used. IgG antibodies can also form immune complexes with different types of antigens and be adsorbed onto red cells and platelets. In vitro, such adsorption is not followed by hemolysis or by phagocytosis of red cells, but in vivo it has been reported to be associated with intravascular hemolysis.

The absorption of IgG-containing immune complexes to platelets is also the cause of drug-induced thrombocytopenia. Quinine, quinidine, digitoxin, gold, meprobamate, chlorothiazide, rifampin, and sulfonamides have been reported to cause this type of drug-induced thrombocytopenia.

Drug Adsorption Mechanism

This mechanism proposes that the adsorbed drug functions as hapten and the RBC as carrier, and an immune response against the drug ensues. The antibodies, usually IgG, are present in high titers, and may activate complement after binding to the drug adsorbed to the red cells, inducing hemolysis (Fig. 3) or phagocytosis. Penicillin (when administered in high doses by

TABLE 7 Correlation between Mechanisms of Red Cell Sensitization and Laboratory Features in Drug-Induced Immuno-Hematological Abnormalities

Mechanism	Prototype drugs	Clinical findings	Serological evaluation	
			Usual direct Coombs' result	In vitro tests for Ab characterization
Immune complex (drug dependent)	Quinidine Phenacetin 3rd generation Cephalosporins	Intravascular hemolysis; renal failure; thrombocytopenia	Positive with anti-C′	Drug + serum + RBC; Ab is often IgM
Drug adsorption to RBC	Penicillins 1–2nd generation Cephalosporins	Extravascular hemolysis associated with high intravenous doses	Positive with anti-IgG	Drug-coated RBC + serum; antibody is IgG
Autoimmune	α-Methyldopa L-dopa Procainamide	Onset of extravascular hemolysis associated with high doses	Positive with anti-IgG	Normal RBC + serum. Auto-antibody to RBC dentical to IgG Ab in warm AIHA

Abbreviations: Ab, antibody; AIHA, auto-immune hemolytic anemia; RBC, red blood cell.

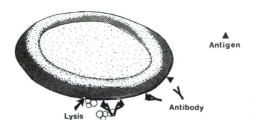

FIGURE 3 Diagrammatic representation of the pathogenesis of drug-induced hemolytic anemia as a consequence of adsorption of a drug to the red cell membrane.

the intravenous route) and cephalosporins can induce this type of hemolytic anemia. Some cephalosporins (such as cephalothin) also have been shown to modify the red cell membrane that becomes able to adsorb proteins nonspecifically, a fact that can lead to a positive direct Coombs' test but not to hemolytic anemia.

Autoimmunity-Induction Mechanism

The drug used as an example of this form of drug-induced hemolytic anemia is α-methyldopa (Aldomet). Ten to fifteen percent of the patients receiving the drug will have a positive Coombs' test, and 0.8% of the patients develop clinically evident hemolytic anemia. It is particularly interesting from the pathogenic point of view in that it is indistinguishable from a true warm autoimmune hemolytic anemia. Alpha methyldopa is unquestionably the trigger for this type of anemia, but the antibodies are of the IgG1 isotype and react with Rh antigens. It is believed that the drug changes the membrane of red cell precursors, causing the formation of antibodies reactive with a modified Rh precursor. Once formed, the antired cell antibodies will react in the absence of the drug, as true autoantibodies. Alpha methyldopa is seldom used clinically because of this complication.

Other drugs such as L-dopa, procainamide, and some nonsteroidal anti-inflammatory drugs can also act by this mechanism. Both α-methyldopa and L-dopa also stimulate the production of antinuclear antibodies.

Treatment

Blood transfusions may be necessary in emergency situations but are made difficult when there are autoantibodies to red cell antigens widely represented in the population. The serum from a patient with cold or warm-type AIHA typically agglutinates all the red cells in an antibody identification panel. It is most important to determine if there are clinically significant under-lying alloantibodies that may be masked by autoantibody. The patient's red cells may be pre-treated in a manner to enhance removal of autoantibody from the serum. After one or more autoadsorptions, the adsorbed serum may be used for alloantibody detection and cross-matching.

Glucocorticoids are the first line of treatment in patients with symptomatic warm AIHA. Other immunosuppressive drugs can be tried in patients not responding to glucocorticoids. Splenectomy can be useful in individuals who do not respond to glucocorticoids, when there is a marked predominance of red cell sequestration in the spleen. In such cases, splenect-omy leads to a longer half-life of the patient's red cells.

Glucocorticoids and splenectomy are generally ineffective in treating cold agglutinin disease. Patients should be kept warm, especially their extremities. If transfusions are to be administered an approved blood warmer may be used.

In cases of drug-induced hemolytic anemia, the offending drug should be withdrawn and hemolysis should resolve.

BIBLIOGRAPHY

Arndt PA, Garratty G. The changing spectrum of drug-induced hemolytic anemia. Semin Hematol 2005; 42:137–144.

Chaudhuri A, Zbrzezna V, Polyakova J, Pogo AO, Hesselgesser J, Horuk R. Expression of the Duffy antigen in K562 cells. Evidence that it is the human erythrocyte chemokine receptor. J Biol Chem 1994; 269:7835–7838.

Harmening DE. Modern Blood Banking and Transfusion Practices. 4th ed. Philadelphia: F.A. Davis Co., 1999.

Leo A, Kreft H, Hack H, et al. Restriction in the repertoire of the immunoglobulin light chain subgroup in pathological cold agglutinins with anti-Pr specificity. Vox Sang 2004; 86:141–147.

Menitove JE. Transfusion practices in the 1990s. Annu Rev Med 1991; 42:297.

Mollison PL, Engelfriet Cp, Contreras M. Blood Transfusion in Clinical Medicine, 10th ed. Oxford: Blackwell Science Ltd, 1997.

Petz LD, Garraty G. Acquired Immune Hemolytic Anemias. New York: Churchill/Livingston Inc., 1980.

Petz LD, Swisher S, Kleinman S, et al. Clinical Practice of Transfusion Medicine. 3rd ed. New York: Churchill Livingstone, 1996.

Rossi EC, Simon TL, Moss GE, Gould SA, eds. Principles of Transfusion Medicine. 2nd ed. Baltimore: Williams & Wilkins, 1996.

Silberstein LE, ed. Molecular and functional aspects of blood group antigens. Bethesda, MD: Amer Ass of Blood Banks, 1995.

Sokol RJ, Booker DJ, Stamps R, Walewska R. Cold haemagglutinin disease: clinical significance of serum haemolysins. Clin Lab Haematol 2000; 22:337–344.

Wells JV, Isbister JP. Hematologic diseases. In: Stites DP, Terr AI, eds. Basic and Clinical Immunology. 7th ed. Norwalk, CT: Lange, 1991:476.

23 | Immune Complex Diseases

Gabriel Virella
Department of Microbiology and Immunology, Medical University of South Carolina, Charleston, South Carolina, U.S.A.

George C. Tsokos
Beth Israel Deaconess Medical Center, Harvard Medical School, Boston, Massachusetts, U.S.A.

INTRODUCTION

The formation of circulating antigen–antibody (Ag·Ab) complexes is one of the natural events that characterize the immunologic response against soluble antigens. Normally, immune complexes (IC) formed by soluble proteins and their respective antibodies are promptly eliminated from circulation by phagocytic cells without any detectable adverse effects on the host. However, there are well-characterized clinical and experimental situations in which it has been proven that IC play a pathogenic role.

In the late 1800s and early 1900s, passive immunization with equine antisera was a common therapy for severe bacterial infections. It was often noted that one to two weeks after administration of the horse antisera, when the symptoms of acute infection had often disappeared, patients complained of athralgias, exanthematous rash, and had proteinuria and an abnormal urinary sediment, suggestive of glomerulonephritis. von Pirquet coined the term serum sickness to designate this condition.

Several decades later, Germuth et al. carried out detailed studies in rabbits in which serum sickness was induced by injection of a single dose of heterologous proteins. As summarized in Figure 1, after the lag time, necessary for antibody production, soluble IC were detected in serum, serum complement levels decreased, and the rabbits developed glomerulonephritis, myocarditis, and arthritis. The onset of disease coincided with the disappearance of circulating antigen, while free circulating antibody appeared in circulation soon after the beginning of symptoms.

Both the experimental one-shot serum sickness and human serum sickness are usually transient and will leave no permanent sequelae. However, if the organism is chronically exposed to antigen (as in chronic serum sickness), irreversible lesions will develop.

The formation of an IC does not have direct pathological consequences. The pathogenic consequences of their formation depend on the ability of those IC that leave the intravascular compartment to become tissue-fixed and activate effector systems, such as the complement system or inflammatory cells that are able to release enzymes and cytokines. Also, IC may form directly in tissues where the antigens are formed or trapped. In either case, the pro-inflammatory properties of IC are related to their physico-chemical characteristics (Table 1).

PHYSICO-CHEMICAL CHARACTERISTICS OF PATHOGENIC IMMUNE COMPLEXES

Size, affinity of the Ag·Ab reaction, and class and subclass of antibodies involved in IC formation are among the most important determinants of the pathogenic significance of IC.

In the case of circulating IC, very large Ag·Ab aggregates containing IgG1 or IgG3 antibodies, will activate complement very effectively, but are usually nonpathogenic. This is due to a combination of facts: very avid ingestion and degradation by phagocytic cells, and difficulty in diffusing across the endothelial barrier. Very small complexes ($Ag_1·Ab_{1-3}$), even while involving IgG1 and IgG3 antibodies, are able to diffuse easily into the extravascular compartment, but are usually nonpathogenic because of their inability to activate complement.

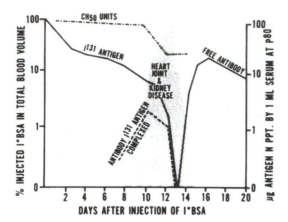

FIGURE 1   Diagrammatic representation of the sequence of events that takes place during the induction of acute serum sickness in rabbits. Six days after injection of radiolabeled bovine serum albumin (BSA) the synthesis anti-BSA antibodies start getting produced and form complexes with the antigen, which is eliminated rapidly with the circulation. The maximal concentration of immune complexes precedes shortly a decrease in complement levels and the appearance of histological abnormalities on the heart, joints, and kidney. After the antigen is totally eliminated, the antibody becomes detectable and the pathological lesions heal without permanent sequelae. *Source*: Reproduced from Cochrane, C.G., Koffler, D. Immune complex disease in experimental animals and man. Adv Immunol 1973; 16:185.

Actually, the most potentially pathogenic circulating IC are those of intermediate size (Ag2–3·Ab2–6), particularly when involving complement-fixing antibodies (IgG1, IgG3) of moderate to high affinity. Under the appropriate circumstances (discussed later), these IC may be deposited in the subendothelial space and trigger inflammatory reactions. On the other hand, IC formed in situ between tissue-fixed antigens and freely diffusible antibodies of the IgG1 and IgG3 class are always likely to be proinflammatory. Due to their large size, IgM antibodies are rarely involved in formation of IC in tissues.

IMMUNE COMPLEX FORMATION AND CELL INTERACTIONS
Immobilization and Deposition of Circulating Immune Complexes

Circulating IC may be deposited in various tissues where they cause inflammation and tissue damage. Characteristically, multiple organs and tissues may be affected and the clinical paradigm is serum sickness. The mechanisms allowing or preventing extravascular deposition of IC are rather complex and involve interactions with a variety of cells and tissues.

TABLE 1   Antigen and Antibody Characteristics
that Affect the Pathogenicity of the Immune Complex

Antibody
Isotype
Valence
Affinity for Fc receptors
Ability to bind and activate complement
Affinity
Charge
Amount
Antigen
Size
Valence
Chemical composition
Charge
Amount

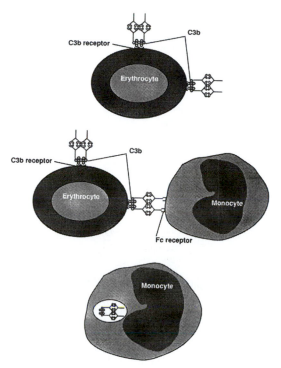

FIGURE 2 Diagrammatic representation of the protective role of erythrocytes against the development of immune complex disease. Erythrocytes can adsorb circulating immune complexes (IC) through C3b receptors or through nonspecific interactions. Red blood cell (RBC)-adsorbed IC persist in circulation until the IC are stripped from the RBC surface by phagocytic cells expressing Fc receptors, which bind the IC with greater avidity. Once taken up by phagocytic cells, the IC are degraded, and this uptake is responsible for their disappearance from circulation.

Adsorption and Transfer of Immune Complexes

Circulating IC can bind to platelets and red cells. Human platelets express Fc receptors, specific for all IgG subclasses and complement receptor (CR) 4, which bind the C3dg fragment of C3. Red blood cells (RBC) express CR1, through which C3b-containing IC can be bound. In addition, IC can bind to RBC through nonspecific interactions of low affinity, which do not require the presence of complement. IC binding to RBC is believed to be an important mechanism for clearance of soluble IC from the systemic circulation. Experimental work in primates and metabolic studies of labeled IC in humans show that RBC-bound IC are maintained in the intravascular compartment until they reach the liver, where they are presented to phagocytic cells. The phagocytic cells have Fc receptors able to bind the IC with greater affinity than the red cells; as a consequence, the IC are removed from the RBC membrane, while the red cells remain undamaged (Fig. 2).

Interactions with Antigen-Presenting Cells and Inflammatory Cells

While the interaction of IC with phagocytic cells can be a protective mechanism, it can also be a pathogenic factor. In systemic lupus erythematosus (SLE), it has been demonstrated that DNA-containing IC bind to CD32 (FcγRIIa) expressed on the surface of plasmacytoid dendritic cells, become internalized, and activate the DNA-binding toll-like receptor 9 (TLR9). Thus, the interaction with a surface receptor (FcγRIIa) and an intracellular receptor (TLR9) cause the activation dendritic cells, which in turn will present antigen to lymphocytes and propagate an unwanted response. C3bi opsonized IC bind to CR3 and FcγR receptors present on polymorphonuclear (PMN) leucocytes (Fig. 3). Binding to these receptors results in the activation of a variety of phospholipases [such as phospholipase A2 (PLA2)] and kinases (e.g., Fyn, Lyn, and Syk). As a consequence of PLA2 activation, platelet-activating factor (PAF) is synthesized and arachidonic acid is released and converted into pro-inflammatory prostaglandins and leukotrienes. The activation of membrane-associated kinases eventually leads to the expression of genes encoding pro-inflammatory cytokines and nitric oxide synthase.

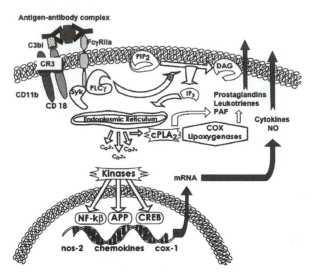

FIGURE 3   Intracellular events triggered following the binding of immune complexes (IC) to Fc and CR binding cells. IC containing immunoglobulin G (IgG) antibodies and associated C3bi bind to Fcγ receptors and CR3 expressed by circulating monocytes, macrophages, polymorphonuclears, and tissue-residing cells. FcγRIIa binding triggers the activation of src kinase Syk and phospholipase γ(PLCγ). CR3 binding activates various kinases including Syk. PLCγ leads to increased release of free calcium (Ca²⁺) in the cytoplasm, which is involved in the activation of various processes. Syk activates a series of kinases including mitogen-activated kinases. Subsequently, cytoplasmic phospolipase A2 followed by activation of lipooxygenase and cyclooxygenases (COX) that lead to the production of leukotrienes and prostaglandings, respectively. In the nucleus, various transcription factors (NFkB, AP1, CREB) become activated and increase the transcription rate of genes such as NOC, COX, and several cytokine and chemokine−encoding genes. Understanding of the involved pathways has prompted investigators to consider additional interventions (such as blocking the activity of Syk or blocking the effect of chemokines) to treat IC-associated diseases. *Abbreviations*: NFκB, nuclear factor κB; AP1, activating protein 1; CREB, cyclic AMP response protein; NOS, nitric oxide synthase 2.

Tissue Deposition of Circulating Immune Complexes

Some of the most frequent localizations of deposited IC are around the small vessels of the skin, particularly in the lower limbs, the kidney glomeruli, the choroid plexus, and the joints. Our understanding of the mechanisms responsible for extravascular deposition of IC is incomplete. A major obstacle to such deposition is the endothelial barrier, which is poorly permeable even to intermediate size IC. The first step in tissue-deposition of IC is likely to be the interaction with vascular receptors. C1q receptors, expressed by endothelial cells, and Fc receptors, expressed on the renal interstitium and by damaged endothelium could play a role in IC immobilization. The frequent involvement of the kidney in IC-associated disease may be a consequence of the existence of C3b receptors in the renal glomerular epithelial cells, Fc receptors in the renal interstitium, and a collagen-rich structure (the basement membrane), which can also be involved in nonspecific interactions with antigens or antibodies. Regional factors may influence the selectivity of IC deposition. For example, the preferential involvement of the lower limbs in IC-related skin vasculitis may result from the simple fact that the circulation is slowest and the hydrostatic pressure highest in the lower limbs.

Any pathogenic sequence involving the deposition of circulating IC has to account with increased vascular permeability in the microcirculation, allowing the diffusion of small to medium-sized soluble IC to the subendothelial spaces (Fig. 4). After IC are immobilized, they are in an ideal situation to activate monocytes or granulocytes, causing the release of vasoactive amines and cytokines. The retention of soluble IC diffusing through the endothelium should be determined by interaction with extravascular structures. For example, in the kidney, C3b receptors of the renal epithelial cells and Fc receptors in the renal interstitium could play the role.

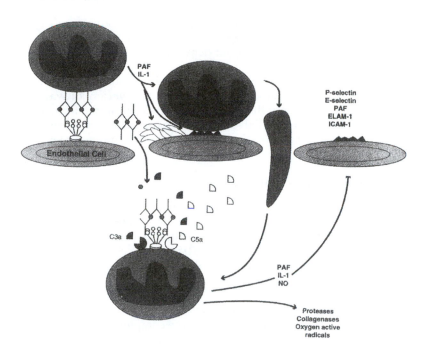

FIGURE 4 The initial stages of circulating immune complex deposition require a sequence of events, which enables circulating immune complexes (IC) and inflammatory cells to cross the endothelial barrier. In this representation of such a hypothetical sequence, the first event is the binding of circulating IC containing IgG antibodies and associated C1q to C1q receptors on the endothelial cell. The immobilized IC are then able to interact with circulating cells expressing Fcγ receptors, such as polymorphonuclear (PMN) leukocytes. Such interaction results in PMN activation and release of mediators, such as platelet-activating factor (PAF) and interleukin (IL)-1. These two mediators have a variety of effects: PAF induces vasodilatation and activates platelets, which form aggregates and release vasoactive amines. The resulting increased vascular permeability allows circulating IC to cross the endothelial barrier. IL-1 activates endothelial cells and induces the expression of selectin molecules that interact with glycoproteins and syaloglycoprotiens on the leukocyte membrane. This interaction slows down PMNs along the endothelial surface, a phenomenon known as "rolling." As endothelial cells continue to receive activating signals they start expressing membrane-associated PAF, which interacts with PAF receptors on neutrophils, ICAM-1, which interacts with leukocyte integrins of the CD11/CD18 family, and VCAM-1, which interacts with VLA-1, upregulated on PMN leukocytes as a consequence of the occupancy of Fc receptors. This promotes firm adhesion of leukocytes to endothelial cells. At the same time the IC that diffuse to the subendothelial space activate complement and generate chemotactic factors, such as C5a and C3a. Adherent PMN leukocytes are attracted to the area and insinuate themselves between endothelial cells, reaching the area of IC deposition. Interaction with those extravascular IC with associated C3b delivers additional activation signals to already primed granulocytes, resulting in the release of metalloproteinases (including proteases and collagenases), oxygen active radicals, and nitric oxide. These compounds can cause tissue damage and can further increase vascular permeability, and in doing so contribute to the perpetuation of an inflammatory reaction. *Abbreviations*: ICAM-1, intercellular adhesion molecule-1; VCAM-1, vascular cell adhesion molecule-1; VLA-2, very late antigen-1.

Formation of Immune Complexes In Situ

Direct injection of antigen into a previously immunized laboratory animal or human can result in local IC formation with circulating antibody. Examples include the Arthus reaction (antigen injected into the dermis binds circulating antibody) and hypersensitivity pneumonitis (antigen inhaled forms IC with circulating antibody).

Other types of IC formed in situ include those formed when antibodies react with antigens present on the cell surface membrane of circulating or tissue cells. IC formed on cell membranes can lead to the destruction of the cell, either by promoting phagocytosis or by causing complement-mediated lysis. This mechanism is responsible for the development of various immune cytopenias.

Autoantibodies may also bind to basement membrane antigens, as in Goodpasture's syndrome, or may react with an antigen that has become adsorbed to a basement membrane due to charge interactions, as seems to be the case of the glomerular deposition of DNA–anti-DNA IC in patients with SLE.

Another example is the formation of IC involving modified low-density lipoprotein (LDL) and corresponding antibodies in vessel walls. LDL is modified in a variety of ways in vessel walls, and although present in circulation (where it becomes involved in the formation of circulating IC), it is also present in the subendothelial space, available to form IC with transudated IgG antibodies. In general, in situ formation of IC appears as the most common mechanism leading to deposition of IC in tissues.

Inflammatory Circuits Triggered by Immune Complexes

The development of inflammatory changes after extravascular formation or deposition of IC is not observed when serum sickness is induced in experimental animals depleted of neutrophils or complement. Activated phagocytic cells and the soluble compounds released as a consequence of their activation also play important roles (Table 2), particularly in chronic conditions (discussed later). Complement components play a significant role as the source of opsonins and chemotactic factors, while activated granulocytes can release a wide variety of proteolytic enzymes that mediate tissue damage.

Activation of the complement cascade results in the generation of chemotactic and pro-inflammatory fragments, such as C3a and C5a (see Chapter 9). These complement components have strong pro-inflammatory effects, mediated by a variety of mechanisms:

1. C5a increases vascular permeability directly as well as indirectly (by causing the release of histamine and vasoactive amines from basophils and mast cells).
2. C5a enhances the expression of the CD11/CD18 complex on neutrophil membranes, increasing their adhesiveness to endothelial cells.
3. C5a and C3a are chemotactic for neutrophils, attracting them to the area of IC deposition and stimulating their respiratory burst and release of granule constituents.

The combination of chemotaxis, increased adherence, and increased vascular permeability plays a crucial role in promoting extravascular emigration of leukocytes. It needs to be stressed that the inflammatory process triggered by IC is usually associated with extravascular granulocyte infiltrates. The migration of neutrophils and other granulocytes is regulated by a series of interactions with endothelial cells, known as the adhesion cascade.

The initial event in the cascade involves the upregulation of selectins (P-selectin and E-selectin) on endothelial cells, which can be caused by a variety of stimuli (e.g., histamine, thrombin, bradykinin, leukotriene C4, free oxygen radicals, or cytokines). The consequence of this upregulation is the slowing down (rolling) and loose attachment of leukocytes (that

TABLE 2   Elements Involved in Immune Complex-Mediated Immunopathology

---
Cells
  PMN leukocytes—PMN depleted animals do not develop arthritis or Arthus reaction
  Monocytes/macrophages—monocyte depletion in experimental glomerulonephritis decreases proteinuria
Soluble factors (circulating and released locally)
  Complement fragments—complement-depleted animals develop less severe forms of serum sickness
  Lymphokines/cytokines—corticosteroids reduce interleukin release and have beneficial effects
    in the treatment of immune complex disease
  Lysosomal enzymes (e.g., matrix metalloproteinases)—the main mediators of PMN-induced tissue damage
  Prostaglandins—important mediators of the inflammatory reaction; their synthesis is inhibited by
    aspirin and most nonsteroidal anti-inflammatory agents
  Nitric oxide and products of the respiratory burst—these compounds can affect vascular permeability
    and induce cell and tissue damage because of their oxidative properties
---
Abbreviation: PMN, polymorphonuclear.

express a third selectin, L-selectin, which binds to membrane oligosaccharides on endothelial cells). These initial interactions are unstable and transient.

The endothelial cells, in response to persistent activating signals, express PAF and ICAM-1 on the membrane. Neutrophils express constitutively a PAF receptor that allows rolling cells to interact with membrane-bound PAF. The interaction of neutrophils with PAF, as well as signals received in the form of chemotactic cytokines such as IL-8 (which can also be released by endothelial cells), activate neutrophils and induce the expression of integrins—CD11a/CD18, leukocyte function antigen (LFA)-1 and related molecules, and VLA-4.

The interaction between integrins expressed by neutrophils and molecules of the immunoglobulin superfamily expressed by endothelial cells (ICAM-1 and related antigens bind LFA-1 and related molecules; vascular cell adhesion molecule (VCAM)-1 binds VLA-4) causes firm adhesion (sticking) of inflammatory cells to the endothelial surface, which is an essential step in leading to their extravascular migration. VLA-4 is also expressed on the membrane of lymphocytes and monocytes, and its interaction with endothelial VCAM-1 allows the recruitment of these cells to the site of inflammation.

The interactions between integrins and their ligands are important for the development of vasculitic lesions in patients with SLE and other systemic autoimmune disorders, and purulent exudates in infection sites. As discussed in Chapter 13, patients with genetic defect in the expression of CD18 and related cell adhesion molecules (CAMs) fail to form abscesses because their neutrophils do not express these molecules and fail to migrate.

The actual transmigration of leukocytes into the subendothelial space seems to involve yet another set of CAMs, particularly one member of the immunoglobulin superfamily known as platelet endothelial cell adhesion molecule (PECAM), that is expressed both at the sites of intercellular junction and on the membranes of leukocytes. PECAM-1 interacts with itself and its expression is upregulated on both endothelial cells and leukocytes by a variety of activating signals. The egression of leukocytes from the vessel wall is directed by chemoattractant molecules released into the extravascular space, and involves diapedesis through endothelial cell junctions.

As leukocytes begin to reach the site of IC formation or deposition, they continue to receive activating signals. Their activation brings about the release of additional chemotactic factors and continuing upregulation of CAMs on endothelial cells, the efflux of phagocytic cells to the subendothelial space will intensify, and the conditions needed for self perpetuation of the inflammatory process are created. All PMN leukocytes express Fcγ receptors and C3bi (CR3) receptors that mediate their binding and ingestion of IC. This process is associated with activation of a variety of functions and with the release of a variety of cytokines, enzymes, and other mediators. As previously mentioned, one important mediator released by activated neutrophils is PAF, which will promote the self perpetuation of the inflammatory process by increasing vascular permeability (directly or as a consequence of the activation of platelets, which release vasoactive amines), inducing the upregulation of the CD11/CD18 complex on neutrophils, and inducing monocytes to release IL-1 and tumor necrosis factor (TNF), which activate endothelial cells and promote the upregulation of adhesion molecules (E and P selectins) and the synthesis of PAF and IL-8.

Furthermore, as granulocytes try to engulf large IC aggregates or immobilized IC, they become activated and release their enzymatic contents, including metalloproteinases with protease and collagenase activity and oxygen active radicals. These compounds can damage cells, digest basement membranes and collagen-rich structures, and contribute to the perpetuation of the inflammatory reaction by causing direct breakdown of C5 and C3 and generating additional C5a and C3a. The formation of C3b promotes the formation of C3 convertase and further activation complement, thus continuing to amplify the pro-inflammatory reaction. As the inflammatory reaction continues to intensify, clinical manifestations emerge. The clinical manifestations of IC disease depend on the intensity of the inflammatory reaction and on the tissue(s) predominantly affected by IC deposition.

While the involvement of neutrophils and complement in acute inflammatory processes induced by IC has been well documented, chronic inflammatory processes, such as the smoldering vascular inflammation characteristic of atherosclerosis, are usually associated with infiltrates of activated macrophages, probably reflecting more complex pathogenic pathways with participation of activated Th1 cells, and predominantly extravascular formation of IC.

HOST FACTORS THAT INFLUENCE THE DEVELOPMENT OF IMMUNE COMPLEX DISEASE

The development of IC disease in experimental animals is clearly dependent on host factors. If several rabbits of the same strain, age, weight, and sex are immunized with identical amounts of a given heterologous protein by the same route, only a fraction of the immunized animals will form antibodies, and of those, only some will develop IC disease. The magnitude of the response primarily depends on genetic factors. The extent of tissue involvement is likely to depend on the general characteristics of the antibodies produced (such as affinity, complement-binding ability, capacity to interact with cell receptors) as well as on the functional state of the reticuloendothelial system (RES) of the animal.

Affinity and Number of Available Fcγ Receptors

The affinity and number of available Fcγ receptors on professional phagocytic cells (PMN leukocytes, monocytes, and macrophages) are important in the expression of IC disease. If IC are predominantly taken up by those cells in tissues where they abound, such as the liver and spleen, the likelihood of developing tissue inflammation is limited. Support given to the importance of Fc-mediated clearance of IC as a protective mechanism was obtained in experiments in which the Fc receptors were blocked. This resulted in decreased IC clearance and increased pathogenicity.

   Patients with SLE and rheumatoid arthritis have decreased ability to clear antibody-sensitized red cells, indicating a general inability to clear circulating IC. Some patients with lupus nephritis have a distinct $Fc_\gamma RII$ allele expression that displays low affinity for IgG that results in poor IC clearance in favor of glomerular deposition.

Ability to Interact with Complement Receptors

The ability to interact with CRs may also be an important determinant of pathogenicity. C1q, C3b, C3bi, C3ċ, and C3d readily associate with IC. This allows IC to bind to cells expressing the corresponding CRs. As mentioned previously, binding of IC to CR1 expressed on the surface membrane of red cells facilitates their clearance for the circulation (discussed earlier). In patients with SLE and other IC diseases the number of CR1 on the surface of red cells is decreased and this contributes to decreased IC clearance. This decreased CR1 expression has been claimed to be genetically determined in SLE. However, it is possible that the decrease may not be numerical, but functional. In other words, in patients with high concentrations of circulating IC CR1 may be saturated and this may result in blocking of the receptors by IC, causes a decrease in the number of available receptors.

DETECTION OF SOLUBLE IMMUNE COMPLEXES

Many techniques have been proposed for the detection of soluble IC. In general these techniques are based either on the physical properties [e.g., precipitation with polyethylene glycol (PEG) or precipitation at cold temperatures] or on the biologic characteristics of the IC. The latter techniques make use of various properties of IC such as their ability to bind C1q or their binding to cells that express CR1 and CR2 (Raji cell assay).

Detection of Cryoglobulins

Circulating IC are often formed in antigen excess, with low affinity antibodies, and remain soluble at room temperature. However, if the serum containing these IC is cooled to 4°C for about 72 hours, the stability of the Ag·Ab reaction increases and eventually there is sufficient cross-linking to result in the formation of large aggregates, which precipitate spontaneously (Fig. 5). Because antibodies are the main constituents of these cold precipitates, and because

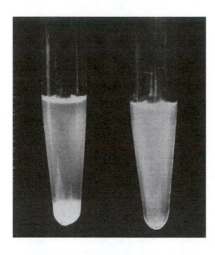

FIGURE 5 Cryoglobulin screening. Two test tubes were filled with sera from a patient (*left*) and a healthy volunteer (*right*). After 48 hours at 4°C, a precipitate is obvious in the patient's serum, but is not present in the control.

antibodies are globulins, the precipitated proteins are designated as cryoglobulins. Serum separated from blood drawn, clotted, and centrifuged at 37°C is used for detection of cryoglobulins. The proper characterization of a cryoprecipitate requires redissolution of the precipitated proteins at 37°C, followed by identification of their constituents by appropriate immunochemical assays. Based on immunochemical characterization, cryoglobulins can be classified in two major types.

Monoclonal Cryoglobulins

Monoclonal cryoglobulins, containing immunoglobulin of one single isotype and one single light chain class, are usually detected in patients with plasma cell malignancies and in some cases of idiopathic cryoglobulinemia. Monoclonal cryoglobulins are essentially monoclonal proteins with abnormal thermal behavior, and their existence has no correlation with IC formation or any special diagnostic significance besides the possibility of creating conditions favorable for the development of the hyperviscosity syndrome (see Chapter 27).

Mixed Cryoglobulins

Mixed cryoglobulins, contain two or three immunoglobulin isotypes, one of which (usually IgM) can be a monoclonal component (with one single light chain type and one single heavy chain class), while the remaining immunoglobulins are polyclonal. Complement components (C3, C1q) can also be found in the cryoprecipitates containing mixed cryoglobulins. Mixed cryoglobulins represent cold-precipitable IC. One of the immunoglobulins present in the precipitate (usually the monoclonal component) is an antibody that reacts with the other immunoglobulin(s) that constitute the cryoglobulin. The most frequent type of mixed cryoglobulin is IgM–IgG, in which IgM is a "rheumatoid factor." It is believed that, at least in some cases, the IgM antibody is directed to determinants expressed by IgG antibodies bound to their corresponding antigens (Fig. 6). Evidence supporting the involvement of infectious agents in the formation of mixed cryoglobulins has been obtained by identifying antigens and/or antibodies in the cryoprecipitates, particularly antigens derived from hepatitis B and C viruses.

Precipitation of Soluble Immune Complexes with Polyethylene Glycol

Low concentrations of PEG (3–4%) cause preferential precipitation of IC relative to monomeric immunoglobulins. As a screening technique, PEG precipitation is nonspecific. But if the antigen involved in IC formation is not precipitated in its soluble form, its finding on a PEG precipitate can be considered as evidence of the presence of circulating IC involving that particular antigenic protein. Also, PEG precipitation is often used as the initial step of IC isolation protocols.

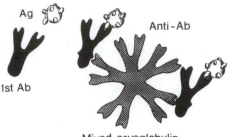

Mixed cryoglobulin

FIGURE 6 Diagrammatic representation of the pathogenesis of mixed cryoglobulins. Initially, an antimicrobial antibody (e.g.,) of the IgG class is produced. This antibody, a consequence of binding to the antigen, exposes a new antigenic determinant, which is recognized by an IgM antiglobulin. The combination of this IgM with the first IgG antibody and the microbial antigen constitutes the mixed cryoglobulin. Viral antigens and corresponding antibodies (e.g., HBsAg and Anti-HBsAg) have been characterized in cryoprecipitates from patients with mixed cryoglobulins, both with and without a history of previous viral hepatitis B infection. It is believed that this mechanism, antiviral IgG combined with an IgM anti-antibody, accounts for over 50% of the cases of essential or idiopathic cryoglobulinemia (cryoglobulinemia appearing in patients without evidence of any other disease). *Abbreviations*: Ab, antibody; Ag, antigen; HBsAg, hepatitis B surface antigen.

Assays Based on Interactions with Complement

One of the most widely used techniques for general screening of IC is based on the binding of C1q. Is usually performed on a solid base platform, in which purified C1q is immobilized in the wells of a microtiter plate and when an IC-containing sample is added to the C1q-coated well the IC contained in the added sample will be bound to the immobilized C1q. To determine whether IC are bound to C1q, enzyme-labeled anti-human IgG antibodies are added to the wells, their retention on the plate is directly proportional to the IC captured by the immobilized C1q.

ROLE OF IMMUNE COMPLEXES IN HUMAN DISEASE
Classification of Immune Complex Diseases

IC have been implicated in human disease either through demonstration in serum or through identification in tissues where lesions are found. Most often, the antibody moiety of the IC is detected, and knowledge about the antigens involved is still very fragmentary. However, one of the most common classifications of IC disease, proposed by a WHO-sponsored committee, is based on the nature of the antigens involved (Table 3).

Clinical Expression of Immune Complex Disease

The clinical expression of IC disease depends on the target organs where the deposition of IC predominates:

1. The kidney is very frequently affected (SLE, mixed cryoglobulinemia, chronic infections, poststreptococcal glomerulonephritis, purpura hypergammaglobulinemica, serum sickness, etc.), usually with glomerulonephritis as the prevailing feature.
2. The joints are predominantly affected in rheumatoid arthritis.
3. The skin is affected in cases of serum sickness, mixed cryoglobulinemia and vasculitis.
4. The large vessels are affected by the subendothelial formation of antigen-antibody complexes containing oxidized LDL and the corresponding antibodies, leading to the development or progression of atherosclerosis.
5. The lungs are affected in extrinsic alveolitis.

The reasons why the target organs can vary from disease to disease are not clear. In some cases, such as in extrinsic alveolitis, the route of exposure to the antigen is a major determinant for the involvement of the lungs. The kidneys, due to their physiological role and to the

TABLE 3 Classification of Immune Complex Diseases According to the Antigen Involved

ICD involving endogenous antigens
    Immunoglobulin antigens, e.g., rheumatoid arthritis, hypergammaglobulinemic purpura
    Nuclear antigens, e.g., systemic lupus erythematosus
    Specific cellular antigens, e.g., tumors, autoimmune diseases
    Modified lipoproteins, e.g., atherosclerosis
ICD involving exogenous antigens
    Medicinal antigens, e.g., serum sickness, drug allergy
    Environmental antigens
        Inhaled, e.g., extrinsic alveolitis
        Ingested, e.g., dermatitis herpetiformes
    Antigens from infectious organisms
        Viral, e.g., chronic hepatitis B and C, HIV/AIDS
        Bacterial, e.g., poststreptococcal glomerulonephritis, subacute endocarditis, leprosy, syphilis
        Protozoan, e.g., malaria, trypanosomiasis
        Helminthic, e.g., schistosomiasis, onchocerciasis
ICD involving unknown antigens
    This category includes most forms of chronic immune complex glomerulonephritis, vasculitis with
        or without eosinophilia, and many cases of mixed cryoglobulinemia

Abbreviation: ICD, immune complex diseases.

existence of complement and Fc receptors in different anatomical structures, appear to be an ideal organ for IC trapping. In rheumatoid arthritis, IC appear to be present not only in the circulation, but also to be present (and probably formed) in and around the joints, and although they do not appear to be the initiating factor for the disease, their potential for perpetuating the inflammatory lesions is unquestionable.

THERAPEUTIC APPROACHES TO IMMUNE COMPLEX DISEASE

The most common types of therapy in IC disease are based on four main approaches:

1. Eradication of the source of persistent antigen production (e.g., infections, tumors).
2. Turning off the inflammatory reaction (using corticosteroids and nonsteroidal agents).
3. Suppression of antibody production using immunosuppressive drugs such as cyclophosphamide, azathioprine, or cyclosporine. This is the mainstay of IC disease treatment, particularly when autoimmune reactions are on its basis.
4. Removal of soluble IC from the circulation by plasmapheresis, a procedure that consists of the removal of blood (up to 5 L each time), separation and reinfusion of red cells, and replacement of the patient's plasma by normal plasma or plasma-replacing solutions. Plasmapheresis appears most beneficial when associated with the administration of immunosuppressive drugs; by itself, it can even induce severe clinical deterioration perhaps related to changes in the immunoregulatory circuits.

In the last few years, there has been considerable interest in applying emerging basic concepts on the pathogenesis of inflammation to the treatment of a variety of conditions in which IC formation or deposition may play an important role. Four major approaches have been tried:

1. Blocking critical cytokines, such as TNF. This has been done either with monoclonal antibodies reacting with pro-inflammatory cytokines, with cytokine receptor antagonists, or with recombinant cytokine receptors (see Chapter 24).
2. Interruption of the interaction between leukocyte integrins and endothelial CAMs. Humanized anti-ICAM-1 (and other cell–cell interaction-facilitating molecules) as well as soluble forms of these molecules have been successfully tested in animal models.
3. Inhibition of the complement activation cascade using soluble forms of regulatory proteins (C1q inhibitor, MCP, DAF, CR1) and antifactor antibodies (anti-C5 antibody) with the goal of inhibiting the production of C3a and C5a (see Chapter 9).

4.   Depletion of B cells using an anti-CD20 antibody to limit the production of antibodies involved in the formation of IC.

BIBLIOGRAPHY

Bielory L, Gascon P, Lawley TJ, Young NS, Frank MM. Human serum sickness: a prospective analysis of 35 patients treated with equine anti-thymocyte globulin for bone marrow failure. Medicine 1988; 67:40.

Dinant HJ, Dijckmans BA. New therapeutic targets for rheumatoid arthritis. Pharm World Sci 1999; 21:49.

Ferri C, Zignego AL, Pileri SA. Cryoglobulins. J Clin Pathol 2002; 55:4–13.

Fleishman RM. Early diagnosis and treatment of rheumatoid arthritis for improved outcomes: focus on etarnacept, a new biological response modifier. Clin Therap 1999; 21:1429.

Hebert LA. The clearance of immune complexes from the circulation of man and other primates. Am J Kidney Dis 1991; XVII(3):352.

Jancar S, Crespo MS. Immune complex-mediated tissue injury: a multistep paradigm. Trends Immunol 2005; 26:48–55.

Lopes-Virella MF, Virella G. The role of immune and inflammatory processes in the development of macrovascular disease in diabetes. Front Biosci 2003; 8:s750–s768.

Luster AD. Chemokines- chemotactic cytokines that mediate inflammation. N Engl J Med 1998; 338:436.

Means TK, Latz E, Hayashi F, Murali MR, Golenbock DT, Luster AD. Human lupus autoantibody-DNA complexes activate DCs through cooperation of CD32 and TLR9. J Clin Invest 2005; 115:407–417.

Mulligan MS, Miyasaka M, Ward PA. Protective effects of combined adhesion molecule blockade in models of acute lung injury. Proc Assoc Am Phys 1996; 108:198.

Nityanand S, Holm G, Lefvert AK. Immune complex mediated vasculitis in hepatitis B and C infections and the effect of anti-viral therapy. Clin Immunol Immunopath 1997; 82:250.

Sansonno D, Dammacco F. Hepatitis C virus, cryoglobulinaemia, and vasculitis: immune complex relations. Lancet Infect Dis 2005; 5:227–236.

Tsai J-F, Margolis HS, Jeng JE, et al. Immunoglobulin- and hepatitis B surface antigen-specific circulating immune complexes in chronic hepatits B virus infection. Clin Immunol Immunopath 1998; 86:246.

Tsokos GC. Lymphocytes, cytokines, inflammation, and immune trafficking. Curr Opin Rheumatol 1995; 7:376.

Wener MH, Mannik M. Mechanisms of immune deposit formation in renal glomeruli. Semin Immunopathol 1986; 9:219–235.

Zimmerman GA, Prescott SM, McIntyre TM. Endothelial cell interactions with granulocytes: tethering and signaling molecules. Immunol Today 1992; 13:93.

24 | Immune System Modulators

Philip D. Hall
Department of Pharmacy and Clinical Sciences, South Carolina College of Pharmacy, Medical University of South Carolina, Charleston, South Carolina, U.S.A.

Gabriel Virella
Department of Microbiology and Immunology, Medical University of South Carolina, Charleston, South Carolina, U.S.A.

INTRODUCTION

Immune system modulators are agents, principally drugs, which adjust the activity of a patient's immune response, either up or down, until a desired level of immunity is reached. The principal targets of immune modulation are the specific components of the immune response, T and B lymphocyte clones, which can hopefully be selectively "fine-tuned" in their function to promote the better health of the patient. Three general clinical scenarios dominate the immunomodulation landscape:

1. Immunosuppressive therapies, utilized when specific T and B lymphocytes of the patient's immune system have become activated against the patient's own body organs, such as in autoimmune diseases (see Chapters 18 and 19) or in organ transplantation (see Chapter 25).
2. Induction of hyporesponsiveness or tolerance that has the advantage of targeting the undesirable immune response rather than inducing a generalized immunosuppression. In some cases, the effect of hyposensitization is truly immunomodulatory, shifting the response from pathogenic to protective or indifferent, as in the case of hyposensitization of patients with IgE-mediated hypersensitivity (see Chapter 21).
3. A third modulator option is to attempt to boost the overall neutrophil, B lymphocyte, and/ or T lymphocyte function of the patient (immunopotentiation)—this can be accomplished either by actively stimulating the patient's own immune system to higher performance levels through immunization techniques or by passively introducing protective immune system components from outside sources, such as gamma globulin, into the patient's body (see Chapter 29).

IMMUNOSUPPRESSION

Suppression of the immune response is at present the only efficient therapy in most autoimmune diseases, in the control of transplant rejection, and in other situations in which the immune system plays a significant pathogenic role. Most of the currently used immunosuppressive drugs have a generalized, nonspecific suppressive effect. Some immunosuppressants have effects practically limited to either humoral or cell-mediated immunity, but they still lead to generalized immunosuppression. More recently, a variety of new biological agents have been tried in different immunosuppressive regimens, including monoclonal antibodies to T cells and their subsets, immunotoxins, IL-2-toxin conjugates, anti-idiotypic antibodies, and so on, with the goal of developing more specific and effective therapies (see Chapter 25). In many cases, these agents are still in the early stages of evaluation, and it is too soon to issue definite judgments about their usefulness. It is, however, unquestionable that they are the prototypes of approaches that will be more and more used in the near future.

Immunosuppressive Drugs: Pharmacological and Immunological Aspects

A variety of drugs, ranging from glucocorticoids to cytotoxic drugs, have been used for the purpose of suppressing undesirable immune responses. While many of these drugs are loosely termed "immunosuppressive," they differ widely in their mechanisms of action, toxicity, and efficacy. The exact mechanisms of action of immunosuppressive drugs are difficult to determine, partly because the physiology of the immune response has not yet been completely elucidated. The target of immunosuppressive therapies are rather diverse, and depending of the agents may include phagocytosis and antigen-processing by macrophages; antigen recognition by lymphocytes; proliferation and/or differentiation of lymphocytes; production of cytokines; and immune effector mechanisms, including the production and release of cytotoxic leukocytes, antibodies, and/or delayed hypersensitivity mediators.

Glucocorticoids

Glucocorticoids or corticosteroids, such as prednisone and prednisolone—the synthetic analogs of the adrenal cortex hormones—are the most widely used immunosupressive agents.

Mechanisms of Action
The mechanisms of actions of glucocorticoids can be divided into three major effects.

Induction of Apoptosis
At certain dosage levels, treatment with glucocorticoids may produce a rapid and profound lymphopenia. This is particularly true in cases of lymphocytic leukemia, and it is a consequence of the induction of apoptosis. The molecular mechanism of glucocorticoid-induced apoptosis hinges on the activation of an endonuclease, which is normally inactive due to its association to a protein. This effect, similar to all other cellular effects of glucocorticoids, including the induction of apoptosis, requires association with a glucocorticoid-cytoplasmic receptor. The glucocorticoid–receptor complex is translocated to the nucleus, where it binds to regulatory DNA sequences (glucocorticoid-responsive elements). At the genetic level, two possibilities have been suggested to account for the enhancement of apopotic processes based on experimental observations: the downregulation of the synthesis of the protein that inactivates the endonuclease and the activation of a cascade of cysteine–dependent aspartate-directed proteases (caspases), which results in the degradation of the endonuclease–inactivating protein.

Downregulation of Cytokine Synthesis
The administration of glucocorticoids is followed by a general downregulation of cytokine synthesis. This effect is secondary to the inhibition of nuclear binding proteins, which activate the expression of cytokine genes. Two mechanisms (not mutually exclusive) have been proposed (Fig. 1).

1. After combining with the glucocorticoid-cytoplasmic receptor, the glucocorticoid–receptor complex is translocated to the nucleus, where it blocks the association of AP-1 with promoter sequences controlling the expression of cytokine genes.
2. The translocated glucocorticoid–receptor complex binds to the promoter of the inhibitory protein that regulates the activity of nuclear factor kappa B (NFκB) (IkB, see Chapters 4 and 11) and induces its expression. The synthesis of abnormally high levels of IkB results in the inactivation of NFκB, thus neutralizing a second nuclear binding protein involved in the upregulation of cytokine genes.

Anti-inflammatory Effects
The anti-inflammatory effect of glucocorticoids is probably the most significant from the pharmacological point of view. Several actions of glucocorticoids combine to induce this anti-inflammatory effect:

1. Downregulation of the synthesis of pro-inflammatory cytokines.

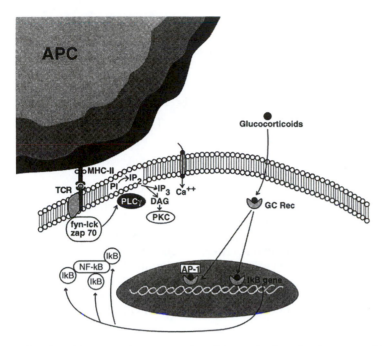

FIGURE 1 Diagrammatic representation of the mechanism of action responsible for the downregulation of cytokine synthesis by glucocorticoids. Once internalized in the cytoplasm, glucocorticoids combine with their receptor and the complex is translocated to the nucleus, where it interacts with the nuclear binding protein AP-1, preventing its interaction with cytokine gene enhancers, and with a glucocorticoid responsive element that upregulates the expression of the IκB gene. The excess of IκB protein prevents the activation of nuclear factor-kappa B, another nuclear binding protein, which normally activates the expression of cytokine genes (see Chapters 4 and 11). *Abbreviations*: APC, antigen-presenting cell; DAG, diacyl glycerol; IP$_3$, inositol triphosphate; MHC, major histocompatibility complex; NF, necrotic factor; PKC, protein kinase C; PLC, phospholipase C; TCR, T cell receptor.

2. Reduced expression of cell-adhesion molecules (CAMs) on the vessel wall, partly as a consequence of the downregulation of cytokine synthesis (pro-inflammatory cytokines upregulate CAM expression) and partly as a consequence of a direct downregulation of the expression of the genes encoding those molecules. The modulation of CAM expression has a marked effect on leukocyte traffic. Neutrophils and T lymphocytes are predominantly affected and remain sequestered on the bone marrow and lymph nodes, impairing their ability to generate both specific immune responses and nonspecific inflammatory responses.

3. The synthesis of phospholipase A2 is downregulated due to the binding of the glucocorticoid–receptor complex to a DNA glucocorticoid-responsive element that has a negative effect on the expression of the phospholipase A2 gene. Consequently, the synthesis of leukotrienes, prostaglandins, and platelet activating factor is also downregulated.

4. The nitric oxide synthase gene is also downregulated; thus, the release of nitric oxide is reduced, eliminating its vasodilator effect.

5. In contrast, glucocorticoids upregulate the expression of lipocortin-1, a protein which has anti-inflammatory effects in part due to its ability to inactivate preformed phospholipase A2.

Nonsteroidal Anti-inflammatory Drugs

Nonsteroidal anti-inflammatory drugs (NSAIDs) are totally unrelated to the corticosteroid family but share certain anti-inflammatory properties. The anti-inflammatory potency of the NSAIDs family appears to directly correlate with its ability to inhibit prostaglandin and thromboxane synthesis from arachidonic acid by inhibiting the enzyme cyclo-oxygenase (COX). There are two isoforms of the COX enzyme. COX-1 is constitutively expressed in most cells while COX-2 is induced in inflamed tissue only. The anti-inflammatory properties of both selective and nonselective NSAIDs appear to be related to their inhibition of COX-2. Some of the adverse effects of the nonselective NSAIDs (e.g., gastrointestinal and renal toxicity) may be related to the inhibition of COX-1. NSAIDs include a large number of prescription and over-the-counter drugs. Common examples of the nonselective COX-1 and -2 inhibitors include aspirin, ibuprofen, indomethacin, naprosyn, and ketorolac, while there are currently only two of the selective COX-2 inhibitors (celecoxib and rofecoxib) available by prescription. NSAIDs do not appear to modulate cytokine release or to alter T and B lymphocyte cell trafficking, and thus have virtually no immunosuppressive effects.

Alkylating Agents and Antimetabolites

Several commonly used immunosuppressants fit into this category. They can be generically classified into two large groups: cell-cycle specific and cell-cycle nonspecific. The choice between the two types of immunosuppressants is both based on clinical experience and on their characteristics. For example, for the treatment of autoimmune diseases that form abnormal immune humoral and cell-mediated immune responses, the goal is to turn off the proliferating auto-reactive lymphocytes, and cell-cycle specific agents with the ability to block DNA synthesis are utilized. On the other hand, plasma-cell malignancies are difficult to treat with cell-cycle specific agents, because the majority of antibody-producing plasma cells are not in cycle, but rather in a prolonged G_1 or G_0 state. In this case, cell-cycle nonspecific agents are most likely to be effective.

Cell Cycle Specific Agents

Cell cycle specific agents cause cell death by interfering with different parts of the cell division cycle. This group includes the antimetabolites methotrexate, azathioprine, and 6-mercaptopurine (6-MP) that appears to act only on cells in the S-phase, when DNA is actively synthesized. Two newer compounds, mycophenolate mofetil and leflunomide, are also included in this group.

Methotrexate

Methotrexate, a folic acid analogue, binds to and inhibits dihydrofolate reductase, thus blocking the formation of the DNA nucleotide thymidine. It is most active against cells in the S-phase of the cell cycle. T lymphocytes after appropriate antigen stimulation begin to proliferate and enter the S-phase of the cell cycle. Therefore, methotrexate is used to block lymphocyte proliferation. Unfortunately, methotrexate also targets other rapidly dividing cells (e.g., bone marrow, gastrointestinal tract, hair follicles) leading to its common side effects (i.e., agranulocytosis and other consequences of bone marrow suppression, diarrhea and other gastrointestinal symptoms, secondary to mucosal damage, and alopecia). Methotrexate is commonly used to treat NSAID-refractory rheumatoid arthritis and malignancies (e.g., breast cancer and acute lymphoblastic leukemia).

Azathioprine

Azathioprine has been used in solid organ transplantation since 1963. After absorption, azathioprine is metabolized by hepatic and red blood cells (RBCs) glutathione to 6-MP. Intracellularly, 6-MP is converted to form thiopurine ribonucleosides and nucleotides that inhibit purine synthesis by both the de novo pathway and salvage pathway, and thereby inhibits the proliferation of T and B lymphocytes. Azathioprine was commonly used with cyclosporin, and prednisone as the "standard" regimen for prevention of solid organ transplant rejection. More recently, mycophenolate has been taking its place in these combinations (discussed later). In addition, azathioprine is used to treat Crohn's disease. 6-MP is mainly used in combination with methotrexate as part of maintenance therapy for acute lymphoblastic leukemia in children.

Mycophenolate Mofetil

Mycophenolate mofetil (MMF, Cellcept) also inhibits lymphocyte proliferation. It acts as a reversible inhibitor of inosine monophosphate dehydrogenase, thus interfering with the de novo pathway of guanine nucleotide synthesis and subsequent DNA replication. T and B lymphocytes are highly dependent on the de novo pathway for the generation of guanosine nucleotides, whereas other cells can use the salvage pathway. Thus, mycophenolate affects T and B lymphocytes with some degree of selectivity over other types of cells. Mycophenolate is used clinically in prophylaxis of organ rejection in solid organ transplantation.

Leflunomide

Leflunomide hinders the proliferation of lymphocytes by inhibiting a different enzyme, dihydro-orotate dehydrogenase. This is a key enzyme in de novo pyrimidine synthesis and activated T lymphocytes primarily to synthesize pyrimidines by this de novo pathway. In three randomized trials, leflunomide appears to exhibit efficacy similar to sulfasalazine (a NSAID) and methotrexate in patients with active rheumatoid arthritis.

Alkylating agents such as cyclophosphamide or radiation therapy, although able to kill cells in cycle to a greater degree than cells not in cycle, can also kill nondividing cells.

Immunosuppressive Effects of Cytotoxic Drugs

The three cytotoxic drugs most widely used for their immunosuppressive effects—cyclophosphamide, azathioprine, and methotrexate—all suppress primary and secondary humoral immune responses, delayed hypersensitivity, skin graft rejection, and auto-immune disease in animals. However, there are some striking differences in the mechanism of the action of these three agents (Table 1).

In studies of the effects of cyclophosphamide, methotrexate, and 6-MP on antibody production in mice, one can compare the dose which kills 5% of the animals within one week (LD_5) with the dose required to reduce the antibody response of the mice by a factor of 2 [inhibitory dose (ID) 2]; a therapeutic index (TI) can be calculated, which is defined as the ratio of the two doses (LD5/ID2). Cyclophosphamide has the highest TI followed by methotrexate and 6-MP (Table 2).

Sharply different effects of azathioprine and cyclophosphamide on humoral antibody production have also been demonstrated, using flagellin as a test antigen. There was a significant suppression of antibody response to flagellin in cyclophosphamide-treated patients, while the responses of azathioprine-treated patients did not differ significantly from those of non-treated control patients. Several investigators have also shown that cyclophosphamide can decrease the production of anti-DNA antibodies, both in NZB mice and humans. This suggests that cyclophosphamide can inhibit an ongoing immune response whereas azathioprine and 6-MP cannot. This, of course, is the situation that one faces in the treatment of patients with autoimmune disease, since the relevant immune responses are already established by the time they are recognized as patients and treated. In patients with systemic lupus erythematosus (SLE), cyclophosphamide treatment can reverse the deposition of immune complexes in the dermo-epidermal junction (which correlates with renal disease), whereas glucocorticoid therapy alone does not.

Studies of the effects of these drugs on cellular immunity have shown that all three depress cellular immunity. However, comparative studies show a greater effect with cyclophosphamide. While both cyclophosphamide and methotrexate are more effective than 6-MP in suppressing a *M. turberculosis* purified protein derivative (PPD) skin test in experimental animals, only cyclophosphamide depletes thymus-dependent areas of the lymph nodes. The in vitro response of lymphocytes to phytohemmaglutin (PHA) and other mitogens is likewise

TABLE 1 Therapeutic Indices of Cytotoxic Agents Inhibiting Antibody Production

Agent	LD_5[a]	ID_2[b]	TI[c]
Cyclophosphamide	300.0	50.0	6.0
Methotrexate	6.3	1.25	5.0
6-Mercaptopurine	240.0	100.0	2.4

[a]LD_5 dose (in mg/kg) killing 5% of animals within one week.
[b]ID_2 dose (in mg/kg) lowering antibody titer to $1/2^2$.
[c]Therapeutic index = LD/ID.

TABLE 2   Summary of Effects of Drugs with Alkylating and Antimetabolite Activity[a]

Effect	Cyclophosphamide	Azathioprine and 6-MP	Methotrexate
Reduced primary immune response	++	++	++
Reduced secondary immune response	++	±	+
Reduced immune complexes	++	0	0
Anti-inflammatory effect	+	++	+
Mitostatic effect	++	++	++
Reduced delayed hypersensitivity	++	+	+
Suppression of passive transfer of cellular immunity	++	±	±
Lymphopenia	++	±	±
Facilitation of tolerance induction	++	+	

[a]On the basis of a combination of experimental and clinical data.

inhibited only by cyclophosphamide. In addition, tolerance induction is much easier to achieve in mice treated with cyclophosphamide than with azathioprine or methotrexate.

Inhibitors of Signal Transduction: Cyclosporin A, Tacrolimus (Prograf, Fk506), and Sirolimus (Rapamycin, Rapamune)

These compounds are fungal metabolites with immunosuppressive properties. Structurally they are macrocyclic compounds; cyclosporin A is a macrocyclic peptide while FK506 and sirolimus are macrocyclic lactones (macrolides). All are virtually devoid of toxicity for leukocyte precursors, and hence, do not cause leukopenia or lymphopenia. Their molecular mechanism of action depends on their binding to cytoplasmic proteins involved in the process of signal transduction essential for lymphocyte activation and/or proliferation (Fig. 2). Because of their ability to bind immunosuppressive compounds these proteins are collectively known as immunophilins.

Cyclosporin A

Cyclosporin A is cyclic undecapeptide obtained from *Tolypocladium inflatum*. It has a uniquely selective effect on T lymphocytes, suppressing humoral T-dependent responses and cell-mediated immune responses. Its mechanism of action involves high affinity binding to cyclophilin. The cyclosporin A–cyclophilin complex, in turn, binds and inactivates calcineurin. This protein, upon activation acquires phosphatase properties and activates the nuclear factor of activated T cells (NF-AT), a nuclear binding protein involved in the control of the expression of the IL-2 gene and other cytokine genes (see Chapter 11) by dephosphorylation. As a consequence of the inactivation of calcineurin, Ca^{2+}-associated T cell activation pathways, such as those triggered by anti-CD3 antibodies or the occupancy of the TcR, are inhibited and there is a general downregulation of the production of IL-2, interferon (IFN)-γ, IL-3, IL-4, Granulocyte-monocyte colony simulating factor (GM-CSF), and tumor necrosis factor (TNF). The expression of the CD40 ligand is also downregulated.

Helper ($CD4^+$) T cells are the chief cellular target for cyclosporin A. Cyclosporin A, but not rapamycin, inhibits the differentiation of Foxp3 T regulatory cells. The activation of cytotoxic T lymphocytes is also inhibited by cyclosporin A, apparently due to both the lack of stimulatory signals provided by IL-2 and IFN-γ, and to a direct inhibitory effect on cytotoxic T cell precursors.

Cyclosporin A has a remarkable ability to prolong graft survival. In experimental animals, even short courses of cyclosporin A can result in significant prolongation of kidney graft survival, suggesting that the drug facilitates the development of low dose tolerance. In humans, used in conjunction with azathioprine or mycophenolate and corticosteroids, it reduces the number of rejection episodes in renal transplantation, even in patients with cytotoxic antibodies and receiving poorly matched organs. It also induces a substantially longer survival of kidney, liver, and especially heart transplants, and reduces the incidence and severity of graft-versus-host disease in bone marrow transplantation. It has also been suggested that the long-term immunosuppression achieved with associations of

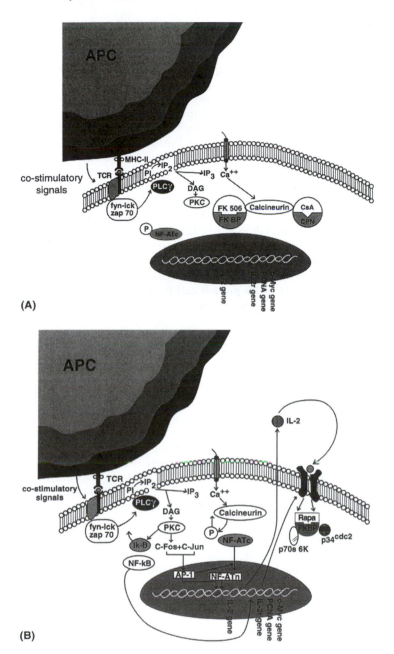

(A)

(B)

FIGURE 2 Diagrammatic representation of the mechanism of action of the inhibitors of signal transduction. Panel A illustrates the mechanism of action of cyclosporin A and tacrolimus (FK506), affecting the main steps of the calcineurin activation pathway. Cyclosporin A associates with cyclophilin (CPN) and the resulting complex binds and inactivates calcineurin. As a consequence, NF–AT remains phosphorylated and inactive. Tacrolimus achieves the same results, but it associates to a different cytoplasmic protein—FKBP. Panel B illustrates the effect of rapamycin, which inhibits the autocrine activation pathway mediated by IL-2. This macrolide combines with the same cytoplasmic protein as tacrolimus (FKBP), and the complex inactivates two protein kinases, p70 s6 and p34^{cdc2}, whose activation appears to be mediated by the interaction of IL-2 and IL-4 with their respective receptors, and are required for cells to progress from G_1 to S. *Abbreviations*: APC, antigen-presenting cell; DAG, diacyl glycerol; IP$_3$, inosital triphosphate; MHC, major histocompatibility complex; NF-AT, nuclear factor of activated T cells; FKBP, FKSO6 (tacrolimus) binding protein; PKC, protein kinase C; PLC, phospholipase C; TCR, T cell receptor.

low-dose cyclosporin A, steroids, and azathioprine or mycophenolate may be preferable to long-term administration of high doses of cyclosporin A, at least in patients with kidney transplants.

The main advantages of cyclosporin A as an immunosuppressant are its selective effect on T lymphocytes and its excellent steroid-sparing effect. The dosages of steroids necessary to achieve effective immunosuppression are considerably lower when steroids are associated to cyclosporin A than when they are associated to other immunosuppressive drugs. As a result, the incidence of infection is substantially reduced, although cytomegalovirus infections are relatively common in cyclosporin A-treated patients. On the other hand, cyclosporin A has many serious side effects, including is nephrotoxicity, a major concern in patients with kidney grafts. The renal toxicity is frequently associated with hypertension, which, in turn, has a negative impact in all patients, but especially in those receiving a heart transplant. Other side effects include hypercholesterolemia, increased hairiness, headaches, tremors, swelling of the gums, and so on. Probably related to hypercholesterolemia is the accelerated atherosclerosis that has been observed in heart transplant recipients surviving for over two years, but the mechanism responsible for this complication is not clear. Finally, after long term administration of cyclosporin A, by itself or in combination with other immunosuppressive agents (e.g., antilymphocyte globulin), there is an increased incidence of lymphoproliferative syndromes, most of them of B cell lineage, probably resulting from the uncontrolled proliferation of the Epstein-Barr virus.

Tacrolimus (Prograf, FK506)

Tacrolimus (Prograf, FK506) is produced by a different fungus (*Streptomyces tsukubaensis*) with a similar mechanism of action to cyclosporin A but is 10 to 100 times more active. The cytoplasmic target of tacrolimus is a different protein, known as FK506 binding protein (FKBP). The tacrolimus–FKBP complex has a very similar effect to the cyclophilin–cyclosporin A complex, inhibiting calcineurin and preventing the activation of NF–AT. Not surprisingly, the cellular effects of FK506 and cyclosporin A are almost identical.

Tacrolimus was first introduced in liver transplantation and was also used early on to reverse rejection in patients unresponsive to other immunosuppressive agents. It has now become a primary immunosuppressant in most types of transplantation because its use has resulted in improved patient survival. Its side effects are similar to those of cyclosporine A, but generally less severe. Neurotoxicity (including rare cases of severe irreversible encephalopathy), gastrointestinal intolerance, and infections (particularly by cytomegalovirus) are the most prominent complications of its use.

Sirolimus (Rapamycin, Rapamune)

Sirolimus (Rapamycin, rapamune), produced by *Streptomyces hygroscopicus*, is structurally similar to tacrolimus, but has a different intracellular target and different pharmacological properties. Sirolimus binds two proteins: FKBP, the same cyclophilin bound by tacrolimus, and the FKBP–sirolimus associated protein (FRAP). The complex formed by cyclophilin, FKBP, and FRAP does not interact with calcineurin, but rather with other cellular targets that are inactivated. The best-characterized targets are two kinases, p70 ribosomal protein S6 kinase and $p34^{cdc2}$. These enzymes appear to be activated by the interaction of IL-2 and IL-4 with their respective receptors, and are required for cells to progress through the replication cycle.

While cyclosporin A and FK506 inhibit the transition of lymphocytes from G_0 to G_1, sirolimus inhibits cell division later in G_1, prior to entry into S phase. Also, sirolimus inhibits both Ca^{2+}-dependent and independent activation pathways, does not inhibit IL-2 synthesis, but inhibits the response of IL-2- and IL-4-sensitive cell lines to exogenous IL-2 or IL-4. Because of the different mechanism of action, sirolimus is effective even when added 12 hours after in vitro mitogenic stimulation of T cells, while cyclosporin A and FK506 are only effective when added to the cultures not later than three hours after the mitogen.

Sirolimus has been approved for the prophylaxis of organ rejection in patients aged 13 years or older receiving renal transplants. It is recommended that sirolimus be used initially in a regimen with cyclosporine and corticosteriods.

Immunosuppressive Polyclonal Antibody Preparations

Polyclonal antibody preparations are commonly used to treat corticosteroid-resistant acute rejection episodes. Currently, there are two preparations available: antithymocyte globulin (equine antiserum) and thymoglobulin (rabbit antiserum) (Table 3). Both antisera are prepared by injecting human T lymphocytes into either a horse or a rabbit. The serum from these animals is then harvested and sterilized for administration into patients. Both preparations have been reported as very effective in reducing the episodes of acute rejection. Unfortunately, these preparations contain not only antibodies directed T lymphocytes but also against neutrophils, erythrocytes, and platelets. Therefore, patients treated with antilymphocyte globulin or with thymoglobulin may experience clinically significant neutropenia, anemia, and thrombocytopenia. In addition, these preparations may cause serum sickness, because even in immunosuppressed patients heterologous proteins are so immunogenic that they end up eliciting a humoral immune response.

Immunosuppressive Monoclonal Antibodies and Other Biological Response Modifiers

Several types of monoclonal antibodies have been used with the purpose of suppressing the immune response. Two basic types of mechanisms of action seem to be involved: blocking of costimulatory signals and delivery of downregulating signals. While murine monoclonal antibodies trigger immune responses that result in loss of efficiency and, in some cases, clinical manifestations of serum sickness, humanized (chimeric) monoclonal antibodies (hybrid molecules containing the variable regions of a murine monoclonal antibody and the Fc regions of a human immunoglobulin) are considerably less immunogenic.

Monoclonal Antibodies that Block Costimulatory Signals

1. Anti-CD2 monoclonal antibodies have been shown to induce prolonged graft survival in experimental animals. Its mechanism of action was initially thought to involve blocking of the CD2/LFA-3 interaction. However, it is also possible that these monoclonal antibodies deliver downregulating signals to T cells.
2. Soluble cytotoxic T cell late antigen (CTLA)-4, CTLA4-Ig, anti-CD80/86, and anti-CD40L monoclonal antibodies have been shown to have immunosuppressive properties, particularly in animal models of autoimmune diseases. The immune suppressive effect is secondary to the blockage of the activation signals mediated by the CD80/86-CTLA4 interaction or by the CD40-CD40L (CD 154) interaction. Abatacept is a CTLA4 Ig fusion protein containing the extracellular domain of CTLA4 and the Fc region of a human immunoglobulin. It has a longer half-life and is more effective than CTLA4. Its mechanism of action involves

TABLE 3 Immunosuppressive Antibody Preparations in Clinical Use

Product	Antigen	Source	Preparation	Comments
ATGAM	Human thymocytes	Equine	Polyclonal	Cross-reacts with neutrophils (neutropenia), RBCs (anemia), and platelets (thrombocytopenia)
Thymoglobulin	Human thymocytes	Rabbit	Polyclonal	Adverse effects similar to ATGAM
Muromonab CD3 (OKT3)	Human CD3	Murine	Monoclonal	Immune response against antibody limits retreatment
Daclizumab (Zenapax®)	IL-2 receptor	Recombinant	Monoclonal	Recombinant antibodies suppress the human immune response more efficiently and are less immunogenic than murine MoAbs
Basiliximab (Simulect®)	α-Subunit (CD25)			

Abbreviations: ATGAM, antithymocyte gamma globulin; RBCs, red blood cells.

inhibition of IL-2R gene expression and blocking of cell division, causing T cells to remain at G_0. In patients with refractory rheumatoid arthritis, abatacept resulted in a significant improvement in disease response especially in patients who did not respond to anti-TNF therapy.

Monoclonal Antibodies that Deliver Inhibitory Signals

Several different monoclonal antibodies against T cell markers (particularly anti-CD3, muromonab CD3) (Table 1) have been successfully used to treat acute graft rejection episodes (see Chapter 28). Muromonab CD3 appears to opsonize T lymphocytes, facilitating their destruction by antibody dependent cellular cytotoxicity (ADCC). Also, the binding of muromonab CD3 to the CD3 protein on T lymphocytes causes the internalization of the complex and anergy of the T lymphocyte. The major limitation in the clinical use of muromonab CD3 is development of human antimurine antibodies. Clinically significant antibody titers to murine immunoglobulins occur in >50% of patients treated with a full course of muromonab CD3, and clinical symptoms of serum sickness often develop in these patients.

Monoclonal Antibodies that Block the Interleukin-2 Receptor

Daclizumab (Zenapax) and basiliximab (Simulect) are humanized and chimeric monoclonal antibodies, respectively, directed against the IL-2 receptor. Humanized antibodies consist of complementarity determining regions (CDR) of a murine antibody incorporated into a human IgG molecule, while chimeric antibodies consist of the murine variable light and heavy chains incorporated into a human IgG molecule. The alpha chain of the IL-2 receptor is an ideal candidate for immunosuppression because it is minimally expressed on resting T cells, and significantly upregulated in activated T lymphocytes. Therefore, basiliximab and daclizumab target mostly activated T-lymphocytes. The proposed mechanism of action is the saturation of IL-2 receptors thereby inhibiting IL-2 driven proliferation, but this may prove to be an oversimplistic explanation. Both basiliximab and daclizumab are used for prophylaxis and reversal of acute rejection episodes in renal, heart, liver, and bone marrow transplantation.

Monoclonal Antibodies Directed Against Cluster of Differentiation (CD) 20

Rituximab (Rituxan) is a chimeric monoclonal antibody targeting CD20 protein expressed on pre-B lymphocytes, mature B lymphocytes, and on subpopulations of dendritic cells (DC) and malignant plasma cells. Administration of rituximab results in the rapid depletion of B lymphocytes, but serum immunoglobulin concentrations remain in the normal range. It is utilized in a variety of B lymphocyte disorders ranging from B-cell lymphomas to autoimmune disorders. For diffuse B-cell lymphomas, clinically aggressive, rituximab added to chemotherapy significantly improves the overall survival of the patients compared to chemotherapy alone. In follicular lymphomas, clinically indolent, rituxumab, is either used alone or with chemotherapy to induce remissions in these patients. Rituximab is also utilized in refractory/relapsed rheumatoid arthritis and idiopathic thrombocytopenia purpura with encouraging results.

Use of Immunosuppressive Drugs In Hypersensitivity and Autoimmune Diseases
Glucocorticoids

Glucocorticoid administration can be life-saving in certain acute disorders, such as bronchial asthma and autoimmune thrombocytopenic purpura and can induce significant improvement in chronic warm autoantibody hemolytic anemia, autoimmune chronic active hepatitis, autoimmune thrombocytopenic purpura, SLE, and a variety of chronic hypersensitivity conditions. Steroids are also part of most immunosuppressive regimens used for preventing the rejection of transplanted organs.

Cytotoxic Agents and Cyclosporin A

Many non-neoplastic diseases, which are either proven or presumed to be immunologically mediated, have been treated with cytotoxic drugs. Results of controlled trials of azathioprine, methotrexate, and cyclophosphamide suggest that these cytotoxic drugs, when given in sufficient quantity, may be capable of suppressing disease activity and eliminate the need for long-term therapy with steroids.

Methotrexate
Methotrexate is the most effective second-line drug for rheumatoid arthritis not controlled by NSAIDs. Methotrexate not only alleviates the signs and symptoms of rheumatoid arthritis but may also increase hemoglobin levels and decrease the erythrocyte sedimentation rate (ESR) in patients. Methotrexate is usually given in weekly oral doses.

Cyclophosphamide
Cyclophosphamide has been demonstrated to be the only effective means of achieving immunosuppression (and sometimes clinical cure) in certain steroid-resistant diseases, such as Wegener's granulomatosis. Cyclophosphamide is also the drug of choice for the treatment of lupus glomerulonephritis and other vasculitides (see Chapters 18 and 23). Interestingly, cyclophosphamide is better tolerated if given as monthly intravenous pulses rather than daily by oral intake.

Azathioprine
Azathioprine has also been used in the treatment of patients with SLE. Controlled studies demonstrated a number of beneficial effects, that is, an increase in creatinine clearance, a decrease in proteinuria, and a decrease in mortality. However, a decrease in glomerular cell proliferation has been noted in renal biopsies of SLE patients receiving azathioprine, and upon discontinuation of treatment, severe exacerbations of the disease have been reported.

Cyclosporin A
Cyclosporin A has not been as widely used in the treatment of autoimmune disorders as azathioprine, methotrexate, and cyclophosphamide, with the exception of type I (insulin-dependent) diabetes and myasthenia gravis. In these conditions, considerable clinical improvement may be seen while the drug is being administered, but relapses occur as soon as Cyclosporin A is suspended.

Combinations of Glucocorticoids and Cytotoxic Agents
Combinations of glucocorticoids and cytotoxic agents have been used in most diseases, which were classically treated with glucocorticoids alone, and although controlled trials are still required to assess overall benefit in many of these diseases, it should be stated that perhaps their major advantage is the possibility of reducing the dose of steroids when such drugs are added to corticosteroid therapy—the previously mentioned "steroid-sparing" effect.

Adverse Consequences of Prolonged Immunosuppression
Bone Marrow Suppression and Neutropenia
Bone marrow suppression is the most common type of toxicity. It is due to the effects on the bone marrow and hemopoiesis, particularly when cytotoxic drugs, such as of methotrexate, azathioprine, 6-MP, and MMF, are used to suppress the immune response.

The degree of bone marrow suppression observed with cytotoxic drugs is usually dose-related and can be modulated by dose changes, although in rare cases, the bone marrow failure may become irreversible. Usually, if a patient's white blood cells (WBC) count falls below 3000 cells/mm^3, any of these drugs should be stopped until the WBC increases to greater than 3000 cells/mm^3, and reinstituted at a lower dose.

When neutropenia develops, severe infections are likely to develop—these infections are extremely difficult to treat, often being the cause of death. For this reason, neutropenia is considered as the most serious side effect of immunosuppression, and continuous monitoring of WBC count is essential in patients treated with these drugs. The availability of recombinant granulocyte-colony stimulating factor (G-CSF) and GM-CSF provides the means to considerably shorten the period of neutropenia (see later).

Infections

Infections are another common adverse effect in patients treated with all types of cytotoxic or immunosuppressive drugs. This is a consequence of global immunosuppression, as reflected by the patient's frequent inability to mount a primary immune response after adequate immunization. Two main features characterize the infections of immunosuppressed patients. First, the infections usually involve low-grade pathogens or opportunistic microorganisms not usually associated with clinical diseases. Second, the extent and distribution of the infection are unusual, differing from those commonly observed in noncompromised hosts.

Because the depression of cellular immunity is the goal pursued when these drugs are used, the patients become more vulnerable to viral infections, such as herpes simplex and varicella, which may disseminate with a fatal outcome. The incidence of herpes zoster (shingles) is increased but the course of the disease is similar to that seen in otherwise normal individuals. The impairment of cell-mediated immunity is also probably responsible for the frequency and severity of opportunistic infections caused by mycobacteria, viruses (e.g., cytomegalovirus, herpes simplex, Varicella-zoster), parasites (e.g., *Toxoplasma gondii*), and fungi (e.g., *Pneumocystis carinii*, *Candida* spp., and *Aspergillus* spp.). Those infections are much more likely to disseminate during immunosuppressive treatment. Systemic candidiasis, measles encephalitis, measles retinitis, progressive multifocal leukoencephalopathy, and cerebral toxoplasmosis are just but a few examples of atypical infections almost exclusively seen in immunocompromised patients (see Chapters 29 and 30).

Increased Incidence of Neoplasms

An increased incidence of neoplasms is a major concern in patients chronically immunosuppressed. Although the precise role of the immune system in eliminating neoplastic clones in a normal individual is not clear, the incidence of malignancies is clearly elevated in patients receiving immunosuppressive drugs. The most frequently seen malignancies in immunosuppressed patients after solid organ transplantation include basal-cell carcinoma, Kaposi's sarcoma, carcinoma of the vulva and perineum, non-Hodgkin's lymphoma (NHL), squamous-cell carcinoma, and hepatobiliary carcinoma. Also, the location and pattern of spread of those malignancies is unusual. For example, primary central nervous system lymphoma (PCNSL) is associated with congenital, acquired, iatrogenic immunodeficiency states, or status post solid organ transplant. The highest incidence of PCNSL occurs in patients with AIDS, 1.9% to 6%. Azathioprine-based immunosuppressive regimens after solid organ transplantation are associated with the highest incidence of cutaneous malignancies. In contrast, high-intensity immunosuppression after solid organ transplantation, especially regimens including antilymphocyte antibody preparations or CD3 antibodies (OKT3, ATGAM). EB virus is believed to be associated with NHL in both immunocompromised as well as immunocompetent individuals because the viral genome is incorporated in the malignant cells. It has been postulated that NHL emerges in individuals carrying the virus in a latent stage as a consequence of a deficient immunosurveillance, which normally would control the proliferation of viral-infected B lymphocytes. Interestingly, the risk of the most common cancers (e.g., breast, lung, prostate, and colon) is not increased over the general population in immunosuppressed patients.

Other Side Effects

Other side effects are secondary to the toxicity of these drugs (particularly of those with cytotoxic properties) over rapidly dividing cells, and include hair loss or alopecia, loss of gonadal function, bloody diarrhea, and so on, as well as constitutional symptoms (e.g., nausea, vomiting, anorexia, malaise, etc.), chromosomal changes, and teratogenic effects.

CYTOKINE MODIFIERS

A new group of biological response modifiers (BRMs) has emerged from efforts to manipulate the immune response using soluble receptors and receptor antagonists to block undesirable effects of pro-inflammatory cytokines. After limited success in sepsis, soluble TNF receptors (sTNFRs) and interleukin-1 receptor antagonists (IL-1RA) are actively being investigated in rheumatoid arthritis.

Tumor Necrosis Factor Antagonists

As discussed earlier, disease-modifying antirheumatic drugs (e.g., methotrexate) do not directly treat the underlying pathophysiology, but rather cause the death of all actively dividing lymphocytes. Although the underlying cause of rheumatoid arthritis is unknown, increasing evidence implicates both IL-1 and TNF in the inflammatory and destructive manifestations of rheumatoid arthritis. Although increased concentrations of both IL-1 inhibitors and soluble TNF receptors are detected in the serum and synovial fluid of patients with rheumatoid arthritis, concentrations of IL-1 and TNF exceed concentrations of their inhibitors.

Soluble Tumor Necrosis Factor Receptors

Soluble TNF receptors (sTNFRs) exist in two forms, 55 kDa (Type B, sTNFRI) and 75 kDa (Type A, sTNFRII). sTNFRs act primarily as inhibitors of TNF by preventing TNF from binding to the membrane-bound TNFRs (Fig. 3). The same effect can be obtained, at least theoretically, with monoclonal antibodies against TNF. Therapeutically, both monoclonal antibodies against TNF and sTNFRs have been approved for clinical use in rheumatoid arthritis. To increase the biologic activity and half-life of sTNFRII, a recombinant protein was developed by combining the sTNFRII with the Fc portion of human IgG$_1$ to form TNFR:Fc (etanercept). In several clinical trials etanercept was shown to cause significant clinical improvement in patients with rheumatoid arthritis not observed with placebo-treated controls.

Infliximab

Infliximab, a IgG1 murine-human chimeric monoclonal anti-TNF antibody, binds to and neutralizes TNF (Fig. 3). Administration of infliximab in conjunction with methotrexate reduces the signs and symptoms of rheumatoid arthritis to a greater extent than methrotexate alone.

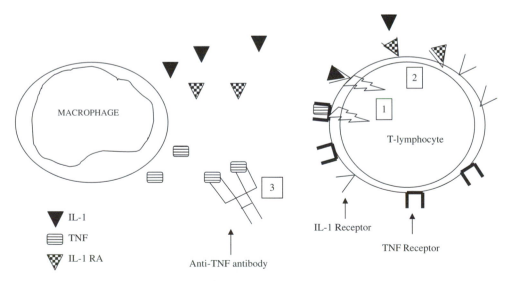

FIGURE 3 Macrophages produce IL-1 and tumor necrosis factor (TNF) that deliver activating signals to T lymphocytes [1,2]. Interleukin-1 receptor antagonist binds to the IL-1 receptor to block IL-1-induced activation [3]. The anti-TNF antibody (infliximab) or soluble TNF receptor (etanercept) bind TNF and prevent it from reaching its receptor. *Abbreviations*: IL, interleukin; TNF, tumor necrosis factor.

Adalimumab

Adalimumab, a fully humanized monoclonal anti-TNF antibody, also binds to and neutralizes TNF (Fig. 3). Both alone and in combination with methotrexate, adalimumab exhibits significant activity in rheumatoid arthritis.

High levels of expression of TNF have been observed in the mucosal and lamina propria cells in patients with active Crohn's disease. In patients with moderate to severe Crohn's disease not responding to conventional therapy, infliximab reduces the disease activity index scores and reduces the number of draining enterocutaneous fistulas. A limitation to infliximab is the fact that after prolonged administration, patients develop antibodies against the murine portion of the antibody.

Interleukin-1 Antagonists

A delicate balance between IL-1 and IL-1RA exists in rheumatoid arthritis. An excess of IL-1 leads to disease progression. It is estimated that only five percent of IL-1 receptors need to be bound by IL-1 to stimulate the cell. Therefore, an excess of IL-1RA is required to block IL-1 and modify the disease process.

Recombinant Human Interleukin-1 Receptor Antagonist

Recombinant human IL-1RA is actively being investigated in rheumatoid arthritis as a modulator of IL-1. When it binds to the IL-1 receptor, IL-1RA does not stimulate the receptor, but blocks IL-1 from stimulating the receptor (Fig. 3). Considering the positive results obtained with separate administration of TNF and IL-1 antagonists, one can anticipate trials combining modulators of IL-1 and TNF in the treatment of refractory rheumatoid arthritis.

IMMUNOPOTENTIATION

Many compounds and biological substances have been used in attempts to restore normal immune system function in clinical conditions in which it is believed to be functionally altered. All of these types of therapeutic interventions fall under the general designation of immunopotentiation, which can be defined as any type of therapeutic intervention aimed at restoring the normal function of the immune system.

Biological Response Modifiers

BRM is a term used to designate a variety of soluble compounds that allow the various elements of the immune system to communicate with one another. This communication network allows for "upregulation" and coordination of immune responses when needed, and "down regulation" of immune responses, when no longer needed by the host.

Structure

All BRM have a surprising degree of structural similarity to one another; this is felt to be reflective of an early gene reduplication event that occurred as the immune system of mammals evolved.

Function

The BRM appear to form a very delicate network of communication signals between the four principal mononuclear leukocyte subsets that participate in the immune response. We are still without a complete understanding as to how these interactions occur; however, the release of these signals appears to be different from hormones. Hormones tend to act at a site far distant from the original cell that secreted the signal; in contrast, BRM appear to work in the immediate vicinity of the cell type, which secretes them. The timing of the release of the BRM coupled with the intensity of their secretion appears to provide the overall balance of signals required to orchestrate the immune response.

Cellular Sources

The most significant sources of BRM compounds are lymphocytes, macrophages, and dendritic cells. T lymphocytes produce a wide range of BRM, including:

1. IL-2, which induces the proliferation of T lymphocytes, B lymphocytes, and natural killer (NK) cells. IL-2 is also capable of upregulating the tumor-killing capabilities of $CD8^+$ T lymphocytes and NK cells.
2. IL-3, a growth factor for stem cells in the bone marrow that stimulates the production of many types of leukocytes from the bone marrow when neded.
3. IL-4, the main determinant of helper T cells 2 (Th2) differentiation; it also stimulates B lymphocytes to proliferate and induces the synthesis of IgE antibodies.
4. IL-5, which has chemotactic and activating properties for eosinophils.
5. IL-10, which downregulates the synthesis of other interleukins and turns-off both Th1 and Th2 activities.
6. GM-CSF, which stimulates the bone marrow to produce both granulocytes and monocytes. It also appears capable of upregulating the spontaneous killing capability of monocytes.
7. IFNγ, the main mediator responsible for the activation of monocytes and macrophages, which is also released by activated NK cells.

NK cells also secrete a series of BRM, particularly IFN-α, an antiviral agent that promotes the activation of NK lymphocytes in vitro. IFN-α is also secreted by monocytes, macrophages, and many other cell types, but its main source has been recently identified as being the lymphoid-derived DC2. In addition to its antiviral and NK-activating properties, IFN-α appears capable of directly inhibiting the growth of certain types of tumor cells, such as the cells that proliferate in hairy cell leukemia (see Chapter 27), chronic myeloid leukemia, and melanoma.

Mononuclear phagocytes (monocytes and macrophages) share with NK lymphocytes the ability to secrete IFN-α. In addition, they secrete several types of interleukins and cytokines. Some of them (IL-6, IL-8, and TNF) are also produced by T lymphocytes.

1. IL-1, also produced by other antigen-presenting cells, promotes the early phases of the B and T lymphocyte activation processes.
2. IL-6, promotes B lymphocyte differentiation and immunoglobulin secretion.
3. IL-8, a chemotactic factor for T lymphocytes and neutrophils.
4. IL-12, responsible for the activation and differentiation of Th1 lymphocytes.
5. TNF has a variety of effects, particularly causing the death of certain types of tumor cells.
6. Two types of colony-stimulating factors, G-CSF and M-CSF. M-CSF promotes the production and activation of monocytes, and G-CSF stimulates the production of granulocytes from stem cells in the bone marrow.

Clinical Applications

Interleukin-2

Of the interleukins, IL-2 has been the most widely used. High-dose IL-2 induces a response in 15% of patients with disseminated melanoma and renal cell carcinoma. Despite the low response rate, the excitement regarding high-dose IL-2 centers around the duration of responses. Seven percent of these responses are complete, meaning that all the tumor and symptoms resolve. These complete remissions are also very durable with median duration of 40 plus months. Unfortunately, high-dose IL-2 is associated with severe side effects (e.g., hypotension, fluid retention, renal failure, mental status changes), which necessitate administration in the hospital. Lower doses of IL-2 that can be administered as an outpatient were extensively investigated in experimental immune reconstitution protocols in AIDS patients (see Chapter 30).

Interferon

IFN-γ has been extensively studied as an inmunomodulator, particularly in patients with chronic granulomatous disease (see Chapter 13).

IFN-α induces antiviral, antitumor, and immunomodulatory effects. It activates their target cells by first binding to specific IFN receptors on cell surface. The binding of IFN-α

induces a signal through secondary messengers to nucleus to induce the synthesis of several effector proteins (e.g., 2′, 5′-oligo-A synthetase, Mx protein, and protein kinase). The upregulation of these effector proteins are important in its antiviral response but may also play a role in its antitumor response. For its antitumor activity, IFN-α may also modulate oncogenes (e.g., c-myc, c-fos) and induce proteins (e.g., indolamine 2,3 dioxygenase) that inhibit macromolecule synthesis essential for the tumor cell survival. IFN-α also has indirect effects by activating macrophages and NK cells and upregulating expression of cell surface proteins (e.g., human leukocyte antigens Class I, CD 80/86, and ICAM-1) on tumor cells. Although the exact mechanism of action of it is unknown in oncology (i.e., direct antiproliferative vs. immunomodulatory effect), IFN therapy is extensively used in the chronic phase of chronic myeloid leukemia, as adjuvant therapy after surgery in patients with a high-risk of recurrence from melanoma, and for the treatment of AIDS-related Kaposi's sarcoma and follicular lymphomas. IFN-α is also used clinically to treat chronic hepatitis B and C. Despite the numerous dosage regimens used in clinical practice, the universal side effects associated with IFN-α therapy are fatigue, flu-like symptoms (i.e., fever and chills, headache), and myalgias.

IFN-β like IFN-α exhibits antiviral, antiproliferative, and immunomodulatory activity. IFN-β is effective in reducing the severity and frequency of exacerbations of multiple sclerosis.

Hematopoietic Growth Factors

Randomized trials using either G-CSF (filgrastim) or GM-CSF (sargramostim) postmyelosuppressive chemotherapy demonstrated not only the ability of these growth factors to accelerate neutrophil recovery but also their ability to reduce the frequency and severity of infections, mainly bacterial, and to decrease antibiotic use. AIDS patients often develop neutropenia, due either to the viral infection itself (by unknown mechanisms) or the side effects of antiretroviral or other antimicrobial drugs. The administration of GM-CSF to these patients may also be beneficial. The ability of G-CSF and GM-CSF to prevent infections is due to two effects (*i*) accelerated generation of neutrophils in the bone marrow, and (*ii*) enhanced activity of neutrophil function.

There is a strong correlation between the nadir of the neutrophil count and length of neutropenia from the chemotherapy with risk of bacterial infections. A neutrophil count less than 500 cells/mm^3 puts a patient at increased risk of infection. However, the length of neutropenia also is critical. Patients with prolonged neutropenia status post chemotherapy (i.e., ≥ 1 week) are much more at risk for an infection than a patient with a short period of neutropenia (i.e., <1 week). In randomized trials, administration of G-CSF or GM-CSF after myelosuppressive chemotherapy has blunted the neutrophil nadir and shortened the period of neutropenia as compared to placebo. Patients receiving G-CSF or GM-CSF typically receive daily injections of the growth factor for 10 to 14 days after chemotherapy. The recent introduction of pegylated G-CSF (PEG-filgrastim) extends the half-life of G-CSF to allow one injection instead of the previously required 10 to 14 injections.

Both G-CSF and GM-CSF improve neutrophil function (phagocytosis, chemotaxis, and superoxide production). Unfortunately, a meta-analysis of randomized clinical trials comparing antibiotics alone to antibiotics plus G-CSF in the treatment of pneumonia did not find a clinical benefit in adding G-CSF. Human GM-CSF is the principal growth factor for the proliferation, maturation, and migration of DC and macrophages. DC and macrophages play a critical role in antigen presentation for primary and secondary T lymphocyte responses. Furthermore, GM-CSF increases the expression of major histocompatibility complex class II, CD 80/86, and adhesion molecules (e.g., ICAM-1) on antigen-presenting cells. Given this critical role of GM-CSF on the proliferation and maturation of DC and macrophages, the possible use of GM-CSF as a vaccine adjuvant has been investigated. Studies in laboratory animals demonstrated increased antibody production using GM-CSF as an adjuvant. Preliminary results of GM-CSF in conjunction with either the hepatitis B or influenza vaccine in humans are encouraging, but further evaluation is necessary.

Two other hematopoietic growth factors available clinically are IL-11 and erythropoietin (Table 4). Platelets are fragments of megakaryocytes that are derived from the pluripotent hematopoietic stem cell, similar to all blood cells (e.g., RBCs, neutrophils). The commitment of a pluripotent hematopoietic stem cell toward a megakaryocyte is under several influences. One of the influences are hematopoietic growth factors, namely IL-11, thrombopoietin, and IL-3. In patients

TABLE 4 FDA-Approved Recombinant Hematopoietic Growth Factors

Cytokine	Generic (trade) name	Source	Maturation	Clinical uses
G-CSF	Filgrastim (Neupogen®) Peg-filgrastim (Neulasta®)	Monocytes/ macrophages, bone marrow stromal cells[a]	Neutrophils	Stimulate neutrophil recovery s/p myelosuppressive chemotherapy; adjunct to antibiotics in severe infections[c]
GM-CSF	Sargramostim (Leukine®)	T-lymphocytes, monocytes, bone marrow stromal cells	Neutrophils, monocytes, eosinophils	Stimulate neutrophil recovery s/p myelosuppressive chemotherapy; adjunct to vaccines[c]; adjunct to antibiotics in severe infections[c]
IL-11	Oprelvekin (Neumega®)	Bone marrow stromal cells, liver	Megakaryocytes, B-lymphocytes[b], neutrophils[b]	Stimulate platelet recovery s/p myelosuppressive chemotherapy
Erythropoietin	Epoetin alfa (Procrit®, Epogen®) Darbepoetin alfa (Aranesp®)	Kidney, liver	RBCs	Stimulate RBC production in patients with anemia of chronic disease (e.g., ESRD, anemia secondary to cancer or its treatment, anemia associated with HIV infection)

[a]Bone marrow stromal cells include fibroblasts and endothelial cells.
[b]In clinical trials, IL-11 does not significantly increase the recovery of neutrophils after myelosuppressive chemotherapy. Its effect on B-lymphocytes *in vivo* is unknown.
[c]Actively under clinical investigation.
Abbreviations: ESRD, end-stage renal disease; G-CSF, granulocyte-colony stimulating factor; GM-CSF, granulocyte-macrophage colony stimulating factor; IL-11, interleukin-11; RBC, red blood cell; s/p, status post.

receiving chemotherapy that causes clinically significant thrombocytopenia, recombinant IL-11 significantly shortened the period of thrombocytopenia (platelet count $<50,000/\mu L$) and the number of platelet transfusions, compared to placebo. It is important to note that most patients who receive myelosuppressive chemotherapy get not only thrombocytopenia but also neutropenia. IL-11 has minimal effects of recovery of neutrophils after chemotherapy. Therefore, it is not uncommon to treat patients receiving severely myelosuppressive chemotherapy with both recombinant IL-11 and G-CSF. In addition, patients with anemia chronic disease (e.g., patients receiving myelosuppressive chemotherapy, or patients with cancer not receiving therapy, or patients with AIDS) may benefit from erythropoietin. Erythropoietin stimulates the production of RBCs from the pluripotent hematopoietic stem cell.

Several BRMs have been used as primary or adjunct agents in the treatment of a variety of malignancies, with variable effects. There have also been many attempts to use BRMs to boost cellular immunity in immunodeficient patients, often with negative or conflicting results.

Intravenous Immunoglobulins

The administration of gammaglobulins as a way to transfer passive immunity to immunodeficient patients is the oldest type of immunotherapy. Earlier preparations were administered intramuscularly, but, later, to circumvent the limitations (e.g., painful injections, inconsistent absorption) of intramuscular immunoglobulin, intravenous immunoglobulin (IVIG) was introduced into clinical practice in the early 1980s. IVIG consists of concentrated polyclonal immunoglobulins, >90% IgG, prepared from pooled plasma collected from donors. In patients with a primary (e.g., common variable immunodeficiency) or secondary humoral immune deficiency (e.g., chronic lymphocytic leukemia), IVIG provides restoration of circulating IgG concentrations. The clinical benefit of restoring IgG concentrations with IVIG is decreased infections and hospitalization of these patients.

Besides providing passive immunity, IVIG can also modulate the immune response. IVIG modulates the immune response by multiple mechanisms. Common uses of IVIG and the proposed mechanism of actions of IVIG are outlined in Table 5.

In many autoimmune disorders, an antibody directed against normal tissues (i.e., autoantibody) binds to tissue and activates complement and ADCC. For example in idiopathic thrombocytopenia purpura, an autoantibody against platelets causes immune destruction of the platelets. IVIG can modulate the autoantibody response by (*i*) saturating Fc receptors on phagocytes (e.g., neutrophils, macrophages) and preventing the engulfment of the autoantibody-coated platelets, and by (*ii*) providing the patient with an anti-idiotype antibody against the autoantibody (Figs. 4 and 5). The anti-idiotype antibody binds the autoantibody in the variable region and prevents it from binding to its antigen, in this example, the platelets. Also, the anti-idiotype antibodies in IVIG may bind the surface immunoglobulin on B lymphocyte producing the autoantibody. The binding of anti-idiotype to the surface immunoglobulin in combination with the binding of IVIG to the Fc receptor on B lymphocyte may induce apoptosis of the B lymphocyte, thus blocking the autoantibody production.

Recently, IVIG has been shown to contain antibodies that bind to and block the Fas receptor, thus interrupting the delivery of apoptotic signals to cells with upregulated Fas. IVIg has been shown to inhibit Fas-mediated cell death both in vitro and in vivo. The clinical applications of this property have yet to be defined.

Active Immunization as an Immunomodulating Intervention

Active immunization can be used for prevention of infectious diseases, as discussed in detail in Chapter 12, or to enhance the immunological defenses in patients already infected. The immunotherapeutic use of vaccines has been the object of experimental protocols in two areas.

Cancer

Anticancer vaccines have been the object of considerable interest and are also the object of ongoing trials (see Chapter 26).

TABLE 5   Common Uses of Intravenous Immunoglobulins

Disease	Proposed mechanism of action	Comments
Primary immunodeficiencies[a]	Replacement of IgG	Standard of care; FDA-approved
Chronic lymphocyte leukemia	Replacement of IgG	FDA-approved; use in individuals with multiple hospitalizations per year due to infections
Pediatric HIV infections	Replacement of IgG	FDA-approved
Status post allogeneic BMT	Replacement of IgG; immunomodulation	FDA-approved; ↓ CMV infections; ↓ acute graft-versus-host disease
Idiopathic thrombocytopenia purpura	Immunomodulation	FDA-approved; second-line therapy for patients failing corticosteroids
Kawasaki syndrome	Immunomodulation	FDA-approved; used in conjunction with high-dose aspirin to decrease coronary artery abnormalities
Guillain-Barré syndrome	Immunomodulation	An alternative to plasma exchange for severe forms
Autoimmune hemolytic anemia	Immunomodulation	Second-line therapy for patients failing steroids
CIPD	Immunomodulation	An alternative to plasma exchange

[a]Common variable immunodeficiency (CVID) and congenital humoral immunodeficiencies (e.g., X-linked agammaglobulinemia, autosomal recessive agammaglobulinemia).
Abbreviations: BMT, blood marrow transplantation; CIPD, chronic inflammatory demyelinating polyneuropathy; CMV, cytomegalovirus.

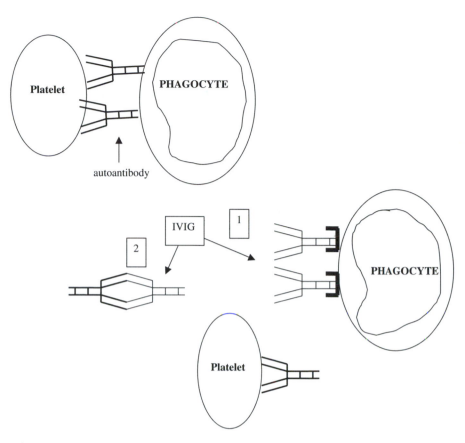

FIGURE 4 In ITP, an autoantibody directed against platelets, opsonizes them. Opsonized platelets are destroyed by phagocytes. The therapeutic effect of IVIg can be explained by two possible mechanisms interfering with phagocytic destruction. (*i*) IVIg can saturate the Fc receptors on phagocytes (e.g., macrophages) so that the macrophage cannot recognize the opsonized platelet. (*ii*) IVIg contains anti-idiotypic antibodies specific for the platelet autoantibody and will block the reaction of the antibody with the platelets. *Abbreviations*: ITP, idiopathic thrombocytopenic purpura; IVIG, intravenous immunoglobulin.

Vaccines to stimulate resistance against antibiotic-resistant bacteria are also under development.

Dialyzable Leukocyte Extracts and Transfer Factor

In a series of classical experiments, Lawrence showed that the injection of an extract of lymphocytes from a tuberculin-positive donor to a tuberculin-negative recipient resulted in acquisition of tuberculin reactivity by the latter. Lawrence coined the term transfer factor to designate the unknown agent responsible for transfer of tuberculin sensitivity. Transfer factor has been used episodically to treat a variety of conditions, and the best results appear to have been obtained in the treatment of chronic mucocutaneous candidiasis, a rare form of cell-mediated immunodeficiency. Because no properly controlled trials have ever been performed with transfer factor, and because its chemical nature remains unknown, its place in immunotherapy remains marginal.

Thymic Hormones

The immunotherapeutic application of thymic hormones has appealed to investigators over the last four decades. Many peptides with thymic hormone-like activities have been isolated and described, including thymosin, facteur thymique serique (serum thymic factor) and thymopoietin. Although better characterized than transfer factor, the successful therapeutic

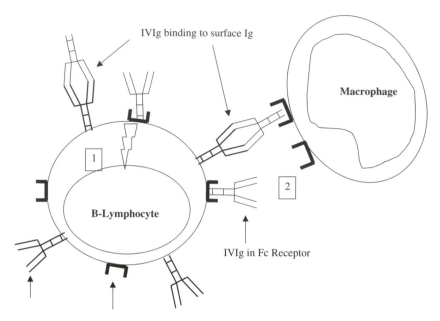

FIGURE 5 Alternative mechanisms of action for IVIg are based on immunomodulatory effects of IVIg. (*i*) Anti-idiotypic antibodies contained in IVIg would recognize surface immunoglobulin in autoantibody-producing B cells. In conjunction, IVIg binds to the FcγRIIb on B lymphocytes. The simultaneous cross-linking of surface immunoglobulins and inhibitory Fc receptors results in apoptosis or functional downregulation of autoantibody-producing B-cell. (*ii*) Binding of anti-idiotypic antibodies contained in IVIg to the surface immunoglobulin on autoantibody producing B lymphocytes may lead to their elimination by phagocytic cells. *Abbreviation*: IVIg, intravenous immunoglobulin.

applications of thimic hormones remain the domain of anecdotal reports. For that reason, thymic hormones have never been recognized as clinically useful.

Bacterial and Chemical Immunomodulators

A variety of killed bacteria, several substances of bacterial origin, and chemical compounds have been used with the goal of activating the immune system in a variety of clinical conditions in which such activation should be beneficial.

Bacterial Immunomodulators
Bacillus Calmette-Guérin and *Corynebacterium parvum* have been extensively used for their adjuvant therapy in therapeutic protocols aimed at stimulating antitumoral immunologic mechanisms (see Chapter 26). At the cellular level, these bacteria appear mainly to activate macrophages.

Chemical Immunomodulators
Levamisole is an antihelminthic drug predominantly used in veterinary medicine that has been found to have immunostimulant properties. In some animal diseases it causes an apparent increase in host resistance to tumor cells. It acts on the cellular limb of the immune system, and can restore impaired cell-mediated immune responses to normal levels but fails to hyper-stimulate the normal functioning immune system. Thus, it shows true immunomodulatory activity.

In humans, levamisole has been reported to restore delayed hypersensitivity reactions in anergic cancer patients and to be of some benefit in the treatment of aphthous stomatitis, rheumatoid arthritis, SLE, viral diseases, and chronic staphylococcal infections. Its most promising application appears to be in patients with resected colo-rectal carcinomas, on whom it appears to increase the duration of disease-free intervals.

Isoprinosine (Inosine Prabonex, ISO) appears to be effective in a wide variety of viral diseases. This is probably due to the fact that this compound has both antiviral and immunostimulating properties. As far as its effects on the immune system is concerned, Isoprinosine potentiates cell-mediated immune responsiveness in vivo; and a major factor in its effectiveness against viral infections appears to be its ability to prevent the depression of cell-mediated immunity that has been shown to occur during viral infection, and to persist for four to six weeks thereafter.

The clinical efficacy of ISO has been well documented in double-blind trials. Its administration results in striking decreases in both the duration of infection and severity of symptoms in a whole host of viral diseases, including viral influenza, rhinovirus infections, herpes simplex infections, herpes zoster, viral hepatitis, rubella, and viral otitis. Of particular interest are the results of ISO therapy in subacute sclerosing panencephalitis (SSPE), a progressive disease due to a chronic measles virus infection, which results in complete debilitation and eventual death of the patient. ISO has been reported to halt the progression of SSPE when given in stages I and II of the disease in 80% of the patients, provided it is administered for at least six months. Indeed, ISO is the only agent to date with documented beneficial effects in SSPE patients.

BIBLIOGRAPHY

Armitage JO. Emerging applications of recombinant human granulocyte-macrophage colony stimulating factor. Blood 1998; 92:4491–4508.

Auphan N, DiDonato JA, Rosette C, et al. Immunosuppression by glucocorticoids: inhibition of NF-kB activity through induction of IkB synthesis. Science 1995; 270:286.

Barnes PJ, Adcock I. Anti-inflammatory actions of steroids: molecular mechanisms. TIPS 1993; 14:436.

Bierer B. Mechanisms of action of immunosuppressive agents: cyclosporin A, FK506, and rapamycin. Proc Assoc Am Phys 1995; 107:28.

Braun W, Kallen J, Mikol V, et al. Three dimensional structure and actions of immunosuppressants and their immunophilins. FASEB J 1995; 9:63.

Brooks PM, Day DO. Nonsteroidal antiinflammatory drugs—differences and similarities. N Engl J Med 1991; 324:1716.

Brown MA. Antibody treatments of inflammatory arthritis. Curr Med Chem 2005; 12:2943–2946.

Burton CM, Andersen CB, Jensen AS, et al. The incidence of acute cellular rejection after lung transplantation: a comparative study of anti-thymocyte globulin and daclizumab. J Heart Lung Transplant 2006; 25:638–647.

Campion GV, Lebsack ME, Lookabaugh J, et al. Dose-range and dose-frequency study of recombinant human interleukin-1 receptor antagonist in patients with rheumatoid arthritis. Arthritis Rheum 1996; 39:1092–1101.

Coenen JJ, Koenen HJ, van Rijssen E, et al. Rapamycin, and not cyclosporin A, preserves the highly suppressive CD27+ subset of human CD4 + CD25+ regulatory T cells. Blood 2006; 107:1018–1023.

D'Amato G. Role of anti-IgE monoclonal antibody (omalizumab) in the treatment of bronchial asthma and allergic respiratory diseases. Eur J Pharmacol 2006; 533:302–307.

Edwards J, Szczepanski L, Szechinski J, et al. Efficacy of B-cell targeted therapy with rituximab in patients with rheumatoid arthritis. N Engl J Med 2004; 350:2572–2580.

Gonzales NR, De Pascalis R, Schlom J, Kashmiri SV. Minimizing the immunogenicity of antibodies for clinical application. Tumour Biol 2005; 26:31–43.

Hall PD. Immunomodulation with intravenous immunoglobulin. Pharmacotherapy 1993; 13:564–573.

Hardinger KL, Schnitzler MA, Koch MJ, et al. Thymoglobulin induction is safe and effective in live-donor renal transplantation: a single center experience. Transplantation 2006; 81:1285–1289.

Hassner A, Adelman DC. Biologic response modifiers in primary immunodeficiency disorders. Ann Intern Med 1991; 115:294.

Lazarus AH, Crow AR. Mechanism of action of IVIG and anti-D in ITP. Transfus Apher Sci 2003; 28:249–255.

Montague JW, Cidlowski JA. Glucocorticoid-induced death of immune cells: mechanism of action. Curr Top Microbiol Immunol 1995; 200:51.

O'Mahony D, Bishop MR. Monoclonal antibody therapy. Front Biosci 2006; 11:1620–1635.

Smith MR. Rituximab (monoclonal anti-CD20 antibody): mechanisms of action and resistance. Oncogene 2003; 22:7359–7368.

25 | Transplantation Immunology

Justin D. Ellett
Department of Surgery, Division of Transplant, Medical University of South Carolina, Charleston, South Carolina, U.S.A.

Gabriel Virella
Department of Microbiology and Immunology, Medical University of South Carolina, Charleston, South Carolina, U.S.A.

Kenneth D. Chavin
Department of Surgery, Division of Transplant, Medical University of South Carolina, Charleston, South Carolina, U.S.A.

INTRODUCTION

The replacement of defective organs with transplants was seemingly one of the impossible dreams of medicine for many centuries. Its realization required a multitude of important steps: surgical asepsis, development of surgical techniques for vascular anastomosis, understanding of the cellular basis of the rejection phenomena, and introduction of drugs and antisera effective in the control of rejection.

By the early 1970s, tissue and organ transplantation emerged as a major area of interest for surgeons and physicians. Solid organ transplants since have become routine in most industrialized countries. Currently, kidney and bone marrow transplants are performed most frequently, followed by liver, heart, pancreas, lung, and small bowel transplants, in order of decreasing frequency. Transplantation of trachea, extremities, and facial tissue are also performed in investigational situations. Other tissues and organs will certainly follow.

The success of an organ transplant is a function of several variables. These include technical advancements, advances in preservation, increased understanding of the immune system, and pharmacologic advances to prevent and treat rejection. However, the magnitude of the immunological response against the graft is the major determinant of acceptance or non-acceptance (rejection) of a technically perfect graft. The likelihood of acceptance or rejection is closely related to the extent of genetic differences between the donor and recipient of the graft. Although transplantation of organs between animals of the same inbred strain or between homozygous (syngeneic) twins is successful and does not elicit an immune rejection response, transplants between distantly related individuals (allogenic) or across species barriers (xenogeneic) are always rapidly rejected.

Thankfully, significant progress in the development of new immunosuppressive drugs and administration regimens has had a very significant impact in transplantation outcome. The very significant increases in graft survival rate are not a consequence of better donor-recipient matching but rather a reflection of better medical management.

DONOR–RECIPIENT MATCHING

Prevention of rejection is more desirable than trying to treat established rejection. This is achieved both by careful matching of donor and recipient and by manipulation of the recipient's immune response peri- and post-transplant. To successfully match donor and recipient, antigenic differences between the two must be avoided. Although many different antigenic systems show allotypic variation, in transplantation practice, only the ABO blood groups and the human leukocyte antigens (HLA) system are routinely typed.

ABO incompatibility is generally considered a contraindication to transplantation since it can lead to an accelerated rejection response, called hyperacute rejection (see later), which likely represents a recipient response to A and B antigens expressed on vascular endothelium of the transplanted organ. However, some groups have reported successful grafting of HLA-compatible but ABO-incompatible organs, after removing anti-A and/or anti-B isohemagglutinins from the recipient by plasmapheresis or by extracorporeal immunoadsorption in conjunction with antibody induction therapy with thymoglobulin. In extremely urgent cases of liver transplantation, ABO matching is sometimes ignored, and reasonable graft function and survival can be seen in this setting as well.

HLA matching is also done routinely, with the goal of matching donor and recipient antigenicity as closely as possible. However, the practical significance of HLA-matching varies depending on the organ to be transplanted. In kidney transplantation, HLA-matching is considered important since there is a positive correlation between the number of HLA antigens common to the donor and recipient and the survival of the transplanted kidney (Table 1). It follows that when grafting kidneys from living relatives, HLA-identical sibling grafts have the best outcome, followed by haploidentical grafts, which, in turn, outperform haplotype-incompatible grafts. Likewise, cadaveric kidney transplants recipient-matched for HLA-A, -B, and -DR achieve survivals similar to those obtained with transplants between two haplotype matched living-related individuals. Major histocompatibility complex (MHC) class II matching appears also to be somewhat important for survival of pancreatic grafts.

Another more important facet of the donor-recipient matching process involves screening the recipient's serum for cytotoxic antibodies directed against the donor's lymphocytes. Presence of these antibodies heralds a recipient who is already immune to potential donor tissue. This screen is achieved by means of a cross-match, in which the recipient's serum is tested against lymphocytes from the potential donor(s) as well as against a cell panel of known phenotypes [known as a Rope test or panel reactive antigens (PRAs)], followed by flow cytometry. This test is useful to prevent rapid rejection of the grafted tissue or organ (discussed later).

In bone marrow transplantation, HLA typing is very important, but this type of transplant presents a unique problem not encountered with solid organ transplants. With bone marrow transplants, it is necessary to avoid both the rejection of the grafted tissue by the host and the damage of host tissue by the transplanted lymphocytes, a phenomenon called graft-versus-host disease (GVHD) (discussed later). A living relative of the recipient is therefore usually the preferred marrow donor. An identical twin is the optimal choice for a donor, followed by an HLA identical sibling (with six identical specificities for HLA-A, -B, and -DR) and a haplotype-identical relative (with three identical specificities for HLA-A, -B, and -DR) in order of preference. Mixed lymphocyte cultures can also be used preoperatively to screen for the GVHD reaction, which can emerge even in HLA-identical siblings due to incompatibilities in nontested, minor antigenic systems. With this technique, cultures are set

TABLE 1   Five-Year Graft Survival Rates Among Various Levels of Human Leukocyte Antigen Mismatched Donors

		N	Average % survival at five years	SEM (%)
Level of HLA mismatch	0	1131	87.4	1.1
	1	601	80.0	1.8
	2	1653	77.6	1.1
	3	2286	76.6	0.9
	4	676	75.9	1.8
	5	678	75.7	1.8
	6	323	78.3	2.4
	Unknown	230	75.4	3.2
Total		7578	78.6	0.5

Notes: 2004 Annual Report of the U.S. Organ Procurement and Transplantation Network and the Scientific Registry of Transplant Recipients: Transplant Data 1994–2003. Department of Health and Human Services, Health Resources and Services Administration, Healthcare Systems Bureau, Division of Transplantation, Rockville, Maryland, U.S.A; United Network for Organ Sharing, Richmond, Virginia, U.S.A; University Renal Research and Education Association, Ann Arbor, Michigan, U.S.A.
Abbreviations: HLA, human leukocyte antigen; SEM, standard error of the mean.

up by mixing the recipient's lymphocytes with lymphocytes from potential donors. A well-matched donor-recipient pair should react minimally to one another and translate into a low probability for GVHD to occur.

In the case of liver transplantation, HLA matching is not important for graft acceptance and survival. This unexpected finding is poorly understood, but may be due to the remarkable regenerative capacity of the liver or to its relatively small antigen load. Unless the recipient has a high PRA level, HLA matching is also not generally performed in the case of heart, lung, and small bowel transplantation because of the scarcity of available donors for these organs.

GRAFT REJECTION

Graft rejection is the consequence of an immune response mounted by the recipient against the graft, due to incompatibility between tissue antigens of the donor and recipient. Cells that express class II MHC antigens (such as passenger leukocytes, in the case of solid organ transplants) play a major role in sensitizing the immune system of the recipient and hightening the potential for graft rejection. These cells also may shed antigen as blood flows through the implanted organ, activating alloreactive helper T lymphocytes from the recipient. This results in the production of interleukin (IL)-2, which leads to clonal expansion, and in turn multiple immunological and inflammatory phenomena—some mediated by activated T lymphocytes and others mediated by antibodies—which can converge to cause graft rejection.

Rejection episodes are traditionally classified as hyperacute, accelerated, acute, and chronic, based primarily on the time-elapsed between transplantation and the rejection episode, and on the type of protein and cellular response, as determined by tissue biopsy of the affected organ.

Hyperacute (Early) Rejection

Hyperacute rejection occurs usually within the first few hours post-transplantation and is mediated by preformed antibodies against ABO or MHC antigens present on the grafted organ. It is also possible that antibodies directed against other alloantigens, such as vascular endothelial antigens, may play a role in this type of rejection. Upon antibody binding to antigen on the transplanted organ, rejection can be caused either by activation of the complement system, which results in the chemotactic attraction of granulocytes and the triggering of inflammatory cascades, and/or by antibody-mediated cellular cytotoxicity (ADCC).

A major pathological feature of hyperacute rejection is the formation of massive intravascular platelet aggregates, which leads to microvascular thrombosis, and ultimately tissue ischemia and necrosis. The formation of platelet thrombi probably results from several factors, including release of platelet activating factor (PAF) from immunologically damaged endothelial cells and/or from activated neutrophils.

Hyperacute rejection episodes are irreversible and uniformly result in graft loss. With proper cross-matching techniques, this type of rejection is almost always avoidable. However, it must be noted that the major limitation to xenogeneic transplantation (e.g., pig to human) is hyperacute rejection by antibodies to cellular, animal-specific, antigens that all humans make, even prior to any known exposure to xenogeneic tissues (natural antibodies).

Acute Rejection

Acute rejection usually occurs within the first few days to months after transplantation. Currently, less than 20% of kidney transplants experience one or more acute rejection episodes. When taking place in the first few days after grafting, it may correspond to a secondary (second set) immune response, implying that the recipient has been previously carried a sensitization to the HLA antigens present in the donated organ as a consequence of a previous antigen exposure, such as transplant, pregnancy, or blood transfusions. This particular phenomenon is known as an accelerated acute rejection. When acute rejection occurs beyond the first week after grafting, it usually corresponds to a first set, or primary, response.

Acute rejection is predominantly mediated by T lymphocytes and by both CD8$^+$ cytotoxic lymphocytes and T helper1 (Th1) CD4$^+$ lymphocytes.

In organs that are undergoing acute rejection, the cellular infiltrates are mostly composed of monocytes and both CD4$^+$ and CD8$^+$ T lymphocytes. The infiltrates also contain small populations of B lymphocytes, natural killer (NK) cells, neutrophils, and eosinophils, all of which contribute to rejection through secretion of inflammatory cytokines. IL-2 and IL-4 signal expansion of specific CD8$^+$ T cells and B cells, interferon (IFN)-γ upregulation of MHC II antigens on the graft, and chemotactic agents, such as IL-8 and complement fragments (C3a and C5a), attract additional immune cells to the transplanted organ.

In most cases, acute rejection if detected early can be reversed by increasing the dose of immunosuppressive agents or by briefly administering additional immunosuppressants.

The initial diagnosis of acute rejection is usually based on clinical suspicion. Abnormal laboratory studies or functional deterioration of the grafted organ are the main bases for considering the diagnosis of acute rejection. Confirmation usually requires a biopsy of the grafted organ. There are established histological criteria (Banff criteria) for the classification of acute rejection in transplanted organs. A hallmark finding in graft undergoing acute rejection is a heavy mononuclear cell infiltration of the affected organ or tissue.

Since biopsy is an invasive procedure with potential complications and pitfalls, several approaches to the noninvasive diagnosis of rejection have been attempted. Currently, the Cylex® system is used to measure immune cell activation. Briefly, this technique allows measurement of ion flow and ATP synthesis as an early activation marker of immune cell activity. Recently, gene array assays have come into favor as noninvasive methods for diagnosing rejection. These allow profiling of gene expression of lymphocytes as a marker of rejection. All of these techniques are experimental, and they are not in clinical use. In addition, these tests have been found to be lacking in sensitivity and specificity. Because of this, tissue biopsy remains the gold standard for the diagnosis of rejection and any other pathologic complications affecting a grafted organ.

Chronic Rejection

Chronic rejection, including chronic allograft nephropathy in the setting of kidney transplantation, is characterized by an insidiously progressive loss of function of the grafted organ. It is not certain if chronic rejection is a unique process or if it represents the final common pathway of multiple injuries occurring over a protracted period of time, such as ischemia/reperfusion injury, and including acute rejection episodes, infection, atherosclerosis, and drug toxicity. Actually, the functional deterioration associated with chronic rejection seems to be due to both immune and nonimmune processes. This is currently the greatest hurdle for advancing longer-term function and graft survival.

The clinical scenario of chronic allograft nephropathy is attributed largely to the chronic use of calcineurin inhibitors. These drugs are known to lead to constriction of the preglomerular arterioles, which leads to decreased glomerular filtration and renal blood flow. They have also been shown to induce the expression of transforming growth factor (TGF)-β and profibrinogenic genes. These factors initially lead to graft fibrosis, which then progresses to chronic allograft nephropathy. This phenomenon has led to the use of calcineurin inhibitor-free regiments (discussed later).

The ultimate cause of chronic rejection remains less clear, but vascular endothelial injury is thought to play a significant role. In fact, this arteriopathy and fibrosis of the graft parenchyma are hallmarks of the chronic rejection process that eventually leads to graft failure. A variety of cells, such as granulocytes, monocytes, and platelets have an increased tendency to adhere to injured vascular endothelium. The expression of PAF on the membrane of endothelial cells may be one of the major factors determining the adherence of neutrophils and platelets. In addition, experimental models have shown the presence of macrophage attractants, such as regulated on activation, normal T cell expressed and secreted (RANTES), which cause these cells to enter tissues and secrete offending proinflammatory cytokines. A variety of ILs and soluble factors are also released by activated leukocytes at the level of the damaged vessel walls, including IL-1, IL-6, tumor necrosis factor (TNF), macrophage chemoattractant protein-1, and platelet-derived growth factor. In addition, growth factors, especially basic fibroblast growth factor and TGF-β are also secreted at the level of the damaged endothelium. A layer of platelets and fibrin covers the damaged endothelium while proliferating fibroblasts and smooth muscle cells can be found in the subendothelial space. The end result is a proliferative lesion in the vessels as consequence of the inflammatory nature of the process, which progresses toward fibrosis and occlusion. Also, the growth factors contribute to progressive vascular hypertrophy. In addition, continuous production of alloantibodies by activated B cells exacerbates the arteriopathy and perpetuates the graft dysfunction. At the same time, the cytokine milieu contributes to the upregulation of MHC II molecules and adhesion molecules, such as intercellular adhesion molecules-1 and vascular cell adhesion molecule (VCAM)-1 that perpetuate the adhesion and damage pathways and continue the chronic rejection cycle.

In summary, although the exact etiology of chronic rejection is not completely understood, a variety of factors are believed to play significant roles. Further research is currently ongoing to define potentially modulate these factors in order to lessen the detrimental effects of the chronic rejection process. However, it should be noted that with the current immunosuppressive therapies available, the number one cause of kidney graft loss is death with a functioning graft.

IMMUNOSUPPRESSION

The ideal transplantation should take place among genetically identical individuals. This is only possible in the rare event of transplantation between identical twins. Thus, the success of clinical transplantation depends heavily on the use of nonspecific immunosuppressive agents that, by decreasing the magnitude of immunological rejection responses, prolong graft survival. Current immunosuppression in transplanted patients is achieved by the use of cytotoxic/immunosuppressant drugs and biological response modifiers, such as antilymphocyte antibodies.

Chemical Immunosuppression

Several drugs are currently used to induce immunosuppression, including glucocorticoids, antimetabolites, cyclosporin A (CsA), sirolimus (rapamycin), and tacrolimus (FK506).

Glucocorticoids
Historically, the first available immunosuppressive drugs used to treat and prevent rejection were glucocorticoids. They have multiple effects on the immune system and are nonspecific with actions that include lymphocyte apoptosis, inhibition of antigen-driven T-lymphocyte proliferation, inhibition of IL-1 and IL-2 release, and inhibition of chemotaxis. Because of the side effects associated with the use of glucocorticoids in relatively large doses for long periods of time (as required in transplantation), they are usually administered together with other immunosuppressant drugs, allowing the reduction of steroid doses below levels causing major side effects. In addition, more recent combination protocols are more frequently being used so as to completely avoid corticosteroids due to their morbidity with chronic use.

Antimetabolites
Antimetabolites are mostly used in the prevention of rejection episodes. All these agents inhibit DNA replication, lymphocyte proliferation, and the expansion of antigen reactive clones of lymphocytes.

Azathioprine (Imuran) undergoes metabolic conversion into 6-mercaptopurine, which inhibits purine nucleotide synthesis and prevents lymphocyte proliferation (both T and B). This therapy is toxic and currently very infrequently used.

Mycophenolate mofetil (CellCept) is converted to mycophenolic acid, which is an inhibitor of inosine monophosphate dehydrogenase, a critical enzyme for the synthesis of guanosine. This process is required for de novo synthesis of purines, upon which lymphocytes are critically dependent for proliferation, whereas other cells can utilize salvage pathways. Therefore, mycophenolate inhibits lymphocyte proliferation and inhibits the production of antibodies. This agent has virtually replaced azathioprine as a maintenance immunosuppressant and is often used in suppression of autoimmune conditions. It has recently been associated with gastro-intestinal (GI) toxicity. Cyclophosphamide (Cytoxan) is an alkylating agent, which modifies DNA and prevents lymphocyte replication. This drug is rarely used in solid organ transplantation. It is used in refractory rejection when more mainstream therapies fail.

Calcineurin Inhibitors (see Chapter 24)

CsA (Sandimmune, Neoral) is used in the prevention and treatment of rejection. The introduction of CsA in 1983 marks the begining of a new era in transplantation and has made possible the transplantation of other solid organs with increasing success. CsA is particularly helpful in the prevention of rejection, usually administered in association with glucocorticoids, because it allows their use in lower doses, or even their discontinuation.

The effects of CsA are mainly related to the inhibition of activity of transcriptional activators controlling the expression of IL-2 and other lymphokine genes in helper T cells, thus curtailing the onset of both cellular and humoral immune responses.

CsA itself has marked toxicity. It is nephrotoxic (and that raises considerable problems in patients receiving kidney transplants, in which it will be necessary to differentiate between acute rejection and CsA toxicity) and commonly causes hypertension. Less frequently causes tremor, hirsutism, and gum hyperplasia. Monitoring of circulating cyclosporine levels is essential to minimize the toxic effects of this drug, as well as monitoring of renal function.

Tacrolimus (Prograf, FK506) has a mechanism of action similar to CsA, although it is ten times more potent. It is able to reverse rejection episodes in patients unresponsive to some other immunosuppressive agents. Tacrolimus is used in a fashion similar to that as CsA, in combination with glucocorticoids and antimetabolites. It also has toxic effects including nephrotoxicity and neurotoxicity. In addition, a form of insulin-dependent post-transplant diabetes mellitus is reported in 20% of patients. This complication is largely reversible but necessitates careful monitoring of blood glucose levels, as well as renal function and potassium levels.

Cell-Cycle Inhibitors

Rapamycin (Sirolimus, Rapamune) is a unique compound that is structurally similar to tacrolimus. However, its mechanism of action seems to be related to cell-cycle inhibition. Rapamycin works by binding to FK506 binding proteins, thereby inhibiting T-cell proliferation by blocking both calcium-dependent and -independent pathways. In addition, it down-regulates the humoral immune response, thereby decreasing potentially cross-reactive antibody formation. Rapamycin is currently used largely in calcineurin inhibitor-free regimens. Sirolimus, in conjunction with mycophenolate and/or steroids subsequent to an immune induction-blocking antibody, has been shown very recently to be less nephrotoxic and reduce the incidence of chronic allograft nephropathy, by reducing the kidney insult induced by the calcineurin inhibitors (see earlier). It should be noted that preliminary evidence has shown that sirolimus can potentiate the nephrotoxic effects of CsA and tacrolimus. However, sirolimus coupled with paradoxically, sirolimus coupled with steroids and/or mycophenolate shows a synergistic effect in preventing chronic allograft nephropathy. Sirolimus is also used in calcineurin inhibitor withdrawal regimens, where immunosuppression is initiated with a calcineurin inhibitor, such as CsA, to prevent early acute rejection. This agent is later withdrawn, and immunosuppression is maintained with sirolimus. It is also currently sometimes used instead of Cellcept or Imuran. However, side effects caused by rapamycin include pancytopenia and hyperlipidemia, and these side effects are often magnified in regimens that include mycophenolate and rapamycin. Of particular interest here is that the hyperlipidemia exacerbates any underlying coronary artery disease, which is the leading cause of death among patients with functioning kidney allografts.

Biological Response Modifiers

This group includes a variety of biological compounds that have been found to be useful in the prevention and treatment of graft rejection. It should be noted that induction therapy is now the standard of care for kidney transplantation, reducing acute rejection percentages to single digits or very low teens. It is also hoped that combinations of biological response modifiers and immunosuppressive agents may lead to tolerization protocols applicable to humans. Tolerance induction to kidney and pancreas grafts, for example, has been successfully accomplished in a variety of animal models, but so far human tolerization remains an elusive target.

Antithymocyte and Antilymphocyte Globulins

Antithymocyte and antilymphocyte globulins were among the earliest successful therapeutic agents used in the management of graft rejection. These reagents are gammaglobulin fractions separated from the sera of animals (rabbits, goats, or horses) injected with human thymic lymphocytes or human peripheral blood lymphocytes. Therefore, they are polyclonal and are directed against numerous cell surface epitopes on platelets, T and B cells, NK cells, macrophages, as well as adhesion molecules. They are very effective in the prevention and reversal of rejection episodes, and their mechanism of action is related to the destruction or inhibition of recipient lymphocytes. Their main drawbacks have been related to difficulty in obtaining standardized preparations, reactivity with other cell types, and frequent sensitization of the patients, which often leads to serum sickness when the globulins are administered repeatedly. However, the serum sickness has been greatly reduced by abandoning the horse preparation in favor of the rabbit preparation. Currently, the rabbit preparation is the most widely used and exhibits less batch variation than preparations from previous species. Thymoglobulin is used in situations where reversal of aggressive rejection is necessary, as well as cases where the patient is resistant to immunosuppression with steroids. Finally, this preparation is also used for pregraft induction, a process that involves suppression of immune cell proliferation prior to host exposure to graft antigens.

Anti-T Cell Monoclonal Antibodies

Anti-T cell monoclonal antibodies derived from mouse B cells and directed against human T cells, particularly those reacting with the CD3 marker (muromonab CD3, OKT3), have been extensively used in the management of transplanted patients. Their mechanisms of action are multiple. CD3 monoclonal antibodies has been reported to cause depletion of $CD3^+$ T lymphocytes, and it is likely that the depletion is due to complement-mediated lysis, opsonization, and ADCC. CD3 monoclonal antibodies also causes down modulation of CD3 on the cell surface of otherwise viable T cells and may induce T-cell anergy.

These antibodies are predominantly used for the treatment of acute rejection. In addition, some groups use the monoclonal antibody as "induction" treatment immediately before transplantation to prevent rejection. As with antilymphocyte and antithymocyte globulins, the possibility of using monoclonal antibodies to treat repeated episodes of rejection is limited by the sensitization of the patients receiving the antibody. It must be noted that in spite of concomitant immunosuppression, up to 30% of patients become sensitized to various antibody preparations. However, changing to a different monoclonal antibody can meet with success in hypersensitive patients. In addition, the modern humanized versions of these antibodies are less immunogenic.

Besides serum sickness, monoclonal and polyclonal antibodies can cause what is known as the cytokine syndrome, which presents with fever, chills, headaches, vomiting, diarrhea, muscle cramps, and vascular leakage and transudation. The main cytokines responsible for this clinical syndrome are TNF, IL-1, IL-6, and IFN-γ. Experiments and data suggest that the syndrome is caused by massive IL release from T cells activated as a consequence of the binding of these antibodies to the lymphocyte membrane. This syndrome can cause pyrexia, hypotension, and rigors similar to systemic sepsis. This condition can lead to life-threatening pulmonary edema if the patient is fluid overloaded or death. The symptoms can be ameliorated by infusion of antihistamines, glucocorticoids, and anti-inflammatory agents prior to the use of CD3 monoclonal antibodies, and continuous infusion throughout the treatment if necessary.

Both monoclonal and polyclonal antilymphocyte antibody preparations are strongly immunosuppressive, so the risk of developing life-threatening infections or post-transplant lymphoproliferative disorder (PTLD) is markedly higher in patients treated with them (see subsequently). This condition is secondary to transformation by Epstein-Barr virus (EBV) and can be life-threatening. As a result, treatment with these agents usually does not exceed 14 days, and repeated courses of antibody treatment are usually contraindicated.

Other Monoclonal Antibodies

1. Anti-IL-2R monoclonal antibodies (Daclizumab/Simulect©, Basiliximab/Zenapax©) are also approved for use in transplantation for the prevention of rejection. Currently, these agents are used in all solid organ transplants. They are used as induction agents, and they are shown to markedly reduce rejection in the vast majority of cases, especially in the instance of kidney transplantation.
2. Anti-CD52 monoclonal antibodies (Alemtuzumab/Campath©). Antibodies directed against the CD52 cell surface protein, found on lymphocytes, NK cells, monocytes, macrophages, and cells of the male reproductive system, are often also used as inductions agents. The specific binding to the surface of the lymphocytes causes their specific lysis, thereby depressing the immune response to antigens encountered in the transplant process. In addition to allowing opportunistic infection and often causing rigors, fever, and nausea, other side effects include, lymphopenia, thrombocytopenia, anemia, and marrow hypoplasia.

Humanized and Chimeric Monoclonal Antibodies

The problem of sensitization can be minimized by the use of genetically engineered monoclonal antibodies of reduced immunogenicity. These antibodies are obtained by combining the antigen-binding regions of a murine monoclonal antibody with the constant regions of human IgG (see Chapter 24). These humanized or chimeric monoclonals can be administered for more prolonged periods of time without the occurrence of sensitization. However, they are considerably more expensive.

Experimental Agents

Currently, cytotoxic late antigen-4 (CTLA-4) immunoglobulin has shown promise in phase II clinical trials, in conjunction with T-cell depletion, to reduce the incidence of GVHD. In addition, Certican (everolimus) inhibits a molecule known as mammalian target of rapamycin (mTOR), which is important in the proliferation signaling pathway. When used in conjunction with CsA, everolimus has been shown to greatly decrease the incidence of cardiac vasculopathy post-transplant.

Total Lymphoid Irradiation

Irradiation of those areas of the body where the lymphoid tissues are concentrated is almost exclusively used to prepare leukemic patients for bone marrow transplantation. In this circumstance, irradiation combines two potential benefits: the elimination of malignant cells and the ablation of the immune system. Another immunosuppressive effect of irradiation is due to the greater radiosensitivity of helper T cells, resulting in the survival and predominance of suppressor/cytotoxic T cells among the residual lymphocyte population after irradiation.

Transplantation preconditioning protocols with total lymphoid irradiation have met with some impressive success: the patients are reported to require very low doses of maintenance immunosuppressive drugs, and in a few cases, it has been possible to withdraw the immunosuppressive drugs completely.

The Transfusion Effect: Stem Cells and Microchimerism

Although blood transfusions were generally avoided in potential transplant recipients due to the fear of sensitization to HLA, blood group, and other antigens, several groups reported, in the early 1980s, that kidney graft survival was longer in patients who had received blood prior to transplantation. This led to attempts to precondition transplant recipients with multiple pretransplant transfusions. Several interesting observations were recorded during these attempts.

1. The effect is more pronounced if MHC-II-expressing cells are included in the transfusion. Thus, the administration of whole blood, packed cells, or buffy coat are more efficient than the administration of washed red cells in improving graft survival.
2. The protection can be induced with a few donor-specific transfusions but usually requires multiple random transfusions. This probably reflects a MHC-specific effect that is obviously easier to achieve when the transfused cells have the same MHC as the graft.
3. The transfusion effect is delayed, usually seen about two weeks after a donor-specific transfusion. Following transfusion, there is a depression of cellular immunity that, according to some studies, seems to become more accentuated and long-lasting with repeated transfusions.

The concept that emerged from these studies was that the transfusion protocols induce a state of at least partial tolerance to the graft. Some investigators suggested that the tolerizing effect of blood transfusions was due to the transfer of donor-derived hematopoietic stem cell precursors. This could lead to the establishment of a low level of donor-derived cells within the recipient bone marrow and peripheral blood and result in a state of microchimerism. The microchimeric state could then induce tolerance to the donor tissues and, consequently, result in improved graft survival. While pretransplant transfusions have been very much abandoned—with improvements in matching and immunosuppression protocols the transfusion effect became less and less evident—there is considerable interest in developing protocols using stem cell administration as a way to induce a more complete tolerance state that could allow suspension or significant dose reduction of immunosuppressive drugs.

Immunosuppression Side Effects

Effective long-term immunosuppression is inevitably associated with a state of immuno-incompetence. Two major types of complications may result from this.

Opportunistic Infections

The immunosuppressed patient is susceptible to a wide variety of infections, particularly caused by infectious agents that are not often seen as pathogens in immunocompetent individuals, such as cytomegalovirus, herpes viruses of the herpes group [EBV, Herpes simplex virus, Varicella-Zoster virus], *Pneumocystis carinii, Toxoplasma gondii*, and fungi (e.g., *Candida albicans* and *Aspergillosis* spp.). The risk of opportunistic infection is highest in the first three months after transplant when the immunosuppression is the highest. Cytomegalovirus (CMV) infections are particularly ominous because this virus can further interfere with the host's immune competence, and may also trigger rejection in a nonspecific way.

The incidence of infections in transplant patients can be reduced by prophylactic therapy with intravenous gammaglobulin, which is part of most post-bone marrow transplant protocols, since those patients are probably the most profoundly immunosuppressed. Bone marrow and solid organ transplant patients also usually receive prophylactic antibiotics such as trimethoprim-sulfamethoxazole (for *Pneumocystis*, urinary tract infections, pneumonia, and cholangitis prophylaxis), ganciclovir or acyclovir (for herpes and CMV prophylaxis), and clotrimazole or fluconazole (for candidiasis). Newer prophylactic therapies, including valgancyclovir (Valcyte), have also allowed the further reduction in opportunistic viral infections.

Malignancies

Either as a consequence of the oncogenic properties of some immunosuppressive agents or as a consequence of disturbed immunosurveillance, the incidence of three main types of malignancy is significantly increased in transplant patients. In patients with survival times following transplantation of 10 years or longer, the frequency of skin cancer (squamous or basal cell carcinoma) may be up to 40%, although the lesions are no more invasive than in normal individuals. Rates of cervical cancer are also increased in immunosuppressed patients. Along with the increased rates of other anogenital cancers, the reasoning behind the increase involves the decreased immune surveillance against transforming oncogenic viruses. An additional 5% of patients may develop other types of malignancies, including EBV-associated post-transplant lymphoproliferative disorder (PTLD), as discussed earlier. Thanks to careful monitoring of EBV infection status, this number has decreased from approximately 20%.

Decreased immune surveillance against transforming oncogenic viruses has been suggested as the reason for the increased incidence of neoplasia in immunosuppressed patients. Thus, the predominance of skin and cervical cancer and PTLD among transplant patient may relate to the inability of the immune system to respond to papilloma viruses and EBV, which are etiologic agents for these malignances, respectively. Some of these PTLDs are reversible with interruption or reduction of immunosuppressive therapy or treatments that include agents such as Rituximab, a monoclonal antibody directed against the CD20 epitope on B cells. Others, however, are true malignant lymphomas that may spread to areas usually spared in non-transplanted patients, such as the brain. Common cancers such as colon, lung, and breast do not show increased frequently in transplant patients. This suggests that immune surveillance does not influence some of the most common cancers.

Other Side Effects

The most widely used immunosuppressive have specific side effects that may have a significant negative impact on the quality of life of transplanted patients. Glucocorticoids can cause, among other side effects, obesity, insulin resistant diabetes, cataracts, avascular necrosis of the femoral head, and thinning of the skin. Antimetabolites are associated with decreased blood counts and bone marrow depression. Cyclosporin and tacrolimus cause hypertension, nephrotoxicity, and neurotoxicity.

The use of combinations of different immunosuppressive drugs usually reduced the incidence and degree of side effects, because each drug that is part of the combination can be used at relatively well-tolerated doses. However, the ultimate goal of transplantation researchers is to develop protocols that would not require maintenance immunosuppression.

GRAFT-VS.-HOST DISEASE

Whenever a patient with a profound immunodeficiency (primary, secondary, or iatrogenic) receives a graft of an organ rich in immunocompetent cells, there is a risk that GVHD may develop. GVHD is a significant problem in infants and children with primary immunodeficiencies, in whom a bone marrow transplant is performed with the goal of reconstituting the immune system, as well as in adults, receiving a bone marrow transplant as part of a therapeutic protocol for aplastic anemia or for a hematopoietic malignancy. Small bowel, heart-lung, and even liver transplantation rank second in risk of causing GVHD, since these organs have a substantial amount of lymphoid tissue. In contrast, transplantation of organs such as the heart and kidneys, poor in endogenous lymphoid tissue, very rarely results in graft-versus-host reaction. The probability of developing GVHD is greatest in the two- to three-month period immediately following transplantation, when immunosuppression is high.

Pathogenesis

Two elements are essential for the development of a GVHD: the immune system of the recipient needs to be severely compromised and the transplanted organ or tissue needs to contain viable immunocompetent cells. The deficiency of the immune system may be congenital or acquired. For example, patients receiving bone marrow transplants receive cytotoxic and immunosuppressive therapy, and their immune system is completely or partially destroyed to avoid rejection of the transplanted bone marrow.

When a graft containing immunocompetent cells is placed into an immunoincompetent host, the transplanted cells can recognize as nonself the host antigens. In response to these antigenic differences, the donor T lymphocytes become activated, proliferate, and differentiate into helper and effector cells that attack the host cells and tissues, producing the signs and symptoms of GVHD. The crucial role played by the donor T cells in GVHD is demonstrated by the fact that their elimination from a bone marrow graft avoids the reactions (see subsequently). However, as the GVHD evolves and reaches its highest intensity, the majority of the cells infiltrating the different tissues affected by the GVH reaction are of host origin and include T and B lymphocytes as well as monocytes and macrophages. The proliferation of host cells is a result of the release of high concentrations of nonspecific mitogenic and differentiation factors by activated donor T lymphocytes.

However, it must be noted that several groups have reported findings suggesting that a low grade GVHD may actually accelerate bone marrow engraftment and has a beneficial impact in patients receiving bone marrow grafts as part of their treatment for leukemia (graft vs. leukemia effect).

Pathology

The initial proliferation of donor T cells takes place in lymphoid tissues, particularly in the liver and spleen (leading to hepatomegaly and splenomegaly). Later, at the peak of the proliferative reaction, the skin, liver, and intestinal walls are heavily infiltrated leading to severe skin rashes or exfoliative dermatitis, hepatic insufficiency, and severe diarrhea or even intestinal perforation. The splenic involvement results in a loss of function not unlike that seen in splenectomized patients. The patients often develop *Streptococcus pneumoniae* bacteremia, and antibiotic prophylaxis may be necessary.

Treatment

All immunosuppressive drugs used in the prevention and treatment of rejection have been used for treatment of GVHD. In addition, thalidomide, the sedative drug that achieved notoriety due to its teratogenic effects, has been used successfully for the control of chronic GVHD unresponsive to traditional immunosuppressants.

Prevention

Once a GVH reaction is initiated, its control may be extremely difficult. Thus, great emphasis is placed on preventing GVH reactions. Besides the administration of immunosuppressive drugs, other approaches have been tried with variable success.

Autologous stem cell transplantation using purified $CD34^+$ cells and allogeneic umbilical cord stem cell transplantation (stem cells obtained from cord blood after delivery) are also associated with a lower risk of GVH reactions. Umbilical cord stem cell transplantation is also associated with reduced graft versus leukemia effect and a higher frequency of relapses.

BIBLIOGRAPHY

Auchincloss H Jr, Sykes M, Sachs DH. Transplantation immunology. In: Paul WE, ed. Fundamental Immunology. 4th ed. Philadelpha, PA: Lippincott-Raven, 1999:1175–1236.
Bakr MA. Induction therapy. Exp Clin Transplant 2005; 3:320–328.
Beniaminovitz A, Itescu S, Lietz K, et al. Prevention of rejection in cardiac transplantation by blockade of the interleukin-2 receptor with a monoclonal antibody. N Engl J Med 2000; 342:613.
Cailhier JF, Laplante P, Hebert MJ. Endothelial apoptosis and chronic transplant vasculopathy: recent results, novel mechanisms. Am J Transplant 2006; 6:247–253.
Dallman MJ. Immunobiology of graft rejection. In: Ginns LC, Cosimi AB, Morris PJ, eds. Transplantation. 1st ed. Malden, MA: Blackwell, 1999:23–42.
Elster EA, Hale DA, Mannon RB, et al. The road to tolerance: renal transplant tolerance induction in non-human primate studies and clinical trials. Transplant Immunol 2004; 13:87–99.
Fugle S. Immunophenotypic analysis of leukocyte infiltration in the renal transplant. Immunol Lett 1991; 29:143.
Ginns L ed. Transplantation. Malden, MA: Blackwell Science, 1999.
Hariharan S, Johnson CP, Bresnahan BA, et al. Improved graft survival after renal transplantation in the United States, 1988 to 1996. N Eng J Med 2000; 342:605.
Hisanga M, Hundrieser J, Boker K, et al. Development, stability, and clinical correlations of allogeneic microchimerism after solid organ transplantation. Transplantation 1996; 61:40.

Kirk AD, Burkly LC, Batty DS, et al. Treatment with humanized monoclonal antibody against CD154 presents acute renal allograft rejection in human primates. Nat Med 1999; 5:686.

Lee TC, Savoldo B, Rooney CM, et al. Quantitative EBV viral loads and immunosuppression alterations can decrease PTLD incidence in pediatric liver transplant recipients. Am J Transplant 2005; 5:2222–2228.

Lechler RI, Sykes M, Thompson AW, Turka LA. Organ transplantation-how much of the promise has been realized. Nat med 2005; 11:605–613.

Lerut JP. Avoiding steroids in solid organ transplantation. Transpl Int 2003; 16:213–224.

Nankivell BJ, Chapman, JR. Chronic allograft nephropathy: current concepts and future directions. Transplantation 2006; 81(5):643–654.

Peggs KS, Mackinnon S. Immune reconstitution following hematopoietic stem cells transplantation. Brit J Haematol 2004; 124:407–420.

Sollinger HW. Mycophenolate mofetil for the prevention of acute rejection in primary cadaveric renal allograft recipients. Transplantation 1995; 60:225.

Yakupoglu YK, Kahan BD. Sirolimus: a current perspective. Exp Clin Transplant 2003; 1:8–18.

26 | Tumor Immunology

Deanne M. R. Lathers
Ralph H. Johnson VAMC and Department of Otolaryngology, Medical University of South Carolina, Charleston, South Carolina, U.S.A.

Sebastiano Gattoni-Celli
Department of Radiation Oncology, Medical University of South Carolina, Charleston, South Carolina, U.S.A.

INTRODUCTION

Cancer is one of the most serious health concerns worldwide. The field of tumor immunology has come of age over the last century, and important lessons have been learned from both the successes and failures of the field. This chapter highlights the concepts that are vital to gain an understanding of the immune responses to tumors.

Almost a century has passed since Paul Erlich first proposed that the immune system has the potential to eradicate cancer even though tumor cells arise from normal cells. In keeping with this proposal, 50 years later the concept of immune surveillance was put forth. The immune surveillance theory suggested that lymphocytes have the capacity to survey and destroy newly arising tumor cells that continuously appear in the body. Although this theory appeared to be disproved in the 1970s, new innovations in the field, including mice with specific genes knocked out, have largely confirmed the immune surveillance theory. The conviction that the immune system can be mobilized as well as manipulated to eradicate tumor cells has invigorated the field of tumor immunology, one of the most active fields in immunology over several decades.

Two important observations in the field occurred, serendipitously, when a group of prominent scientists interested in cancer genetics began breeding inbred strains of mice that were susceptible to a high frequency of neoplasms, such as mammary tumors and leukemias, with those that had a low susceptibility to neoplasms. These experiments led to the discovery of a genetic background of mice that allowed for the multiplication of endogenous, cancer-causing retroviruses as well as identification of the responsible viruses. A second unforeseen outcome was the identification of the loci associated with the mouse major histocompatibility complex (MHC). These experiments coincided with the identification of the human leukocyte antigen (HLA) loci in humans. These discoveries have shaped the progress of immunology to the present day.

These parallel discoveries of histocompatibility antigens in humans and mice are good examples of how studies in animal models and humans may correspond. Animal studies have allowed the evaluation of multiple parameters in tumor immunology studies that are not possible in clinical studies. This is mainly a consequence of using inbred animals, which represent a well-controlled environment in which to study specific parameters. Human clinical studies, on the other hand, are by necessity carried out in individuals of very diverse genetic background. This is a significant cause of divergence between human and animal studies. Nonetheless, animal studies continue as a basis for important advances in tumor immunology even though the translation to human clinical trials has often been disappointing.

Animal studies and clinical observations have led to several recent breakthroughs in the field of tumor immunology. These observations include (*i*) the discovery of immune stimulatory and immune suppressive cytokines; (*ii*) the ability to expand tumor-specific effector cells; (*iii*) the identification of tumor-associated antigens; (*iv*) the observation that dendritic cells are key antigen-presenting cells (APC) in the induction of antitumoral responses; and (*v*) recognition of the ability of tumors to evade and actively suppress the immune system. Each of these concepts will be discussed in detail in the context of tumor immunology and the development of immunotherapies for the treatment of cancer.

IMMUNOGENICITY OF TUMORS

The immunogenicity of tumors has been a major topic of debate for several decades. In a seminal study on the immune response induced by spontaneous tumors, none of 27 different spontaneous murine tumors were reported to exhibit detectable immunogenicity. These results contrasted with prior studies demonstrating that chemically-induced rodent tumors elicit an immune response causing rejection of tumor grafts in syngeneic animals. We now know that even spontaneously occurring tumors induced in laboratory animals are immunogenic when tested under appropriate experimental conditions.

Rejection Antigens

Rejection antigens were originally defined as those responsible for induction of an effective immune response against murine tumors induced by the chemical carcinogen, methylcholanthrene. Similar observations were subsequently made with other chemical carcinogens. Rejection antigens appear to vary among different carcinogens and between individual animals given the same carcinogen, demonstrating that rejection antigens are unique to each individual tumor. These observations suggested that a mutational mechanism, not necessarily directed to the same genetic target, might be responsible for the generation of antigenic entities easily recognized by the host immune response. At the same time, tumor rejection was shown to be mediated by activated T cells. In vitro studies utilizing tumor-specific T cells also revealed that the recognition of antigenic entities by lymphocytes did correlate with tumor rejection in vivo. It is important to understand that the antigenicity of a tumor may not be sufficient to mediate immunological rejection of the same tumor because they may be only weakly immunogenic and fail to elicit an effective immune response.

Tumor Antigens

Numerous tumor antigens have been identified in human and mouse cancers as potential targets for antitumor immunotherapies. These tumor antigens can be further divided into two major categories; tumor-specific antigens and tumor-associated antigens.

Tumor-Specific Antigens

Tumor-specific antigens are defined as gene products that are specifically expressed in tumors, such as the mutant *ras* oncogene-encoded proteins and the mutant *p53* suppressor gene-encoded proteins. These mutational changes provide the tumor cells with growth advantages but are not immunogenic. Thus, these tumor-specific antigens are not tumor-rejection antigens. However, they are currently being tested as gene therapy targets in several clinical studies.

Tumor-Associated Antigens

Tumor-associated antigens are normal cellular proteins overexpressed in certain cancers. Several of these proteins have been identified and characterized in great detail in human melanoma, which represents the best-studied tumor from an immunological perspective. This interest is largely due to the extensive clinical and biological evidence that the host immune response can have a measurable impact on its natural disease progression. Examples of melanoma tumor-associated antigens are melanoma antigen recognized by T cells-1 (MART-1), GP100, and tyrosinase. These gene products are also lineage-specific, meaning that their expression is limited to melanocyte lineage and their overexpression correlates with neoplastic development.

Melanoma-Associated Antigen

This family of melanoma antigens represents a separate set of melanoma-associated antigens (MAGEs) that result from overexpression of normal cellular genes. These proteins are not lineage-specific, as they are normally expressed in the testes. However, these antigens are tumor-associated because they are often overexpressed not only in melanoma, but in several other epithelial cancers. Results of several clinical studies suggest that well-defined MAGE epitopes can induce effective antitumor responses following injection into melanoma patients.

Carcinoembryonic Antigen

Additional studies have led to the identification of tumor-associated antigens in several tumor types. The primary example is carcinoembryonic antigen, an oncofetal antigen, which is overexpressed in adenocarcinomas of the gastrointestinal tract as well as some head and neck squamous cell carcinomas.

Prostate-Specific Antigen

Another important example is prostate-specific antigen, a protease expressed by prostate gland cells that becomes elevated in hypertrophic and cancerous prostate tissue.

Alpha-Fetoprotein

A third example is alpha-fetoprotein that becomes elevated in patients with cancer of the liver or testes. These tumor-associated antigens are often overexpressed and may provide useful markers for monitoring the course of disease, as they can be measured in serum.

EFFECTOR MECHANISMS IN TUMOR IMMUNITY

The importance of immune effector cells was demonstrated by the results of studies performed in animals following exposure to chemical carcinogens. Immunity was transferred among mice of the same strain through intravenous injection of immune cells, but not through transfer of serum.

Tumor-Specific Cytotoxic T Cells

Subsequent studies have demonstrated the importance of tumor-specific cytotoxic T cells (CTL) that are MHC-restricted $CD8^+$ lymphocytes. CTL kill target cells through recognition of an antigenic epitope bound to an appropriate MHC-I molecule, expressed on the surface of tumor cells.

Until recently, the main focus of antitumor immune responses has been CTL responses based on the expression of MHC-I and lack of MHC-II expression on tumor cells. Numerous animal studies have now demonstrated that $CD4^+$ helper T cells (Th) are crucial to antitumor immunity. In mice, of the two functional T helper populations, the Th1 population seems to be more effective in antitumor immune responses, because Th1 cells activate both CTL and APC (i.e., dendritic cells) and favor the switch to immunoglobulin (Ig) G2a synthesis, a biologically potent IgG isotype that enhances antibody dependent cell-mediated cytotoxicity (ADCC) and phagocytosis of tumor cells. Th2 cells assist exclusively the humoral response, which is much less effective as an antitumor protective mechanism. The importance of Th1 cells in the development and activation of CTL has been demonstrated in animal models. In tumor-bearing animals infused with Th1 cells, an increased CTL-mediated antitumor response was observed. One hypothesized mechanism for this response is that Th1 cells produce cytokines for CTL development and activation. Interferon (IFN)-γ, secreted by Th1 cells, may be the key to this effect because it upregulates MHC-I expression on tumor cells, increasing their sensitivity to CTL killing. IFN-γ also activates APC, which further stimulates Th1 and CTL responses to mediate tumor cell killing. Other studies have demonstrated that direct cell–cell contact between Th1 and CTL results in enhanced proliferation and survival during antitumor immune responses. The direct interaction of costimulatory molecules and receptors on the Th1 cells and CTL, respectively, are suggested to mediate these enhanced responses. The most significant conclusion from numerous studies is that HLA-restricted CTLs are the most effective killers of autologous tumor cells.

APC, such as dendritic cells, are a central element in antitumor immune responses. Dendritic cells are the most potent APC known with the unique ability to stimulate naïve T cell responses. Dendritic cells express both MHC-I and MHC-II molecules, which allow presentation of tumor antigen to both CTL and $CD4^+$ Th cells. In addition, dendritic cells express costimulatory molecules (i.e., CD80, CD86) required to stimulate the differentiation of $CD8^+$ T cells into antitumor CTL as well as the activation of Th cells. Importantly, dendritic cells have been recognized to confer immunogenicity to antigenic entities that would otherwise have been nonstimulatory and counterproductive to tumor immunity.

Macrophages

In addition to their ability to phagocytize and present tumor antigen, macrophages also have the capacity to kill tumor cells directly through release of toxic soluble molecules, such as lysosomal enzymes, reactive oxygen intermediates, and nitric oxide. Activated macrophages also secrete tumor necrosis factor (TNF) that directly kills tumor cells. Although the mechanism by which macrophages recognize tumor cells is unknown, the formation of complex, interdigitating interfaces with the target tumor cells creates optimal conditions for tumor cell killing through these toxic soluble molecules.

Antibodies

Antibodies may contribute to killing tumor cells by activating complement or by ADCC, in which Fc receptor-bearing macrophages or natural killer (NK) cells mediate the killing. Elimination of tumor cells by antibodies has been demonstrated in vitro. However, little evidence exists demonstrating that antibodies control tumor growth and spread in vivo. Nonetheless, several monoclonal antibodies are currently being assessed as therapeutics for numerous human cancers.

Cytokines

Cytokines play very important roles as mediators of antitumor immunity. The type and concentration of cytokines, as well as the cytokine receptor expressed, directs the immune response toward stimulation or tolerance. As discussed earlier, TNF directly kills tumor cells. In addition, Th responses are directed by cytokines. In the presence of interleukin (IL)-12, an antitumor Th1 response will develop. However, in the presence of IL-4, a much less effective Th2 response ensues. Finally, several cytokines are known to augment antitumor immunity.

Interleukin-2
IL-2, a well-known activator of T cell immunity, stimulates Th cells to proliferate and become activated following interactions with APC. With the right sequence of costimulatory signals, the IL-2-induced proliferation of undifferentiated Th cells results in a predominant Th1 response, which assists activation and differentiation of CTL, thus promoting the killing of target tumor cells.

Interleukin-12
IL-12, a pleiotropic immunomodulatory cytokine secreted by APC, has an essential role in innate and adaptive antitumor immune responses. In addition to directing toward a Th1 response, IL-12 activates Th1 and CTL to secrete IFN-γ leading to enhanced cell-mediated antitumor immune responses.

Granulocyte-Macrophage Colony-Stimulating Factor
Granulocyte-macrophage colony-stimulating factor (GM-CSF) is known to promote the recruitment and activation of dendritic cells and other APC. Following APC activation, tumor antigen can be processed and presented to stimulate antitumor T cells responses (e.g., Th and CTL). The use of these and other immunostimulatory cytokines in anticancer therapies is discussed in the Immunotherapy section.

GREAT ESCAPE: IMMUNE EVASION OF TUMORS

Despite a reasonable understanding of antitumor effector mechanisms, clinical studies investigating spontaneous antitumor immune responses have yet to lead to reproducible or consistent tumor regression. Thus, the question of why tumors continue to grow and metastasize in immunological competent cancer patients remains unanswered. Several observations have demonstrated that tumors evade and actively suppress the immune system. Tumor evasion of the immune system, termed immune escape, may occur through several mechanisms, including *(i)* tolerance or anergy induction; *(ii)* the genetic instability of tumors; *(iii)* modulation of tumor antigens; and *(iv)* decreased MHC-I expression. In addition to evasion of the immune system, tumors actively suppress the immune system directly through production of immune suppressive cytokines and indirectly through the induction of immune inhibitory cells.

Tolerance or Anergy Induction

Tumor cells present antigens bound to MHC molecules expressed on their cell surface. As discussed in Chapter 4, costimulation is required to initiate T cell responses. Tumor cells do not express costimulatory molecules (e.g., CD28), a requirement for engagement of the B7 (CD80, CD86) molecules on APC. This results in inadequate T cell activation leading to tolerance or anergy of potential effector cells and diminished antitumor immune responses.

Genetic Instability of Tumors and Modulation of Tumor Antigens

The heterogeneity and instability, both genetically and phenotypically, of tumors may also contribute to their evasion of the immune system. The expression of tumor antigens is frequently lost due to the genetic instability of tumors. From an immunological standpoint, antigen-negative tumors have a distinct growth advantage. Several studies have supported this concept as loss of tumor antigens correlated with increased tumor growth and metastasis.

Decreased Major Histocompatibility Complex-I Expression

In addition to tumor antigen modulation, MHC-I molecules may be downregulated or completely lost. Decreased synthesis or alterations in MHC-I molecules, β_2-microgobulin and/or transporter proteins associated with antigen processing and presentation may all contribute to alterations in MHC-I expression on tumor cells. An inability of CTL to recognize tumor antigens and kill tumor cells is a direct consequence of decreased MHC-I expression, as CTL only recognize tumor-derived antigenic epitopes when bound to the extracellular portion of MHC molecules.

Immunoediting

Selective pressure by the immune system also contributes to the growth and metastasis of tumors. Not only are tumors derived from self-cells, their high mitotic rate and genetic instability contribute to phenotypic diversification. One consequence of the specificity of immune responses is selective killing of tumor cell clones that express high levels of tumor antigen, as well as tumor cell clones that express normal levels of MHC molecules. Thus, cells that express low levels of MHC or do not express tumor-associated antigens survive the assault of the immune system. The selection of tumor variants that better survive in an immunologically intact environment has been termed immunoediting and results in the generation of tumor cells with a greater resistance to antitumor immune effector mechanisms.

Suppression of Antitumor Immune Responses

In addition to immune evasion, tumors actively suppress antitumor immune responses. Numerous tumor types in both animal models and cancer patients secrete a variety of cytokines and other soluble factors that can be immunosuppressive, such as transforming growth factor (TGF)-β, IL-10, and prostaglandins. This secretion of soluble factors is thought to contribute to the Th2 skewed immune responses observed in cancer patients. One important immunosuppressive factor secreted in large quantities by many tumor types is TGF-β, one of the most potent immunosuppressive molecules known. Proliferation and activation of both lymphocytes and macrophages are inhibited by TGF-β. In addition, in vitro studies suggest that TGF-β induces the development of $CD4^+CD25^+$ T regulatory cells. The ability of these cells to suppress CTL effector function has been demonstrated in cancer patients. This could be a key mechanism explaining how tumors can indirectly suppress antitumor immunity.

Tumor burden roughly correlates with the degree of immunosuppression observed in cancer patients. This has led to the concept that immunotherapeutic modalities may be more appropriate for patients with small tumor burdens, who are more likely to respond to stimulation than those with very profound immunosuppression. Immunotherapeutic modalities may also be more appropriate for patients who have undergone surgical excision of their tumors to prevent recurrence of cancer and stimulate antitumor immunity to eliminate residual micrometastases.

Generalized Suppression of the Immune Response in Cancer Patients

The immunosuppression associated with malignancies can be specific for the autologous tumor or extend to other aspects of the immune response, such as decreased reactivity to viral and bacterial recall antigens. This more generalized type of immunosuppression is often the consequence of treating patients with anticancer agents such as chemotherapeutic drugs or ionizing radiation, as neutrophils and lymphocytes are highly susceptible to these agents. Additional exogenous causes of immunosuppression include alcohol abuse, poor nutritional status, glucocorticoid administration, as well as surgery, which induces prostaglandin release. These are important considerations when assessing the potential efficacy of immunotherapeutic regimens administered to patients. Another factor to consider is age, which is also associated with a generalized decline of immune functions. Since cancer often strikes older people, a weaker immune response may make them more vulnerable to the disease and less likely to benefit from immunotherapy.

IMMUNOTHERAPY

The advent of tumor immunotherapy dates back more than one hundred years when the intratumoral application of bacteria was observed to induce a strong inflammatory response and, at times, regression of neoplastic lesions. For quite some time, clinical investigators attempted this type of nonspecific immunotherapy based on the administration of inactivated/attenuated bacteria. Success was obtained in eliciting a strong delayed-type hypersensitivity response. Unfortunately, severe toxicities of local necrosis and ulcerations were also elicited.

Since these historic studies were performed, a wide array of immunotherapeutic approaches has been tested for the treatment of cancer. This is an area of tumor immunology that has been plagued by failure, even when treatments in mouse tumor models showed promise. Each failed therapy has provided new information from which to design more effective approaches.

Expansion and Activation of Tumor-Infiltrating Lymphocytes

Pioneering work in cell-mediated antitumor immunotherapies was centered on the expansion and activation of lymphocytes recovered from tumors, tumor-infiltrating lymphocytes (TIL). In patients with melanoma, TIL were obtained by expanding lymphocyte populations present in surgically excised tumors in vitro, in the presence of IL-2 and appropriate antigenic stimulation. The resulting cells represented an enriched population of CTL capable of recognizing and killing autologous tumor cells. Following infusion of IL-2 and large numbers of the patients' expanded TIL (10^{11} to 10^{13}), some clinical benefit was observed as measured by tumor regression. However, a combination of technical complexity and variable results has led most groups to abandon this approach except in combination with partial bone marrow ablation. These studies have provided an important building block for the highly experimental approach of partially ablating the bone marrow using whole body radiation treatments or chemotherapies followed by infusion of highly antitumor reactive T cells to colonize the bone marrow in cancer patients. The goal of this partial ablation is to allow the infused cells room to expand in the bone marrow and maintain a longer lasting appearance of the tumor-reactive CTL leading to the clinical response of tumor regression.

Activated Natural Killer Cells

The antitumor potential of NK cells has been the object of considerable interest. NK cells are a specialized subset of $CD3^-CD56^+$ lymphocytes that preferentially recognize target cells, which are low- or nonexpressors of MHC molecules. Tumor cells frequently have low levels of MHC-I expression, which facilitates escape from recognition by host CTL. Several recent studies have focused on the interactions of NK cells and dendritic cells, a key APC, as a potential immunotherapeutic approach to cancer vaccines. Reciprocal activation of dendritic cells and NK cells occurs via dendritic cell activation of NK cells through secretion of type I IFN and NK cell activation of dendritic cells through ligand interactions and IFN-γ secretion. Importantly, these interactions lead to the activation of both innate and adaptive antitumor immune responses. This ability to augment antitumor immune responses may lead to the inclusion of NK cells in future vaccination strategies.

Tumor Vaccines

Tumor vaccines have been the object of numerous trials with the goal of stimulating antitumor immune responses by active immunization. A wide variety of antigens has been used, ranging from killed tumor cells to purified tumor antigens. Autologous cell-based vaccines are made from the patient's own tumor cells. Allogeneic cell-based vaccines are obtained from a mixture of tumor cells that are not derived from the patient to be vaccinated. Autologous tumor cell vaccines are specific but difficult to generate, while allogeneic vaccines can be produced in large quantities but are not patient-specific. Allogeneic vaccines are generally made of several established cell lines with the objective of encompassing a wide variety of antigenic specificities for that particular tumor type. Cell-based vaccines appear to be more effective when combined with an adjuvant that enhances the immunogenicity of the antigens associated with tumor cells. In several tumor vaccine studies, synthetic peptides specific for antigenic tumor epitopes formulated with incomplete Freund's adjuvant were given in combination with immune stimulatory cytokines, such as IL-2. The goal of these protocols was to stimulate the host immune response to recognize tumor-associated antigenic complexes and promote the destruction of autologous tumor cells. The role of the immune stimulatory cytokines is to stimulate proliferation and activation of Th1 cells and CTL. Treatment requires repeated administration of these therapeutic synthetic vaccines to establish a sustained antitumor immune response. In recent trials, cancer patients were treated with multiple infusions of dendritic cells pulsed with synthetic peptides specific for antigenic tumor epitopes or killed tumor cells. The unique capacity of dendritic cells to traffic to secondary lymphoid tissue as well as to activate a multitude of immune effector cells, including Th cells, CTL, and NK cells, makes dendritic cells an attractive immunotherapeutic approach to the treatment of cancer. Infusion of dendritic cells pulsed with tumor cell lysates, tumor protein extracts, or irradiated tumor cells have also been tested in clinical studies with some efficacy. Although this cell-mediated vaccination strategy has shown some promise in clinical studies, not all tumor types regress in response to vaccinations. Efforts continue to optimize vaccination strategies to improve antitumor immune responses.

Immunostimulatory Cytokines and Chemokines

One such effort in vaccination strategies is their use with other therapies such as surgery, radiation therapy, chemotherapy, or other immunotherapies. Several immunostimulatory cytokines and chemokines are potential components of these combined therapies. Because of its role in the early stages of cell-mediated immune responses, IL-2 has become the focus of intense study, leading to its approval as an immunotherapeutic agent for both melanoma and renal-cell carcinoma. Although high dose therapy with IL-2 can cause fevers and vascular leak, systemic low doses and localized intratumoral delivery of IL-2 have shown promise as adjuvants in immunotherapeutic approaches to cancer treatments.

IL-15 is a recently cloned member of the IL-2 family that has been tried as both an immunotherapeutic agent and as an adjuvant for antitumor vaccines. Numerous studies in mouse tumor models have demonstrated increased antitumor immunity as well as tumor regression following administration of IL-15. This cytokine induced a central memory phenotype in CD8$^+$ T cells expanded in vitro that delayed tumor growth and increased survival, following infusion into tumor-bearing mice. Treatment with IL-15 also results in an expansion of a population of activated NK cells. Recently, early clinical studies began at the National Cancer Institute, Bethesda, MD, U.S.A, to test IL-15 as an adjuvant in antitumor vaccine studies based on its ability to activate both NK and CTL.

GM-CSF has shown efficacy as an immunotherapeutic approach to increase the efficiency of tumor vaccines. Tumor cells were engineered to express and release GM-CSF as a means to recruit host APC to the tumor site, where tumor antigen expression is optimal. The expectation is that the vaccine-containing tumor cells will "educate" the immune response to recognize and subsequently kill autologous tumor cells. Histological analyses of metastatic lesions in many patients enrolled in these clinical studies have confirmed the validity of this approach. Numerous lesions were heavily infiltrated by lymphocytes and often had extensive areas of hemorrhagic necrosis. The clinical product of these experiments, GVAX^{TM}, has demonstrated efficacy in several large trials for multiple cancer types, such as lung, prostate, and pancreatic cancers.

The in vivo efficacy of IL-12 treatments to enhance antitumor immune responses has been demonstrated in several studies using animal tumor models. This efficacy is primarily attributed to the ability of IL-12 to direct and augment Th1 responses as well as CTL responses. Unfortunately, this promising preclinical data in mouse tumor models has not come to fruition in a clinical setting. Cancer patients treated with recombinant IL-12 suffered severe toxicities with limited clinical responses. However, IL 12 has potent adjuvant activity, likely, due to its ability to recruit and activate APC. Its use as an adjuvant to tumor immunotherapies is under intense investigation in clinical studies.

C-C chemokine ligand (CCL21) is one member of the chemokine family that shows promise as an antitumor immunotherapy. CCL21 specifically attracts naïve T cells and dendritic cells and also has a positive effect on Th1 responses. These properties led to the testing of CCL21 treatments in a mouse model of lung cancer to induce colocalization of T cells and dendritic cells intending to reverse tumor-induced immune suppression and elicit cell-mediated immunity. The results of these studies demonstrated that CCL21, delivered through CCL21 transfected dendritic cells, was able to stimulate Th1 cytokine expression and generate systemic antitumor immune responses. The use of chemokines to stimulate antitumor immune responses shows significant therapeutic potential and will likely advance to clinical studies in the near future.

Heterogenization

Heterogenization, which can be achieved by *(i)* infecting tumor cells with a virus; *(ii)* transfecting tumor cells with foreign MHC-I or II molecules; or *(iii)* fusing tumor cells with various allogeneic cells, is another approach to increase the immunogenicity of a tumor. The purpose of heterogenization is to force the host immune response to recognize tumor-associated antigens in the context of allogeneic MHC-I or II molecules or in proximity of strong nonself antigens. The allogeneic/nonself antigen would provide a strong costimulatory signal to enhance antitumor immune responses.

Antitumor Monoclonal Antibodies

Another important immunotherapeutic tool that has been tried against some types of cancer is passive immunization, through the administration of monoclonal antibodies targeting tumor-associated antigens. Some of the monoclonals used in tumor immunotherapy are specific for molecular structures expressed on tumor cell surfaces. Others are equivalent to anti-idiotypic antibodies, which represent surrogate antigens, since they are the internal image of tumor antigens.

Antitumor antibody therapies have had marked success in reducing both death and recurrences in cancer patients. One example of this is trastuzumab, a molecularly engineered antibody that is a chimera of a human monoclonal antibody and the antigen-binding site of a murine antibody. Trastuzumab recognizes the extracellular domain of human epidermal growth factor receptor 2 (HER2), a protein overexpressed in breast cancer. This treatment has shown significant efficacy in HER2-positive metastatic breast cancer. Two recently completed trials demonstrated even greater efficacy of treatment with trastuzumab when combined with adjuvant chemotherapy. Other monoclonal antibodies, such as anti-CD20 (Rituximab), have been used successfully (usually in combination with chemotherapeutic agents) in the treatment of B lymphocyte malignancies (see Chapter 27). These studies highlight a new horizon in tumor immunology, namely combining immunotherapy with other therapies to treat aggressive disease.

FINAL CONSIDERATIONS

As our understanding of tumor biology and antitumor effector mechanisms increases, immunotherapeutic modalities are becoming more widely studied and accepted as an integral part of cancer therapy. While success has been limited, immunotherapy is likely to play an increasingly important role in cancer treatment. Tumor immunology appears to be on the verge of a new era as new tumor antigens are identified, novel strategies are developed to improve vaccine potency against weak tumor antigens, high-avidity CTL to clear tumors more effectively are selected, and the importance of overcoming tumor-induced immune suppression is recognized. The full realization of its apparent potential will require much more experimental work. This work will improve our understanding of the factors influencing the outcome of immunotherapeutic interventions. Extensive clinical trials will test the potential impact of these new treatments. Using combination therapies to concurrently stimulate antitumor immune reactivity, while diminishing tumor-induced immune suppression, is likely to require a reduction in tumor burden as well as a multi-pronged immunotherapeutic approach.

BIBLIOGRAPHY

Abbas AK, Lichtman AH. Cellular and molecular immunology. 5th ed. Philadelphia: Elsevier Science, 2003.

Berzofsky JA, Terabe M, Oh S, et al. Progress on new vaccine strategies for the immunotherapy and pr vention of cancer. J Clin Invest 2004; 113:1515.

Boon T, van derBruggen P. Human tumor antigens recognized by T lymphocytes. J Exp Med 1996; 183:725.

Colombo MP, Trinchieri G. Interleukin-12 in anti-tumor immunity and immunotherapy. Cytokine Growth Factor Rev 2002; 13:155.

Diab A, Cohen AD, Alpdogan O, Perales M-A. IL-15: targeting CD8$^+$ T cells for immunotherapy. Cytotherapy 2005; 7:23.

Dranoff G, Jaffee E, Lazenby A, et al. Vaccination with irradiated tumor cells engineered to secrete murine granulocyte-macrophage colony-stimulating factor stimulates potent, specific, and long-lasting antitumor immunity. Proc Natl Acad Sci 1993; 90:3539.

Giuntoli RL, Lu J, Kobayashi H, et al. Direct costimulation of tumor-reactive CTL by helper T cells potentiate their proliferation, survival and effector function. Clin Cancer Res 2002; 8:922.

Kalinski P, Giermasz A, Nakamura Y, et al. Helper role of NK cells during the induction of anticancer responses by dendritic cells. Mol Immunol 2005; 42:535.

Knutson KL, Disis ML. Tumor antigen-specific T helper cells in cancer immunity and immunotherapy. Cancer Immunol Immunother 2005; 54:721.

Li C-Y, Huang Q, Kung H-F. Cytokine and immuno-gene therapy for solid tumors. Cell Mol Immunol 2005; 2:81.

Old LJ, Boyse EA, Clarke DA, et al. Antigenic properties of chemically-induced tumors. Ann N Y Acad Sci 1962; 101:80.

Piccart-Gebhart MJ, Procter M, Leyland-Jones B, et al. Trastuzmab after adjuvant chemotherapy in HER2-positive breast cancer. N Engl J Med 2005; 353:1659.

Romond EH, Perez EA, Bryant J, et al. Trasruzmab plus adjuvant chemotherapy for operable HER2-positive breast cancer. N Engl J Med 2005; 353:1673.

Rosenberg SA. Adoptive cellular therapy in patients with advanced cancer. Biol Ther Cancer Updat 1991; 1:1.

Rosenberg SA, Yang JC, Schartzentruber DJ, et al. Immunologic and therapeutic evaluation of a synthetic peptide vaccine for the treatment of patients with metastatic melanoma. Nat Med 1998; 4:321.

Smyth MJ, Cretney E, Kershaw MH, Hayakawa Y. Cytokines in cancer immunity and immunotherapy. Immunol Rev 2004; 202:275.

Yang S-C, Hillinger S, Riedl K, et al. Intratumoral administration of dendritic cells overexpressing CCL21 generates systemic antitumor responses and confers tumor immunity. Clin Cancer Res 2004; 10:2891.

27 | Lymphocyte and Plasma Cell Malignancies

Gabriel Virella
Department of Microbiology and Immunology, Medical University of South Carolina, Charleston, South Carolina, U.S.A.

INTRODUCTION

Lymphocytes are frequently affected by neoplastic mutations, perhaps as a consequence of their intense mitotic activity. Lymphocyte malignancies can be broadly classified into B-cell and T-cell malignancies. B-cell malignancies (or dyscrasias) can be identified by the production of abnormal amounts of homogeneous immunoglobulins (or fragments thereof), resulting from the monoclonal proliferation of immunoglobulin-secreting B cells or plasma cells, or by the proliferation of lymphocytes expressing specific B-cell markers. T-cell malignancies (or dyscrasias) are usually defined as proliferations of lymphocytes expressing T-cell membrane markers.

B-CELL DYSCRASIAS

Malignant proliferations of immunoglobulin-producing cells usually produce abnormally homogeneous immunoglobulins that are designated as monoclonal proteins (Fig. 1). The conditions associated with detection of monoclonal proteins are generically designated as monoclonal gammopathies, plasma cell dyscrasias, or B-cell dyscrasias (from the Greek *dyskrasis*, meaning "bad mixture," often used to designate hematological disorders affecting one particular cell line).

Monoclonal proteins or paraproteins, in practical terms, are defined by the fact that they are constituted by large amounts of identical molecules, carrying one single heavy chain type and one single light chain type or, in some cases, by isolated heavy or light chains of a single type. It must be noted that monoclonal proteins may be detected in patients without overt signals of malignancy (some mutations may lead to clonal expansion without uncontrolled cell proliferation).

Diagnosis of B-Cell Dyscrasias
Plasma Cell and Plasma Cell Precursor Dyscrasias
In general, the diagnosis of a plasma cell or a plasma cell precursor dyscrasia relies on the demonstration of a monoclonal protein. Secreted paraproteins are detected by a combination of methods.

Classically, the initial screening involved the electrophoretic separation of serum and urine from the suspected case (Fig. 2). To be sure that urinary proteins were not overlooked because of their low concentration, the urine sample was concentrated.

However, as stated previously, a monoclonal protein has to be defined by its homogeneity in heavy and/or light chains, and this information can only be obtained through immunochemical techniques, such as immunofixation (Fig. 3). It has become an accepted practice to perform the immunofixation study both as a screening and confirmatory test, skipping serum electrophoresis as initial screening. Immunofixation is also the method of choice to diagnose specific B-cell dyscrasias, such as light chain disease, Waldenström's macroglobulinemia, or the heavy chain diseases, discussed later in this chapter.

In some instances, plasma cell dyscrasias do not result in the secretion of paraproteins. In rare cases of multiple myeloma, for example, the neoplastic mutation alters the synthetic process so profoundly that no paraproteins are produced (nonsecretory myeloma).

In the majority of cases, the finding of a monoclonal protein does not give a very precise diagnostic indication. For example, the isolated finding of homogeneous free light chains (Bence-Jones protein) in the urine may correspond to one of the following B-cell dyscrasias: (*i*) light chain disease; (*ii*) chronic lymphocytic leukemia (CLL); (*iii*) lymphocytic

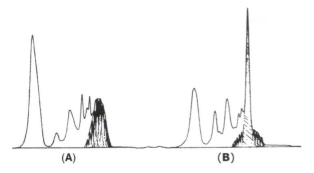

FIGURE 1 Concept of monoclonal gammopathy: In normal sera or reactive plasmacytosis, the gammaglobulin fraction is made up of the sum of a large number of different antibodies, each one of them produced by a different plasma cell clone **(A)**; if a B-cell clone escapes normal proliferation control and expands, the product of this clone, made up of millions of structurally identical molecules, will predominate over all other clonal products and appear on the electrophoretic separation as a narrow-based, homogeneous peak in the gammaglobulin fraction **(B)**.

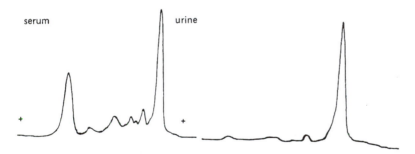

FIGURE 2 Electrophoresis of serum and urine proteins from a patient with multiple myeloma. The serum, shown on the left, depicts a very sharp peak in the gammaglobulin region with a base narrower than that of albumin, corresponding to an IgG monoclonal component. The urine, shown on the right, indicates a sharp fraction in the gamma region with only traces of albumin, meaning that the monoclonal peak is constituted by proteins smaller than albumin, able to cross the glomerular filter. This monoclonal protein in the urine was constituted by free κ-type light chains (κ type Bence-Jones protein).

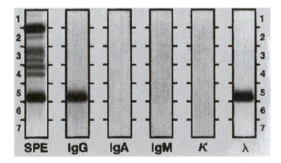

FIGURE 3 Immunoblot of the serum protein of a patient with multiple myeloma. The lane labeled serum protein electrophoresis was fixed and stained after electrohophoresis and shows a homogeneous fraction in the gamma globulin region, near the bottom part of the separation region. The remaining lanes were blotted with the following antisera: anti-IgG, anti-IgA, anti-IgM, anti-kappa chains (κ), and anti-lambda chains (λ). Notice that the antisera specific for IgG and for λ chains reacted with the homogeneous fraction, which therefore was identified as an IgGλ monoclonal protein. *Abbreviations*: Ig, immunoglobulin; SPE, serum protein electrophoresis. *Source*: Immunoblot courtesy of Dr. Sally Self, Department of Pathology and Laboratory Medicine, Medical University of South Carolina, Charleston, SC, U.S.A.

lymphoma; or (*iv*) "benign" or "idiopathic" monoclonal gammopathy. The precise diagnosis depends on a combination of clinical and laboratory data, as discussed in detail later in this chapter.

B-Cell Malignancies

B-lymphocyte malignancies may or may not be associated with the synthesis of monoclonal proteins.

1. CLLs are B-cell proliferations in the vast majority of cases, but only one-third show paraproteins; the remainder have monoclonal cell surface immunoglobulins only.
2. B-cell acute lymphocytic leukemias show rearrangements of their immunoglobulin heavy chain genes in chromosome 14, and the malignant cells may synthesize μ chains, but they remain intracytoplasmic and there is no detectable monoclonal protein in serum or urine.

Physiopathology of B-Cell Dyscrasias
Direct Pathological Consequences of Malignant B-Cell Proliferation

Depending on the type of proliferating B cell, patients may present with a variety of symptoms directly resulting from the expansion of a malignant B-cell population, including:

1. Enlargement of lymph nodes, spleen, and liver, as seen in lymphomas and some leukemias.
2. Leukemic invasion of peripheral blood, characteristic of B-cell leukemias.
3. Compressive and obstructive symptoms resulting from the proliferation of plasma cells in soft tissues. Oropharyngeal plasmocytomas often lead to obstructive symptoms. Heavy chain-producing intestinal lymphomas, when grossly nodular, can lead to intestinal obstruction.
4. Intestinal malabsorption, typical of α-chain disease. It results from extensive infiltration of the intestinal submucosa by malignant B cells, causing total disruption of the normal submucosal architecture.

General Metabolic Disturbances

General metabolic disturbances are responsible for some major pathological manifestations of B-cell dyscrasia, such as bone destruction, renal insufficiency, anemia, and secondary immunodeficiency.

Bone Destruction

Bone destruction results from a combination of osteoclast hyperactivity and depressed osteoblast function. Malignant plasma cells attach to bone marrow stromal cells, stimulating several events that result in osteoclast proliferation and activation. Among the factors that have been proposed to play these roles are the ligand for the receptor activator of NFκB (RANKL), macrophage colony-stimulating factor (M-CSF), interleukin (IL)-6, IL-11, IL-1β, and lymphotoxin-α (TNF-β). On the other hand, the production of osteoprotegerin, which inhibits the effects of the ligand for the receptor for the activator of NFκb, is depressed. Malignant plasma cells produce additional osteoclast activating factors, including IL-3 and macrophage inflammatory protein-1α. At the same time, conditions for osteoblast proliferation and differentiation are adverse, as a result of the release of soluble factors by malignant plasma cells that suppress osteoblast differentiation. The end result of this imbalance is localized or disseminated bone reabsorption.

Renal Insufficiency

Renal insufficiency can result from a diversity of factors, such as hypercalcemia (secondary to bone reabsorption), hyperuricemia, deposition of amyloid substance in the kidney, clogging of glomeruli or tubuli with paraprotein (favored by dehydration), and plasmocytic infiltration of the kidney.

Anemia

Anemia (normochromic, normocytic) is frequent and is basically due to decreased production of red cells. A moderate shortening of red cell survival is also common.

Immunodeficiency

Immunodeficiency is a paradoxical feature of many B-cell malignancies. It often develops in patients that have marked increases in their concentrations of circulating immunoglobulins. This is particularly obvious in patients with multiple myeloma, who have an increased tendency for pyogenic infections. In reality, if the levels of residual normal immunoglobulins are measured, they are found to be low. Also, these patients show decreased antibody production after active immunization. The depression of the immune response in patients with multiple myeloma appears to be multifactorial.

1. In IgG myeloma, the large amounts of IgG secreted by the malignant cells are likely to have a negative feedback effect, depressing normal IgG synthesis (see Chapter 6).
2. A more general mechanism of suppression of the humoral response seems to be mediated by phagocytic monocytes (and to a lesser extent T cells). The immunosuppressor properties of these cells can be demonstrated by coculturing peripheral blood mononuclear leukocytes from normal donors and from myeloma patients. The coculture results in impairment of the function of the normal B lymphocytes. Recent, but unconfirmed, data suggest that patients with multiple myeloma have an expansion of $CD4^+CD25^{high}$, $FoxP3^+$ T regulatory cells, which could be an important factor in causing a generalized state of immunodepression.
3. Other abnormalities that may contribute to the predisposition to infections are defects in neutrophil responses and impairment of $Fc\gamma$ receptor functions in phagocytes, which are more likely to exist in patients with renal failure. Anemia also seems to predispose to infections, for unknown reasons.

In CLL, in addition to a depression of humoral immunity (milder than that seen in multiple myeloma), there is a depression of T-cell counts and function. Viral and fungal infections, as well as cases of disseminated infection after administration of live attenuated viral vaccines, have been reported in patients with this type of leukemia. Recent studies have demonstrated that T cells from patients with CLL stimulated with anti-CD3 plus IL-2 in vitro express the costimulatory molecule CD28 at lower levels and for a shorter time than cells from normal controls, whereas they express higher levels for longer periods of time of the downregulatory molecule CTLA-4 (CD152). These findings could explain why CLL patients have impaired cell-mediated immune responses.

Serum Hyperviscosity

Some plasma cell dyscrasias may present with a constellation of symptoms known as the hyperviscosity syndrome. This is a direct result of increased serum viscosity caused by high concentrations of monoclonal proteins. Serum viscosity is directly related to protein concentration. IgM and polymeric IgA, due to their molecular complexity and high intrinsic viscosity, lead to disproportionate increases of blood viscosity (Fig. 4). Not surprisingly, the hyperviscosity syndrome is a frequent manifestation of Waldenström's macroglobulinemia, a B-cell dyscrasia defined by the synthesis of monoclonal IgM. However, the hyperviscosity syndrome is also observed in multiple myeloma patients, mainly in those with polymeric IgA paraproteins, and occasionally in IgG myeloma, when the concentrations of IgG are very high. The symptoms of serum hyperviscosity are related to high protein concentration, expanded plasma volume, and sluggishness of circulation. Table 1 lists the main signs and symptoms of the syndrome. Typical fundoscopic changes are shown inC Figure 5.

Pathological Consequences of the Immunological Activity of a Paraprotein

Most paraproteins have unknown and inconsequential antibody activities, but in some exceptional cases, the reactivity of a monoclonal protein may be directly responsible for some of the manifestations of the disease.

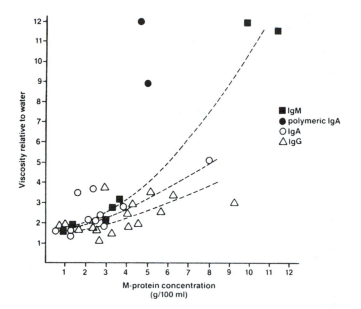

FIGURE 4 Plot of relative serum viscosity versus monoclonal protein concentration in sera containing IgG, IgA, and IgM monoclonal proteins. The highest viscosity values were determined in sera containing IgM or polymeric IgA monoclonal proteins.

Cold Agglutinin Disease

Cold agglutinin disease results from the synthesis of large concentrations of monoclonal IgM (IgMκ in more than 90% of the cases) with cold agglutinating properties. Those monoclonal cold agglutinins react with the "I" antigen expressed by the erythrocytes of all normal adults. Because the affinity of IgM antibodies is low, its reactivity with red cells is enhanced by cold temperatures (for this reason, these autoantibodies are known as cold agglutinins). Clinical disease is seen during the winter months, when the temperatures of cold exposed areas drop below 37°C. The sera of patients with suspected cold agglutinin disease is tested at 4°C on a direct hemagglutination test, using O positive red cells as antigens.

TABLE 1 Clinical Manifestations of the Hyperviscosity Syndrome

Ocular
    Variable degrees of vision impairment
    Fundoscopic changes
    Dilation and tortuosity of retinal veins ("string-of-sausage" appearance)
    Retinal hemorrhage and "cotton-wool" exudates
    Papilledema
Hematologic
    Mucosal bleeding (oral cavity, nose, gastrointestinal tract, urinary tract)
    Prolonged bleeding after trauma or surgery
Neurological
    Headaches, somnolence, coma
    Dizziness, vertigo
    Seizures, EEG changes
    Hearing loss
Renal
    Renal insufficiency (acute or chronic) due to clogging of the glomerular
        vessels with paraprotein and diminished concentrating and diluting abilities
Cardiovascular
    Congestive heart failure secondary to expanded plasma volume

Abbreviation: EEG, electroencephalogram.
Source: Modified from Bloch KJ, Maki DG. Hyperviscosity syndromes associated with immunoglobulin abnormalities. Sem Hematology 1973; 10:113.

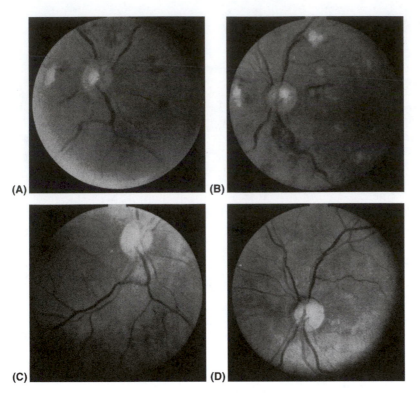

FIGURE 5 Fundoscopic examination of a patient with hyperviscosity syndrome. **(A)** and **(B)** are pictures obtained from the right and left eyes, respectively, at the time of admission. Flame-shaped hemorrhages, "cotton-wool" exudates, and irregular dilation of retinal veins are evident. **(C)** and **(D)** are pictures obtained from the same eyes after five months of therapy, showing total normalization. *Source*: Reproduced from Virella G, Valadas PR, Graça F. Polymerized monoclonal IgA in two patient with myelomatosis and hyperviscosity syndrome. Brit J Haematol 1975; 30:479.

Monoclonal cold agglutinins can be detected in cases of IgM-producing B-cell malignancy (Waldenström's macroglobulinemia, see later), when the IgM paraprotein behaves as a cold agglutinin. The titers of cold agglutinins in such cases are very high, and usually the patient will have symptoms attributable to the cold agglutinin. In patients with symptomatic cold agglutinin disease the cold agglutinin titers may be equally high, but there is no evidence of B-cell dyscrasia other than the presence of the monoclonal anti-I cold agglutinin and an increase in the numbers of lymphoplasmocytic cells in the bone marrow.

The clinical manifestations of cold agglutinin disease fall into two categories: cold-induced hemolytic anemia and cold-induced ischemia. Hemolysis in patients with cold agglutinin disease is usually mild. In mild cases, the cold agglutinins are present in relatively low titers and have low thermal amplitude; that is, do not react at temperatures close to normal body temperature, and hemolysis is due to opsonization of red cells through C3b receptors. In severe cases, when cold agglutinins are present in high titers and react at temperatures close to normal body temperature, they cause intravascular hemolysis. The release of large concentrations of hemoglobin can lead to acute renal failure. Cold-induced ischemia is caused by massive intracapillary agglutination in cold-exposed areas.

Hyperlipidemia
A pronounced increase in serum lipid and lipoprotein levels can be detected in patients with monoclonal gammopathies. In exceptional cases, the monoclonal protein has antibody activity to lipoproteins. It has been demonstrated that the binding of antibodies to the lipoprotein molecules alters the uptake and intracellular processing of the lipoprotein, resulting in hyperlipidemia and in increased accumulation of cholesterol in macrophages.

Clinical Presentations of B-Cell Dyscrasias
Multiple Myeloma

The most frequent presenting clinical symptoms of multiple myeloma are (*i*) bone pain and "spontaneous" or "pathological" fractures; (*ii*) fatigue and weakness, secondary to anemia; and (*iii*) recurrent infections. Less frequently, the patients may present with malaise, headaches, or other symptoms related to hyperviscosity. Renal failure usually develops later in the disease.

Frequently, anemia is the leading feature, and the diagnosis is established when the cause of anemia is investigated. Hemoglobin levels below 7.5 g/dL are usually associated with poor prognosis. Other cases are first seen in a rheumatology outpatient clinic, due to "bone pains." If there is advanced bone destruction, the diagnosis may be prompted by a fracture after minimal trauma (known as "pathological" fractures). Symptoms related to hyperviscosity (Table 1) may also lead to hospitalization.

Recurrent infections and renal failure, which are more frequent in advanced stages of the disease, are among the most common causes of death. Infection is associated with an increased risk of death, and the prognosis of a multiple myeloma patient with renal failure, particularly when his blood urea nitrogen exceeds 80 mg/dL, is also poor.

Laboratory Diagnosis

A typical case of multiple myeloma will present at least two elements of the following diagnostic triad: (*i*) bone lesions, (*ii*) monoclonal protein in serum and/or urine, and (*iii*) bone marrow plasmacytosis.

Bone Lesions. Bone lesions are typically osteolytic (appear in the X ray as punched-out areas without peripheral osteosclerosis) and multiple (several punched-out areas appear in the same bone and can be seen in a number of bones in the same patient) (Fig. 6). Practically all bones can be affected. In advanced cases, pathological fractures can occur in the long bones, skull, or spinal column. Rarely, a single bone lesion may be detected in one patient; however, such a "solitary bone plasmacytoma" is in fact rarely solitary, and bone marrow aspiration will reveal diffuse plasmacytosis in most cases. Exceptionally, a patient with monoclonal gammopathy and diffuse plasmacytosis can present with no evident bone lesions or with generalized osteoporosis. In those cases, anemia, hypercalcemia, and renal failure can be considered as part of the triad, indicating bone/bone marrow involvement (in multiple myeloma kidney, damage is most often a consequence of hypercalcemia).

Monoclonal Proteins in Serum and/or Urine. A monoclonal protein can be detected in 97% of the cases of multiple myeloma if proper techniques are used. The distribution of monoclonal

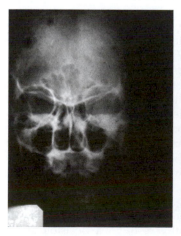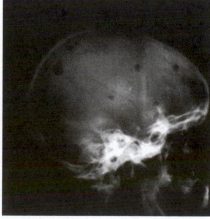

FIGURE 6 X ray of the skull of a patient with multiple myeloma, showing typical osteolytic lesions. *Source*: Courtesy of Dr. S. Richardson, Department of Hematology, Medical University of South Carolina, Charleston, SC, U.S.A.

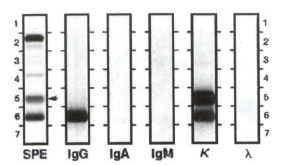

FIGURE 7 Immunoblot study of the urinary proteins of a patient with multiple myeloma. The serum protein electrophoresis (SPE, *left lane*) of the urine reveals several proteins, including albumin (*top*) and two homogeneous fractions (*bottom*), suggesting a moderate degree of kidney insufficiency. The bottom fraction on SPE reacted both with an antiserum specific for IgG heavy chains and anti-κ chains, and is thus identifiable as complete IgGκ. The second homogeneous protein seen in SPE (*arrow*) reacted only with anti-κ chains. Thus, this fraction is identifiable as free κ chains (Bence-Jones protein, κ type). *Abbreviations:* Ig, immunoglobulin; SPE, serum protein electrophoresis. *Source:* Immunoblot courtesy of Dr. Sally Self, Department of Pathology and Laboratory Medicine, Medical University of South Carolina, Charleston, SC, U.S.A.

proteins among the different immunoglobulin classes closely parallels the relative proportions of those immunoglobulins in normal serum: 60% to 70% of the proteins are typed as IgG, 20% to 30% as IgA, 1% to 2% as IgD and, very rarely, one monoclonal protein can be typed as IgE. A single light chain type is found in these paraproteins. For example, IgG paraproteins can be either κ or λ. The finding of a heterogeneous increase of IgG or any other immunoglobulin (i.e., an increase of both IgGκ and IgGλ molecules) is not compatible with a diagnosis of multiple myeloma.

In the urine, the most frequent finding is the elimination of free light chains, κ or λ (Bence-Jones proteins, Fig. 7). These light chains are usually found in addition to a monoclonal immunoglobulin detectable in serum, but in about 20% to 30% of patients with multiple myeloma, the only abnormal proteins to be found are the free monoclonal light chains in the urine. Some authors give the designation of light chain disease to the form of multiple myeloma, in which the paraprotein consists of free light chains.

Very rarely (about 3% of cases), no monoclonal paraprotein is detected in the serum or urine of a patient with a typical clinical picture or multiple myeloma. This situation is designated as nonsecretory myeloma. In most nonsecretory myelomas, immunofluorescence studies have demonstrated intracellular monoclonal proteins that are not secreted into the extracellular spaces. Nonsecretory myelomas have a very poor prognosis.

Bone Marrow Plasmacytosis. This is the third element of the diagnostic triad for multiple myeloma. Bone marrow aspirates show increased numbers of plasma cells (>10% of bone marrow cells) with a more or less mature appearance (Fig. 7). The plasma cell infiltration can be massive, with sheets of plasma cells occupying the bone marrow. However, it must be stressed that an increase in the number of plasma cells in the bone marrow, even when associated with morphological aberrations, is not sufficient to differentiate between malignant and reactive plasma cell proliferation. The differential diagnosis between malignant and reactive plasma cell proliferation should be based on the immunochemical characteristics of the patient's immunoglobulins. Although a patient with a malignant B-cell dyscrasia will show either a monoclonal protein or low immunoglobulin levels (if it is a case of nonsecretory myeloma), reactive plasmacytosis is invariably associated with a polyclonal increase of immunoglobulins.

Management
The management of a patient with a monoclonal gammopathy rests on a decision about whether the malignancy is dormant or aggressive. Multiple myeloma is, in the vast majority of cases, an aggressive malignancy, and its management is usually based on staging.

Staging. The most recent staging system takes only two parameters in consideration: serum albumin and beta-2 microglobulin levels. The serum albumin concentration reflects the general metabolic state of the patient, and the levels of circulating beta-2 microglobulin are an apparent indicator of the B-cell proliferation rate. Serum albumin levels >3.5 g/dL and beta-2 microglobulin levels <3.5 mg/L are associated with the best prognosis (median survival of 62 months), whereas beta-2 microglobulin levels >5.5 mg/L (irrespectively of the serum albumin level) are indicative of poor prognosis (median survival of 29 months). Other parameters indicative of poor prognosis (survival <12 months) are beta-2 micro-globulin levels >10 mg/L, serum creatinine >4 mg/dL, serum albumin <2.5 g/dL, and platelet count <130,000/μL. Cytogenic studies can also give prognostic indications, particularly deletion of chromosome 13 by florescence in situ hybridization analysis, associated with poor prognosis.

Therapy. Therapy of multiple myeloma is less than satisfactory and, for that reason, is in a state of evolution. Autologous stem cell transplantation after induction with dexamethasone in combination with thalidomide (because of its anti-angiogenic properties) is a popular approach for patients with standard risk. An alternative for induction is the association of lenalinomide (an immunomodulatory analog of thalidomide) and dexamethasone, which seems more effective and less toxic. The goal of induction therapy is to reduce the tumor burden prior to stem cell transplantation. Once induction is achieved, the patients are conditioned with high doses of melphalan (an alkylating agent) plus GM-CSF and CD34$^+$ stem cells are harvested from the patient's blood. Stem cell transplantation is considered successful when the level of monoclonal protein is reduced by >90%. To achieve this goal, a second stem cell transplantation may be required. Maintenance therapy after the transplant is still uncertain. Most commonly, prednisone and thalidomide plus pamidronate (a biphosphonate, see later) are being evaluated. Recombinant RANK-Fc proteins and humanized monoclonal antibodies to RANKL are also being evaluated, with encouraging preliminary results. The classical association of melphalan and prednisone is reserved for patients who are not good candidates for stem cell transplantation or patients who relapse after stem cell transplantation, although combinations of thalidomide, dexamethasone, and cyclophosphamide are also used in relapses. A new agent that is being evaluated, by itself or in association with other agents, in high risk and relapsing multiple myeloma is bortezomib, a proteasome inhibitor. Hypercalcemia is usually treated with glucocorticoids, but biphosphonates, such as pamidronate and zoledrenic acid, have been found to be highly effective. Biphosphonates are also used successfully to reduce bone destruction and avoid pathological fractures. Recent reports of severe oral adverse effects, especially painful necrosis of the jaw bones, associated with several products of this group in patients receiving chemotherapy, raise issues about the long-term use of biphosphonates in patients with multiple myeloma and other malignancies affecting the bones.

Plasmapheresis. In plasmapheresis, indicated in cases with hyperviscosity, the patient's plasma is replaced by normal plasma or by a plasma-replacing solution. The reduction on viscosity secondary to the reduction in the circulating levels of monoclonal protein caused by chemotherapy takes time, and the rapid correction of hyperviscosity may be essential for proper management. The rapidly beneficial effects of plasmapheresis are illustrated in Figure 4, which shows the normalization of retinal changes observed after plasmapheresis.

Other supportive measures include hemodialysis or peritoneal dialysis in cases with renal insufficiency, and antibiotic therapy and prophylactic administration of gammaglobulin in patients with recurrent infections.

Plasma Cell Leukemia

Plasma cell leukemia is the designation applied to cases in which large numbers of plasma cells can be detected in the peripheral blood (exceeding 5–10% of the total white blood cell count). Besides the leukemic picture in the peripheral blood, the remaining clinical and laboratory features of plasma cell leukemia are usually indistinguishable from those of multiple myeloma. The prognosis is generally poor; this may reflect a higher degree of de-differentiation on the part of malignant plasma cells that abandon their normal territory.

Monoclonal Gammopathy of Unknown Significance

The designations of monoclonal gammopathy of unknown significance, as well as of benign or idiopathic monoclonal gammopathy, are used when a monoclonal protein is found in an asymptomatic individual or in a patient with a disease totally unrelated to B lymphocyte or plasma cell proliferation (solid tumors, chronic hepatobiliary disease, different forms of non-B cell leukemia, rheumatoid arthritis, etc.).

Scandinavian authors conducting extensive population studies have given an average figure for the incidence of idiopathic monoclonal gammopathies of about 1%, by far the most common form of B-cell dyscrasia. The incidence seems to increase in the elderly, up to about 20% in 90-year-old and older individuals.

The clinical significance of the finding of a benign or idiopathic monoclonal gammopathy lies in the need to make a differential diagnosis with a malignant B-cell dyscrasia in its early stages (such as what is known as a "smoldering multiple myeloma"). Several criteria for the differential diagnosis between benign and malignant plasma cell dyscrasias have been proposed (Table 2).

Management

A good practical rule is to assume that any monoclonal gammopathy detected unexpectedly during the investigation of a condition not clearly related to a B-cell malignancy, or during screening of a normal population (particularly in individuals of advanced age), should be considered as benign until proven otherwise. The best attitude in such cases is to withhold cytotoxic therapy and follow the patients closely, every three to six months, measuring the amount of paraprotein; malignant cases show a progressive increase, whereas in benign cases, the levels remain stable. Patients with benign gammopathy have to be observed at least yearly after the first two years of follow-up, since there are documented cases of malignant evolution after five or more years of "benign" behavior. Early treatment before frank progress has not been observed to improve the survival rate of those cases that show malignant evolution.

Waldenström's Macroglobulinemia

This is a B-cell proliferative disorder characterized by bone marrow infiltration and IgM monoclonal gammopathy. It was first described by a Swedish physician, Dr. Jan Waldenström, after whom the disease was named.

TABLE 2 Laboratory Features that Have Been Proposed for the Differentiation Between Malignant and Idiopathic Monoclonal Gammopathies

Feature	Benign	Malignant
Paraprotein	Complete molecule; little or no Bence-Jones protein	Bence-Jones proteinuria >0.6 g/day
Normal immunoglobulins	Conserved	Depressed
Serum paraprotein	<1 g/100 mL	>1 g/100 mL
Serum albumin	>3 g/100 mL	<3 g/100 mL
Hemoglobin	>10 g/100 mL	<10 g/100 mL
Serum urea	<80 mg/100 mL	>80 mg/100 mL
Serum β_2-microglobulin	<7mg/L	>7mg/L
Nonspecific proteinuria	Absent	Present
Numbers of B cells in peripheral blood	Normal	Decreased
Labeling index	Normal	Increased

Clinical Features

Waldenström's macroglobulinemia is clinically characterized by a constellation of symptoms that include weakness and anemia, fever, night sweats, weight loss, hyperviscosity-related symptoms (Table 1), hepatomegaly, splenomegaly, and lymphadenopathy.

Symptoms suggestive of multiple myeloma, such as bone pain, bone lesions, or "spontaneous" fractures, are rare. The immunosuppression is also milder than in multiple myeloma. Hypercalcemia, leukopenia, thrombocytopenia, and azotemia are rarely seen. Renal insufficiency, when present, is usually a manifestation of serum hyperviscosity and can be reversed by plasmapheresis and/or peritoneal dialysis. In general, the disease has a much more benign evolution than multiple myeloma, with median survival rates ranging from 5 to 10 years.

Diagnosis

The two main diagnostic features of Waldenström's macroglobulinemia are the presence of an IgM monoclonal protein (Fig. 8) and the pleomorphic infiltration of the bone marrow with predominance of small lymphocytes, plasmocytoid cells, and mature plasma cells. Mast cells can also be prominent. Most infiltrating lymphocytes and lymphoplasmocytic cells express B-cell markers (CD19, 20, and 22).

Management

Waldenström's macroglobulinemia frequently follows a benign course. Poor prognosis is associated with a variety of parameters, such as age (≥ 65), anemia, and high beta-2 microglobulin levels. In patients with high levels of circulating IgM, serum hyperviscosity can be the cause of a variety of complications, some of them life-threatening (Table 1). In such cases, repeated plasmapheresis is often sufficient to keep the patient asymptomatic, avoiding the use of cytotoxic drugs and their side effects. Cytotoxic therapy may be required, due to the severity of the symptoms or the impossibility of keeping the patient on repeated plasmapheresis. Chlorambucil (leukeran) has been most widely used, usually given in a continuous low dosage. Rituximab, a CD20 monoclonal antibody, has been showed to be effective in cases refractory to cyclophosphamide. It is also significant to note that some trials using the combination of cyclophosphamide with rituximab as the initial treatment of Waldenström's macroglobulinemia have better outcomes than the treatment with each agent alone, so this combination may become more widely used in the future.

Heavy Chain Diseases

Some B-cell dyscrasias are associated with the exclusive production of heavy chains (or fragments thereof) or with the synthesis of abnormal heavy chains that are not assembled as complete immunoglobulin molecules and are excreted as free heavy chains. Both types of abnormality can be on the basis of a heavy chain disease. The heavy chain diseases are classified according to the isotype of the abnormal heavy chain as γ, α, μ, and δ (one single case of δ chain disease has been reported, and ε chain disease has yet to be described).

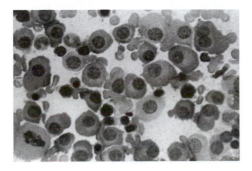

FIGURE 8 Plasma cell infiltration of the bone marrow in a patient with multiple myeloma. Note the binucleated plasma cell in the upper right corner of this figure.

α-Chain Disease

This is the most common and best defined heavy chain disease. It affects patients in all age groups, even children, and is more frequent in the Mediterranean countries, particularly affecting individuals of Jewish or Arab ancestry.

Clinically, it is indistinguishable from the so-called Mediterranean-type abdominal lymphoma, characterized by diarrhea and malabsorption unresponsive to gluten withdrawal, with progressive wasting and death. Intestinal X-ray changes is suggestive of diffuse infiltration of the small intestine, such as thickened mucosal folds. Intestinal biopsy reveals diffuse infiltration of the submucosa by reticulolymphocytic cells.

Diagnosis relies on the demonstration of free α chains, usually in serum. Routine electrophoresis usually fails to show a monoclonal component, but immunofixation shows an abnormal IgA band that does not react with antisera specific for light chains.

γ-Chain Disease

This was the first form of heavy chain disease discovered. Clinically, it appears as a lymphoma with lymphadenopathy, splenomegaly, and hepatomegaly. Bone marrow and lymph node biopsies show lymphoplasmocytic proliferation. The diagnosis is based on the immunochemical demonstration of free γ chains in the serum and/or urine.

μ-Chain Disease

This variant of heavy chain disease is less frequent than either γ- or α-heavy chain diseases. Clinically, it is indistinguishable from CLL or lymphocytic lymphoma, with marked Bence-Jones proteinuria and small amounts of free μ chains detectable in the serum and sometimes also in the urine.

LEUKEMIAS AND LYMPHOMAS
Nomenclature

The malignant proliferation of leukocytes can be classified by a variety of criteria. One first important distinction is made between leukemia and lymphoma. It should be noted that it is not rare for a patient to have features of both types of processes, but the clinical classifications of lymphocyte malignancies are useful and widely used.

Leukemia refers to any malignant proliferation of leukocytes, in which the abnormal cell population can be easily detected in the peripheral blood and in the bone marrow. Leukemias may involve any type of hematopoietic cell, including granulocytes, red cells, and platelets. Leukemias are often classified as acute or chronic, based on their clinical evolution and morphologic characteristics that are closely related. Acute leukemias follow a very rapid progression toward death if left untreated. Many immature and atypical cells can be seen in the peripheral blood of patients with acute leukemias. Chronic leukemias have a more protracted evolution; differentiated cells predominate in the peripheral blood of patients with chronic leukemia. Leukemic states may evolve from a chronic form to an acute disease, and the type of proliferating cell may also change during the course of the disease. For example, transition from a chronic granulocytic stage to an acute and very often fatal lymphoblastic leukemia is characteristic of chronic myelocytic leukemia.

Lymphoma refers to localized lymphocyte malignancies, often forming solid tumors, predominantly affecting the lymph nodes and other lymphoid organs. Lymphomas are always lymphocytic malignancies.

Classification of Lymphocytic Leukemias and Lymphomas

All malignant proliferations of cells identifiable as lymphocytes are classified as either T- or B-cell malignancies, based on a variety of characteristics:

1. Identification of the malignant cells as immunoglobulin-producing cells allows their classification as B-cell malignancies.
2. Cell membrane markers are widely used to classify malignant lymphocyte proliferations.

3. Cytogenetic studies and molecular genetic procedures are the basis of further subclassifications with prognostic and therapeutic implications. The classifications have increased in complexity, and their full discussion can be found in specialty publications and hematology textbooks. In this chapter, we will limit our discussion to paradigmatic entities, and we will center our discussion in aspects that tie together basic and clinical science.

Chronic Lymphocytic Leukemia

CLL is a B-cell malignancy and the most common form of leukemia in the Western hemisphere. The disease usually has a late onset (median age of diagnosis is 65 years) and relatively benign course (median survival of 10 years). In the vast majority of cases, the leukemic cells are small or medium-sized lymphocytes, expressing CD5 and CD23 and low levels of surface immunoglobulins (low levels of sIgM can be detected in >95% of the patients). Central to its pathogenesis seems to be an overexpression of the *bcl-2* gene, which inhibits apoptosis.

Clinical Symptoms

Clinical symptoms are often absent or very mild. Malaise, fatigue, or enlargement of the lymphoid tissues felt by the patient are the most frequent presenting complaints. Physical diagnosis shows enlargement of the lymph nodes, spleen, and liver. Viral infections, such as herpes and herpes zoster, and fungal infections are frequent in these patients, pointing to a T-cell deficiency, which is confirmed by the finding of reduced numbers of T cells and reduced responses to T-cell mitogens. The prognosis is determined by the frequency of severe opportunistic infections. Recent data suggest that patients with mutated immunoglobulin variable heavy chain gene or expressing a specific heavy chain variable region gene (VH3-21) have significantly lower survivals, probably reflecting cells with higher degrees of biological abnormalities, less likely to respond to therapy.

Diagnosis

Diagnosis is established by a variety of approaches, including morphological studies and identification of specific cell membrane markers (CD5, CD23). Bence-Jones proteins can be detected in the concentrated urine of approximately one-third of the patients. Rarely, IgM monoclonal proteins may be detected in serum. Most patients are hypogammaglobulinemic.

Management

The combination of two cytotoxic drugs, fludarabine and cyclophosphamide, is very effective. Allogeneic stem cell transplantation after myeloablative conditioning has also been found to be curative in a significant number of patients.

Hairy Cell Leukemia
Clinical Features

Hairy cell leukemia is a rare lymphoid B-cell malignancy, predominantly affecting middle age males (median age of diagnosis: 55 years). The clinical presentation is nonspecific, and includes malaise, fatigue, and frequent infectious episodes. The physical examination usually shows splenomegaly and sometimes generalized lymphadenopathy. Laboratory data show pancytopenia, anemia being most frequent, followed by thrombocytopenia, and leukopenia. The diagnosis is based on the finding of atypical lymphocytes with numerous finger-like (or hairy) projections in the peripheral blood (the name of the disease derives from the morphological characteristics of the abnormal lymphocytes). The abnormal cells express surface immunoglobulins, often of several isotypes (IgG3 often predominating), and also express classical B-cell markers (CD19, CD20, CD22).

Management

Interferon-α is therapeutically useful in hairy cell leukemia. This seems to result from a direct antiproliferative effect that is attributed to the ability of interferon-α to promote redifferentiation of malignant cells, stopping their uncontrolled multiplication. However, the remissions obtained with interferon-α are usually partial and temporary. Better results are obtained with nucleoside analogues, such as 2-chlorodeoxyadenosine and deoxycoformycin. Rituximab (monoclonal antibody to CD20) and immunotoxins based on CD22 mononoclonal antibodies have also been tried successfully (particularly rituximab) in patients with relapsed hairy cell leukemia.

Acute Lymphoblastic Leukemia
General Characteristics
Acute lymphoblastic leukemia (ALL) is the result of a wide array of mutations that affect hematopoietic stem cells and result in the proliferation of lymphoblasts, which spill into the peripheral blood. At the same time normal hematopoiesis is negatively affected, and the patients develop anemia, neutropenia, and thrombocytopenia. Bone marrow failure is the most frequent cause of morbidity and mortality.

ALL is most common in childhood, and the majority of cases occur between 2 and 10 years of age. Childhood ALL generally responds well to chemotherapy (overall cure rates of 80%, expected to rise to 90% in the near future), but the same is not true for adults with ALL.

Death usually occurs as a consequence of the massive lymphocytic proliferation in the bone marrow, where the proliferating cells overwhelm and smother the normal hematopoietic cells.

Classification and Prognosis
ALL can be classified by immunophenotyping (Table 3). The large majority (about 95%) of acute ALL are B-cell derived, because the proliferating cells express the CD19 B-cell marker and have rearranged immunoglobulin genes. Overall, the precursor B-cell leukemia is the most common form of ALL. The remaining 5% of these leukemias are of the T-cell type, express T-cell markers (CD3, CD4, CD8), and have rearranged TcR genes. In addition, leukemic cells of patients with ALL may express enzymes of the purine salvage pathway, particularly terminal deoxynucleotidyl transferase (Tdt), not expressed by mature B lymphocytes but re-expressed in about 80% of all cases of this type of leukemia, when the proliferating populations correspond to earlier stages of T-cell and B-cell differentiation. The measurement of the expression of Tdt is clinically useful, because its levels fall during remission and increase again before a clinically apparent relapse.

T-cell acute lymphocytic leukemia has usually a worse prognosis than B-cell acute lymphocytic leukemia. In addition, the two main types of ALL (B cell and T cell) respond differently to cytotoxic drugs.

Chromosomal and genetic abnormalities are common in ALL and some of them have defined prognostic implications. For example, hyperdiploidy, trisomy 4,10,17, and translocation t(12,21), the most common translocation, are associated with good prognosis, whereas hypodiploidy, trisomy 5, and rarer translocations such as t(1;19) and t(9:22)—the Philadelphia chromosome more frequently associated with acute myeloid leukemia—are associated with poor prognosis. The coexpression of myeloid and lymphoid characteristics by the leukemic cells was also considered as a poor prognosis indicator, but therapeutic progress has blunted the differences. In the end, prognosis is established based on a sum of clinical, immunological, and genetic data.

TABLE 3 Classification of Acute Lymphoblastic Leukemia Based on Immunophenotyping

Group gene	Marker									
	Tdt	HLA-DR	CD19	CD20	sIg	Ig gene rearrangement	CD3	CD5	CD4/CD8	TcR gene rear rearrangement
Early pre-B cell	+	+	+	−	−	+	−	−	−	−
Pre-B cell	+	+	+	+	−	+	−	−	−	−
Mature B cell	−	+	+	+	+	+	−	−	−	−
T cell	+	−	−	−	−	−	+	+	+	+

Management

Chemotherapy with a glucocorticoid, vincristine, and a third agent (asparaginase or anthracy-cline) is commonly used to induce remission with great success (98% rate of complete remission in children and 85% in adults). Once normal hematopoiesis is restored, the patients are placed under intensification therapy, which usually involve methotrexate, 6-mercaptopurine, and pegylated recombinant asparaginase. Allogeneic hematopoietic stem cell transplantation has been used in adults with ALL, but its value is still debated. Finally, continuation treatment with methrotexate and mercaptopurine for at least two years is instituted in most patients with ALL. Newer forms of therapy still in their initial evaluation stages involve drugs aimed at abnormal molecular targets identified in patients with ALL and the use of monoclonal antibodies directed against antigens commonly expressed in ALL, such as CD20 (rituximab) and CD22 (apratuzumab).

Adult T-Cell Leukemia
Etiology

Adult T-cell leukemia (ATL) has the unique feature of being caused by an infectious agent, the human T-lymphotrophic virus 1 (HTLV-1) human retrovirus. It has a very unique geographic distribution, closely associated to the prevalence of HTLV-1 in the population, with particularly high incidence in Japan and the Caribbean basin (where the rates of infection reach endemic proportions); the virus has also been reported, although with lower frequency, in southeastern United States as well as in Central and South America.

HTLV-1 is predominantly transmitted through infected cells, and there are three main routes of transmission—breast feeding, sexual transmission, and parenteral transmission through blood or blood products containing live infected cells. The receptor for HTLV-1 is the glucose transporter type 1, whose expression on T cells is enhanced by transforming growth factor-β. After penetrating T cells, the virus integrates and the infected cell number increases, because the virus promotes proliferation and inhibits apoptosis. The HTLV-1-associated T-cell leukemia develops 10 to 20 years after infection with the virus, but it only develops in a small fraction of the HTLV-1-infected individuals (4–5% of the seropositive individuals).

Pathogenesis

HTLV-1 is an exogenous retrovirus, fully able to replicate and to be transmitted horizontally. Its genome contains a transforming gene, *tax*, whose gene product (Tax protein) is a transcriptional activator of the viral long terminal repeat, thus promoting *HTLV-1* gene expression and genomic replication. In addition, Tax activates the nuclear binding protein NFkB, leading to the permanent overexpression of IL-2 receptors (CD25), and it also induces the activation of the IL-2 promoter. IL-13, IL-15, and IL-15Rα are also upregulated. These changes, associated with direct activating effects of Tax on cyclin-dependent kinases that control cell cycle, could explain the T-cell proliferation associated with HTLV-1. In addition, Tax removes controls that normally would counteract this effect, by inactivating p53 and the Rb gene product. Thus, Tax has both proliferative and antiapoptotic effects. However, the long latency between HTLV-1 and the detection of ATL suggests that other factors must be involved in the final transforming events, which seems to be due to DNA damage caused by Tax. Of note is the fact that fully transformed cells often do not express Tax, suggesting that once the cells have become immortalized and chromosomal aberrations have developed, Tax is no longer required.

Clinical Presentation and Diagnosis

ATL can present as an acute or chronic condition, with or without lymphomatous characteristics. The acute presentation is the most common. The chronic, as well as smoldering forms, usually evolve to assume acute characteristics. Clinical findings include lymphadenopathy, hepatosplenomegaly, osteolytic lesions, and hypercalcemia, secondary to osteoclast activation caused by the excessive release of monocyte-CSF by leukemic cells, and skin lesions. The most common skin lesions are erythroderma and skin ulcerations, and are associated with a dense lymphocytic infiltration of the dermis and epidermis. It is believed that increased venous permeability, probably caused by an increased local concentration of IL-2 and other interleukins, are responsible for the formation of cellular infiltrates, which, in turn, interfere with proper oxygenation of tissues, leading to localized ischemia and necrosis. Some patients present with Sézary syndrome, an exfoliative erythroderma with generalized lymphadenopathy and circulating atypical cells. The skin is the original site of malignant cell proliferation, and the phase of cutaneous lymphoma can last many years with little evidence of extracutaneous dissemination. The leukemic evolution is associated with the invasion of the peripheral by malignant cells. Occasionally, the skin lesions are similar to those that are classically described as mycoses fungoides, where the infiltrating cells in the skin are also CD4$^+$ but no leukemic stage seems to develop.

Patients with ATL are often immunocompromised, as a consequence of several factors, including the shedding of IL-2 receptors from the membrane of the leukemic cells that adsorb IL-2 and block its activating effect on normal T cells. In addition, in ATL, the proliferating CD4$^+$ cells function as suppressor-inducers and turn on cells with suppressor activity.

Diagnosis is based on morphological and phenotypic characteristics of the malignant lymphocytes and confirmation of HTLV-1 infection. The peripheral blood lymphocytes in the more aggressive forms of disease include Sézary syndrome with leukemic evolution; the circulating malignant lymphocytes are often large, with a characteristic polylobulated nucleus (Sézary cells, flower cells).

The phenotype of ATL malignant cells is characterized by the expression of activated T-cell markers, including CD2, CD3, CD4, CD25, and MHC-II complex. Tdt is not expressed.

Management

Chemotherapy with cyclophosphamide, adriamycin, vincristine, and prednisolone is the standard first line therapy, but the response is not very good with complete remissions usually below 20% and survivals ranging from 5.5 to 13 months in patients presenting with acute leukemia or lymphoma.

T-Cell and B-Cell Lymphomas

Most lymphomas are B-cell derived, and they can be grouped into three large groups: Burkitt's lymphoma, Hodgkin's lymphoma, and non-Hodgkin's lymphoma. All groups can be subclassified by a variety of criteria. We refer the readers to hematology publications for the full details about classification and management of lymphomas.

Hodgkin's Lymphoma

Hodgkin's lymphoma has been finally classified as a B-cell lymphoma in the vast majority of the cases, based on evidence of B-cell receptor rearrangement of the Reed–Sternberg cells characteristic of the disease, which are very dedifferentiated and do not express markers that allow their phenotypic definition as B cells. T cell Hodgkin's lymphomas also exist, but are a rarity—1% to 2% of the cases.

The Reed–Sternberg cells show constitutive expression of NFkB and are resistant to apoptosis, as a consequence of the expression of the products of at least two antiapoptotic genes and of a mutated Fas protein (CD95). In addition, these cells produce IL-13 and express the corresponding receptor, creating conditions for an autocrine proliferation circuit. In about 40% of the cases of classical Hodgkin's lymphoma, there is evidence of infection with the Epstein–Barr virus (EBV), and two of the viral-encoded transforming proteins of the EBV [latent membrane protein (LMP1) and LMP2a] are expressed by infected Reed–Sternberg cells. Thus, at least in this 40% of cases, it is possible that EBV infection may play a role in the oncogenic transformation.

A significant feature of Hodgkin's lymphoma is the formation of large cellular infiltrates around the Reed–Sternberg cells, which follow different morphological patterns (basis of the classification of the disease into four subtypes). The infiltrating cells are nonclonal and seem to be attracted by chemokines released by the Reed–Sternberg cells. There is a close interaction between the Reed–Sternberg cells and the infiltrating nonclonal cells, which is essential for the continuing proliferation of the malignant cells.

Non-Hodgkin's Lymphoma

Non-Hodgkin's lymphoma is a designation that encompasses a very heterogeneous group of malignancies affecting the lymphoid tissues. Although they can be divided into B-cell and T-cell lymphomas, the vast majority (90%) are B-cell malignancies. They can be classified by a variety of criteria. The two most common histological entities are follicular lymphoma and diffuse large B-cell lymphoma. Burkitt's lymphoma is usually discussed separately because of the clear association of its African endemic form with EBV.

Follicular lymphomas are usually indolent, presenting with lymphadenopathy, and, as the disease progresses, fever, high sweat, and weight loss may develop. The bone marrow is usually infiltrated, and normal hematopoiesis may be compromised. Hepatosplenomegaly is frequently detected. Large B-cell lymphomas are more aggressive, and although lymphadeno-pathy is present in most patients, extranodal proliferation (gastrointestinal tract, skin, sinuses, thyroid, central nervous system) is common. Systemic symptoms are also more frequent in patients with this type of lymphoma.

Chromosomal translocations are common in non-Hodkin's lymphoma, and usually associated with the expression of antiapototic genes and/or genes that promote cell proliferation.

Management depends largely on staging, which is based on the histological features and the extent of diffusion of the malignancy. Positron emission tomography is the preferred technique for staging. Treatment involves radiation therapy and/or chemotherapy in a variety of combinations according to the extent of lymphatic tissue involvement. Patients with follicular lymphomas usually experience long survival, but only a minority is truly cured. Diffuse large B-cell lymphomas are treated with combinations of chemotherapeutic agents and rituximab. The rate of cure is about 50%.

Burkitt's Lymphoma

Burkitt's lymphoma, endemic in certain areas of Africa and sporadic in the United States, has been characterized as a B-cell lymphoma expressing monotypic surface IgM. Endemic Burkitt's lymphoma is epidemiologically linked to infection of the B lymphocytes with the EBV. The malignant B cells in Burkitt's lymphoma usually express a single EBV gene product, the nuclear antigen EBNA-1, which is essential for establishment of latency, but has no known transforming properties. It is possible that the EBV infection has as its main role promoting a state of active B-cell proliferation that may favor the occurrence of the translocations involving the region of chromosome 8 coding for *c-myc*. Similar translocations are also found in sporadic Burkitt's lymphoma, not linked to EBV infection. A common consequence of the translocations is the overexpression the *c-myc* gene, often mutated, which is believed to be a major factor contributing to the uncontrolled B-cell proliferation characteristic of this disease.

Clinically, Burkitt's lymphoma is usually characterized by the development of a large tumor, either in the angle of the jaw and neck (epidemic form) or in the abdomen (endemic form). Burkitt's lymphoma responds well to chemotherapy, and most adults with the disease are cured.

B-Cell Lymphomas in Immunocompromised Patients

B-cell lymphomas are frequently detected in immunodeficient or iatrogenically immunosuppressed patients. In post-transplant situations [post-transplant lymphoproliferative disorder (PTLD)], the overall incidence is 1% to 2%, with highest rates after heart, heart–lung, intestinal transplantation, and allogeneic stem cell transplantation in T-cell depleted patients. In the majority of these cases, there is evidence of association with viral infection, particularly EBV. A variety of EBV-coded proteins may be expressed on the malignant cells, including six different nuclear antigens and three different membrane proteins. Of the proteins coded by nuclear antigens, EBNA-2 protein has immortalizing properties, transactivating the *cyclin-2* gene and others; EBNA-LP impairs the function of the products of two tumor suppressor genes, p53 and the retinoblastoma gene product; and the LMP-1 is considered as a transforming gene whose activity seems to be mediated by the activation of a Ca^{2+}/calmodulin-dependent protein kinase. In addition, host cell molecular alterations are present in PTLD, including translocation and overexpression of *c-myc*, rearrangement of *BCL-6*, and *p53* mutations.

Patients with AIDS are at increased risk for the development of common as well as some rare types of lymphomas. The risk seems not to be as high for Hodgkin's disease, as it is for non-Hodgkin's lymphoma. Among the rare types of lymphomas that affect AIDS patients, it is worth mentioning the association with Kaposi's sarcoma and primary effusion lymphoma, both caused by the human herpes virus type 8 . The incidence of lymphoma is related to the degree of immunodepression of the patient, and since the introduction of highly active antiretroviral therapy (HAART), the frequency of HIV-infected patients with very low CD4 counts has decreased; with this, there has been an associated decrease in the frequency of lymphoid malignancies. Furthermore, patients that develop lymphoid malignancies but are treated with HAART can tolerate chemotherapy, and their survival is close to that of the general population.

BIBLIOGRAPHY

Bataille R. New insights in the clinical biology of multiple myeloma. Semin Hematol 1997; 34(suppl 1):23–28.

Capello D, Rossi D, Gaidano G. Post-transplant lymphoproliferative disorders: molecular basis of disease and pathogenesis. Hematol Oncol 2005; 23:61–67.

Carbone A, Gloghini A. AIDS related lymphomas: from pathogenesis to pathology. Br J Haematol 2005; 130:662–670.

Dimopoulos MA, Kyle RA, Anagnoistopoulos A, Treon SP. Diagnosis and management of Waldenstrom's macroglobulinemia. J Clin Oncol 2005; 23:1564–1577.

Frydecka I, Kosmaczewska A, Bocko D, et al. Alterations of the expression of T-cell-related costimulatory CD28 and downregulatory CD152 (CTLA-4) molecules in patients with B-cell chronic lymphocytic leukaemia. Br J Cancer 2004; 90:2042–2048.

Gentile M, Mauro FR, Guarini A, Foa R. New developments in the diagnosis, prognosis and treatment of chronic lymphocytic leukemia. Curr Opin Oncol 2005; 17:597–604.

Grassmann R, Aboud M, Jeang K-T. Molecular mechanisms of cellular tranformation by HTLV-1 tax. Oncogene 2005; 24:5976–5985.

Greipp PR, San Miguel J, Durie BGM, et al. International staging system for multiple myeloma. J Clin Oncol 2005; 23:3412–3420.

Hari P, Pasquini MC, Vesole DH. Cure of multiple myeloma—more hype, less reality. Bone Marrow Transplant 2006; 37:1–18.

Klein B. Cytokine, cytokine receptors, transduction signals, and oncogenes in human multiple myeloma. Semin Hematol 1995; 32:4.

Lim ST, Levine A. Recent advances in acquired immunodeficiency syndrome (AIDS)—related lymphoma. CA Cancer J Clin 2005; 55:229–241.

Pui C-H, Evans WE. Treatment of acute lymphoblastic leukemia. N Engl J Med 2006; 354:166–178.

Rajkumar SV, Kyle RA. Multiple myeloma: diagnosis and treatment. Mayo Clin Proc 2005; 80:1371–1382.

Randolph TR. Advances in acute lymphoblastic leukemia. Clin Lab Sci 2004; 17:235–245.

Ravandi F, O'Brien S. Chronic lymphoid leukemias other that chronic lymphocytic leukemia: diagnosis and treatment. Mayo Clin Proc 2005; 80:1660–1674.

Stone MJ, Merlini G, Pascual V. Autoantibody activity in Waldesntrom's macroglobulinemia. Clin Lymphoma 2005; 5:225–229.

Taylor GP, Matsuaka M. Natural history of adult T-cell leukemia/lymphoma and approaches to therapy. Oncogene 2005; 24:6047–6057.

Terpos E, Dimopoulos M-A. Myeloma bone disease: pathophysiology and management. Ann Oncol 2005; 16:1223–1231.

Wahner-Roedler DL, Kyle RA. Heavy chain diseases. Best Pract Res Clin Haematol 2005; 18:729–746.

28 | Diagnosis of Immunodeficiency Diseases

John W. Sleasman
Department of Pediatrics, Division of Allergy, Immunology, and Rheumatology, University of South Florida, St. Petersburg, Florida, U.S.A.

Gabriel Virella
Department of Microbiology and Immunology, Medical University of South Carolina, Charleston, South Carolina, U.S.A.

INTRODUCTION

Immunodeficiency diseases are a major cause of mortality and morbidity worldwide. Immune deficient states can be subdivided into primary immune deficiency diseases due to a hereditary or intrinsic defect in the immune system, or secondary immune deficiency as the result of infection, such as HIV, administration of cytotoxic drugs, as with cancer chemotherapy, or metabolic states, such a malnutrition, that compromise the immune system. Primary immune deficiency diseases provide valuable insight into the nature of the immune response and the physiology of the human immune system.

CLINICAL SIGNS AND SYMPTOMS OF IMMUNE DISORDERS

Most immune deficient states can be classified on the basis of the major component of immunity that are primarily impacted. In general, the immune response can be subdivided into the innate and adaptive immune responses. Innate immune responses consist primarily of nonspecific defense mechanisms mediated by a variety of antimicrobial substances, phagocytic cells, and the complement system (see Chapter 14), while adaptive immunity is antigen specificity, has "memory," and can be subdivided into humoral and cellular immune responses. Defects in each of these components are associated with characteristic clinical presentations that provide clues into the nature of the disorder. A careful and systematic assessment of the clinical history and laboratory evaluation will often lead to the precise nature of the immunodeficiency, and will allow the prompt and effective initiation of a therapeutic intervention.

General Considerations

The clinical diagnosis of a probable immunodeficiency disease is based on a variety of criteria (summarized in Table 1), such as history of recurrent infections, the pattern of infections, length of time to clear the infections, types of infecting organism(s), particularly when involving opportunistic or unusual organisms, and responses to antibiotic therapy. The clinical history should include a complete family history to determine if there are patterns of inheritance such as autosomal codominant, X-linked, or autosomal recessive disease patterns. Questions should include infant deaths due to infections, familial patterns of autoimmune disease, recurrent pneumonia, or spontaneous angioedema among family members. The physical exam should explore findings associated with immune disorders such as failure to thrive and growth retardation, eczema, easy bruising or bleeding, abnormal hair and dentition, skeletal abnormalities, congenital heart disease, history of neonatal tetany, or albinism. One should consider possible causes of secondary immune deficiency, such as HIV infection, as well as the possibility of nonimmune causes of recurrent infections (e.g., cystic fibrosis, occult malignancy, congenital heart disease, and sickle cell anemia). Laboratory results should be interpreted in the context of the patient's age. Finally, if no obvious diagnosis can be made after the initial evaluation is complete, a followup plan for evaluation and further referral should be implemented.

Over half of patients evaluated for recurrent infections will be found to have normal immune systems. Most of these cases will be due to exposures to infections in day care settings or in the work environment. About 30% of patients with recurrent sinopulmonary infections will be found to have underlying allergic disorders and 10% will have a nonimmune chronic condition that predisposes them to infection. Only about 10% of patients evaluated for recurrent infections will be found to have a known primary immune deficiency disease.

Antibody Deficiency

Defective antibody production is the most common cause of primary immunodeficiency accounting for over half of all cases (see Chapter 29). Clinical manifestations of a congenital antibody deficiency are primarily recurrent of severe bacterial sinopulmonary infections beginning after the first year of life as passively acquired maternal antibody wanes. Infections with *Haemophilus influenzae*, *Streptococcus pneumoniae*, and other encapsulated bacterial organisms are most common. Other clinical manifestations include chronic *Giardia* enteritis, *Pseudomonas* sepsis, or chronic inflammatory arthritis.

Cellular Immune Deficiency

Clinical symptoms resulting from primary defects in cellular immunity or combined defects in cellular and antibody immunity begin during the first year of life. Symptoms consist of failure to thrive, chronic mucocutaneous candidiasis, chronic viral infections such as cytomegalovirus or herpes simplex virus, *Pneumocystis jiroveci (carinii)* pneumonia, and unexplained graft-versus-host disease. Children and adults with defective cellular immunity are at increased risk for malignancy, particularly B cell lymphomas or lymphoproliferative diseases driven by Epstein-Barr virus. Defects in cellular immunity should be suspected in infants, and children will also have dysmorphic facies, congenital heart disease, or skeletal abnormalities.

Phagocytic Cell Deficiency

Defective phagocytic cell function commonly is associated with recurrent or chronic infections of the soft tissues such as cellulitis, lymphadenitis, and osteomyelitis. Abscesses and granulomas of the liver, lung, and spleen are also common. Many times, the initial clinical presentation will consist solely of fever of unknown origin until the occult infection can be identified. Oral and periodontal disease is common among patients with phagocytic disorders including chronic necrotizing gingivitis, oral ulcers, and dental abscesses. Poor wound healing and delayed separation of the umbilical cord (more than six weeks after birth) is characteristic of primary phagocytic cell defects. Systemic infections with *Staphylococcus aureus*, *Serratia* spp., *Aspergillus* spp., *Escherichia coli*, and *Pseudomonas aeruginosa* are commonly diagnosed.

Complement Deficiency

Hereditary deficiencies in the complement system have highly variable clinical manifestations that are associated with the particular component of the complement cascade impacted. Defects in regulatory proteins, such as C1 inhibitor, can present with angioedema and are associated with an increased risk for autoimmune disease. Individuals with defects in the early components of the classical complement cascade have and increased risk for bacterial infection and commonly develop autoimmune disease such as systemic lupus erythematosus, rheumatoid arthritis, and glomerulonephritis. Defects in the terminal components of the complement cascade will often develop chronic or recurrent infections by *Neisseria* spp. and also have an increased risk for autoimmune disease (Table 1).

LABORATORY ASSESSMENT OF IMMUNITY

The effective laboratory investigation of an immunodeficiency consists of a step-by-step assessment that correlates with the clinical manifestations of the immune disorder. In order to optimize the use of the clinical laboratory, testing should first focus on quantitative and qualitative

TABLE 1 Clinical Features Suggestive of Primary Immunodeficiency

Defect in antibody-mediated immunity
Recurrent bacterial sinopulmonary infections, particularly involving encapsulated   organisms (e.g., *Haemophilus influenzae, Streptococcus pneumoniae*)
Chronic enteroviral gastroenteritis
Chronic giardiasis
Pseudomonas sepsis
Polyarticular arthritis
Clinical features suggestive of a defect in cell-mediated immunity
Recurrent Viral Infection
Failure to Thrive
Mycotic infections (e.g., fungal pneumonia, mucocutaneous candidiasis)
Pneumocystis jiroveci (formerly *carinii*) pneumonia
Unexplained graft-versus-host disease
Clinical features suggestive of a defect in phagocytic function
Poor wound healing
Delayed separation of the umbilical cord
Soft tissue abscesses and lymphadenitis
Chronic gingivitis and periodontal disease
Mucosal ulcerations
Infections with catalase positive microorganisms (e.g., *Staphyococcus aureus, Serratia marcescens,*   *Aspergillus* spp., *Candida* spp.)
Clinical features suggestive of a defect in the complement system
Angioedema of face, hands, GI tract
Autoimmune disease (e.g., glomerulonephritis, rheumatoid arthritis)
Recurrent pyogenic infections
Recurrent disseminated neisserial infections
Chronic urticaria
Family history suggestion of autosomal dominant inheritance

screening evaluations followed by more expensive and complex testing to pinpoint the precise nature of the disorder and confirm the suspected diagnosis (Fig. 1).

Diagnosis of Antibody Deficiency Diseases

Patients with recurrent bacterial infections are often suspected of having antibody deficiency disease. However, optimal clearance of bacterial pathogens requires not only immunoglobulin synthesis but also cellular phagocytosis, and in some cases, complement activation plays a key role. Furthermore, allergic conditions such as asthma and systemic conditions such as cystic fibrosis often lead to recurrent bacterial pneumonias that mimic antibody deficiency states. A reasonable strategy for screening a patient with suspected antibody deficiency would be to evaluate total antibody levels by measuring immunoglobulin G (IgG), IgA, and IgM and performing a complete blood count with differential to verify that neutrophil and lymphocyte counts are normal. A total IgE to evaluate for elevations that would be associated with allergy, and a total hemolytic complement level to evaluate the complement cascade are part of the initial screening evaluations.

Determination of Serum Immunoglobulin Levels

Immunoglobulin levels must be interpreted in the context of the patient's age since infants and children have lower levels of IgG and IgA when compared to adolescents and adults and, therefore, normal values vary with age (Table 2).

Immunoglobulin assay is a fundamental element in the classification of immunodeficiencies (Table 3). A quantitative depression of one or more of the three major immunoglobulin isotypes is considered as compatible with a diagnosis of humoral immunodeficiency. If all immunoglobulin classes are depressed, the condition is designated as hypogammaglobulinemia. If the depression is very severe, and the combined levels of all three immunoglobulins are below 200 mg/dL, the patient is considered as having severe hypogammaglobulinemia or agammaglobulinemia.

Diagnostic Steps in Evaluating for Primary Immunodeficiency Disease

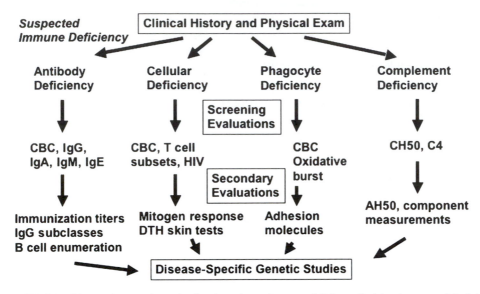

FIGURE 1 Diagnostic steps in evaluating for primary immune deficiency first involve a careful clinical history and physical exam to determine the principal component of the immune system impacted by the disorder. Screening evaluations for antibody, cellular, phagocytic, and complement disorders represent the first steps, and secondary evaluations are preformed based on the screening results. Definitive diagnosis is made on the basis of disease-specific genetic screening. *Abbreviations*: AH50, alternative hemolytic complement 50; CBC, complete blood count; CH50, total hemolytic complement 50.

IgG subclasses can also be measured and the results of the assay may reveal subclass deficiencies. Total IgG concentration might be normal to slightly depressed and one or two of the minor subclasses be deficient. Low or absent IgG4 is common in healthy individuals and its deficiency is not considered to be clinically significant.

Measurement of Functional Antibody

The determination of serum immunoglobulin levels is inadequate to fully evaluate humoral immunity. Measurement of functional antibody is an essential component to the accurate diagnosis of antibody deficiency diseases. These assessments are generally carried out by measuring antibody titers before and after a standard immunization, or measuring isohemagglutinins

TABLE 2 Normal Values for Human Immunoglobulins

	IgG	IgA	IgM
Newborn	636–1606	0	6–25
1–2 months	250–900	1–53	20–87
4–6 months	196–558	4–73	27–100
10–12 months	294–1069	16–84	41–150
1–2 yrs	345–1210	14–106	43–173
3–4 yrs	440–1135	21–159	47–200
5–18 yrs	630–1280	33–200	48–207
8–10 yrs	608–1572	45–236	52–242
Greater than 10 yrs	639–1349	70–312	57–352

Note: In mg/dL, as determined by immunonephelometry in the Department of Laboratory Medicine, Medical University of South Carolina, South Carolina, U.S.A.

TABLE 3 Immunoglobulin Levels in Immune Deficiency (in mg/dL)

Patient	IgG	IgA	IgM	Interpretation
A	850	2.8	128	IgA deficiency
B	1990	39.4	145	IgA deficiency
C	131	28.2	Traces	Severe hypogammaglobulinemia
D	690	16.0	264	IgA deficiency
E	154	60.0	840	Hyper IgM syndrome

Abbreviation: Ig, immunoglobulin.

in the form of anti-A and anti-B antibodies to red blood cell antigens. On the other hand, the need to identify the etiologic agents in patients with recurrent and unusual infections cannot be overstressed. Besides providing very useful treatment for the selection of the most adequate antimicrobial(s), it allows to carry out the most informative test for the diagnosis of a humoral immunodeficiency, that is, the assay of antibodies against the infectious agent. If the patient fails to produce antibodies, the diagnosis is obvious.

Assay of Antibodies After Antigenic Challenge
The response to immunization may be primary or secondary, and the immunogens used to elicit the response are either T-cell dependent or T-cell independent (see Chapter 4). Common T-cell dependent antigens are suitable for use as diagnostic tests include tetanus and diphtheria toxoids and conjugated pneumococcal polysaccharide antigens. Unconjugated *S. pneumoniae* polysaccharides are suitable for the evaluation of the T-independent immune response.

Protective levels to diphtheria and tetanus toxoids are titers greater than 0.01 IU/mL. The usual postimmunization response exceeds 1.0 IU/mL, and when pre-immunization titers are measurable, a four-fold rise above pre-immunization levels is expected. Protective levels to conjugated *H. influenzae* vaccine are greater than 0.15 μg/mL, and the usual postimmunization levels exceed 1.0 μg/mL. Even preterm infants are able to mount antibody responses to T-dependent antigens.

Given the lack of information concerning normal postimmunization values for many antibodies, and the fact that the abnormality searched for is the lack of an active response rather than a low level of antibody, the best approach is to measure pre-immunization titers prior to a boosting with the corresponding antigen and repeat the study with a sample collected three to four weeks later. Following this protocol, we detected active responses in all but two of a group of children randomly selected from the population of a rural county of South Carolina (Fig. 2). The existence of normal nonresponders needs to be considered when evaluating a patient suspected of having an immunodeficiency.

An interesting example of the application of tetanus toxoid immunization is the followup of the humoral immune response after a hematopoietic stem cell transplant. The patients receive immunosuppressive treatments prior to transplantation to prevent graft-versus-host disease, and continue to be immunosuppressed, at least for the first few months, after transplant (see Chapter 27). When myeloid cells are reconstituted and there is no evidence of graft-versus-host disease, immunosuppression is stopped and the patient is then immunized for tetanus toxoid to determine whether the immune function has reconstituted. As illustrated in Figure 3, this recovery may only be observed several months after the suspension of immunosuppressive therapy. It needs to be noted that the immunoglobulin levels may be normal while the patient shows a complete lack of response to immunization.

The antibody response to T-independent antigens is usually measured using the poly-valent (23 serotypes) pneumococcal polysaccharide vaccine. Titers exceeding 2.0 μg/mL or a four-fold rise in at least three serotypes are considered a normal response. Normal children under the age of two cannot respond to T-independent antigens. The results to polysaccharide vaccination should be interpreted cautiously in children who have previously received the conjugated pneumococcal vaccine that includes serotypes—the seven most common invasive serotypes causing infection in the United States and Europe.

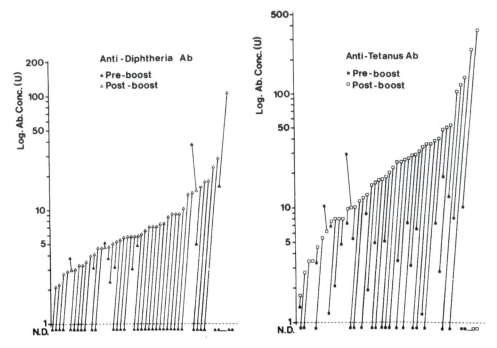

FIGURE 2   Pre- and post-booster antibody titers to diphtheria and tetanus toxoid determined in 46 healthy children between 16 and 33 months of age. *Source*: Reproduced from Virella G, Fudenberg HH, Kyong CU, Pandey JP, Galbraith RM. Z Immunitatsforsch 1978; 155:80.

Induction of a Primary Immune Response

When patients are receiving immune globulin therapy it is difficult of evaluate antibody production in vivo since the majority of circulating antibodies will be passively acquired from the gammaglobulin donor pool. In this case, or if measurement of response to a

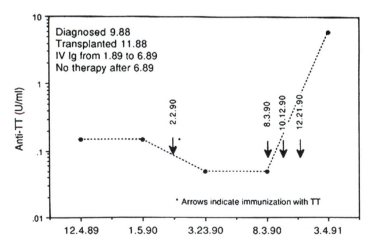

FIGURE 3   Graphic representation of a longitudinal study of the serum levels of anti-tetanus toxoid (anti-TT) antibodies in a patient who received a bone marrow graft in December 1988. The patient received intravenous gammaglobulin from January to June 1989, as anti-infectious prophylaxis. The clinical evolution was excellent, and all therapy (immunosuppressive and immunoprophylactic) was discontinued in June 1989. The first assay of anti-TT antibody in December 1989 showed that the patient had low levels of antibody (0.15 U/mL). A first immunization with TT in February 1990 was followed by a paradoxical decrease of anti-TT antibody concentration. Only after three additional boosters given between August and February of 1991 was there a significant increase in anti-TT antibody concentration. At that time, the patient could be judged as immunologically recovered.

primary immunogen is needed, immunization with an antigen to which natural exposure is highly unlikely is of clinical value. Antibodies to these antigens will not be present in the donor pool so that any detectable antibody will be from the patient being immunized. The bacteriophage ϕX-174 is a highly immunogenic T-cell dependent neoantigen used in vivo to assess both primary and secondary antibody responses, and designated by WHO Committee on Primary Immunodeficiency as a standard, potent, and safe antigen for assessment of immune response in humans (Fig. 4). Antibodies to ϕX-174 produced by the immunized subject are used to neutralize the phage in a reverse lytic plaque assay. Phage immunization has been carried out by several groups in different countries and has been proven to be a nonpathogenic and harmless. A second alternative that has had limited use is keyhole limpet hemocyanin; a large protein extracted from a mollusk, which is strongly immunogenic even when injected without adjuvant. A significant advantage of this antigen is that antibody assay can be done by a conventional enzymoimmunoassay.

Enumeration of B Lymphocytes

The finding of an immunoglobulin deficiency or of the inability to mount a humoral immune response does not give many clues as to the pathogenesis of the defect. Besides the possibility of dealing either with a primary or a secondary immunodeficiency, which implies the need

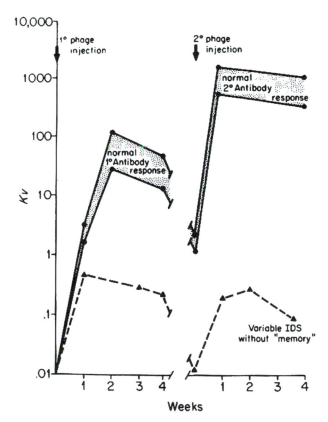

FIGURE 4 Primary and secondary antibody responses elicited by immunization with bacteriophage ØX 174 in a patient with suspected humoral immunodeficiency. The shaded area between the solid lines indicates the range for normal responses. The patient's response, indicated by the interrupted line, showed a definite but diminished antibody response; the secondary response was not greater than the primary—no memory/ amplification occurred. The immunoglobulin class of antibody in both primary and secondary responses was entirely IgM. *Source*: Reproduced from Wedgewood RJ, Ochs, HD, Davis SD. The recognition and classification of immunodeficiency disease with bacteriophage phiChi 174. Birth Defects: Original Article Series 1975; 11:331.

to investigate known causes of secondary immunodeficiency, primary humoral immunodeficiencies may result from a variety of defects, such as absence or lack of differentiation of B cells, defects in intracellular synthesis, assembly, or secretion of immunoglobulins, deficient helper T cell function, and other causes discussed in greater detail in Chapter 29.

The number of B lymphocytes in the peripheral blood is determined by using cytometry analysis to calculate the percentage of peripheral blood lymphocytes (PBL) with specific B lymphocyte markers (usually CD19 or CD20). B cells usually represent between 4% and 10% of the circulating lymphocytes, corresponding to a range of 96–421 CD19$^+$ cells/μL. If the number of B cells in the peripheral blood is significantly depressed, the immunodeficiency is most likely the result of deficient B cell differentiation, particularly in infantile agammaglobulinemia (see Chapter 29). Studies of B cell differentiation in vivo can be accomplished by examining tissues for germinal centers and immunoglobulin-producing plasma cells in a lymph node tissues or rectal biopsy.

Enumeration of T Helper Cells and Cells Expressing the CD40 Ligand

The number of CD4$^+$ T lymphocytes in the peripheral blood is also a critical parameter that needs to be determined, because in some types of common, variable, immunodeficiency and of combined immunodeficiency the main defect may be a deficient CD4 T cell population.

The determination of the number of T cells expressing the CD40 ligand (CD40L, gp39), one of the membrane molecules involved in T–B cell interactions and signaling, is critical for the diagnosis of the hyper-IgM syndrome (see Chapter 29).

Investigation of B-Cell Function In Vitro

The investigation of B cell function in vitro requires separation of PBL and their stimulation with substances known to induce the proliferation and/or differentiation of B lymphocytes. Several substances have been used as B cell mitogens, but pokeweed mitogen (PWM), a plant lectin that induces proliferation and differentiation of T and B lymphocytes, is the most widely used. The effects of this mitogen on B lymphocytes are T-cell dependent but when immunoglobulin synthesis is used as the endpoint, the assay measures PWM-induced functional differentiation of B lymphocytes.

Laboratory Assessment of Cell-Mediated Immunity

Screening evaluations for patients suspected of having defects in cell-mediated immunity consist of a total lymphocyte count, enumeration of CD3, CD4 and CD3, CD8 T cell subsets, functional testing using delayed hypersensitivity skin testing, and assessment of HIV antibody status to ensure that there is no evidence of secondary T-cell deficiency as a result of HIV infection.

Flow Cytometry of T Cell Subpopulations

Using flow cytometry T cell subpopulations can be accurately enumerated in the clinical laboratory. In healthy children and adults CD3$^+$ T cells make up 60% to 70% of the total lymphocyte count. Children have higher lymphocyte counts and high absolute T-cell counts when compared to adults. The normal ratio of CD4 to CD8 T cells is greater than 1.0 and generally approaches 2:1. B cells make up less than 10%, and the remaining lymphocytes are natural killer (NK) cells and gamma/delta T cells. The sum of these cells should roughly add up to 100% and represent the total lymphocyte number. Other useful T cell markers include CD45RA and CD62L, which identify naïve T cells that have recently left the thymus, CD45RO which identifies memory T cells, and activation markers such as human leukocyte antigens (HLA)-DR, CD38, and CD25 (a marker for the IL-2 receptor). NK cells are identified by the surface markers of CD16 and CD56. The normal distribution of lymphocyte subpopulations in a normal adult is shown in Table 4. Quantitative abnormalities may range from complete absence or pronounced deficiency of all T cells, as detected with CD3 antibodies, to low CD4$^+$ T cells and elevated CD8 T cells, as is seen during HIV infection.

TABLE 4 Distribution of the Major Human Lymphocyte Subpopulations in Peripheral Blood, as Determined by Flow Cytometry

CD marker	Lymphocyte subpopulation	Normal range (%)	Normal range (absolute count)
CD19, CD20	B lymphocytes	4–20	96–421 cells/μL
CD3	T lymphocytes	62–85	700–2500 cells/μL
CD2	T lymphocytes; NK cells	70–88	840–2800 cells/μL
CD4	Helper T cells	34–59	430–1600 cells/μL
CD8	Cytotoxic T cells	16–38	280–1100 cells/μL

Note: Values obtained at the Flow Cytometry Laboratory, Department of Pathology and Laboratory Medicine, Medical University of South Carolina, Charleston, SC, U.S.A.
Abbreviations: CD, cluster of differentiation; NK cells, natural killer cells.

In Vivo Testing of Delayed-Type Hypersensitivity

Delayed hypersensitivity responses, are discussed in greater detail in Chapter 20. Primarily, they are mediated by activated T lymphocytes migrating to the dermis where the antigen is associated to dermal dendritic cells. The result is a hyperstimulation of cell-mediated immunity in a localized area where the antigen was injected. Using controlled conditions, it is possible to challenge individuals with antigens known to cause this type of reactions as a way to explore their cell-mediated immunity. The two classical approaches to measure delayed-type hypersensitivity responses in vivo are skin testing and induction of contact sensitivity.

Skin Testing

Skin testing, first described by Koch in 1891, is based on eliciting a secondary response to an antigen to which the patient was previously sensitized. A small amount of soluble antigen is injected intradermally on the extensor surface of the forearm. The antigens used are usually microbial in origin [e.g., purified protein derivative of tuberculin, tetanus toxoid, mumps antigens, and a variety of fungal extracts, including Candidin (from *Candida albicans*), coccidioidin (from *Coccidioides immitis*), and histoplasmin (from *Histoplasma capsulatum*)].

The area of the skin receiving the injection is observed for the appearance of erythema and induration, which are measured at 24 and 48 hours after the injection. A positive skin test is usually considered to be associated with an area of induration greater than 10 mm in diameter, but in patients with acquired immunodeficiency disease induration greater than 5 mm in diameter is considered positive. If no reaction is observed, the test may be repeated with a higher concentration of antigen.

If a patient has no reaction after being tested with a battery of antigens, it is assumed that a state of anergy exists. Anergy can be caused by immunological deficiencies, infections (such as measles or chronic disseminated tuberculosis), but it can also be the result of errors in the technique of skin testing.

Although these tests have the theoretical advantage of testing the function of the T-cell system in vivo, they meet with a variety of problems. On one hand, skin tests are difficult to reproduce, due to the difficulty in obtaining consistency among different sources and batches of antigens, and to variations in the technique of inoculation among different investigators. On the other hand, the interpretation of negative tests has to be carefully weighed. Negative results after challenge with antigens to which there is no record of previous exposure can always be questioned, while a negative result with an antigen extracted from a microbial agent, which has been documented as causing disease in the patient, has a much stronger diagnostic significance, implying a functional defect in cell-mediated immunity.

In Vitro Assays of T-Cell Function

There are limitations to the interpretation of numerical data, given the very loose correlation between membrane markers and biological function. However, numerical data are simpler and cheaper to obtain than functional data, which usually requires cell isolation and which is obtained in conditions that are anything but physiological (see Chapter 15). Human lymphocytes can be stimulated in vitro by specific antigens or by mitogenic substances.

Mitogenic Stimulation Assays

Cellular responses to mitogens are more quantitative and reproducible than delayed hypersensitivity responses elicited by skin testing. Mitogens activate nonspecifically large numbers of lymphocytes to induce cellular proliferation that can be quantitatively estimated by measuring the uptake of tritiated thymidine [^{3}H-Tdr] in the in vitro culture system by the stimulated cells. The most commonly used T lymphocyte mitogens are plant lectins such as phytohemagglutin and concanavalin A, which activate T cells only, and pokeweed mitogen, which activates both T and B lymphocytes. Cross-linking T cell signaling pathways with immobilized monoclonal antibodies directed at CD3 and CD28 induce similar responses. Thymidine uptake by cells activated by the mitogen is compared to proliferation of lymphocytes incubated in media alone. Results are expressed as a stimulation index that divides the optimal [^{3}H-Tdr] uptake in the presence of the mitogen by the unstimulated control. In normal individuals the mitogen stimulation index is 10- to 20-fold greater than the media control. Defects in T cell signaling pathways result in mitogen responses many fold lower than those of normal individuals. Lymphocyte proliferation responses to mitogens are very useful in the diagnosis of many of the T cell immune disorders discussed in Chapter 29.

Response to Antigenic Stimulation

The study antigen-specific T cell responses of lymphocytes in vitro may be more relevant, but the proportion of responding T cells is much lower, generally less than 1% of the cells in culture. As a result, proliferation response and [^{3}H-Tdr] update is lower, and a normal stimulation index to recall antigens is only three to five times above the media control.

The probabilities of obtaining a measurable response can be increased if the lymphocytes are stimulated with antigens to which the lymphocyte donor has been previously exposed, and the cultures are incubated with the antigen for five to seven days prior to addition of ^{3}H-Tdr.

Diagnostic Evaluation of Phagocytic Cell Function

Phagocytic cell function tests have been discussed in detail in Chapter 13. Basically, three sets of tests are commonly used to evaluate a possible phagocytic cell deficiency. A complete blood count with differential is essential because the most common phagocytic cell deficiency is iatrogenically induced neutropenia. The expression of CD11/18 markers on neutrophil and monocyte cell membranes is the most efficient way to rule out adhesion molecule deficiencies, which are extremely rare. Finally, a variety of tests can be used to measure the superoxide burst after ingestion of opsonized particles to investigate killing defects, such as those associated with chronic granulomatous disease—by far the most common form of primary phagocytic cell deficiency.

Diagnostic Evaluation of Complement Function

The complement system can be activated by three different pathways, as discussed in Chapter 9. All three pathways utilize C3 and the membrane attack complex (MAC), and the common effects of complement activation are opsonization, chemotaxis, and cell lysis.

Primary screening tests for complement deficiencies include the CH50 and AH50 assays. The total hemolytic complement assay (CH50) utilizes sheep erythrocytes coated with rabbit antisera. When complement is added and binds to the antibody coating the sheep blood cells, the classical pathway is activated, the red cells are lysed, and hemoglobin is released into the supernatant, which can be measured using a spectrophotometer. A standard dilution of complement, used as reference, causes hemolysis of 50% of the red cells in the test. Since all complement components are necessary for the MAC any absent factor in the classical or alternative pathway will prevent activation of the lytic sequence and the result of the CH50 assay will be 0%. If any component is low, but not absent, such as in states of complement consumption or in heterozygous individuals with genetic complement deficiencies, the concentration of patient sera needed to achieve 50% lysis of red cells will be much higher than controls and the calculated CH50 will be lower than normal. The alternative pathway hemolytic 50 (AH50) is based on the same principal except that red cell lysis is induced in the absence of antibody by rabbit erythrocytes, which are potent nonspecific activators of the alternative complement cascade. The results of the CH50 and AH50 assays can be used to identify which component of the complement cascade is deficient. Defects in C3 or the membrane attack complex, common to both pathways, will result in abnormal AH50 and CH50. A low CH50 with normal AH50 points to a defect in the initial components of the classical pathway. A low AH50 with normal CH50 points to an abnormality in the initial components of the alternative pathway. The next step is to use specific assays for different complement components and their fragments; to determine which complement component is deficient.

Molecular Genetic Studies

The genes involved in most of the characterized primary immune deficiency diseases have been identified and mapped. Confirming the genetic mutation is essential for the initiation of a rationale treatment plan, the identification of carriers, and in effective family counseling. While some primary immune deficiencies, such as DiGeorge syndrome, can be diagnosed on the basis of chromosomal cytogenetic studies (see Chapter 29), the majority of primary immune disorders are the result of single gene mutations, deletions, or duplications that require careful sequencing of the genetic regions and cannot be detected by karyotyping alone. The advent of DNA and RNA based techniques now allow clinicians to accurately diagnosis the majority of primary immune disorders if the patient has been sufficiently characterized by the laboratory-based assays described in this chapter. Many patients may lack a strong family history for the suspected underlying genetic mutation because as many as 40% of newly diagnosed patients with known primary immune disorders represent new mutations within the family. All family members at risk should be screened based on the family history and in suspected mode of inheritance. Diagnosis is usually based on the sequencing of DNA or cDNA obtained from DNA amplified, using polymerase chain reaction amplification.

BIBLIOGRAPHY

Barclay AN et al. The Leukocyte Antigen Facts Book. Oxford (U.K.): Academic Press, 1993.

Conley ME, Notarangelo LD, Eizioni A. Diagnostic criteria for primary immunodeficiencies. Clin Immunol 1999; 93:190–197.

Cooper MD, Lanier LL, Conley ME, Puck JM. Immunodeficiency disorders. Hematology (Am Soc Hematol Educ Program) 2003; 314–330.

Denny TN, Oleske JM. Flow cytometry in pediatric immunologic diseases. Clin Immunol Newsletter 1991; 11:65.

Gergen P, McQuillan GM, Kiely M, Ezzati-Rice TM, Sutter RW, Virella G. Serologic immunity to tetanus in the U.S. population: Implications for national vaccine programs. N Engl J Med 1995; 332(12):761–766.

Hanson LÅ, Sodertrom R, Nilssen DE, et al. IgG subclass deficiency with or without IgA deficiency. Clin Immunol Immunopathol 1991; 61(part 2):S70.

Lim MS, Elenitoba-Johnson KSJ. The molecular pathology of primary immunodeficiencies. J Mol Diagn 2004; 6:59–83.

Lougaris V, Badoloato R, Ferrari S, Plebani A. Hyper immunoglobulin M syndrome due to CD40 deficiency: clinical, molecular, and immunological features. Immunol Rev 2005; 203:48–66.

Rose NR, de Macario EC, eds. Manual of Clinical Immunology, 4th ed., Am Soc Microbiol, Washington, DC, 1992.

Wen L, Atkinson JP, Giclas PC. Clinical and laboratory evaluation of complement deficiency. J Clin Immunol 2004; 113:585–593.

29 | Primary Immunodeficiency Diseases

John W. Sleasman
*Department of Pediatrics, Division of Allergy, Immunology, and Rheumatology,
University of South Florida, St. Petersburg, Florida, U.S.A.*

Gabriel Virella
*Department of Microbiology and Immunology, Medical University of South Carolina,
Charleston, South Carolina, U.S.A.*

INTRODUCTION

Primary immunodeficiencies can be classified by a variety of criteria, such as the main limb of the immune system affected, the spectrum of infections, their primary or secondary nature, and, in the case of hereditary primary immunodeficiencies, their mechanism of genetic transmission (Table 1). Most of the known primary immunodeficiency diseases, as classified by the International Union of Immunological Societies, are listed in Table 2. This chapter reviews some of the more common and well-characterized primary immune disorders, in order to discuss their clinical relevance and to review their mechanism of disease. Many of these disorders have provided great insight into the function of the normal human immune response.

HUMORAL IMMUNODEFICIENCIES

Humoral immunodeficiencies are those in which antibody synthesis is predominantly impaired. The general characteristics of the most common primary immunodeficiencies included in this group are summarized in Table 3. Patients with primary humoral immunedeficiency generally do not develop clinical symptoms until after the first year of life and the disappearance of maternally derived IgG. As summarized in Chapter 28, the most frequent clinical symptoms of defective antibody production are recurrent sinopulmonary infections with encapsulated bacterial pathogens, such as *Haemophilus influenzae* and *Streptococcus pneumoniae*.

X-Linked Infantile Agammaglobulinemia

This is the prototype of "pure" B-cell deficiency. The defective gene is located on Xq21.2–22, the locus coding for the B-cell progenitor kinase or Bruton's tyrosine kinase (Btk). Patients may have mutations at different sites within the locus, resulting in either the lack of synthesis of the kinase or in the synthesis of a nonfunctional protein. Btk plays an important role in B-cell differentiation and maturation, and is also a part of the group of tyrosine kinases involved in B-cell signaling. Most mutations affecting Btk are associated with infantile agammaglobulinemia, but some patients with similar mutations have mild forms of immunodeficiency with variable levels of immunoglobulin production. These findings suggest that B-cell differentiation may depend on additional factors, not yet identified. There are other more rare forms of infantile agammaglobulinemia. These defects are autosomal recessive, and some have been associated with deletions of genes encoding parts of either the Vλ region or of the Cμ heavy chain region. Such deletions are associated with a total lack of differentiation of B lymphocytes, similar to the defect seen in patients with Btk deficiency.

Pathogenesis

The hallmark of infantile agammaglobulinemia is the lack of B lymphocytes in blood and tissues. This B-cell maturation arrest, early in development, differentiates it from other

TABLE 1 Criteria for Classification of Immunodeficiency States

By their range
  Broad spectrum
  Restricted ("antigen-selective")
By their etiology
  Primary
  Secondary
By the limb of the immune system predominantly affected
  Humoral immune deficiencies
  Cellular immune deficiencies
  Combined immune deficiencies
  Phagocyte dysfunction syndromes
  Complement deficiencies
By the mechanism of transmission
  Genetically transmitted
    X-linked
    Autosomal recessive
    Autosomal dominant
  Sporadic

forms of antibody deficiency. Quantitative immunoglobulin levels are low for all isotypes, although some "leaky" patients have been described who produce low levels of immunoglobulins. Histological examination of lymphoid tissues shows lack of germinal centers and secondary follicles in lymph nodes and peri-intestinal lymphoid tissues. Plasma cells are absent both from peripheral lymphoid tissues and from bone marrow. Adenoids, tonsils, and peripheral lymph nodes are hypoplastic. The thymus has normal structure and the T-cell dependent areas in peripheral lymphoid organs are normally populated. In BtK deficiency, normal numbers of B-cell precursors can be demonstrated in the bone marrow, indicating that the basic defect is a maturation block, restricted to B-cell development. Total peripheral blood lymphocyte counts, T lymphocyte cell subsets, and T lymphocyte function are normal.

Clinical Presentation

Infectious symptoms usually begin early in infancy, generally after the first year, as maternally acquired IgG disappears. The patients most commonly suffer from repeated infections of the sinopulmonary system caused by common pyogenic bacteria (*S. pneumoniae, Pseudomonas aeruginosa, and H. influenzae*). Pyoderma, purulent conjunctivitis, polyarticular arthritis, otitis media, sinusitis, and bronchitis are common clinical findings. Severe, life-threatening infections, such as pneumonia, empyema, meningitis, and septicemia, are frequent. Without gammaglobulin replacement therapy, chronic obstructive lung disease and bronchiectasis develop as a consequence of repeated bronchopulmonary infections. Chronic diarrhea and malabsorption caused by infection with *Giardia lamblia* are seen more frequently in these patients than in the general population. Arthritis of the large joints develops in about 30% to 35% of the cases, and is sometimes associated with infection by *Ureaplasma urealyticum*. Patients are at risk of developing paralytic polio after vaccination with the live attenuated polio vaccine. They also are at risk of developing chronic viral meningoencephalitis and other clinical manifestations of systemic infection by echovirus, particularly ECHO 11.

Diagnosis

The lack of B lymphocytes in peripheral blood (less than 2% of the circulating lymphocytes are CD19$^+$), as determined using flow cytometry, is sufficient to confirm the diagnosis. The serum levels for the three major immunoglobulins (IgG, IgA, and IgM) are greater than 2 standard deviations (SD) below the normal level for children of the same age, although, in infants, low IgG levels are often masked by the presence of maternal antibody. However, infants will fail to develop isohemagglutinin antibodies. Usually, the sum of the three major

TABLE 2   Classifications of Primary Immunodeficiencies

Predominant antibody defects
  X-linked agammaglobulinemia
  Autosomal recessive agammaglobulinemia
    Kappa chain deficiency
    Immunoglobulin heavy chain deletions
  Hyper IgM syndromes
    X-linked
    AID defect
    CD40 deficiency
  Common variable immunodeficiency
  Selective IgA deficiency
  IgG subclass deficiency
  Selective deficiency of other immunoglobulin isotypes
  Antibody deficiency with normal or hypergammaglobulinemia
  Transient hypogammaglobulinemia of infancy
Combined antibody and cellular immunodeficiency
  $T^- B^+$ SCID
    X-linked γ-chain deficient
    JAK 3 deficiency
  $T^- B^-$ SCID
    RAG deficiency
    Adenosine deaminase deficiency
  Omenn syndrome
  MHC class I deficiency (TAP-2)
  MHC class II deficiency
  T cell receptor signaling defects
    CD3γ or CD3ε deficiency
    CD8 deficiency (ZAP 70 deficiency)
  Purine nucleoside phosphorylase deficiency
Other cellular immunodeficiencies
  DiGeorge's Anomaly
  Wiscott Aldrich syndrome
  Ataxia-telangiectasia
Phagocytic dysfunction
  Chronic granulomatous disease
  Leukocyte adhesion deficiency
  Severe congenital neutropenia (Kostmann syndrome)
  Cyclic neutropenia (elastase deficiency)
  Leukocyte mycobacterial defects
    Interferon-γ receptor deficiency
    IL-12 receptor deficiency
    STAT 1 deficiency
Immunodeficiencies associated with lymphoproliferative disease
  X-linked lymphoproliferative disease
  Fas ligand deficiency
  Complement deficiency
  C1 inactivator deficiency (hereditary angiodema)
    Inherited deficiency of complement classical pathway component: C1q, C1r, C1s, C4, C3,
      C5, C6, C7, C8, and C9
    Inherited deficiency of complement alternative pathway component: factor I (C3b inactivator)
      deficiency; factor P; factor D

Abbreviations: AID, activation-induced (cytosine) deaminase; MHC, major histocompatibility complex; SCID, severe, combined immunodeficiency; TAP, transporters associated with antigen processing.
Source: Modified from Chapel H, Geha R, Rosen F, and the IUIS PID (Primary Immunodificiencies) Classification committee. Primary immunodeficiency diseases: an update. Clin Exp Immunol 2003; 132:9–15.

immunoglobulin isotypes is less than 100 mg/dL, and electrophoresis fails to show a gamma globulin peak.

    Criteria for the definitive diagnosis of X-linked agammaglobulinemia requires at least one of the following: (*i*) DNA sequencing that detects of Btk mutations, (*ii*) absence of Btk mRNA or lack of Btk protein in monocytes or platelets by Western blot analysis, or (*iii*) maternal male relatives with less than 2% CD19$^+$ B cells.

TABLE 3 Summary of the Main Characteristics of Primary Humoral Immune Deficiencies

Characteristic	Infantile agammaglobulinemia	Hyper-IgM syndrome[a]	Common variable immunodeficiency[b]	IgA deficiency[c]	Transient hypogammaglobulinemia of infancy
Genetics	Usually X-linked	Usually X-linked	Variable	?	?
Molecular basis	Lack of Bruton's tyrosine kinase	Lack of expression of CD40L	Variable	Variable	Unknown
Lymphoid tissues	Lack of development of B-cell territories (follicles)	Normal	Follicular necrobiosis, reticulum cell hyperplasia	Normal	Normal
B lymphocytes	Very low to absent	Normal or elevated numbers	Normal or increased numbers, abnormal differentiation or function	Normal numbers	Normal numbers
Serum immunoglobulins	Very low	Low IgG and IgA, high IgM	Low to very low levels	IgA <10 mg/dL	Low for age
Infections	Bacterial (pyogenic), parasitic (*Giardia*), viral (enteroviruses)	Bacterial, fungal (*Pneumocystis*), parasitic (*Cryptosporidium*)	Bacterial, viral (enteroviruses), parasitic (*Giardia*)	Bacterial, parasitic (*Giardia*)	Bacterial
Treatment	IVIg	IVIg, GCSF, prophylactic antibiotics, stem cell transplantation	IVIg	IVIg (when associated to IgG subclass deficiency)	IVIg (if the infant suffers from severe infections)

[a]Impaired cell-mediated immunity and neutropenia are associated with the B-cell deficiency.
[b]About one-third of patients have abnormal T cell numbers and/or function; autoimmune disease, granulomatous infections, and gastrointestinal malignancy are increased in incidence.
[c]Often associated with gastrointestinal disease and/or autoimmune disease.
Abbreviations: GCSF, granulocyte colony stimulating factors; IVIg, intravenous gammaglobulin.

Therapy

The primary strategy in therapy of infantile agammaglobulinemia is the prevention of infections using replacement gammaglobulin therapy (see later). Aggressive treatment of infections with antibiotics and clinical monitoring for the known complications of agammaglobulinemia is the standard medical care. The administration of live attenuated vaccines is contraindicated in these patients.

Hyper-Immunoglobulin M Syndrome

The hyper IgM syndrome results from the failure of B cell to undergo immunoglobulin class switch, resulting in low levels of IgG, IgA, and IgD in association to an elevation of IgM. In about 70% of the cases, the molecular abnormality is an X-linked inherited mutation of the CD40 ligand (CD40L, CD159) gene, located on Xq26–27. As a consequence, T cells do not express CD40L, and the signals mediated by CD40L–CD40 interactions are not delivered. This signal is essential for B-lymphocyte differentiation and switching from IgM synthesis to the synthesis of other immunoglobulin classes. In addition to the failure to switch from IgM to IgG (IgA, IgE) synthesis during an immune response, germinal centers do not differentiate in the peripheral lymphoid tissues.

There are three autosomal recessive variants of hyper IgM syndrome. Two of the variants have been described due to defects in activation-induced cytidine deaminase or uracil nucleoside glycosylase. These enzymes are involved in the processes of isotype switching and somatic hypermutation of immunoglobulin genes. A third variant is due to the absence of CD40 on B lymphocytes.

Clinical Presentation

Symptoms develop during the first five years of life. The most common manifestation is an increased frequency of pyogenic infections. There is also associated neutropenia that increases the predisposition for pyogenic and other opportunistic infections. Unlike other humoral immunodeficiencies, patients with defective CD40L or CD40 consistently have impaired cell-mediated immunity. They carry a high increased risk for *Pneumocystis jerovici (carinii)* pneumonia, chronic malabsorbtion, and diarrhea due to cryptosporidium. Aplastic anemia following infection with parvovirus B19 infection has been reported. Production of autoantibodies is common and patients have an increased risk for lymphoproliferative syndromes, biliary carcinomas, and biliary cirrhosis.

Diagnosis

The association of normal or high IgM levels with low IgG and IgA levels is the most consistent diagnostic clue among all types of hyper IgM syndrome. The numbers of T and B cells are normal or elevated. T-cell proliferation responses to mitogens are normal, but the cytokine release patterns are usually abnormal. B cells also respond to mitogenic stimulation, but produce IgM only. Definitive diagnosis of the different forms of X-linked hyper IgM syndrome can be made either by the examination of gene sequences bearing CD40L mutations or by assessment of CD40L expression on T cells. To diagnose the variant forms, it is necessary to detect either the defects of uracil nucleoside glycosylase and activation-induced cytidine deaminase or lack of CD40 on B cells.

Therapy

Replacement gammaglobulin therapy can correct the antibody deficiency but does not correct all of the immune defects associated with the hyper IgM syndrome. Neutropenia can be treated with granulocyte colony stimulating factors (G-CSF) and prophylaxis with trimethoprim-sulfamethoxazole is indicated to prevent *Pneumocystis* pneumonia. When feasible, hematopoietic stem cell (HSC) transplant should be considered.

Common, Variable Immunodeficiency or Acquired Hypogammaglobulinemia

This immunodeficiency derives its designation as the most common form of hypogamma-globulinemia diagnosed in adults and its variable pathogenesis. The disorder is extremely heterogeneous in its etiology but all forms share hypogammaglobulinemia, with the presence of B cells, and variability in the age of onset (usually after two years of age, most frequently between 15 and 35 years of age). The clinical signs and symptoms are similar to agammaglobulinemia.

Physiopathology

Most variants of common, variable immunodeficiency (CVID) have normal or increased numbers of B lymphocytes in peripheral blood, but the B cells often express immature maturation markers and their differentiation into plasma cells is defective. About a third of patients have abnormal T-cell numbers and function, including inverted CD4/CD8 T-cell ratios, increased activation markers, and decreased response to mitogenic stimulation. Recently, genetic defects in the inducible costimulatory molecule and genes in the TNF receptor family transmembrane activator and calcium-modulator and cyclophillin ligand interactor , which mediates isotype switching in B cells, were found to present in 10% to 20% of patients with CVID. It is likely that new genetic defects in B-cell signaling will be discovered to elucidate the etiologies of CVID.

Clinical Presentation

Similar to other disorders of antibody production, sinopulmonary infections with encapsulated bacteria such as *H. influenzae, Moraxella catarrhalis*, and *S. pneumoniae* are common and often lead to chronic obstructive pulmonary disease and bronchiectasis. Similarly, the risk for chronic giardiasis is increased, and can lead to malabsorption. In addition, celiac disease is commonly associated with CVID. About 10% of the patients develop granulomatous lympho-cytic interstitial lung disease, hypersplenism, and granulomatous hepatitis that can lead to portal hypertension and liver failure. Clinical features that differentiate common variable immunodeficiency from infantile agammaglobulinemia and other forms of hypogammaglobulinemia are the increased incidence of autoimmune disease, as well as of malignancy, particularly within the gastrointestinal system. The most frequent autoimmune conditions diagnosed in these patients include idiopathic thrombocytopenic purpura and autoimmune hemolytic anemia. Other autoimmune diseases associated with CVID include pernicious anemia, arthritis, inflammatory arthritis, sprue, autoimmune thyroiditis, and polymyositis. The development of inflammatory complications and maligancies has been reported to be more frequent among patients with CVID, with low to absent numbers of memory B cells.

Diagnosis

The main diagnostic criteria for CVID are antibody deficiency developing after two years of age with poor functional antibody, as measured by the response to both polysaccharide and protein vaccines, or lack of isohemagglutinins. Other causes of hypogammaglobulinemia need to be excluded. Serum immunoglobulin levels are variably depressed. Measurement of IgG and IgA greater than 2 SDs below the normal level for age is necessary for a probable diagnosis of CVID, but some patients may only show a significant decrease in only one of the major immunoglobulin isotypes (IgG, IgA, or IgM).

In contrast to what is observed in infantile agammaglobulinemia, these patients have normal or increased numbers of B lymphocytes in peripheral blood, and those B cells can often be stimulated in vitro to produce immunoglobulins. Lymphoid tissues and tonsils, lymph nodes, and spleen may be enlarged. Lymph node biopsies show morphological changes including necrobiosis of the follicles (also seen in the spleen) and/or reticular cell hyperplasia (which may be the major contributing factor for the development of lymphadeno-pathy and splenomegaly).

Treatment

Overall, therapy is similar to that for congenital agammaglobulinemia. Special emphasis should be directed toward preventing pneumonia and progression to bronchiectasis. Gamma-globulin therapy should be administered at a dose to maintain levels at greater than 600 mg/dL at all times (see gammaglobulin therapy). Frequent monitoring for malignancy, autoimmunity, and infections is the standard medical care for these patients.

Selective Immunoglobulin Deficiencies

Together, these are the most common of the antibody deficiency disorders. They have variable clinical manifestations; from asymptomatic to recurrent infections requiring immunoglobulin replacement therapy. IgA and IgG subclass deficiency are most common while selective IgM and IgE deficiency are rare.

Selective Immunoglobulin A Deficiency

The most common antibody deficiency has a frequency of approximately 1 out of 600 to 800 normal Caucasian individuals. The criterion used to define selective IgA deficiency is based on the sensitivity of the methods used to measure IgA but in general it is below 7 to 10 mg/dL, as measured by immunonephelometry. The pathogenesis of IgA deficiency appears to be heterogeneous. In some cases, phenotypic studies of circulating B cells show patterns similar to those of cord blood B lymphocytes, suggesting a differentiation abnormality, sometimes reflected by a defect in secretion of intracytoplasmic IgA. In other cases, there is evidence for immunoregulatory defects. For example, there are individuals who have IgA deficiency with concomitant IgG2 and IgG4 subclass deficiency and normal levels of IgG1 and IgG3. Anti-IgA antibodies reacting with isotypic or allotypic determinants of IgA can be detected in about one-third of the patients with selective IgA deficiency, suggesting that autoantibodies may play a role in the development of the deficiency. When present in high titers, anti-IgA antibodies can trigger potentially fatal reactions upon transfusion of IgA-containing blood products.

Clinical Presentation

Although many cases of selective IgA deficiency are asymptomatic, recurrent bacterial upper respiratory infections, in particular sinusitis, and gastrointestinal infections with *G. lamblia* are common. Allergic diseases such as eczema, food allergies, and asthma are more frequent when compared to individuals with normal IgA.

IgA deficiency can also be associated with a number of gastrointestinal diseases including celiac disease, nodular hepatitis, pernicious anemia, ulcerative colitis, and regional enteritis. Autoimmunity is more common than in the general population, particularly rheumatoid arthritis, idiopathic thrombocytopenia, and systemic lupus erythematosus (SLE). There is also an increased risk for gastrointestinal malignancy including gastrointestinal lymphoma, adenocarcinoma of the stomach, and nodular lymphoid hyperplasia. All patients with anti-IgA antibodies carry an increased risk for anaphylactoid reactions to IgA containing blood products, including plasma and intravenous gammaglobulin (IVIg).

Diagnosis

Any patient over the age of four years with less than 10 mg/dL of serum IgA and normal levels of IgG and IgM fulfills the diagnostic criteria. Certain drugs, such as phenytoic and valpropic acid, can induce IgA deficiency that corrects when the drugs are discontinued. Symptomatic patients with selective IgA deficiency should be evaluated for IgG subclass deficiency. Ataxia-telangiectasia can also be associated with selective IgA deficiency (see later).

Therapy

There is no effective replacement therapy for selective IgA deficiency. Treatment is usually targeted to treat infections and decrease allergies symptoms and inflammation. Replacement therapy with intravenous immunoglobulin (IVIg, see later) is not indicated, and can induce anaphylaxis due to the small amounts of IgA contaminating the products. Administration of

IVIg with minimal amounts of IgA is indicated in patients with combined IgA and IgG subclass who would benefit from replacement therapy due to recurrent and severe bacterial infections. IgA-deficient patients who require blood transfusions should be given red blood cells extensively washed with saline. If plasma infusions are needed, it should be provided by an IgA-deficient donor or an alternative therapy should be considered. Patients should be educated about their increased risk of reactions to blood products.

Transient Hypogammaglobulinemia of Infancy

This disorder is an accentuation of a normal physiologic phenomenon. Passively acquired maternal IgG has a half-life of approximately one month, and, as it is catabolized, the infant's IgG production fails to maintain adequate levels. As a result, infantile IgG levels are normally significantly lower than adults and older children. The IgG nadir normally occurs between three and six months of age. This process is more pronounced in pre-term infants whose IgG levels are low at birth, as the transport of IgG across the placenta is greatest during the third trimester of gestation.

There are some infants whose IgG nadir drops below 2 SD for age, and thus fulfils the criteria for transient hypogammaglobulinemia of infancy. Most of these patients are evaluated because of an increased frequency and/or severity of infections. Differentiation from more severe forms of humoral immunodeficiency is based on functional tests and enumeration of B cells. Peripheral blood B lymphocytes are usually normal in number; in most cases, a deficiency of CD4 helper T cell function may play a role in the pathogenesis. Antigen-specific antibody production following immunization is normal and is the most effective way to confirm the diagnosis.

Therapy

Most infants do not require therapy. Treatment with IVIg is unnecessary unless the infant suffers from severe infections and should only be administered until the child's immunoglobulin levels normalize.

GAMMAGLOBULIN REPLACEMENT THERAPY

Severe antibody deficiency diseases such as infantile agammaglobulinemia, CVID, IgG subclass deficiency, and the hyper IgM syndrome can be effectively treated with regular repeated infusions of passive immunoglobulin. Most commonly, this is done using IVIg infused at monthly intervals. IVIg consists of purified polyclonal human IgG obtained from the pooled plasma from healthy plasma donors. Generally, the donor pool reflects the immunoglobulin from 3000 to 60,000 different individuals. Serum IgA and IgM are removed in the fractionation process. Hepatitis C virus is screened in plasma before isolation of IVIg, and positive plasma is discarded. In addition, IVIg is also treated with a detergent to minimize the risks of infection by other blood-borne viruses. An alternative to IVIg is the use of subcutaneously administered gammaglobulin. With this administration, the monthly dose is divided into four equal aliquots and administered weekly in the abdominal subcutaneous tissues using a small gauge needle. This process minimizes some of the adverse reactions associated with IVIg and does not require intravenous access. The dosing of gammaglobulin is 200 to 600 mg/kg per month or the amount needed to maintain total IgG troughs at greater than 600 mg/dL.

IVIg primarily remains in the plasma and tissue compartment. Adverse reactions to IVIg include aseptic meningitis that is associated with severe headaches. Anaphylactoid reactions can occur and can be treated by slowing the infusion rate or by using a low IgA containing product in patients with anti-IgA antibodies. IgG crosses the blood brain barrier poorly. Viral infections in the central nervous system may require infusions with intraventricular gammaglobulin. Chronic infections of the gastrointestinal tract sometimes require the use of human or bovine colostrum or oral gammaglobulin, because IgG is not transported by mucosal cells.

CONGENITAL THYMUS APLASIA (DIGEORGE SYNDROME)

The DiGeorge syndrome (DGS) can be considered as the paradigm of a pure T-cell deficiency. The syndrome is a spectrum of anomalies that include thymic hypoplasia, resulting in T-cell deficiency, hypoparathyoidism, facial dysmorphism, and conotruncal cardiac defects. All are believed to be the result of abnormal migration of neural crest cells that form the third and fourth pharyngeal arches during the fourth week of gestation that ultimately contribute to the development of the thymus, the parathyroid gland, the heart, and the face.

Etiology and Pathogenesis

Approximately 90% of patients with DGS have an underlying genetic abnormality of a micro-deletions of chromosomal region 22q11.2. A number of critical genes in this chromosomal region are thought to play a role in the clinical spectrum of the anomalies associated with the syndrome. Other genetic defects that result in a DiGeorge phenotype have been described in deletions in chromosome 10p13 and 17p13. Approximately 5% of DGS have no detectable genetic abnormality. Overall, most cases are sporadic, but 10% of cases will have an affected parent.

Clinical Presentation

The clinical features of DGS track with the embryonic defects. Conotruncal cardiac defects, including truncus arteriosus, tetralogy of Fallot, interrupted aortic arch type b, and aberrant right subclavian artery, are the most frequent cardiac features. Facial dysmorphy include prominent nasal root with bulbous tip, protuberant ears, cup-shaped helices, and small, carp-like mouth. Cleft lip and palate and velopharyngeal insufficiency result in speech abnormalities. Hypoparathyroidism leads to hypocalcemia, often associated with neonatal tetany. Mental retardation, speech and language delay, learning difficulties, and neuropsychiatric problems are common.

From the immunological point of view, the most important feature is thymic hypoplasia. Complete DGS results in no detectable thymus or T cells and early death due to opportunistic infections. More often, there are low T cell numbers, elevated CD4 to CD8 T cell ratios, and low numbers of naïve T cells in the blood. The immune deficiency slowly corrects with age, but antibody abnormalities, including poor response to immunizations, selective IgA deficiency, and hypogammaglobulinemia, can persist throughout life in some patients.

Diagnosis of Immunological Abnormalities

A hallmark finding is the absence or extreme reduction in size of the thymic image on an anti-posterior chest X ray or on a magnetic resonance imaging. T cells are characteristically reduced in numbers (less than $500/\mu L$ CD3$^+$ T cells), and there is poor to null response of peripheral blood mononuclear cells to T-cell mitogens, such as phytohemagglutinin. However, in some patients there are residual T lymphocytes and/or partial thymus functions (partial DGS). Definitive diagnosis requires the presence of two out of three other abnormalities besides T-cell deficiency, including (*i*) conotruncal cardiac defects, (*ii*) persistent hypocalcemia, or (*iii*) deletion of chromosome 22q11.2.

Therapy

If T cells are detectable at birth (>50 cells/μL), slow but progressive normalization of immune functions will occur. In early infancy, treatment should focus on correction of the cardiac and parathyroid defects and prevention of opportunistic infections with prophylactic antibiotics.

Complete DGS can be successfully corrected with HSC transplant of thymic transplant. Thymic tissues obtained during elective cardiac surgery can be implanted and has been successfully carried out without human leukocyte antigen (HLA) matching or the risk of graft versus host disease. In infancy, all patients should receive prophylaxis with sulfamethoxazole-trimethoprim to prevent infections by *P. carinii*. Those patients with antibody deficiency benefit from the administration of IVIg. Irradiated blood products to prevent graft versus host disease should be used if heart surgery is performed before correction of the conotruncal heart defects.

COMBINED ANTIBODY AND CELLULAR IMMUNODEFICIENCIES

Combined immunodeficiencies are those in which both cell-mediated immunity and humoral immunity are impaired. The common classification of these disorders is summarized in Table 2. The general characteristics of this group are summarized in Table 4.

Severe, Combined Immunodeficiency

Severe, combined immunodeficiency (SCID) is a group of heterogeneous disorders associated with lack of both T- and B-cell function. The name is derived from the overall poor prognosis associated with the disorders. Subtype classification is based on the predominant arm of immunity impacted, arrest in T cells with normal B cell numbers (T^-, B^+ SCID) or arrest of both T- and B-cell development (T^-, B^- SCID). Most forms are due to an inheritable disorder, which can be inherited as an X-linked recessive form or as an autosomal recessive form. The frequency of SCID is estimated to be 1:50,000 to 1:100,000 births.

Pathogenesis
There are several predominant pathogenic mechanisms in SCID. First, defects in cytokine receptors, which result in impaired T-cell signal transduction pathways triggered by the

TABLE 4 Summary of the Main Characteristics of the DiGeorge Syndrome and Combined Immune Deficiencies

Characteristic	DiGeorge syndrome[a]	Severe combined immune deficiency	MHC deficiencies
Genetics	Microdeletions of chromosomal region 22q11.2; 90% of the cases are sporadic	X-linked or autosomal recessive	Mutations affecting the TAP genes or a TAP-binding protein
Embryologic/molecular basis	Lack of differentiation of the third and fourth pharyngeal arches during the fourth week of gestation	Deficient interleukin receptor common γ chain (X-linked SCID) RAG mutations Deficient ZAP-70 kinase Deficient TCR/CD3 complex ADA and PNP deficiencies	Lack of expression of MHC-I (bare lymphocyte syndrome) or MHC-II
Lymphoid tissues	Thymic hypoplasia or aplasia	Thymic aplasia; general atrophy of lymphoid organs	Normal
T lymphocytes	Low T cell numbers; high CD4/CD8 ratio	Very low in X-linked SCID; normal in number and deficient in function in ZAP-70 deficiency	Low (low CD4 counts in MHC-II deficiency)
B lymphocytes	Normal numbers, deficient function	Low or undetectable; normal or high in X-linked SCID	Normal numbers, deficient function
Serum immunoglobulins	Low levels; IgA deficiency	Usually low	Low levels
Infections	Bacterial, fungal (*Pneumocystis*)	All types	Bacterial, fungal (*Pneumocystis*, *Candida*), parasitic (*Cryptosporidium*)
Treatment	Prophylactic antibiotics; stem cell transplantation	Prophylactic antibiotics; stem cell transplantation PEG-ADA, gene therapy	Stem cell transplantation; IVIg (if pyogenic infections predominate)

[a]Other associated abnormalities affect the heart and large vessels and parathyroids. Facial dysmorphy and mental retardation are common features of the syndrome.
Abbreviations: ADA, adenosine deaminase; MHC, major histocompatibility complex; PEG, polyethylene glycol; PNP, purine nucleoside phosphorylase; RAG, recombinase-activating genes; SCID, severe, combined immunodeficiency; TAP, transporters associated with antigen processing; TCR, T cell receptor; ZAP, zeta-associate protein.

occupation of cytokine receptors and lack of T-cell differentiation within the thymus. Second, there are defects impacting the differentiation of lymphoid progenitor cells, most commonly due to mutations in the recombinase-activating genes (RAG); examples include RAG deficiency and Omenn's syndrome. A third form of SCID occurs due to defects in the T cell receptor (TCR) signaling cascade either in the TCR/CD3 complex or downstream of this complex, as is seen is zeta-associated protein (ZAP)-70 deficiency. Defects due to abnormal enzymes involved in purine metabolism lead to the accumulation of intracellular toxins that block T- and B-cell differentiation. Finally, defective expression of major histocompatibility complex (MHC) class I and MHC class II leads to impaired intrathymic development of CD8 and CD4 T cells, respectively.

Deficiencies in Cytokine Receptors

Deficiency of the interleukin receptor common γ chain, the most common form of SCID, is X-linked, due to a mutation in the γ chain of the IL-2 receptor (IL-2Rγc or γc). The γc cell surface protein is present in several other cytokine receptors and mediates signals through several interleukins including IL-2, IL-4, IL-7, IL-11, and IL-15. Mutations in IL-2Rγc result in absent down stream cell surface signaling through the JAK/STAT signal transduction cascade, a critical component of interleukin induced T-cell activation. JAK-3 deficiency predictably results in a nearly identical SCID phenotype. Mutations in JAK-3 are inherited in an autosomal recessive pattern.

Children with SCID secondary to IL-2Rγc or JAK-3 deficiency have no circulating mature CD3$^+$ T cells because of maturation arrest of T-cell development within the thymus. B cells are present in normal or increased numbers but are deficient in function, presumably due to a lack of T helper cell function. Natural killing (NK) cell numbers and function are also deficient.

IL-7 receptor α chain deficiency results in lack of T-cell differentiation, proving the key role of IL-7 in human T-cell differentiation. NK cells, however, are less affected than in the other forms of SCID described earlier.

Defects Impacting the Differentiation of Progenitor Cells

Mutation of RAG 1, 2, and/or 3 genes control the V(D)J recombination essential for the differentiation of membrane immunoglobulins and TCRs (see Chapters 7 and 10). These patients lack both T and B cells, because those two cell populations cannot fully be differentiated in the absence of their defining antigen receptors. Those patients are severely immune compromised. Inheritance is autosomal recessive.

ZAP-70 is a critical kinase involved in signal transmission after occupation of the TCR on mature T lymphocytes (see Chapters 4 and 11). In addition, it plays a critical role in CD8$^+$ T-cell differentiation, and patients with ZAP-70 mutations have large numbers of CD3$^+$ and CD4$^+$ T cells but low numbers of CD8$^+$ T cells. In addition, these patients' T cells fail to proliferate in vitro when activated by mitogens.

Defects in the TCR/CD3 complex can also lead to SCID. While defects of the γ and ε chains are associated with classical SCID or T cell deficiency, defects in the σ chain cause a different set of abnormalities. The thymus is normal in size, is populated with T lymphocytes, but the lymphocytes fail to develop normally, and circulating T cells are functionally abnormal.

Deficiencies of Purine Salvage Enzymes

The most common of these disorders are adenosine deaminase (ADA) and purine nucleoside phosphorylase deficiencies. Both lead to the intracellular accumulation of metabolites with toxic effects on T cells.

ADA catabolizes the deamination of adenosine and 2'-deoxyadenosine, converting these compounds into inosine. Therefore, the lack of ADA causes the intracellular accumulation of adenosine and 2'-deoxyadenosine. 2'-deoxyadenosine is phosphorylated intracellularly and the activity of the phosphorylating enzyme is greater than the activity of the dephosphorylating enzyme. Consequently, there is a marked accumulation of deoxyadenosine triphosphate (deoxyATP), which has a feedback inhibition effect on ribonucleotide reductase, an enzyme required for normal DNA synthesis. As a consequence, DNA synthesis will be greatly impaired, and no cell proliferation will be observed after any type of stimulation. In addition,

2'-deoxyadenosine is reported to cause chromosome breakage and this mechanism could be the basis for the severe lymphopenia observed in these patients. The reason why lymphocytes are predominantly affected over other cells that also produce ADA in normal individuals is that immature T cells are among those cells with higher ADA levels (together with brain and gastrointestinal tract cells).

Purine nucleotide phosphoralase deficiency is a similar but not as severe disorder of purine metabolism. This enzyme converts inosine and guanosine into hypoxanthine, and its deficiency causes an accumulation of deoxyguanosine, which is triphosphorylated to deoxy guanosine triphosphate (deoxyGTP). Similarly, to deoxyATP, deoxyGTP has toxic effects on T lymphocytes, causing their selective depletion.

Clinical Presentation
In all forms of SCID, symptoms start very early in life, usually by four months of age. Survival beyond the first year of life is rare without aggressive therapy. Frequent clinical presentations include persistent infections of the lungs, often caused by opportunistic agents such as *P. jerovici (carinii)*, severe mucocutaneous candidiasis, chronic, untractable diarrhea, and failure to thrive. In most cases physical examination shows absence of all lymphoid tissues: atrophic tonsils, very small or undetectable lymph nodes, signs of pulmonary infection, evidence of poor physical development, and oral thrush. A chest X-ray will reveal absent thymic shadow, bony abnormalities of the ribs in patients with ADA deficiency. Approximately 20% of infants with SCID will develop graft-versus-host disease as a consequence of the transplacental transfer of maternal T lymphocytes late in gestation. The maternal T lymphocytes that enter the fetal circulation are not destroyed because of the infant's deficient cell-mediated immunity. The maternal T cells can proliferate in the skin, gastrointestinal tract, and liver. Symptoms of graft-versus-host disease include rash, jaundice, hepatitis, and chronic diarrhea. Severe cases of graft-versus-host disease are often fatal. Children with SCID and other T-cell deficiencies can also develop graft-versus-host disease following blood transfusions containing viable mononuclear cells. Children with SCID carry an increased risk of malignancy, particularly lymphomas positive for the Epstein-Barr virus.

Diagnosis
The general laboratory parameters seen in the various forms of SCID can be found in Chapter 28. In most forms of SCID these patients have very low lymphocyte counts. In X-linked SCID more than 75% of the residual lymphocyte population are $CD19^+$ B cells, while $CD3^+$ T cells and $CD16/56^+$ NK cells usually represent less than 10% and 2% of the residual population, respectively. The deficiency in cell-mediated immunity is reflected by negative skin tests, delayed rejection of allogeneic skin grafts, and lack of response of cultured mononuclear cells to T-cell mitogens and CD3 monoclonal antibodies. Neutropenia can also be seen in some patients. In cases of ZAP-70 deficiency, lymphocyte counts may be normal or close to normal, and the T lymphocytes do not respond to stimulation with mitogens. However, T cells can be activated by a mixture of CD3 and phorbol esters, which will cause the phosphorylation of downstream kinases, bypassing the ZAP-70 defect.

Immunoglobulins are usually low (levels more than 2 SD below the normal level for age), but in some cases can be normal or irregularly affected. B cells and plasma cells are low or undetectable in ADA deficiency and RAG deficiency. In all forms of SCID, antibody responses are very low to absent.

The definitive diagnosis and identification of the cause of SCID often requires evaluation at the molecular level to identify the genetic defect(s) underlying the immunodeficiency. The diagnosis of ADA deficiency can be made through enzymatic analysis of red blood cells, lymphocytes, fibroblasts, amniotic cells, fetal blood, or chorionic villous samples.

Therapy
Most cases of SCID lead to a fatal outcome due to infections or malignancy unless treated early in life. Prophylaxis with trimethoprim-sulfamethoxazole to prevent *Pneumocystis* pneumonia should be initiated by the first month of life. If blood transfusions are necessary, they should receive irradiated blood products to prevent graft-versus-host disease and leukocytes should

be depleted. Blood products should be received from donors who test negative for viral infections such as cytomegalovirus to minimize the risk of transfusion-acquired infections. Exposure to all pathogens should be limited, although implementation is not easy (as reflected by the term "bubble baby"). Children with SCID and other defects in T cell function should not receive immunizations with live attenuated vaccines.

Hematopoietic Stem Cell Transplantation

All forms of SCID can be corrected with HSC transplantation. Best results are obtained with stem cells obtained from an HLA-matched related donor. If such a donor is not available, alternative strategies include transfusion of T-cell depleted haploidentical bone marrow cells from a parent, an HLA-matched unrelated bone marrow donor, or umbilical cord blood leukocytes from an unrelated donor. The risk for GVH varies depending on the degree of HLA mismatch and the number of mature T cells within the transplanted cells. Preconditioning chemotherapy generally improves the chances of engraftment but increases overall morbidity and mortality. A unique feature of HSC transplantation in SCID is that it can be successfully performed without conditioning to ablate pretransplant immunity. Administration of immunosuppressive drugs following transplant is usually required to make sure that GVH does not develop.

ADA deficiency can be effectively treated by the administration of bovine ADA plus polyethylene glycol (PEG). The addition of PEG results in decreased immunogenicity and increased half-life of the bovine ADA.

Gene Therapy

Both the X-linked form of SCID and ADA deficiency have been corrected by gene therapy. ADA deficiency was actually the first human disease to be successfully treated by gene therapy. The original protocol involved: harvesting peripheral blood T lymphocytes from the patients, transfecting the ADA gene using a retrovirus vector, expanding the transfected cells in culture, and re-administering them to the patient. In the first treated patient, normal peripheral blood T lymphocyte counts and clinical improvement were seen after several such infusions. The infusions needed to be periodically repeated, since the ADA^+ T-lymphocyte population eventually declines. The normalization of T-cell counts probably reflects the fact that the transfected ADA^+ cells will produce excess ADA, which will diffuse into genetically deficient cells unable to synthesize it. All patients treated with this protocol had to continue receiving PEG-ADA to maintain a relatively symptom-free status.

Gene therapy using transfected stem cells was successfully used for the first time for the correction of SCID secondary to IL-2Rγc deficiency. Two children with this form of immunodeficiency received their own $CD34^+$ stem cells after ex vivo transfection of the defective gene by means of a murine retroviral vector. In contrast with ADA gene therapy, the patients with IL2Rγc deficiency have shown long-term immune reconstitution. The recovery of immune functions in these two children was basically complete—T, B, and NK cell counts and function became undistinguishable from those of normal age-matched controls, and so did the capacity of mounting antigen-specific responses. The series was expanded to 10 patients, nine of whom were successfully reconstituted. The successfully treated children were able to live free of infections without prophylactic measures. However, long-term follow-up of these children have revealed that the retroviral insertion result in lymphocytic leukemia, apparently caused by overexpression of the LMO-2 transcription factor, induced by the insertion of the retroviral vector near the 5′ end of its coding domain. This protocol is currently on hold until an alternative approach can be developed.

Other Forms of Combined Immune Deficiency
Deficient Expression of Major Histocompatibility Complex Molecules

The lack of expression of either MHC-I or MHC-II molecules is associated with combined immunodeficiency.

Major Histocompatibility Complex-I Deficiency (Bare Lymphocyte Syndrome)
MHC-I deficiency is a rare condition characterized by a deficient expression of HLA-A, B, and C markers and absence of β_2-microglobulin on lymphocyte membranes. The underlying genetic defects affect the genes coding for the "Transporters Associated with Antigen Processing" (TAP-1, TAP-2) or for a TAP-binding protein. Both TAP proteins and TAP-binding proteins are essential for proper intracellular assembly of the MHC-I molecules (see Chapter 4).

Although some patients with this syndrome may be asymptomatic, most suffer from infections. In some cases, the infection pattern, involving fungi and *P. jerovici (carinii)*, is consistent with combined immunodeficiency; in other patients, the symptoms are mainly due to infections with pyogenic bacteria. The link between the lack of expression of MHC-I markers and humoral immunodeficiency is unclear.

Laboratory findings include lymphopenia, poor mitogenic responses, low immunoglobulin levels, and lack of antibody responses. B cells are usually detected, but plasma cells are absent.

Major Histocompatibility Complex-II Deficiency
MHC class-II deficiency is inherited as an autosomal recessive trait, resulting from mutations in genes involved in the transcription of MHC-II genes. It is associated with a severe form of combined immunodeficiency, with absent cellular and humoral immune responses after immunization. These patients have low number of $CD4^+$ helper T lymphocytes, which results in lack of differentiation of B lymphocytes into antibody-producing cells. This syndrome provides strong support to the theory that suggests that the interaction between double positive $CD4^+$, $CD8^+$ thymocytes, and MHC-II molecules is the essential stimulus for the differentiation of $CD4^+$ helper T lymphocytes.

The patients often have protracted diarrhea, secondary to infections with *Candida albicans* or *Cryptosporidium parvum*, leading to malabsorption and failure to thrive. Pulmonary infections are also frequent. Residual cytotoxic T cell function is reflected by the ability of these children to reject grafted cells and tissues. The prognosis is very poor. Death tends to occur before the second decade of life, unless the deficiency is corrected by bone marrow transplant.

Laboratory findings include normal counts of $CD3^+$ lymphocytes associated to low numbers of $CD4^+$ cells. The expression of MHC-II molecules in monocytes and/or B cells is absent or very low (less than 5% of normal). Molecular genetic studies are required to characterize the responsible gene mutations.

Immunodeficiency with Ataxia-Telangiectasia
Genetics and Physiopathology
Ataxia-telangiectasia is genetically transmitted by an autosomal inheritance pattern. It is believed that the disease may result from a deficiency of DNA repair enzymes, as suggested by the high frequency of lymphoreticular malignancies. In addition, the enzyme defect seems to result in a generalized defect in tissue maturation, affecting many tissues, but with particular significance the brain capillary vessels. Persistently increased levels of serum α-fetoprotein and carcinoembryonic antigen in many patients with this disease support this last postulate.

Clinical Presentation
The initial symptoms are of progressive cerebellar ataxia beginning in early childhood associated with insidiously developing telangiectasia (first appearing as a dilation of the conjunctival vessels). The capillary abnormalities are systemically distributed, and involve the cerebellum, causing the motor difficulties characteristic of ataxia. In late childhood, recurrent sinobronchial infections start to manifest, leading to bronchiectasis.

Associations of thymic hypoplasia, T-cell deficiency, and low immunoglobulin levels characterize this immunodeficiency. Low or undetectable IgA is reported in 80% of the patients.

Therapy
The prognosis is poor and there is no effective therapy. Correction of the immune deficiency through bone marrow transplant does not alter the course of the central nervous system

deterioration. Death usually occurs before puberty, most frequently as a consequence of lymphoreticular malignancies or of the rupture of telangiectatic cerebral blood vessels.

Immunodeficiency with Thrombocytopenia and Eczema (Wiskott-Aldrich Syndrome)
Genetics and Pathogenesis
This is another immune disorder with an X-linked recessive pattern of inheritance. The associated gene has been located to Xp11.23, which encodes the protein known as Wiskott-Aldrich Syndrome Protein (WASP). This protein is expressed by hematopoietic cells and appears to play a role in actin polymerization and cytoskeleton arrangement. The mutations are associated with either lack of synthesis or with synthesis of an abnormal WASP. In the absence of functional WASP, hematopoietic cells demonstrate abnormal size, shape, and function that is most apparent in platelets and lymphocytes. Platelets are small in size, aggregate poorly, and are sequestered and destroyed in the spleen. T lymphocytes are also smaller than normal and show disorganization of the cytoskeleton and loss of microvilli. Abnormal expression of Th2 cytokines and expression of costimulatory molecules (see Chapters 4 and 11) contribute the severe eczema and autoimmunity observed in these patients.

Clinical Presentation
Eczema, thrombocytopenia, and frequent infections characterize the Wiskott-Aldrich syndrome. Most frequently, the infections are caused by viruses, such as herpes simplex, Varicella-Zoster, and molluscum contagiosum. Increased frequency of infections with encapsulated pyogenic bacteria, such as *S. pneumoniae*, *Neisseria meningitidis*, and *H. influenzae*, can also be seen. Later in life, the patients can suffer from all types of opportunistic infections, reflecting a deterioration of both cell-mediated and humoral immune functions. There is an increased frequency of autoimmune diseases, particularly autoimmune hemolytic anemia and rheumatoid arthritis. Hemorrhage is the most frequent cause of death, but some children develop opportunistic infections or lymphoreticular malignancies that can have a fatal evolution.

Laboratory Findings
The finding of profound thrombocytopenia with small-sized platelets very early in life is often the first clinical sign of Wiskott-Aldrich Syndrome. Platelets are characterized as small and dysmorphic. There are several laboratory abnormalities characteristic of this immune deficiency. These include low IgM levels (the levels of the other immunoglobulin isotypes may be low, normal, or elevated), and failure to respond to polysaccharide vaccines or to immunizations with neoantigens such as bacterial phage øx174 (see Chapter 15). Lymphocyte count and function are normal in early infancy, but deficient mitogenic and mixed lymphocyte culture responses develop over time. Definitive diagnosis requires either molecular studies revealing mutations of the WASP gene, or absence of the WASP mRNA, or WASP protein, in peripheral blood lymphocytes.

Therapy
Thrombocytopenia improves following splenectomy. The immunological defects can be corrected by stem cell transplantation. Replacement therapy with IVIg has been used in some patients.

PHAGOCYTIC CELL DEFICIENCIES

Cell findings in patients with phagocytic disorders include infections of soft tissues, cellulitis, and chronic recurrent lymphadenitis. Recurrent abscesses in organs such as lung, liver, and bone are also frequent. Commonly, these infections are due to *Staphylococcus* sp., *Pseudomonas* sp., *Candida* sp., and *Aspergillus* sp. Chronic or recurrent oral ulcers, poor wound healing, periodontal disease, and delayed separation of the umbilical cord is an early hallmark of deficiencies in phagocytic cell function or numbers. Phagocytic dysfunction can result from either quantitative or qualitative defects in phagocytic cells. Figure 1 diagrammatically

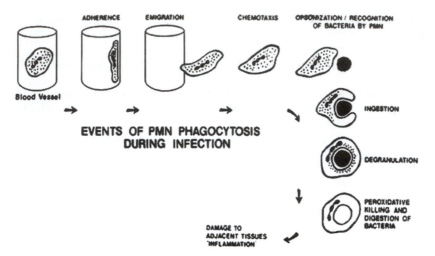

FIGURE 1   Diagrammatic representation of the major primary functional derangements of neutrophils that have been characterized in man. *Source*: Reproduced from Wolach B, Baehner RL, Boxer LA. Review: clinical and laboratory approach to the management of neutrophil dysfunction. Israel J Med Sci 1982; 18:897.

illustrates the aspects of polymorphonuclear (PMN) function that can be affected in different pathological situations.

Disorders of Leukocyte Adherence

The most common among these very rare disorders is the lack of expression of the CD11/CD18 complex, and affects phagocytic cells and T lymphocytes. This disease is inherited as an autosomal recessive trait. Initial clinical manifestations include a delayed separation of the umbilical cord and chronic leukocytosis. During childhood, these individuals suffer from repeated pyogenic infections and, with less frequency, from fungal infections. Severe necrotizing gingivitis and periodontal disease is common.

Job's Syndrome (Hyper-Immunoglobulin E Syndrome)

The clinical characteristics of Job's syndrome include chronic severe atopic dermatitis, very high levels of serum IgE, chronic eczematous dermatitis with frequent staphylococcal superinfection, pyogenic infections of the upper airways, and opportunistic infections, such as lung infections involving *Aspergillus* spp. and disseminated molluscum contagiosum. Chronic candidiasis can also be associated with this syndrome. Inheritance is usually autosomal dominant, but cases of autosomal recessive inheritance have been published.

The mechanism of this disease has not been well defined. A defect of monocyte chemotaxis has been reported in most patients, but the severity is quite variable. It is unlikely that this is the primary defect leading to immunedeficiency. The high levels of IgE correspond, at least in part, to the production of IgE anti-*S. aureus* antibodies. In contrast, IgA antibodies to *S. aureus* are abnormally low, and other indices of humoral immune function (responses to toxoid boosters and to in vitro stimulation with PWM) are also depressed.

Chronic Granulomatous Disease

Chronic granulomatous disease (CGD), although rare, is the most frequent primary phagocytic cell deficiency. The majority of cases are inherited as an X-linked trait, but autosomal recessive inheritance is involved in 25% to 35% of the cases.

Molecular Basis

The molecular basis of CGD is heterogeneous. The X-linked form is the result of a mutation in the alpha chain (91 Kd) phosophoprotein (gp91phox) of cytochrome b558. Molecular genetic studies have shown that in about half of the cases of X-linked CGD, there is a failure to express mRNA for the gp91phox protein, and, in the remainder cases, mRNA is present but there is a failure to transport or properly insert the protein in the cytoplasmic membrane. The remaining cases of CGD are inherited as autosomal recessive traits, involving other proteins involved in the assembly of nicotiamide adenine dinucleotide- phosphate (NADPH) oxidase, such as neutrophil cytosolic factors 1 (p47phox) and 2 (p67phox), or the beta chain (22 Kd) of cytochrome b558 (p22phox).

All of the cytochrome B deficiencies result in a lack of functional NADPH oxidase at the cell membrane level. There is a failure to generate superoxide and H_2O_2 and, consequently, intracellular killing is defective. Both types of phagocytic cells (PMN leukocytes and monocytes) are affected.

The killing defect leads to infections with catalase positive organisms such as *Staphylococci, Serratia marscecens, Klebsiella* sp., *Aerobacter* sp., *Salmonella* sp., *Chromobacterium violaceum, Burkholderia cepacia, Nocardia* sp., and *Aspergillus sp.* Catalase negative organisms (such as *S. pneumoniae)*do not usually cause infections in these patients. The lack of involvement of catalase negative organisms results from the fact that when ingested by phagocytic cells continue to generate H_2O_2 that they cannot degrade. The H_2O_2 generated by the bacteria progressively accumulates in the phagosome, eventually reaching bactericidal levels.

Clinical Manifestations

The clinical manifestations are dominated by recurrent bacterial and fungal infections. The most frequent infection sites are the lungs, lymph nodes, liver, skin, and soft tissues. The infections are characterized by the formation of microabscesses and noncaseating granulomas. Suppurative lymphadenitis, pyoderma, pneumonia with suppurative complications, liver abscesses, osteomyelitis, and severe periodontal disease are among the most frequently seen infections. Generalized lymphadenopathy and hepatosplenomegaly are frequently found on physical examination. Because the infectious agents are often sequestered within leukocytes or walled-off in granulomas, it is common for blood or tissue cultures to be negative. Most patients have elevated levels of the major immunoglobulins (hypergammaglobulinemia).

Diagnosis

Diagnosis is usually confirmed by flow cytometry analysis of oxidative burst by neutrophils or using a quantitative variant of the nitroblue tetrazolium reduction test (see Chapters 14 and 28). These assays can also be used for the detection of female carriers.

Treatment

Infections are treated with antimicrobials chosen on the basis of susceptibility studies if bacteria have been recovered from infection sites. Prophylactic administration of trimethoprim-sulfamethoxazole is generally recommended. Interferon-γ administration has been found to result in a decrease of the frequency of infectious episodes in same patients with CGD. Early trials suggested that interferon-γ enhanced the neutrophil respiratory burst and that the effect was more pronounced in patients with the autosomal variants of CGD.

The identification of the genes coding for the different molecular components of the oxidase system has led to trials of gene therapy, by using retroviral vectors to insert the gp91phox gene into the puripotent stem cells. Also, nonmyeloablative HSC from HLA matched donors has become a viable treatment alternative for CGD. This approach resulted in low but adequate engraftment of normal neutrophils and normalization of granulocyte function.

Chediak-Higashi Syndrome

This rare disease is due to abnormalities in the lysosomal trafficking modulator that is essential for the assembly of cytoplasmic granules and their fusion with phagosomes, to form the phagolysosme. The PMN leukocytes are able to ingest microorganisms, but the cytoplasmic granules tend to coalesce into giant secondary lysosomes, with reduced enzymatic contents, which are inconsistently delivered to the phagosome. As a consequence, intracellular killing is slow and inefficient. NK-cell function has also been reported to be impaired.

Clinical Manifestations

Mucocutaneous albinism, recurrent neutropenia, unexplained fever, and peripheral neuropathy characterize patients with this syndrome. Many patients develop hepatosplenomegaly and lymphadenopathy associated with recurrent bacterial and viral infection, fever, and prostration. End-stage disease is associated with a poor prognosis.

Diagnosis

The finding of morphological abnormalities in the PMN leukocytes (giant lysosomes) supports the diagnosis. Phagocytic cells killing tests show impaired intracellular killing.

Treatment

Infections are treated symptomatically with antibiotics. Ascorbic acid administration has been shown to increase bactericidal activity in some patients. This improvement may be related to an effect of ascorbic acid on membrane fluidity, which is abnormally high in the patient's PMN leukocytes and is normalized by ascorbic acid.

COMPLEMENT DEFICIENCIES

Deficiencies of virtually all components of the complement cascade have been reported. Clinical findings associated with complement deficiencies are highly variable and dependent on the location of the defect within the complement cascade. Symptoms range from an increased risk for the development of autoimmune disease to recurrent infections. The deficiencies can be grouped as early component (C1, C2, and C4) deficiencies, late component (C5 to C9) deficiencies, C3 deficiency, and defects in the alternative complement cascade. The characteristics of these groups are summarized in Table 5.

TABLE 5 Summary of the Main Characteristics of Primary Complement Deficiencies, Using Common Variable Immunodeficiency as a Term of Reference

Characteristic	Common variable immunodeficiency	Early complement component deficiencies	C3 deficiency	Late complement component deficiencies
Genetics	Variable	Autosomal codominant	Autosomal recessive	Variable
Molecular basis	Variable, ill defined	Lack of synthesis	Lack of synthesis	Lack of synthesis
Lymphoid tissues	Follicular necrobiosis, reticulum cell hyperplasia	Normal	Normal	Normal
B lymphocytes	Normal numbers, abnormal differentiation or function	Normal	Normal	Normal
Serum immuno-globulins	Low to very low levels	Normal to high	Normal to high	Normal to high
Infections	Bacterial, parasitic (Giardia)	Pyogenic bacteria	Pyogenic bacteria	Capsulated bacteria, especially *N. meningitiis*
Autoimmunity	Rheumatoid arthritis	Systemic lupus erythematosis-like syndrome	Vasculitis, glomerulonephritis	None

Early Component Deficiencies

Deficiencies of C1, C2 and C4 can be asymptomatic, can be associated with predisposition to infections, or, most frequently, can be associated with clinical symptoms suggestive of auto-immune disease. C2 and C4 deficiencies are inherited as an autosomal codominant trait and are often associated with a syndrome mimicking SLE, although the clinical evolution is more benign, and renal dysfunction is less frequent. Patients with homozygous C2 or C4 deficiency often have associated defects in factor B. Recurrent viral and bacterial infections are common. Persistent levels of circulating immune complexes are often found in patients with C2 or C4 deficiency, probably as a result of altered dynamics of immune complex clearance. As a result of low levels of C2 or C4 and due to the interruption in the activation sequence, these patients do not generate normal amounts of C3b.

Primary C3 Deficiency

Primary C3 deficiency is a rare condition, transmitted as an autosomic recessive trait. Patients with C3 deficiency have an inability to opsonize antigens and suffer from recurrent pyogenic infections from early in life, with a clinical picture similar to that of X-linked infantile agamma-globulinemia with normal B- and T-cell function. This is not surprising, given the pivotal role played by C3 in complement activation and in opsonization of microbial agents. Furthermore, C3-deficient patients may present manifestations of immune complex disease, such as glomer-ulonephritis and vasculitis.

Factor I (C3b Inactivator) and Factor H Deficiencies

Factor I (C3b inactivator) and factor H deficiencies result on a deficiency of C3 secondary to a fourfold increase in the catabolic rate of this complement component. Patients are prone to recurrent pyogenic infections, particularly with encapsulated bacteria such as *S. pneumoniae* and *N. meningitidis*. They are also prone to the development of immune complex disease. "Anaphylactoid" reactions secondary to the spontaneous generation of C3a are also frequently observed in these patients.

Late Component Deficiencies

Deficiencies of C5, C6, C7, C8 and C9, complement compounds that make up the membrane attack complex, have been reported to be associated with increased frequency of infections, most commonly due to bacteria with polysaccharide-rich capsules such as *Neisseria* sp.

BIBLIOGRAPHY

Advances in Primary Immunodeficiency (The Jeffrey Modell Immunodeficiency Symposium). Clin Immunol Immunopathol 1995; 76(3 Pt 2):S145.

Bayry J, Hermine O, Webster DA, Levy Y, Kaveri SV. Common variable immunodeficiency: the immune system in chaos. Trends Mol Med 2005; 11:371–376.

Bonilla FA, Geha RS. Primary immunodeficiency diseases. J Allergy Clin Immunol 2003; 111:S571–S581.

Bonilla FA, Geha RS. Update on primary immunodeficiency diseases. J Allergy Clin Immunol 2006; 117:S435–S441.

Buckley RH. Molecular defects in human severe combined immunodeficiency and approaches to immune reconstitution. Annu Rev Immunol 2004; 22:625–655.

Castigli E, Geha RS. Molecular basis of common variable immunodeficiency. J Allergy Clin Immunol 2006; 117:748–752.

Cavazzana-Calvo M, Hacein-Bey S, de Saint Basile G, et al. Gene therapy of human severe combined immunodeficiency (SCID)-X1 disease. Science 2000; 288:669.

Chapel H, Geha R, Rosen F, and the IUIS PID (Primary Immunodeficiencies) Classification committee. Primary immunodeficiency diseases: an update. Clin Exp Immunol 2003; 132:9–15.

Conley ME, Notarangelo LD, Eizioni A. Diagnostic criteria for primary immunodeficiencies. Clin Immunol 1999; 93:190–197.

Cooper MD, Lanier LL, Conley ME, Puck JM. Immunodeficiency disorders. Hematology Am Soc Hematol Educ Program 2003; 314–330.

Goldacker S, Warnatz K. Tackling the heterogeneity of CVID. Curr Opin Allergy Clin Immunol 2005; 5:504–509.

Knight AN, Cunningham-Rundles C. Inflammatory and autoimmune complications of common variable immunodeficiency. Autoimmun Rev 2006; 5:156–159.

Ko J, Radigan L, Cunningham-Rundles C. Immune copetence and switched memory B cells in common variable immunodeficienncy. Clin Immunol 2005; 116:37–41.

Lekstrom-Himes JA, Gallin JI. Immunodeficiency diseases caused by defects in phagocytea. N Engl J Med 2000; 343:1702–1712.

MacCarthy L, Gaspar HB, Wang Y-c, et al. Absence of expression of the Wiskott-Aldrich syndrome protein in peripheral blood cells of Wiskott-Aldrich syndrome patients. Clin Immunol Immunopathol 1998; 88:22–27.

Ochs HD. The Wiskott-Aldrich syndrome. Semin Hematol 1998; 35:332.

Taubenheim N, von Hornung M, Durandy A, et al. Defined blocks in terminal plasma cell differentiation of common variable immunodeficiency patients. J Immunol 2005; 175:5498–5503.

Weiler CR, Bankers-Fulbright JL. Common variable immunodeficiency: test indications and interpretation. Mayo Clin Proc 2005; 80:1187–1190.

30 | AIDS and Other Acquired Immunodeficiency Diseases

John W. Sleasman
Department of Pediatrics, Division of Allergy, Immunology, and Rheumatology, University of South Florida, St. Petersburg, Florida, U.S.A.

Gabriel Virella
Department of Microbiology and Immunology, Medical University of South Carolina, Charleston, South Carolina, U.S.A.

INTRODUCTION

Many factors influencing the function of the immune system can lead to variable degrees of immunoincompetence. Infections, exposure to toxic environmental factors, physical trauma, and therapeutic interventions can all be associated with immune dysfunction (Table 1). In some cases, the primary disease that causes the immunodeficiency is very obvious, while in others a high degree of suspicion is necessary for its detection. The pathogenic mechanisms are very clear in some cases, and totally obscure in others. The following is a brief summary of some of the most common secondary immunodeficiencies, followed by a more detailed discussion of acquired immunodeficiency syndrome (AIDS).

SECONDARY IMMUNODEFICIENCIES
Immunodeficiency Associated with Malnutrition

Immunodeficiency secondary to malnutrition has been reported in association with generalized malnutrition or in association with vitamin, mineral, and trace element deficiencies. Severe protein–calorie malnutrition is primarily associated with a depression of cell-mediated immunity. Different groups have reported anergy, low T lymphocyte counts, depressed lymphocyte reactivity to phytohemagglutinin (PHA), and depressed cytokine release in malnourished populations. In kwashiorkor, which is due to a combination of protein–calorie malnutrition and deficiency in trace elements and vitamins, the degree of immunodeficiency seems to be more profound. Affected children seem to have a delayed maturation of the B cell system and often have low levels of mucosal IgA, without apparent clinical manifestations. Efforts to study the humoral immune response to active immunization have yielded variable results. The complement system and neutrophil functions have been reported as depressed, but the phagocytic impairment is mild and depressed complement levels seem to be primarily a result of consumption as a consequence of infections.

Several causes for the immune deficiency associated with malnutrition have been suggested, including general metabolic depression, thymic atrophy with low levels of thymic factors, depressed numbers of helper T lymphocytes (which could account for the variable compromise of humoral immunity), and impaired cytokine release. A practical consideration to bear in mind is that malnourished children should not be vaccinated with live, attenuated vaccines, which are generally contraindicated in immunodeficient patients. It is also believed that malnutrition is a contributing factor to the high mortality among human immunodeficiency virus (HIV)-infected patients in Austral Africa.

Immunodeficiency Associated with Zinc Deficiency

The significance of zinc deficiency for the normal functioning of the immune system is underlined by observations performed in patients with acrodermatitis enteropathica, a rare

TABLE 1 Causes of Secondary Immunodeficiency

Malnutrition
Systemic disorders
      Immunoglobulin hypercatabolism
      Excessive loss of immunoglobulins
      Renal insufficiency
      Extensive burns
Drug induced
      Cytotoxic drugs
      Glucocorticoids
      Antimalarial agents
      Captopril
      Carbamazepine
      Fenclonefac
      Gold salts
      Phenytoin
      Sulfasalazine
      Alcohol, cannabinoids, opiates
Surgery
Malignancies
      B cell and plasma cell malignancies
      Immunodeficiency with thymoma
      Non-Hodgkin lymphoma
Infectious diseases
      HIV
      Congenital rubella
      Congenital cytomegalovirus infection
      Congenital toxoplasmosis
      Epstein-Barr virus

congenital disease in which diarrhea and malabsorption (affecting zinc, among other nutrients) play a key pathogenic role. Affected patients often present with epidermolysis bullosa and generalized candidiasis, associated with combined immunodeficiency that can be corrected with zinc supplementation.

Secondary zinc deficiencies are considerably more frequent and can develop as a consequence of low meat consumption, high fiber diet, chronic diarrhea, chronic kidney insufficiency, anorexia nervosa and bulimia, alcoholism, diabetes, psoriasis, hemodialysis, parenteral alimentation, and so on. The depletion caused by these conditions, however, does not seem to be severe enough to cause symptomatic immunodeficiency, but may be one of several factors adversely affecting the immune system.

The basis for the depression of cell-mediated immunity in zinc deficiency is not fully known, but it has been proposed that zinc may be essential for the normal activity of cellular protein kinases involved in signal transduction during lymphocyte activation.

Immunodeficiency Associated with Vitamin Deficiencies

Several vitamin deficiencies are associated with and are presumably the cause of abnormalities of the immune response, particularly when associated with protein–calorie malnutrition. The molecular mechanisms underlying these deficiencies have not been defined. Deficiencies of pyridoxine, folic acid, and vitamin A are usually associated with cellular immunodeficiency. Panthotenic acid deficiency is usually associated with a depression of the primary and secondary humoral immune responses. Vitamin E deficiency is associated with a combined immunodeficiency. Vitamin D3 deficiency is associated with higher frequency of inflammatory diseases.

Immunodeficiency Associated with Renal Failure

Patients with renal failure have depressed cell-mediated immunity, as reflected in cutaneous anergy, delayed skin graft rejection, lymphopenia, and poor T lymphocyte responses to mitogenic stimulation. Humoral immunity can also be affected, particularly in patients with the nephrotic syndrome, who may lose significant amounts of IgG in their urine. Several factors seem to contribute to the depression of cell-mediated immunity in patients with renal failure:

1. Release of a soluble suppressor factor, as shown by experiments demonstrating that plasma or serum from uremic patients suppresses the mitogenic responses of normal lymphocytes in vitro. The responsible factors have a molecular weight less than 20,000, and it has been suggested that methylguanidine and "middle molecules" (molecular weight 1200) are responsible. These molecules can be isolated from uremic sera and have been shown to suppress in vitro mitogenic responses of normal T lymphocytes.
2. In end-stage renal disease the circulating levels of tumor necrosis factor (TNF), interleukin (IL)-6, and IL-10 are increased, and the balance seems to be in favor of the proinflammatory cytokines. Indeed, these patients have a high prevalence of wasting and cardiovascular disease, suggesting that a persistent systemic inflammatory response is taking place.
3. Fc-mediated phagocytosis is impaired in patients with severe renal failure, perhaps secondary to increased levels of endogenous glucocorticoid levels. There is also evidence of a compromise of the capacity of monocytes to function as antigen-presenting cells (APC). These abnormalities are reproducible when normal monocytes are incubated with uremic serum. Dialysis may accentuate the problem as a consequence of complement activation in the dialysis membranes, which causes a poorly understood downregulation of the expression of cell adhesion molecules by phagocytic cells.
4. Patients with chronic renal failure secondary to autoimmune diseases are often treated with immunosuppressive drugs that further compromise the immune system.

Burn-Associated Immunodeficiency

Bacterial infections are frequent and severe complications prevail in burn patients, often leading to death. There are several factors that may contribute to the incidence of infections in burned patients, including the presence of open and infected wounds, a general metabolic disequilibrium, and a wide spectrum of immunological abnormalities.

Depressed Neutrophil Function

Depressed neutrophil function is a major factor contributing to the lowered resistance to infection. Defective chemotaxis and reduced respiratory burst are the most prominent abnormalities. Several factors may contribute to this depression:

1. Exaggerated complement activation (mostly by proteases released in injured tissues) causes the release of large concentrations of C5a that may disturb proper chemotactic responses and cause massive activation of granulocytes. When the already activated granulocytes reach the infected tissues, they may no longer be responsive to additional stimulation.
2. Bacterial endotoxin, prostaglandins, and β-endorphins have been suggested as additional factors that adversely affect neutrophil functions. The involvement of prostaglandins has been supported by studies in experimental animals, in which administration of cyclooxygenase blockers normalize phagocytic cell functions.
3. Another contributing factor seems to be the low opsonizing power of the burn blister fluid, which has very low levels of both complements and immunoglobulins.

Macrophage Activation

Macrophages harvested from patients with burn injury appear to be in a state of activation, releasing increased amounts of IL-1, TNF, IL-6, transforming growth factor (TGF-β), and prostaglandin E2 (PGE$_2$) after in vitro stimulation. These cytokines are measured in increased levels in the circulation of patients with severe burns. Of these cytokines, IL-6 has been shown to be the one that is consistently elevated after thermal injury. It has been proposed that this state of activation increases the response of macrophages to other stimuli, such as endotoxin, thus increasing the susceptibility of burn patients to sepsis.

Depressed Cell-Mediated Immunity

Impairment of cell-mediated immunity is suggested by a prolongation of skin homograft survival and depressed delayed hypersensitivity responses. Laboratory studies shown have documented low responses to mitogenic stimuli and depressed mixed lymphocyte culture reactions. A major functional abnormality of T lymphocytes isolated from burned patients is their depressed release of IL-2 after mitogenic stimulation. This depression may be secondary to the release of immunosuppressive factors by the burned tissues, including a 10 kDa glycopeptide, a 1000 kDa lipid–protein complex, and PGE_2 is released by overactive monocytes and causes an increase of intracellular cAMP in T cells, inhibiting their proliferation. In addition, the circulating levels of tumor growth factor-β (TGF-β) are elevated six to eight days postinjury. Given the immunosuppressive effects of TGF-β on both T and B cells, it is not surprising that some investigators have suggested that TGF-β plays a significant role in causing immunosuppression in patients with severe burns.

Iatrogenically-Induced Immune Deficiencies

A wide range of therapeutic interventions has been shown to cause functional depression of the immune system. On top of the list is the administration of cytotoxic/immunosuppressive drugs (see Chapter 26), but many other medical procedures have unexpected effects on the immune system.

Neutropenia

The reduction of the total number of neutrophils is the most frequent cause of infection due to defective phagocytosis. Although there are rare congenital forms of neutropenia of variable severity, most frequently neutropenia is secondary to a variety of causes (Table 2). Administration of cytotoxic drugs is almost inevitable followed by neutropenia (see Chapter 24), but a variety of drugs of other groups may cause idiosyncratic neutropenia with variable frequency.

Postsurgery Immunodeficiency

Both surgery and general anesthesia are associated with transient depression of immune functions, affecting the mitogenic responses of peripheral blood lymphocytes (PBL), cutaneous hypersensitivity, and antibody synthesis. Multiple factors seem to contribute to the depression of the immune system (Fig. 1): a transient severe lymphopenia that can occur in the immediate postoperative period; the exaggerated release of PGE_2 due to the post-traumatic activation of inflammatory cells; depressing of T lymphocyte and accessory cell functions; blood loss that can be associated with a reduction of IL-2 release by activated T lymphocytes and of major histocompatibility complex (MHC)-II expression by accessory cells and with reduced B lymphocyte responses to antigenic stimulation; transfusions that have a poorly understood

TABLE 2 Causes of Neutropenia

Congenital
Secondary (acquired)
Depressed bone marrow granulocytosis
Drug-induced
Tumor invasion
Nutritional deficiency
Unknown cause (idiopathic)
Peripheral destruction of neutrophils
Autoimmune (Felty's syndrome)[a]
Drug-induced

[a]An association of rheumatoid arthritis, splenomegaly and neutropenia.

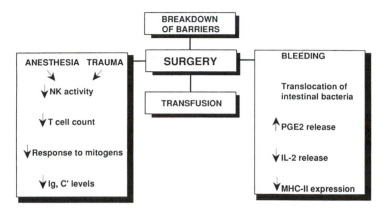

FIGURE 1 Diagrammatic representation of the different factors contributing to the immune suppression associated with surgery.

immunosuppressive effect; anesthesia and administration of opiates (as painkillers), which can lead to a depression of phagocytic cell functions and to a reduced activity of natural killer (NK) cells.

Complete normalization of immune function may take 10 days (for mitogenic responses) to a month (for delayed hypersensitivity reactions and the humoral immune response).

It also needs to be kept in mind that postsurgical infection is facilitated by a variety of factors associated with surgery, which even in its simplest form is traumatic to the patient. For example, the surgical incision disrupts the integrity of the skin—a very important barrier against infection. Special types of surgery, such as intestinal surgery, promote spreading of bacteria from a highly contaminated organ into the surrounding tissues. The introduction of intravenous lines and catheters, often associated with surgical procedures, opens new routes for the penetration of opportunistic agents into the skin. Severe blood loss during surgery can cause massive entrance of intestinal bacteria into the portal circulation, and subsequently, into the systemic circulation (phenomenon known as bacterial translocation). If one adds a depressed immune system to these factors, it is easy to understand the clinical significance of postsurgical infection.

Splenectomy

Splenectomy deserves special reference as a cause of immune depression. The removal of the spleen represents the loss of an important filtration organ, very important for the removal of circulating bacteria. In addition, the spleen plays a significant role in recruiting immunocytes in the initial phases of the immune responses. Splenectomized patients are weakly responsive to polysaccharides and if we add this fact to the inability to remove bacteria, particularly those with polysaccharide capsules, from circulation it is easy to understand why splenectomized patients are prone to severe septicemia. The most commonly offending organisms include *Streptococcus pneumoniae* (50% of the cases), *Haemophilus influenzae*, and *Neisseria meningitidis*—all of them pyogenic bacteria with antiphagocytic polysaccharide capsules. Other organisms involved as frequent causes of infection in splenectomized patients include *Staphylococcus aureus* and group A *Streptococcus*. It has also been demonstrated that about one-third of the cases of human infection by *Babesia*, an intracellular sporozoan, occur in splenectomized patients.

Similar defects are noticed in patients with sickle cell anemia, who develop splenic atrophy as a consequence of repeated infarctions and fibrosis (autosplenectomy). Noteworthy is the fact that patients with sickle cell anemia are particularly prone to develop salmonella bacteremia involving strains of *Salmonella enteritidis*, which do not disseminate in the blood stream of normal individuals. This allows *S. enteritidis* to spread to organs other than the intestine, namely the bones (*S. enteritidis* is the most frequent cause of osteomyelitis in patients with sickle cell anemia).

Thymectomy

Thymectomy is frequently done in neonates with congenital heart disease, to ensure proper surgical access. It is generally believed that thymectomy after birth has few (if any) effects on the development of the immune system of humans and there is no conclusive evidence suggesting otherwise.

Immunosuppression Associated with Drug Abuse

There is considerable interest in defining the effects of drug abuse on the immune system. Unfortunately, most data concerning the immunological effects of drugabuse are based on in vitro experiments or on studies carried out with laboratory animals, which may or may not reflect the in vivo effects of these compounds in humans.

Alcohol

Chronic alcoholism is associated with a depression of both cell-mediated and humoral immunity, but it could be argued that factors other than ethanol consumption, such as malnutrition and vitamin deficiencies, could be the major determinants of the impairment of the immune system. A direct effect of ethanol is supported by animal experiments, in which both T lymphocyte functions and B lymphocyte responses to T-dependent antigens are compromised after eight days of ethanol administration.

Cannabinoids

There is little concrete evidence for an immunosuppressive effect of cannabinoids in humans, except for depressed results in vitro T-lymphocyte function tests and for an increased incidence of *Herpes genitalis* among young adults who use cannabinoids. In laboratory animals, cannabinoid administration predominantly affects T and B lymphocyte functions, increases the sensitivity to endotoxin, and increases the frequency of infections by intracellular agents, such as *Listeria monocytogenes*. However, the conditions of administration of these compounds to laboratory animals are rather different than the conditions surrounding their use as recreational drugs.

Opiates
Cocaine

Cocaine has been shown to have direct effects over human T lymphocytes in vitro, but the required concentrations greatly exceed the plasma levels measured in addicts. The results of studies carried out in addicts have been contradictory.

Intravenous Heroin

Intravenous heroin use is associated with a high frequency of infections. In many instances, the infection (thrombophlebitis, soft tissue abscesses, osteomyelitis, septic arthritis, hepatitis B and D, and HIV infection) seems clearly related to the use of infected needles, but in other cases (bacterial pneumonia, tuberculosis), the infection could result from a depression of the immune system. However, to this date no conclusive evidence supporting a depressive effect of heroin over the immune system has been published.

Immunosuppression Associated with Infections

A wide variety of infectious agents have acquired the ability to thwart the immune system in a variety of ways, and in doing so, ensuring their ability to survive in the host for at least the time necessary for their replication.

Bacterial Infections

Disseminated mycobacterial infections are often associated with a state of anergy. The patients fail to respond to the intradermal inoculation of tuberculin and other antigens, and their in vitro lymphocyte responses to phytohemagglutinin (PHA) and to mycobacterial antigens are depressed. The mechanisms leading to anergy are poorly understood and probably involve more than a single factor:

1. An increased production of IL-10 and IL-4 could reduce the activity of Th1 helper lymphocytes, thus depressing cell-mediated immunity.
2. *Mycobacteria* infect phagocytic monocytes, and intracellular infection is associated with a depression of both the antigen-presentation capacities and the ability to deliver costimulatory signals to T lymphocytes (e.g., the expression of the CD80/86 molecules is depressed). In addition, infected monocytes/macrophages may release nitric oxide, which inactivates lymphocytes in the proximity of the infected cells.

The release of soluble immunosuppressor compounds has been demonstrated for several bacteria. Several different substances, including enzymes (ribonuclease and asparaginase), exotoxins (such as staphylococcal enterotoxins), and other proteins have been shown to have immunosuppressive properties, although probably their effects are limited to reducing the specific anti-infectious immune response. The staphylococcal enterotoxins are part of a group of bacterial proteins known as superantigens (see Chapter 13). In vitro, most superantigens have stimulatory properties, but when administered in vivo, induce generalized immunosuppression (perhaps as a consequence of indiscriminate nonspecific T cell activation).

Parasitic Infections
Parasitic infections due to protozoa seem to be often associated with suppression of the immune response to the parasite itself. In some cases, however, there is evidence of the induction of a more generalized state of immunosuppression. For example, acute infections with *Trypanosoma cruzi* are associated with cell-mediated immunity (CMI) depression that can be easily reproduced in laboratory animals. Both in humans and experimental animals, there is a reduced expression of IL-2 receptors, which can be interpreted as resulting from a downregulation of Th1 cells, either by cytokines or by suppressor compounds released by the parasite. Similar mechanisms seem to account for the generalized immunosuppression observed in experimental animals infected with *Toxoplasma, Schistosoma, Leishmania*, and *Plasmodia*.

Viral Infections
The AIDS epidemic has certainly focused our attention in the interplay between viruses and immunity. However, HIV is certainly not the only virus able to interfere with the immune system. Classical example are the temporary immunosuppression associated with viral influenza, which facilitates secondary bacterial infections, particularly in the lungs, and the development of a transitory state of anergy during the acute stage of measles, which was first reported by Von Pirquet in 1908.

The mechanisms responsible for the transitory state of anergy associated with measles were revisited in modern times. We now know that during the three to four weeks following the acute phase of measles, patients show lymphopenia and the residual population of PBL shows poor responses to mitogens and antigens such as PHA and *Candida albicans*. The function of APCs, including dendritic cells is also impaired, with reduced release of IL-12. This state of anergy seems to be caused by the release of viral proteins by infected cells that have immunosuppressive properties. A viral nucleoprotein interacts with the FcγR on dendritic cells and viral envelope glycoproteins interact with the viral hemagglutinin receptor, CD46. Other targets of viral proteins are CD150, TLR2, and FcγRII.

Other viruses, such as cytomegalovirus (CMV) and the rubella virus, can cause immunosuppression. CMV mainly depresses the specific response to the virus, while the rubella virus induces a generalized immunosuppression, similar to that caused by the measles virus. Viruses can also release suppressor factors (Herpes simplex virus secretes a protein similar to IL-10, which can downregulate cytokine release by activated T lymphocytes) and interfere with antigen presentation (adenovirus infection is associated with a depressed expression of MHC-I molecules). However, patients infected with these viruses do not develop generalized immunosuppression, so it seems likely that the significance of these mechanisms is mostly related to promoting conditions favorable for the persistence of the infection.

ACQUIRED IMMUNODEFICIENCY SYNDROME

AIDS was recognized as a novel clinical entity in 1981–1982, when the association of severe immunodepression with increased incidence of *Pneumocystis carinii* pneumonia and Kaposi's sarcoma in homosexual men was first recognized as representing possible variations in the spectrum of a new immunodeficiency disease.

The infectious nature of the syndrome was established in 1983, when Drs. Françoise Barre-Sinoussi and J. C. Chermann, at the Pasteur Institute in Paris, isolated a new retrovirus from the lymph node of a patient with disseminated lymphadenopathy and other symptoms that usually precede the development of AIDS. The new virus was initially named lymphade-nopathy-associated virus (LAV) and later received the designation of HIV.

HIV belongs to the *Lentiviridae* family of retrovirus. Two major variants of the virus have been identified. HIV-1, the first to be isolated, exhibits remarkable genetic diversity, and the different variants have been grouped into seven different families or clades, differing by 30% to 35% in their primary structures. HIV-2, prevalent in West Africa, was isolated a few years later. HIV-2 is less virulent than HIV-1, rarely causes a full-blown AIDS syndrome, and it is not spreading so widely and rapidly as HIV-1. Both viruses are derived from simian immune deficiency virus (SIV) and there is now strong genetic data to support that HIV is derived from the chimpanzee form of SIV.

General Characteristics of Human Immunodeficiency Virus

Structurally, HIV-1 and HIV-2 are constituted by two identical strands of (+) RNA associated with matrix proteins, a double protein capsid, and a lipid envelope with inserted glycoproteins. The integrated form of HIV-1 (provirus) is approximately 9.8 kilobases in length. Both ends of the provirus are flanked by a repeated sequence known as the long terminal repeats. The genes of HIV are located in the central region of the proviral DNA. There are three major genes, common to all retroviruses—*gag, pol,* and *env.*

The *gag* gene encodes structural proteins. It gives rise to a 55-kilodalton (kDa) Gag precursor protein (p55). During translation, the N terminus of p55 is myristylated, triggering its association with the cytoplasmic aspect of cell membranes. The membrane-associated Gag polyprotein recruits two copies of the viral genomic RNA along with other viral and cellular proteins that trigger the budding of the viral particle from the surface of an infected cell. After budding, p55 is cleaved by the virally encoded aspartic protease (discussed later) during the process of viral maturation into four smaller proteins designated MA [matrix (p17)], CA [capsid (p24)], NC [nucleocapsid (p9)], and p6.

The *pol* gene encodes a protein which, in its native form, functions as a reverse transcriptase, but after fragmentation can function as a ribunuclease and an endonuclease, involved in the integration into the host chromosome.

The *env* gene encodes the envelope glycoproteins. The transcript of the *env* gene is a gp160, which is cleaved by a cellular protease into gp120 and gp41. The gp41 moiety contains the transmembrane domain of Env, while gp120 is located on the surface of the infected cell and of the virion through noncovalent interactions with gp41. The gp120 protein mediates the viral attachment between HIV and the CD4 molecule and one of the HIV coreceptors. One highly variable region of gp120, the V3 loop, interacts with the second class of HIV coreceptors, the chemokine receptors, CXCR4 and CCR5. The V3 loop is also the principal target for neutralizing antibodies that block HIV-1 infectivity, but it has a high degree of mutational variation, due the lack of copyediting properties of the reverse transcriptase. The gp41 moiety contains an N-terminal fusogenic domain that mediates the fusion of the viral and cellular membranes, thereby allowing the delivery of the virion inner components into the cytoplasm of the newly infected cell.

In addition, the HIV genome codes for a protease and several regulatory proteins. The protease is essential to split polyprotein precursors into structural, regulatory, and accessory proteins.

The main function of the regulatory proteins encoded by noncontiguous segments of the genome, in some cases read in alternative frames, is to promote the transcription and transport to the cytoplasm of integrated viral genomes. They are also required for viral replication. The accessory proteins interfere with cell functions that would represent impediments to persistent infection, facilitate viral progeny assembly and release, and increase the infectivity of the progeny virions.

Epidemiology of HIV/AIDS

By the end of 2004 it was estimated that about 40 million people lived with HIV/AIDS worldwide, and that approximately five million people had been infected during that year. The highest numbers of infected people are estimated in Sub-Saharan Africa (25 million), followed by South and Southeast Asia (6.5 million), Latin American (1.6 million), Eastern Europe and Central Asia (1.3 million), and North America (1 million). The highest infection rates are estimated to occur in Sub-Saharan Africa (7.5%) and the Caribbean (2.3%). During 2003 it is estimated that a total of three million people died worldwide as a consequence of HIV infection. In North America (United States and Canada) the prevalence of HIV/AIDS is estimated at 0.6%. About half of the 40,000 new infections/year occur among African Americans, with an increasing proportion of women infected through unprotected sex with HIV-positive men.

In the United States, the type of sexual contact with greatest risk is male to male, followed by male to female, and female to male (Table 3). Heterosexual transmission is considerably more common in third world countries but is on the rise in the United States. Factors associated with increased risk of venereal transmission include receptive anal intercourse, IV drug-using partner, presence of genital ulcers, and multiple partners. The main modes of transmission are sex between men (42%), heterosexual contact (33%), and injecting drug use (25%). In many instances, a given individual may be involved in multiple high-risk activities. For example, the proportion of infected African-American men who consider themselves heterosexual but admit bisexuality is about 34%.

Vertical transmission is a major problem in underdeveloped countries where prophylactic antiretroviral therapy is not widely available. The infection is most frequently acquired intrapartum (about 80% of the cases). Intrauterine transmission occurrence in about 20% is next in frequency. It usually takes place late in pregnancy and the infection is acquired either transplacentally or as a consequence of prolonged rupture of the amniotic membranes. The risk of transplacental or perinatal transmission is directly related to the magnitude of the viral load. Transmission by breastfeeding is estimated to range between 5% and 12% of babies nursing from HIV-infected mothers; the risk is directly related to the viral load and to the duration of breastfeeding. In the developed world, HIV-infected women are advised to avoid breast-feeding but in the developing world the risk of death from diarrhea is actually higher in nonbreast fed infants.

HIV and the Immune System
Viral Life Cycle

The primary cellular targets of HIV are CD4$^+$ cells, particularly the helper T cells. Most infected CD4$^+$ lymphocytes co-express the CD45RO marker, considered as actively dividing memory helper T lymphocytes. It thus appears that activated CD4$^+$ T cells are most susceptible to infection, but productive infection of resting CD4$^+$ T cells has also been demonstrated.

The initial interaction of HIV and CD4$^+$ cells involves specific regions of gp120 and the CD4 molecule. It is believed that, this interaction results in a conformational change of gp120, which allows it to interact with a coreceptor. Two β-chemokine receptors (see Chapter 11) play the role of principal coreceptors. One, CCR-5 is the receptor for three

---

TABLE 3   Adult AIDS Cases by Exposure Group (End of 2002)

Men who have sex with men (55%)
Injecting drug use (22%)
Men who have sex with men and inject drugs (8%)
Heterosexual contact cases (5%)[a]
Other/risk not reported or identified (9%)

[a]42% among women.

chemokines—RANTES, macrophage inhibitory proteins 1α (MIP-1α), and 1β (MIP-1β). CCR-5 is expressed primarily by macrophages and activated T cells. The second, CXCR-4 (fusin), is expressed primarily by T lymphocytes.

The interaction between the CD120 and the coreceptor molecules results in exposure of the fusogenic domain of gp41 that can then interact with the cell membrane. This, in turn, results in the fusion of the membrane and the viral envelope, and penetration of the nucleocapsid into the cytoplasm.

Different HIV strains seem to show different coreceptor specificities. Macrophage-tropic HIV strains (which predominate in the early stages of infection) use CCR-5 as coreceptors, while CD4 lymphotropic strains use CXCR-4 as coreceptor. Some strains that can infect both CD4 T lymphocytes and macrophages use CCR5 to infect macrophages, and a third chemokine receptor, CCR2b to infect lymphocytes. Mucosal transmission involves the infection of both submucosal CD4$^+$ T cells and Langerhans cells, followed by rapid spread to the regional lymph nodes, where it propagates to other CD4$^+$ cells, including helper T cells, macrophages, and dendritic cells. When the virus is directly introduced into the blood stream, it will most likely be filtered in the spleen, where its ultimate fate will depend on its affinity for the different coreceptors mentioned previously.

During HIV infection, the expression of coreceptors may be upregulated in cell populations that normally do not express them, and that may allow HIV to infect those cell populations. However, some cell populations infected by HIV (e.g., intestinal cells) are not known to express CD4. The infection of mucosal epithelial cells is believed to be acquired from infected T cells and probably involves penetration through alternative receptors.

Once HIV enters a cell, its RNA is reverse transcribed into proviral DNA and is transported to the nucleus to integrate into the host genome using the viral-encoded enzyme *integrase*. Virus can remain within latently infected cells for months to years depending on the degree of cellular activation. The next phase of the viral life cycle is viral expression that depends on cellular activation. Several mechanisms of T cell activation leading to enhanced replication of integrated HIV have been proposed, but all rely on extrinsic factors leading to T cell activation. Viral replication is initiated by the transcription of viral genomic RNA and in the transcription and translation of viral proteins. Viral polypeptides are cleaved as the virus is assembled, and buds from infected cell by the HIV proteases results in a viable virion.

HIV-Specific Immune Response

The initial HIV-specific immune response to control viral replication is predominately mediated by host cellular immunity that can be detected by the third week of infection. There is a hierarchy of MHC-I restricted CD8$^+$ T lymphocytes, which recognize a variety of epitopes expressed by MHC-I–associated peptides derived from *gag, env, tat, nef,* and *pol* HIV proteins. Cell-mediated cytotoxic reactions seem to be especially prominent in HIV positive individuals that remain asymptomatic for prolonged periods of time, and the status of CMI is the principal determinant of disease progression. CD8 lymphocytes are also able, at least in vitro, to release cytokines (particularly RANTES, MIP-α and β, and IL-16) which appear to act by blocking the chemokine coreceptors used by HIV to penetrate noninfected CD4$^+$ cells. In addition, a soluble factor released by CD8$^+$, CD28$^+$ T cells inhibits the replication of integrated HIV. Thus, cell-mediated immunity seems to be able to either block infection or to reduce viral replication to tolerable levels.

The role of helper T cells is less well defined, but there is data suggesting that they may play a significant role. For example, some individuals who remain symptom-free and keep low viremia levels without therapy often have strong T helper responses to HIV-1 *gag* protein. The T cells of these individuals release the same type of inhibitory cytokines that are released by CD8$^+$ T cells.

As HIV replicates, a vigorous anti-HIV immune response is elicited. A strong humoral immune response against HIV can be detected in most patients. Neutralizing antibodies, which inhibit the infectivity of free HIV in vitro, directed against epitopes of gp120 and gp41, can be demonstrated. Also potentially protective are antibody dependent cellular cytotoxicity (ADCC)-promoting antibodies that react with gp160, expressed on the membrane of infected cells. The rate of progression to AIDS and the mortality rate are considerably higher in individuals lacking neutralizing antibodies. However, neutralizing antibodies do not prevent infected individuals from eventually developing AIDS, partly due to the high frequency of mutations in gp120, which result in the developing of mutants not neutralized by previously existing antibodies. It has also been reported that highly variable and glycosylated regions in gp120 shield the most effective antibody epitopes from B-cell recognition. The virus does not expose the immunodominant regions of gp120 in vivo, thus preventing the effective reactivity of gp120 antibodies.

HIV Escape Mechanisms

Most HIV-infected patients develop disease progression in spite of evidence of a strong antiviral antibody and cytotoxic T lymphocytes (CTL) responses. Loss of immunologic recognition or "immune escape" results in increased viral replication, and is the best predictor of progression to AIDS within the next five years.

Several factors contribute to HIV escape from the immune response. HIV mutates at a much faster rate than most other viruses. The error rate of HIV reverse transcriptase is about 1 in 10^4 base pairs or approximately one new nucleotide per new virion. This high mutation rate coupled with the 10^9 new virions produced each day results in a high degree of variability within the replicating pool of viruses. Viruses that have mutations in CTL and antibody epitopes have a selective advantage for ongoing replication. As HIV replicates, it alters its coreceptor use allowing it to expand. In many patients with advanced disease the predominant replicating virus utilizes CXCR4 and replicates most effectively in T cells.

HIV causes downregulation of human leukocyte antigens (HLA)-A and HLA-B expression without affecting the expression of HLA-C and HLA-E. In this way the infected cells may escape detection by CTL and are not affected by NK cells. Humoral immune responses are relatively inefficient in eliminating viral-infected cells. ADCC and lysis of viral-infected cells after exposure to antibody and complement have been observed in vitro, but it is questionable that these may be significant defense mechanisms in vivo, partly because of escape secondary to viral mutations, partly because the epitopes recognized by HIV antibodies are directed against structures not exposed in the circulating virus.

CD4$^+$ T Lymphocyte Depletion

As the infection persists and progresses there is a steady decline in the numbers of CD4$^+$ cells (Fig. 2). This T cell depletion affects predominantly the CD4, CD45RO$^+$ population, and is the direct cause of the profound immunodepression seen in AIDS patients. Several factors have been suggested to account for the depletion of CD4$^+$ T cells:

1. Direct cytotoxicity caused by virus replication is believed to be the most important cause of T cell death.
2. The cross-linking of CD4 molecules by gp120 is believed to prime T lymphocytes for apoptosis. In this case, active infection may not be essential, since apoptosis-primed T cells can undergo apoptosis when activated by some other stimulus, at least in vitro.
3. The expression of gp120 with unique sequences of the V_1 to V_2 and of the V_3 regions of gp120 on the membrane of infected T cells facilitates the formation of syncytia by interaction and fusion with the membranes of noninfected cells expressing CD4. The formation of syncytia allows direct cell−cell transmission of the virus and contributes to the reduction in the number of viable T cells. The emergence of strains with the syncytia-inducing sequences in infected patients is usually a late event in the course of an HIV infection, and associated with a faster progression to AIDS (median of 23 months), partly because these HIV strains are more apt to infect CD4 T cell precursors.
4. The immune response against viral-infected T cells (mediated both by cytotoxic T cells and by ADCC mechanisms) may also contribute to CD4$^+$ T cell depletion.
5. Co-infection of HIV-infected T cells with other microorganisms, such as CMV or *Mycoplasma fermentans*, has synergistic effects in the induction of viral replication and cell death.

Besides excessive CD4$^+$ T cell death, HIV has been shown to be able to infect T lymphocyte precursors and impair T cell production in the thymus. A major consequence of the

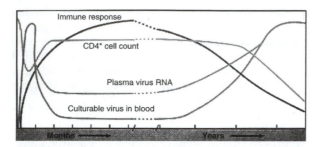

FIGURE 2 Diagrammatic representation of the longitudinal evolution of laboratory parameters during the course of an untreated HIV infection. *Source*: Adapted from Saag MS, Holodniy M, Kuritzkes DR, et al. HIV viral load markers in clinical practice. Nature Medicine 1996; 2:625.

infection of these targets is a significant decrease in the ability to repopulate the peripheral CD4 T lymphocyte pool under attack by HIV. The combination of excessive loss and of lack of production of CD4 cells is a marked decrease in their absolute numbers.

Other Factors Contributing to AIDS-Associated Immune Depression

Several other factors beyond the depletion of CD4$^+$ cells seem to contribute to the state of marked immunodepression associated with full-blown AIDS:

1. A reduction of the T cell receptors (TcR) β variable region repertoire on T cells, reducing the number of immunogenic peptides to which the patient can mount an adequate immune response.
2. An imbalance of the Th1 and Th2 subsets is been reported by some groups to precede the evolution toward AIDS. Several factors have been suggested as causing the dysfunction, particularly lack of expression of CD80/86 by HIV-infected APCs. The lack of costimulatory signals involving CD80/86 and CD28 would interfere with Th1 differentiation and lead to predominant Th2 activity. Th2 cells release IL-4 and IL-10, which would further downregulate Th1 cells and could induce the release of suppressor cytokines by CD8$^+$ T lymphocytes. It must be noted that clear evidence for predominant Th2 activity in patients evolving toward symptomatic HIV infection has not been substantiated by a variety of investigators.
3. Release of soluble gp120 by infected cells. Soluble gp120 binds to CD4, and may block the interaction of this molecule with MHC-II antigens, thereby preventing the proper stimulation of helper T cells by APCs. In addition, the interaction between gp120 and CD4 induces apoptosis of the CD4$^+$ T lymphocyte.
4. Immune complexes involving viral antigens and the corresponding antibodies may also play a role in depressing immune responses. For example, binding of gp120–anti-gp120 complexes to CD4$^+$ molecules of normal lymphocytes results in blocking T cell activation via the TcR.
5. Infected monocytes are functionally abnormal, unable to perform chemotaxis, synthesize cytokines, and present antigens to helper T cells.

Of note is the fact that humoral immune responses become severely dysfunctional in patients with AIDS. These patients are unable to respond to antigenic challenges, while, at the same time, produce a variety of autoantibodies (including antinuclear autoantibodies and autoantibodies directed against platelets and lymphocytes). The synthesis of autoantibodies is probably a consequence of a state of permanent polyclonal activation of the B-cell system, probably as a result of increased release of IL-6 by activated APC and T cells. At the same time, the de novo induction of protective immune responses is compromised by the lack of adequate T cell help.

In contrast with the cytotoxic effect of HIV infection on activated T cells, the infection of resting memory T cells, monocytes, macrophages, and related cells is not cytotoxic, and the infected cells become HIV reservoirs. Monocytes, macrophages, and related cells undergo chronic productive infection and perpetuate the infection in lymphoid tissues (lymph nodes and peri-intestinal lymphoid tissue). In contrast, HIV does not replicate in resting memory T cells. These cells can harbor the virus for long periods of time, are not affected by antiretroviral therapy, but are perfectly able to support HIV replication when activated. This is the principal reason why even in patients whose antiretroviral therapy suppresses the viral load to undetectable levels, HIV will rebound when therapy is discontinued.

Natural History of an HIV Infection

In the early stages of HIV infection, the virus appears to replicate at a very low level and both a transient decrease of total $CD4^+$ cells and a rise in circulating HIV-infected $CD4^+$ T cells may be detected. As early as 5 to 10 days after infection, infectious viral particles, viral mRNA, as well as soluble p24 protein can be detected in the circulation (Fig. 2). Viral replication as measured by RNA copies in the blood, usually peaks 10 to 20 days after infection, and remains high until seroconversion (i.e., the point of time when free anti-HIV antibody becomes measurable in the patient's serum). In the period preceding seroconversion, there is an extensive $CD4^+$ T cell attrition in the lymphoid tissues (primarily in the gut lymphoid tissues) and a high degree of $CD8^+$ T cell activation. This coincides with a peak of the viremia. As immunity controls viral replication, an equilibrium exists between ongoing viral replication and the capacity of the immune response to control it. Immune activation, as measured by the percentage of $CD4^+$ T cells and number of activated $CD8^+$ T cells, declines and $CD4^+$ T cells rebound (although to levels lower than those prior to infection).

HIV infected patients remain asymptomatic for variable periods of time, often exceeding 10 to 15 years (the average length of the asymptomatic period is currently of 14 years). During that period of time the virus replicates actively, and both integrated and soluble viral genomes continue to be detectable by several nucleic acid amplification techniques (Table 4). There is a marked difference between the amount of circulating viral RNA (viral load) and the number of recoverable infectious particles, suggesting either that most infected cells die before viral assembly is completed or that the viral progeny is predominantly constituted by defective particles. The magnitude of the viral load during this period (known as "set point") is proportionally related to the rate of decline of the $CD4^+$ T cell population and to the rate of progression to AIDS.

A steady state for the $CD4^+$ cell population is reached in which the number of dying $CD4^+$ T cells is roughly equivalent to the number of $CD4^+$ T cells differentiated in the primary lymphoid tissues. There is evidence suggesting that the rate of $CD4^+$ cell differentiation does not change during the asymptomatic stages of the disease, but it declines, eventually, when T cell precursor cells become infected.

Long-Term HIV Survivors

Understanding why some HIV-infected individuals are long-term survivors while others develop AIDS rather swiftly is a major priority in AIDS research. At this point it appears as if both host and microbial factors are involved.

TABLE 4   Techniques for the Assay of the Number of HIV Genome Copies in Plasma

AMPLICOR assay
Uses RT to obtain a cDNA and PCR to amplify cDNA
Sensitivity: 40 copies/mL
Nucleic acid based sequence amplification assay (NASBA)
Uses a mixture of RT and RNA polymerase to convert RNA into cDNA and copy the cDNA back into RNA
Sensitivity: 80 copies/mL
Branched DNA assay (QUANTIPLEX)
Uses branched DNA to detect a "captured" HIV RNA fragment
Sensitivity: 50 copies/mL

Abbreviations: PCR, polymerase chain reaction; RT, reverse transcriptase.

On the host side, the genetic constitution of the individual may be critical. Differences in MHC repertoire and transporters associated with antigen processing (TAP) proteins are emerging as related to the evolution of HIV infection. For example, it has been found that the HLA-B*5701 allele is associated with nonprogressive infection because the antigenic epitopes presented to T cells elicit a more broadly reactive CTL response making immune escape less likely. In addition, genetic variants in the chemokine receptor structure have also been linked to the duration of the asymptomatic phase. As a rule, individuals homozygous for mutant forms of CCR5 lacking a 32 base-pair segment (CCR5δ32) remain free of infection; heterozygous individuals for CCR5δ32 that become infected tend to be slow progressors. Also, probably, under genetic control may be the development of a strong cytotoxic reaction directed against viral infected cells, a major correlate of long-term survival in most HIV-infected individuals.

On the virus side, the route of exposure and the nature of the infective strain are significant factors. Mucosal exposure to low virus loads seems to induce protective CMI at the mucosal level, and the individuals may remain seronegative in spite of repeated exposures. On the other hand, some long-term survivors seem to be infected by strains of reduced pathogenicity, which replicate less effectively, and are associated with lower viral loads.

All the factors associated with long-term survival have an effect on viral load. Indeed, there is an inverse correlation between the number of HIV-1 RNA copies in plasma and the duration of the asymptomatic period. It has been reported that only 8% of HIV-infected patients with less than 4350 copies of viral RNA/mL of plasma at the time of diagnosis developed AIDS after five years of follow up. In other words, low virus loads are associated with prolonged survival. The monitoring of viral load and CD4$^+$ lymphocyte counts is considered as the best approach for the follow up of HIV infected patients (Fig. 2), as well as for monitoring the effects of antiretroviral therapy.

Clinical Stages of HIV Infection

When the infection is left to follow its natural course, most HIV-infected patients will develop AIDS. The asymptomatic period that precedes the diagnosis of AIDS may extend for several years, and the onset of clinical manifestations of AIDS may be gradual or abrupt. Many alternative classifications of the clinical stages of HIV-induced disease have been proposed, one of which is as follows:

1. Acute retroviral infection (usually a mononucleosis-like syndrome with fever and adenopathy)
2. Asymptomatic infection (no symptoms with the exception of the presence of lymphadenopathy)
3. Early symptomatic infection (non-life threatening infections, chronic or intermittent symptoms)
4. Late symptomatic infection (increasingly severe symptoms; life threatening infections; malignancies)
5. Advanced infection (high frequency of "opportunistic infections"; increased death risk)

Acute Illness Associated with Seroconversion (Acute Retroviral Syndrome)

The typical incubation time is estimated to be two to four weeks between exposure and onset of symptoms. Viremia (often exceeding 10^6 copies/mL) occurs at that time and virus transmission can take place before antibodies are detected. The clinical picture is similar to infectious mononucleosis or flu-like fever. Fever, sore throat, myalgias, headache, malaise, and a *maculopapular rash* are the most predominant symptoms. Although these symptoms may be rather frequent (it is estimated that 30%–70% of the patients present them), their lack of specificity leads to frequent misdiagnoses both on the part of the patient and of the physician. Less frequently, the presenting symptoms are those of acute hepatitis or of aseptic meningitis. Most patients recover completely from the acute infection, although in some, headaches and adenopathy may persist.

The results of immunoassays for HIV antibody during this stage are often negative. Seroconversion usually occurs six weeks after infection (antibodies to gp120 and gp41 are usually detected first, followed by antibodies to p24). Thus, if a patient suspected of being infected with HIV is seronegative, but definitely classified as belonging to a high-risk group, the serological studies should be repeated after six additional weeks. In rare cases, seroconversion can be significantly delayed (sometimes for one year or longer).

With the availability of highly effective therapy, there is a strong current of opinion emphasizing the need for early diagnosis to monitor disease progression. Rapid diagnosis of HIV infection can be best achieved by detection of viral RNA by polymerase chain reaction (PCR). This is also the best available approach to diagnosis in a child born from an HIV-infected mother. All children born to infected women will have positive results from the HIV enzyme-linked immunosorbent assay (ELISA) and Western blot assays due to the placental transfer of IgG antibodies. These maternal antibodies persist for over a year. The only way to differentiate between infected and uninfected infants is to use one of the sensitive molecular-based assays that can detect viral RNA in the baby's blood.

Asymptomatic Infection

The patient remains seropositive with minimal or no symptoms (diffuse reactive lymphadenopathy and headache may be present at this stage) for variable periods of time (between nine and 11 years, as an average, probably exceeding 20 years in some individuals). Disseminated lymphadenopathy, believed to represent a reactive response of all the nodal elements, is prominent in some patients and less obvious in others. Both T and B cell populations are expanded and virus is not present in the reactive B lymphocytes.

Considerable interest has been focused on the study of laboratory parameters that may be associated with the progression of HIV-infected individuals toward clinically significant immunodeficiency. Determination of the viral load is considered as the most reliable parameter for prognostic evaluation of any given patient. The CD4 count should also be followed closely, as an index of the degree of immunocompromise.

It is important, in this asymptomatic stage, to evaluate the patient for other diseases that may be seen in HIV-infected patients, such as syphilis, hepatitis B, and tuberculosis, and treat any such condition that may be diagnosed. Toxoplasma serology is also recommended, since it may help screen the patients at risk for developing severe toxoplasmosis at later stages of the disease. In HIV$^+$ females, biannual PAP smears are indicated, due to increased frequency of infection with papilloma viruses and increased risk for the development of cervical carcinoma. Prophylactic measures to avoid infections that are known to occur with increased frequency in HIV$^+$ patients (tuberculosis, viral influenza, pneumococcal pneumonia) are best medical practice.

Early Symptomatic HIV Infection

Fever, night sweats, fatigue, chronic diarrhea, and headache in the absence of any specific opportunistic disease in a previously asymptomatic HIV$^+$ patient mark the transition toward symptomatic disease. Diarrhea in these patients is most likely due to direct infection of the GI mucosa by the HIV virus.

Mucosal candidiasis is a frequent presenting symptom. In adult men, oral candidiasis is very rare other than in HIV positive patients. In HIV positive women, recurrent vaginal candidiasis is a frequent cause for seeking medical attention.

With time, anergy and other laboratory evidence of immunodeficiency may develop, and some opportunistic infections may start affecting these patients, particularly recurrent mucosal candidiasis, oral leukoplakia (often asymptomatic), upper and lower respiratory tract infections, and periodontal disease.

Late Symptomatic and Advanced HIV Disease

With the progressive decline of CD4$^+$ counts, the risk for development of opportunistic infections increases. The onset of opportunistic infections is considered as the clinical hallmark for diagnosis of full-blown AIDS.

Acquired Immunodeficiency Syndrome

The designation of AIDS is applied when an HIV positive patient (determined by positive serological tests, isolation of the virus, or detection of viral genomic material by PCR) presents one or more of the following features:

1. Opportunistic infections (a list of the most common is shown in Table 5). Of particular concern among opportunistic infections are *Pneumocystis jerovici (carinii)* pneumonia, whose frequency increases significantly when the $CD4^+$ lymphocyte count falls below 200/mm³, and toxoplasmosis, which in AIDS patients often affects the brain. With lower CD4 counts (<100/mm³) infections with *Mycobacterium avium-intracellulare*, CMV, esophageal candidiasis, cryptococcal pneumonitis and meningitis, recurrent herpes simplex, and wasting disease increase in frequency.
2. Progressive wasting syndrome (known as "slim disease" in Africa) in adults and failure to thrive in infected infants, probably related to the exaggerated release of TNF (Cachectin) by activated macrophages.
3. Unusually frequent or severe infections not considered as opportunistic, such as recurrent bacterial pneumonia or pulmonary tuberculosis. Recurrent bacterial infections are the most common infectious presentation of AIDS in infants and children. In women, recurrent vaginal candidiasis is a very frequent presentation (presenting symptom in 24% to 71% of the cases, depending on the series).
4. Specific neoplastic diseases, such as Kaposi's sarcoma, AIDS-related lymphoma, and invasive cervical carcinoma.

AIDS-related lymphoma is a consequence of long-term stimulation and proliferation of B cells caused by HIV itself, as well as by reactivation of EBV infections secondary to HIV-induced immune depression. Translocations involving chromosomes 8 and 14, as well as overexpression of EBV's late membrane protein (LMP)-1 are often detected in these lymphomas. The incidence of AIDS-related lymphoma has not decreased after the introduction of effective antiretroviral therapy. Lymphomas can be located in any anatomical area of the body, are usually diagnosed late in the disease, and are the cause of death in 12% to 16% of patients with AIDS. The prognosis in patients with AIDS-related lymphoma depends on a variety of criteria: $CD4^+$ count below 100/μL, history of opportunistic infections preceding the lymphoma, age greater than 35 years, history of injectable drug use, elevated serum lactic dehydrogenase (LDH), are associated with poor prognosis. Some cases may respond to vigorous antiretroviral therapy, but in general require the administration of cytotoxic agents and/or irradiation.

Kaposi's sarcoma is caused by a virus of the Herpes family (human herpes virus 8). Infections with this virus in HIV^+ patients seem to be associated with exaggerated release of IL-6, IL-1,

---

TABLE 5 Opportunistic Infections Characteristically Associated with AIDS

Pneumocystis carinii pneumonia
Chronic *cryptosporidiosis* or Isosporiasis causing untractable diarrhea
Toxoplasmosis
Extra-intestinal strongyloidosis
Candidiasis (oral candidiasis is common as a prodromal manifestation and is considered as a
    marker of progression toward AIDS; esophageal, bronchial, and pulmonary candidiasis are
    pathognomonic)
Cryptococcosis
Histoplasmosis
Infections caused by atypical mycobacteria, such as *M. avium intracellulare*
Pulmonary and extrapulmonary tuberculosis (often resistant to therapy)
Disseminated cytomegalovirus infection (may affect the retina and cause blindness)
Disseminated herpes simplex infection
Multidermatomal herpes zoster
Recurrent *Salmonella bacteremia*
Progressive multifocal leukoencephalopathy
Invasive nocardiosis

TNF, and oncostatin M by activated macrophages, which would act synergistically in promoting the development of the vascular proliferative lesions typical of the tumor. The frequency of Kaposis's sarcoma has decreased after introduction of effective therapeutic modalities.

1. Neuropsychiatric diseases such as encephalopathy (dementia) and progressive multifocal leukoencephalopathy (due to reactivation of an infection with the JC virus) or significant developmental delays or deterioration in children.
2. Lymphocytic interstitial pneumonitis in infants and children.
3. A CD4$^+$ cell count below $200/mm^3$ or representing less that 14% of the total lymphocyte count.

HIV may affect many different organ systems during the course of AIDS. Cardiomyopathy and nephropathy (which may progress to renal failure) may occur at any time during the progression of HIV infection. Bone marrow suppression, peripheral neuropathy, and encephalopathy occur later in the course of AIDS.

The evolution of concurrent chronic infections is also altered by HIV infection. This is particularly evident in the case of chronic hepatitis B or C, which have faster rates of progression to hepatic failure and cirrhosis, and poorer response to therapy.

Serological Diagnosis of HIV Infection

The initial screening of anti-HIV antibodies is done by an ELISA test, using HIV antigens obtained either from infected cells or by recombinant technology. Since this is a screening test, used to screen blood on blood banks, its cutoff is set for maximal sensitivity (it is preferable to discard some false positive blood units than to transfuse contaminated units with low antibody titers that otherwise could be considered safe.

Any positive result on ELISA needs to be confirmed, first by repeating the ELISA to rule out errors or technical problems. If the repeat test is positive, the result should be confirmed by Western blot (immunoblot). A Western Blot is considered positive if antibodies to structural proteins (e.g., p24), enzymes (gp41), and envelope glycoproteins (gp41 or gp120) are simultaneously detected. The accuracy of the combined tests (ELISA and Western blot) is better—more than 99.5%. A positive viral load test can also be considered confirmatory.

Therapy

The antiretroviral agents currently in use can be divided into several different pharmacological groups, acting at different levels of the viral replication cycle (Fig. 3).

Reverse transcriptase inhibitors, which can be subclassified into three groups:

1. *Nucleoside analogs*, including zidovudine (azidodideoxythymidine, ZDV), the most widely used antiviral agent for treatment of HIV infections, and several other compounds [zalcitabine (2′,3′-dideoxycytidine, ddC), didanosine (2′,3′-dideoxyinosine, ddI), stavudine (2′3′-didehydro-3′deoxythymidine, d4T), lamivudine (2′-deoxy-3′-thiacytidine, 3TC) emtricitabine (FTC), and abacavir (ABC)]. All these drugs are phosphorylated by cellular thymidine kinases and are taken up preferentially by the HIV reverse transcriptase. DNA transcription is blocked by at least two mechanisms: binding to the reverse transcriptase, which blocks its active site, and termination of DNA synthesis when the activated nucleosides are incorporated into nascent viral DNA and block further elongation.
2. *Nucleotide analogs*, such as adefovir and tenofovir, are compounds that terminate DNA elongation upon incorporation into nascent DNA chains. One significant advantage of tenofovir is its long half-life that allows effective treatment with a single pill given once daily. It is also equally effective against HIV-1 and HIV-2.
3. *Non-nucleoside reverse transcriptase inhibitors (NNRTI)*, such as nevirapine, delavirdine, and efavirenz, bind to a hydrophobic pocket of the reverse transcriptase at a site different from active site, but still block the activity of the enzyme by steric hindrance. Because of the different binding sites, strains of HIV resistant to nucleoside reverse transcriptase inhibitors are not cross-resistant to NNRTIs.

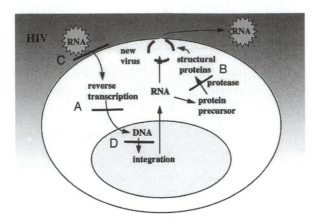

FIGURE 3 Diagrammatic representation of the HIV life cycle and the points of action of antiretroviral agents. The first antiretrovirals introduced were the reverse transcriptase inhibitors, which block the first step of viral replication after the virus has penetrated into a competent cell (A). The second generation of antiretrovirals were the protease inhibitors, which prevented the processing of viral proteins, a step essential for the assembly of viral progeny (B). The last antiretroviral approved by the FDA in the USA prevents the penetration of HIV into competent cells (C). Agents able to inhibit viral DNA integration (D) are currently being evaluated.

Protease inhibitors, such as saquinavir, ritonavir, indinavir, nelfinavir, lopinavir, atazanavir, and amprenavir, are synthetic, nonhydrolyzable synthetic peptides that compete as substrates for the HIV protease. HIV-infected cells exposed to these compounds accumulate *gag* polyprotein precursors that are not cleaved due to the inhibition of protease activity. This results in cell death.

Inhibitors of Viral Penetration

Several compounds have been tried for the treatment of HIV infections by preventing HIV penetration in noninfected cells. Anti-CD4 antibodies and humanized copies of gp120 tetrapeptides that bind to CD4 and block viral adsorption were the first to be tried, without clinical success. A synthetic peptide (enfurtivide) that blocks the interaction of gp41 with the plasma membrane has been approved by the FDA. It has some significant drawbacks, such as being an injectable.

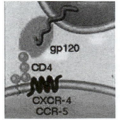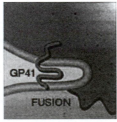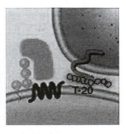

FIGURE 4 Diagrammatic representation of the point of action of T-20, a peptide inhibitor of HIV penetration. The penetration of HIV into a competent cell involves several steps. First, gp120 interacts with CD4 and with a chemokine coreceptor (CXCR-4 or CCR-5). These interactions result in the exposure of fusogenic domains in gp41 otherwise sterically hindered by gp120. The functional activation of gp41, in turn, results in the fusion of the viral envelope with the plasma membrane, required for the intracellular release of the viral nucleocapsid. This process can be blocked by compounds that bind to the chemokine-coreceptors or by compounds, such as enfurtivide, that bind to gp41. *Source*: Adapted from Dynamics of HIV Infection: A special report. Science & Medicine 1998; 5:38.

New Antiretroviral Agents

New antiretroviral agents under development include additional inhibitors of HIV penetration, such as RANTES analogs that block the interaction with CCR5, integrase inhibitors, and reverse transcriptase inhibitors designed to be effective against drug-resistant mutants.

Highly Active Antiretroviral Therapy

Administration of three or more different antiretrovirals, known as highly active antiretroviral therapy (HAART), is the current standard recommendation for HIV therapy. Most combinations include two reverse transcriptase inhibitors with different binding sites in the polymerase (e.g., ZDV and 3TC). The rationale for the association is to combine nucleoside analogues that require different HIV mutations for resistance to develop. The probability of emergence of a double mutant polymerase retaining functional activity is relatively low.

The third component of a HAART regimen can be a member of any of the available drug classes, but most commonly would be a nonnucleoside reverse transcriptase or a protease inhibitor. As a rule, a NNRTI is preferred because of simpler dosing schemes, lower pill burden, fewer side effects, and less drug–drug interactions. On the negative side, when a virus becomes resistant to a NNRTI, the resistance extends to all other members of the class and, unlike protease inhibitors, few mutations are needed to confer resistance. It has also been noted that African Americans are more susceptible to side effects of at least one of the NNRTI (Efavirenz), perhaps as a consequence of slower metabolism of the drug.

HAART in any of its modalities induces remarkable reductions in viral load after 12 weeks of administration—very frequently below the detection level of the most sensitive assays in compliant patients (which is the desirable goal of therapy). The reduction in viral load is usually associated with increases in $CD4^+$ T cell counts, averaging 120 to 150 over the pretreatment levels after the first month of therapy. In addition, several immune function parameters show improvement after combination therapy: skin test reactivity, mitogenic responses, $IFN\gamma$ and IL-2 synthesis, and CD28 expression (both by $CD4^+$ and $CD8^+$ cells). At the same time, IL-6 and TNF levels decrease, reflecting a lower degree of T cell activation.

The increase in CD4 T cell numbers (affecting both 45RA and 45RO subpopulations) is usually not associated with an immediate increase in the repertoire of TcR $V\beta$ regions. In fact, the immediate expansion of CD4 T cells seems to involve the residual memory and naïve T-cell clones that survived the effects of HIV infection. Progressive, but slow, increases in CD4 counts are often seen during the following years. Recovery of normal T cell counts may take six or more years, assuming HIV replication is suppressed during that period. The rate of T cell recovery and restoration of the T cell repertoire is primarily a thymic function output. Children and adults with intact thymic function restore T cell immunity faster than those whose thymus continues to be impaired. It is noteworthy that when HAART succeeds in reducing the viral load to undetectable levels, HIV-specific CD4 and CD8 responses remain depressed, suggesting that specific HIV immunity not only requires regeneration of lymphocyte pools, but also antigenic exposure. Some groups advocate periodic interruptions of antiretroviral therapy to allow for a burst of HIV replication that may then induce specific immunity, but the real therapeutic value of these protocols is yet to be established.

In spite of all these limitations, patients successfully treated with any modality of HAART are able to mount immune responses when properly immunized, and show both a decrease in the frequency of opportunistic infections and a remarkable significant reduction in mortality. These beneficial effects are observed even in the absence of a complete regeneration of the TcR repertoire (it has been estimated that effective immune responses can be generated with 10% of the original TcR repertoire).

Effective HAART is not associated with emergence of mutant viruses. Interruption of treatment is usually followed by the re-emergence of the original viral strains characterized before this type of therapy was initiated. In patients who develop strong anti-HIV cytotoxic responses during HAART, suspension of therapy is not immediately followed by increase in viral load. As a rule, however, the viral load will eventually rebound to high levels after interruption.

TABLE 6 DHHS Guidelines to Initiate Therapy in HIV$^+$ Patients (May 2006)

Antiretroviral therapy is recommended for all patients with history of AIDS-defining illness or severe symptoms of HIV infection regardless of CD4$^+$ T cell count

Antiretroviral therapy is also recommended for asymptomatic patients with less than 200 CD4$^+$ T cells/mm^3

Asymptomatic patients with CD4$^+$ T cell counts of 201–350 cells/mm^3 should be offered treatment

For asymptomatic patients with CD4$^+$ T cell counts >350 cells/mm^3 and plasma HIV RNA >100,000 copies/mm^3 most experienced clinicians defer therapy but some clinicians may consider initiating treatment

Therapy should be deferred for patients with CD4$^+$ T cell counts >350 cells/mm^3 and plasma HIV RNA <100,000 copies/mm^3

Source: Adapted from Guidelines for the Use of Antiretroviral Agents in HIV-1-Infected Adults and Adolescents (http://AIDSinfo.nih.gov).

Indications for Antiretroviral Therapy and Problems Encountered on its Implementation

Therapy is unquestionably indicated for symptomatic HIV positive patients, even if not fulfilling the AIDS diagnostic criteria—for HIV infected patients with CD4$^+$ T cell counts below 350/mL, or for HIV infected patients with viral loads greater than 100,000, irrespective of CD4 counts and clinical symptoms. Treatment recommendations are regularly issued by several organizations, including Department of Health and Human Resources (DHHS) in the USA (Table 6).

The treatment with multiple drug combinations, including those needed to treat or prevent opportunistic infections (discussed in the next paragraph) raises serious problems, such as cost, compliance, and drug interactions. Compliance is made difficult not only by the number of drugs involved, but also by complicated administration schedules. Furthermore, the side effects may be so distressing that some patients cannot tolerate the therapy.

Drug interactions become a very significant problem when multiple potent drugs are simultaneously administered. The interactions happen at many different levels. For example, not all combinations of anti-retroviral drugs are adequate, some can interfere with each other and reduce the efficiency of the treatment. Zidovudine (ZDV) and high doses of trimethoprim-sulfamathoxazole (TMP/SMX) should not be administered at the same time because both drugs can cause bone marrow depression. Rifamycins upregulate the metabolism of protease inhibitors, and as a consequence therapeutic levels of protease inhibitors are difficult or impossible to reach. Some protease inhibitors inhibit the effect of tuberculostatics. Some members of the azole group of antifungal drugs reduce the metabolic elimination of protease inhibitors. Detailed knowledge of potential drug interactions is essential for the proper treatment of these patients.

Prevention of Materno-Fetal Transmission

The risk of materno-fetal transmission of HIV is estimated to be around 25% to 30%, with a direct correlation with the viral load of the infected mother. The risk can be reduced by a variety of antiretroviral regimens that should contain ZDV. Some antiretrovirals, such as efavirenz, should not be given to pregnant women. Zidovudine should be administered as part of a HAART regimen and according to the guidelines shown in Table 7. Administration of ZDV

TABLE 7 Guidelines for Use of Zidovudine (ZDV, AZT) in Pregnancy

During pregnancy
    ZDV, 200 mg p.o. TID
    Begin after 14 weeks of gestation
During delivery
    ZDV, 2 mg/kg IV over 1 hr
    Thereafter, ZDV, 1 mg/kg by continuous infusion until delivery
Neonatal
    Oral ZDV syrup, 2 mg/kg q 6 hr × 6 weeks
    Can give ZDV IV if p.o. not possible

Notes: Give ZDV, during delivery even if patient has had none during pregnancy.
Give ZDV, to neonate even if mother has had none.

alone reduces the risk of HIV transmission to 8%. Further reductions (to about 2%) are possible by using ZDV-containing HAART. Delivering newborns by elective C-section also reduces the risk of transmission but not significantly more than HAART therapy alone.

Resistance to Antiretrovirals

The high mutation rate of HIV associated with the selective pressure exerted by antiretrovirals results in the rapid emergence of resistant strains. The likelihood of such strains emerging is reduced when several antiretrovirals are used in combination and the patient complies with the prescribed schedule of administration. To better decide what antiretrovirals to use, particularly when trying to decide the most adequate combination of antiretrovirals to be given to a patient who has developed resistance, two basic methods of determining antiretroviral susceptibility of HIV have been introduced. One is a phenotypic assay, based on testing the ability of HIV isolated from a given patient to replicate in permissive cells in the presence of different antiretrovirals. The other approach is a genotypic test, which consists of analyzing the nucleic acid of a patient's isolate to determine the presence of mutations known to be associated with resistance to different antiretrovirals (Fig. 5). Neither approach is perfect, because the sensitivity is such that viral populations representing less than 20% of the total HIV load will not be detected.

Biological response modifiers have also been widely used in patients with AIDS, with a variety of goals. Erythropoietin and granulocyte colony stimulating factor have been administered to patients with neutropenia or red cell aplasia secondary to the administration of ZDV to promote the proliferation of red cell and neutrophil precursors. Interferon-α has been approved for administration to patients with Kaposi's sarcoma. IL-2 and IL-12 are being evaluated for the capacity to accelerate the restoration of immune functions in AIDS patients. High doses of IL-2 induce increases in CD4 counts in patients in whom antiretrovirals have significantly reduced the viral load, but the side effects are considerable. Lower doses are better tolerated but not as effective. In either modality, the beneficial effects of IL-2 can be detected for several weeks after administration. One of the potential adverse effects of IL-2 administration is the activation of infected resting T cells and promotion of viral replication, although clinical trials using IL-2 in patients with optimal viral suppression on HAART has not revealed significant viral breakthrough.

Another avenue explored by several groups trying to boost the immune system of HIV$^+$ individuals is the immunization of infected patients with the purpose of accelerating the immune reconstitution of patients successfully treated with HAART. Killed HIV, gp120-depleted HIV, recombinant gp160, and recombinant canary pox vaccines have been used for that purpose. Overall, the data suggest that when the vaccines succeed in generating a strong cell-mediated response to HIV, some degree of virological suppression is achieved.

Mutations Associated with Resistance to Nucleoside and Nucleotide HIV ReverseTranscriptase Inhibitors

	41	50	65	67	69	70	74	75	115	151	184	215	219	333	
ddI															ddI
d4T															d4T
3TC												ZDV/			3TC
ZDV												3TC			ZDV
Abacavir															Abacavir
ddC															ddC
Adefovir															Adefovir
	41	50	65	67	69	70	74	75	115	151	184	215	219	333	

FIGURE 5 Diagrammatic representation of the different mutations in the HIV reverse transcriptase associated with resistance to nucleoside and nucleotide reverse transcriptase inhibitors. The *shaded boxes* represent substitutions associated with resistance to specific drugs—*dark shading* represents a higher degree of resistance than light shading. Notice that mutations affecting position 151 of the reverse transcriptase result in resistance to all the nucleoside and nucleotide HIV reverse transcriptase inhibitors. *Source*: Adapted from Gene Chart, published by the Academy of Continuing Education Programs, 1999.

Recent reports also suggest that a Tat vaccine may be worth developing. Antibodies to the Tat protein have several potential useful effects, such as reducing the level of HIV replication and transmission and preventing some of the immunosuppressive effects of the virus. In a monkey model this vaccine reduced HIV viremia to undetectable levels and prevented $CD4^+$ T cell decrease.

Immunoprophylaxis

The development of an effective HIV vaccine is a highly desirable and very elusive goal in the global efforts to contain the AIDS pandemic. Different groups are exploring a variety of approaches. Recombinant viral particles made by inserting HIV glycoprotein genes in vaccinia virus or canary poxvirus genomes, for example, have been shown to induce neutralizing antibodies in animals. These vaccines also seem to be prone to stimulate the differentiation of HIV-specific HLA class I-restricted cytotoxic lymphocytes. Component vaccines have been prepared using isolated gp120, polymerized gp120, or gp120 peptides representing more conserved regions (such as the CD4-binding domain). Recent evidence suggests that a monoclonal antibody to a unique epitope of gp120 has neutralizing activity, thus raising some hope that gp120-based vaccines tailored to induce antibodies to the epitope recognized by those monoclonal antibodies may be effective. Recently, Tat protein vaccines have been proposed, with the rationale that antibodies to this protein will prevent the intercellular transactivation of HIV replication mediated by soluble Tat protein. Gag protein vaccines have also been tried and reported to be more effective in inducing T cell-mediated immunity than other types of vaccines. Finally, DNA vaccines also appear to induce HIV-specific HLA class I-restricted cytotoxic lymphocytes and have been found to induce protection in primates. However, DNA vaccines are weakly immunogenic in humans. Phase 3 clinical trials were recently concluded for a recombinant gp120 vaccine, but the results were very disappointing. Several other vaccines, including combinations of canary pox and DNA vaccines are in clinical evaluation, but, so far, the results are not promising.

Difficulties in evaluation of candidate vaccines, due to the relative inadequacy of animal models, and by the lack of adequate indices of protection in humans, are responsible for a considerable part of the problems faced by vaccine developers. Most commonly, the assessment of the efficacy of a vaccine is based on the assay of protective antibodies. However, antibodies are not truly protective in the case of HIV; in most cases the antibodies induced by gp120 do not neutralize primary HIV isolates because gp120 is not fully exposed in the virion.

All evidence point to the fact that an efficient vaccine should stimulate the differentiation of HIV-specific CTL, which may be the only way to eliminate or control virally-infected cells that apparently can be involved in the transmission of HIV infection. Macaques immunized with plasmid DNA vaccines or recombinant poxvirus vaccines, and then challenged with a human-simian HIV (SHIV) recombinant became infected, but the vaccinated animals had substantially lower levels of viral mRNA in circulation than nonimmunized macaques. The animals developed CTL and neutralizing antibodies and survived for as long as 1.5 years after SHIV infection. Other experiments using plasmid DNA vaccines potentiated with IL-2 showed suppression of viremia for even longer periods. So, at the present time it appears that the most successful vaccines may not prevent infection, but rather induce a state of resistance to HIV resulting in low viremia, preservation of $CD4^+$ T cells, delaying or preventing the onset of clinical disease.

BIBLIOGRAPHY

Andiman WA. Transmission of HIV-1 from mother to infant. Curr Opin Pediatr 2002; 14:78–85.

Brand J-M, Kirchner H, Poppe C, Schmucker P. The effects of general anesthesia on human peripheral immune cell distribution and cytokine production. Clin Immunol Immunopathol 1997; 83:190.

Chandra RK. Nutrition and the immune system: an introduction. Am J Clin Nutr 1997; 66:460S.

Chun T-W, Engel D, Mizell SB, et al. Effect of interleukin-2 on the pool of latently infected, resting the $CD4^+$ T-cells in HIV-1-infected patients receiving highly active anti-retroviral therapy. Nat Med 1999; 5:651.

Connors M, Kovacs JA, Krevat S, et al. HIV infection induces changes in CD4$^+$ T-cell phenotype and depletions within the CD4$^+$ T-cell repertoire that are not immediately restored by antiviral or immune-based therapies. Nat Med 1997; 3:533.

Cunningham-Rundles S, McNeeley DF, Moon A. Mechanisms of nutrient modulation of the immune response. J Allergy Clin Immunol 2005; 115:1119–1128.

Field CJ, Johnson IR, Schley PD. Nutrients and their role in host resistance to infection. J Leukoc Biol 2002; 71:16–32.

Friedman H, Eisenstein TK. Neurological basis of drug dependence and its effects on the immune system. J Neuroimmunol 2004; 147:106–108.

Goulder PJR, Walker BD. The great escape - AIDS viruses and immune control. Nat Med 1999; 5:1233.

Grieco M, Virella G. Acquired Immunodeficiency Syndrome. Principles and Practice of Medical Therapy in Pregnancy. 3rd ed. Stemford: Appleton & Lange, 1998.

Hanson K, Hicks C. New antiretroviral drugs. Curr HIV/AIDS Rep 2006; 3:93–101.

Harris BH, Gelfand JA. The immune response to trauma. Semin Pediatr Surg 1995; 4:77.

Hulsewe KWE, Van Acker BAC, von Meyenfeldt MF, Soeters PB. Nutrional depletion and dietary manipulations: effects on the immune response. World J Surg 1999; 23:536.

Kerdiles YM, Sellin CI, Druelle J, Horvat B. Immunosuppression caused by measles virus: role of viral proteins. Rev Med Virol 2006; 16:49–63.

Marie JC, Kehren J, Trescol-Biémont M-C, et al. Mechanism of measles virus-induced suppression of inflammatory immune responses. Immunology 2001; 14:69.

McMichael AJ, Hanke T. Is an HIV vaccine possible? Nat Med 1999; 5:612.

Migueles SA, Sabbaghian MS, Shupert WL, et al. HLA B*5701 is highly associated with restriction of virus replication in a subgroup of HIV-infected long term nonprogressors. Proc Natl Acad Sci USA 2000; 97:2709.

Pavia CS, La Mothe M, Kavanagh M. Influence of alcohol on antimicrobial immunity. Biomed Pharmacother 2004; 58:84–89.

Saag MS, Holodniy M, Kuritzkes DR, et al. HIV viral load markers in clinical practice. Nat Med 1996; 2:625.

Schwacha MG. Macrophages and post-burn immune dysfunction. Burns 2003; 29:1–14.

Sleasman JW, Goodenow MG. HIV. J Allergy Clin Immunol 2003; 111:S582–S592.

Stenvinkel P, Ketteler M, Johnson RJ, et al. IL-10, IL-6, and TNF-alpha: central factors in the altered cytokine network of uremia–the good, the bad, and the ugly. Kidney Int 2005; 67:1216–1233.

Trkola A, Kuster H, Rusert P, et al. Delay of HIV-1 rebound after cessation of antiretroviral therapy through passive transfer of human neutralizing antibodies. Nat Med 2005; 11:615–622.

Zahng A-Q, Schuler T, Zupanic M, et al. Sexual transmission and propagation of SIV and HIV in resting and activated CD4$^+$ T cells. Science 1999; 286:1353.

Index

About the Editor

Gabriel Virella is professor of microbiology and immunology and vice chairman of education, microbiology, and immunology, Medical University of South Carolina, Charleston, South Carolina, U.S.A. Dr. Virella has published three textbooks and 226 articles on topics related primarily to immunology, with particular emphasis on immunoglobulin structure and abnormalities, immune complex diseases, and the involvement of autoimmune phenomena in the pathogenesis of atherosclerosis. He is a fellow of the American Academy of Microbiology, a member of the Clinical Immunology Society, and a section editor for *Clinical Immunology*. He is also a member of the editorial boards of the *Journal of Clinical Laboratory Analysis* and *Clinical and Diagnostic Laboratory Immunology*. Dr. Virella received the M.D. and Ph.D. degrees from the University of Lisbon School of Medicine, Lisbon, Portugal.